Advanced Cardiac Imaging

Advanced Cardiac Imaging

Editor: Ava Riley

FOSTER ACADEMICS

www.fosteracademics.com

www.fosteracademics.com

FOSTER ACADEMICS

Cataloging-in-Publication Data

Advanced cardiac imaging / edited by Ava Riley.
p. cm.
Includes bibliographical references and index.
ISBN 978-1-63242-969-8
1. Heart--Imaging. 2. Heart--Diseases--Diagnosis.
3. Cardiovascular system--Diseases--Diagnosis. 4. Diagnostic imaging. I. Riley, Ava.
RC683.5.I42 A38 2020
616.120 75--dc23

Foster Academics,
118-35 Queens Blvd., Suite 400,
Forest Hills, NY 11375, USA

ISBN 978-1-63242-969-8 (Hardback)

Contents

Preface

This book has been an outcome of determined endeavour from a group of educationists in the field. The primary objective was to involve a broad spectrum of professionals from diverse cultural background involved in the field for developing new researches. The book not only targets students but also scholars pursuing higher research for further enhancement of the theoretical and practical applications of the subject.

Cardiac imaging is a non-invasive imaging technique used for the diagnosis of a heart condition. The use of magnetic resonance imaging (MRI), ultrasound, computed tomography (CT) and nuclear medicine imaging allows the visualization of the heart. Transthoracic echocardiography is the most common imaging tool that allows the non-invasive evaluation of heart function and the blood flow through the heart. It applies ultrasonic waves to examine the heart chambers and blood movement. Using multidetector CT, cardiac images can be obtained in a matter of few seconds, which are reconstructed using algorithms. Such CT techniques have facilitated the diagnosis of cardiac artery disease in a non-invasive way. MRI allows soft tissues to be differentiated and permits the quantitative assessment of morphology, size, function and tissue characteristics. Constant research in these techniques will help to ensure better cardiac imaging for the diagnosis of cardiovascular diseases. This book discusses the fundamentals as well as modern approaches of cardiac imaging. The topics included herein are of utmost significance and bound to provide incredible insights to readers. A number of latest researches have been included to keep the readers up-to-date with the global concepts in this area of study.

It was an honour to edit such a profound book and also a challenging task to compile and examine all the relevant data for accuracy and originality. I wish to acknowledge the efforts of the contributors for submitting such brilliant and diverse chapters in the field and for endlessly working for the completion of the book. Last, but not the least; I thank my family for being a constant source of support in all my research endeavours.

Editor

1

Early decrease in carotid plaque lipid content as assessed by magnetic resonance imaging during treatment of rosuvastatin

Ruixue Du[1†], Jianming Cai[2†], Xue-Qiao Zhao[3], Qing-Jun Wang[2], Dan-Qing Liu[2], Wen-Xiu Leng[1], Peng Gao[1], Hong-Mei Wu[1], Lin Ma[2*] and Ping Ye[1*]

Abstract

Background: Statin therapy has shown to deplete atherosclerotic plaque lipid content and induce plaque regression. However, how early the plaque lipid depletion can occur with low-density lipoprotein cholesterol (LDL-C) lowering in humans *in vivo* has not been fully described.

Methods: We enrolled 43 lipid treatment naïve subjects with asymptomatic carotid atherosclerosis and LDL-C ≥ 100 and ≤ 250 mg/dl. Rosuvastatin 5–20 mg/day was used to lower LDL-C levels to < 80 mg/dl. Lipid profile and carotid MRI scans were obtained at baseline, 3, 12, and 24 months. Carotid plaque lipid-rich necrotic core (LRNC) and plaque burden were measured and compared between baseline and during treatment.

Results: Among the 32 subjects who completed the study, at 3 months, an average dose of rosuvastatin of 11 mg/day lowered LDL-C levels by 47% (125.2 ± 24.4 mg/dl vs. 66.7 ± 17.3 mg/dl, $p < 0.001$). There were no statistically significant changes in total wall volume, percent wall volume or lumen volume. However, LRNC volume was significantly decreased by 7.9 mm^3, a reduction of 7.3% (111.5 ± 104.2 mm^3 vs. 103.6 ± 95.8 mm^3, $p = 0.044$). Similarly, % LRNC was also significantly decreased from 18.9 ± 11.9% to 17.9 ± 11.5% ($p = 0.02$) at 3 months. Both LRNC volume and % LRNC continued to decrease moderately at 12 and 24 months, although this trend was not significant.

Conclusions: Among a small number of lipid treatment naïve subjects, rosuvastatin therapy may induce a rapid and lasting decrease in carotid plaque lipid content as assessed by MRI.

Keywords: Atherosclerosis, Plaque lipid content, Statin, Magnetic resonance imaging

Background

Atherosclerosis alone is thought to be a relatively benign disease and progresses with aging; however, it is frequently complicated by acute thrombosis, usually triggered by the rupture or erosion of an atherosclerotic plaque which is determined by plaque morphologic characteristics, local composition and inflammation [1,2]. Plaque rupture or erosion can lead to major cardiovascular events such as acute coronary syndromes and strokes. The cardiovascular events reduction with statin therapy demonstrated in the past 2 decades is most likely induced by improved plaque stability that is determined by lipid core size, fibrous cap thickness and the level of inflammatory infiltrates and activity.

Development of high-resolution magnetic resonance imaging (MRI) techniques in recent years has made it possible to directly assess plaque composition. Numerous studies have shown that MRI creates high contrast for internal features of plaques and that the combined information from multiple contrast weightings is critical for distinguishing all plaque components [3]. The accuracy and reproducibility of carotid MRI has been extensively validated, using histological analysis of lesions [4,5]. Thus, carotid MRI can accurately assess plaque tissue contents.

* Correspondence: cjr.malin@vip.163.com; yeping301@sina.com
†Equal contributors
[2]Department of Radiology, Chinese PLA General Hospital, No. 28, Fuxing Road, Beijing 100853, China
[1]Department of Geriatric Cardiology, Chinese PLA General Hospital, No. 28, Fuxing Road, Beijing 100853, China
Full list of author information is available at the end of the article

Previous studies have demonstrated that low-density lipoprotein cholesterol (LDL-C) lowering with statin induced plaque regression [6,7] and plaque lipid content reduction [8,9]. However, how early the plaque lipid depletion can occur with intensive LDL-C lowering in humans *in vivo* has not been fully described.

Thus, we designed and conducted a prospective study, Rosuvastatin Evaluation of Atherosclerotic Chinese Patients, (REACH study, NCT00885872), to test the hypothesis that statin therapy induces rapid plaque lipid depletion as assessed by MRI.

Methods

Research subjects

Subjects were recruited and enrolled to the REACH study if they met the following inclusion criteria: 1) age 18 to 75 years; 2) carotid stenosis 16 - 69% by ultrasound; 3) the maximum wall thickness ≥ 3 mm, an intact fibrous cap as assessed by MRI; 4) LDL-C ≥ 100 mg/dl and ≤ 250 mg/dl; 5) triglycerides ≤ 353 mg/dl; and 6) no history of statin or other lipid treatment. 7) The patients who were willing to be enrolled have to remain on the low cholesterol dietary before the screening. Exclusion criteria were: 1) uncontrolled hypertension; 2) severe heart disease; 3) peripheral arterial disease; 4) liver disease; 5) renal dysfunction; 6) hypothyroidism; 7) uncontrolled hyperglycemia with an HbA1c > 9%; 8) familial hypercholesterolemia; 9) history of any lipid-lowering agents.

As shown in Figure 1, among 1108 subjects screened by ultrasound, 103 were identified to have stenosis of 16 - 69% and suitable for carotid MRI scans. 46 subjects were confirmed to meet the above MRI requirements. Of the 46 subjects, 43 qualified for lipids and without any liver and renal abnormalities and enrolled in the REACH study. During the study, 1 patient was withdrawn for protocol violations, 2 withdrew consent, 2 experienced adverse events (one for increases in alanine aminotransferase and aspartate aminotransferase, the other for increases in creatine kinase), and 6 were excluded from the final analyses for poor image quality or missing one or more scans. Thus, 32 subjects completed the study with matched serial MRI scans and acceptable image quality.

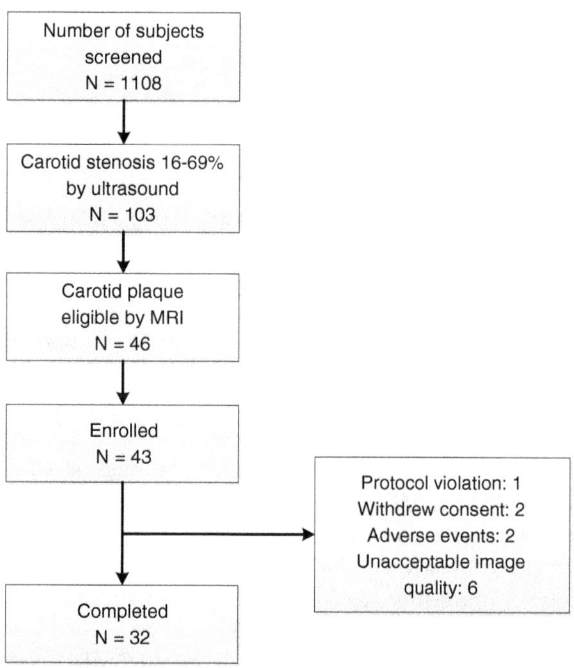

Figure 1 REACH study recruitment, enrollment and completion.

The REACH study was carried out at the People Liberation Army (PLA) General Hospital (Beijing, China) between March 29th, 2009 (first patient enrolled) and February 26th, 2012 (last patient completing the study). All procedures were performed according to the Declaration of Helsinki, and the study protocol was approved by the PLA General Hospital's institutional review board. All patients provided a written informed consent.

Statin therapy and follow-up

All subjects received an initial treatment of rosuvastatin 10 mg daily. Dose adjustment was performed after 4 weeks according to the Chinese guidelines for the prevention and treatment of adult dyslipidemia [10]. If LDL-C levels were ≥ 80 mg/dl, or if HDL-C were < 40 mg/dl, rosuvastatin dose was increased to 20 mg. If LDL-C levels < 80 mg/dl, rosuvastatin dose was maintained at 10 mg. Rosuvastatin dose was decreased to 5 mg when LDL-C levels were < 50 mg/dl. The dose determined at 4 weeks was maintained during the rest of the 24-month.

After the study initiation, regular clinic visits were scheduled every 1 to 3 months over the 24-month follow-up period. At each visit, vital signs, physical examination, dietary counseling, adverse events monitoring and medication compliance calculation were performed. Serum lipids, liver functions, kidney functions and muscle enzymes were assessed at 3, 12, and 24 months.

Magnetic resonance imaging protocol

High-resolution and multicontrast bilateral carotid MRI scans were performed using a 3.0-T MRI scanner (Signa Echo Speed, GE Healthcare, Waukesha, WI, USA) at baseline, and at 3, 12, and 24 months. All follow-up MRI scans were performed using the same imaging protocol and carefully matched for scan coverage using the carotid bifurcation as an internal landmark. An index artery with the worse maximum wall thickness was identified at the baseline scan.

A standardized protocol was used to obtain 3-dimensional time-of-flight (TOF), proton-density-weighted (PDW), T2-weighted (T2W) and T1-weighted (T1W) images. Twelve axial images, centered at the bifurcation of the index artery, were acquired with a 2-mm slice thickness for a total longitudinal coverage of 24 mm without gap. Gadolinium contrast material (Magnevist at 0.1 mmol/kg) was then administrated intravenously and the T1-weighted scan was repeated 5–7 minutes after contrast administration. Total acquisition time for all images was approximately 40 minutes.

MRI analysis of plaque morphology and composition

All images were analyzed by experienced reviewers at IBMarker Company, Seattle, WA, USA. An experienced reviewer matched the axial images from all 4 time points according to the distance from the carotid bifurcation. Then, two experienced reviewers, who were blinded to the order of MR scans, evaluated and interpreted all images with matched locations of the index artery by reaching a consensus opinion. This image review process was blinded to laboratory results and clinical course.

Using a custom-designed image analysis tool (CASCADE, IBMarker Company, Seattle, WA, USA), the lumen and outer wall boundaries were identified [4,11]. The total vessel area and lumen area (LA) were quantified by placing contours around the outer wall boundaries and the lumen of the carotid artery, respectively. Wall area (WA) was calculated by subtracting the lumen area from the total vessel area. Wall, lumen volumes and total vessel volumes were obtained by adding the areas across slices and multiplying by the slice thickness (2 mm). Percent wall volume (PWV), which is similar to percent atheroma volume described in the IVUS literature, was calculated as: (wall volume/total vessel volume) × 100%.

Lipid-rich necrotic core (LRNC) was identified and automatically quantified using previously published histologically-validated MRI criteria [4,5,11]. Specifically, LRNC was identified using multicontrast weightings plus post-contrast T1W images. LRNC usually appears as isointense to hyperintense on the TOF and pre-contrast T1W images, has variable signal intensity on PDW and T2W images, and has no or slight contrast enhancement compared with the surrounding tissue on post-contrast T1W images. Total LRNC volume was measured by multiplying the slice thickness by the sum of the LRNC areas. The proportion of LRNC relative to the wall volume (% LRNC) was calculated as: (LRNC volume/wall volume) × 100%. Both LRNC volume and % LRNC were calculated using images containing LRNC.

According to previous studies, the reproducibility of measuring plaque burden (ICC ranging from 0.96-0.99) and LRNC size (ICC ranging from 0.94-0.99) with automatic analysis is good to excellent [4,8,12].

Endpoints

The primary endpoint was the carotid plaque lipid content presented as LRNC volume and %LNRC as measured by MRI. The secondary endpoint was the plaque burden presented as PWV.

Statistical analysis

The sample size was estimated according to previous similar study [8]. For the change in % LRNC at baseline, a sample size of approximately 26 patients was required for 90% power and a 2-sided level of 0.05 to detect an expected change of 2.7%, assuming an SD range from 2.5% to 5.3%. If approximately 25% of patients discontinued from the study, then 35 patients allocated to study medication would result in 26 patients completing the study, which would provide sufficient power to assess the primary end points.

Descriptive statistics are presented as mean ± SD. Changes over time in lipids were compared to baseline using the Wilcoxon's signed-rank test (non-normally distributed variables) or the paired *t*-test (normally distributed). Changes over time in plaque measurements were compared to baseline using the paired *t*-test when data presented normally distributed. Otherwise, data were logarithmically transformed to normalize their distributions. Associations test of plaque lipid content changes were assessed using the Spearman rank correlation coefficient. Analysis was carried out using SPSS 17.0 (SPSS Inc. Chicago, IL, USA). A p-value < 0.05 was considered statistically significant.

Results

Patient baseline characteristics

Baseline demographic characteristics for the 32 subjects who completed the trial are summarized in Table 1. The mean age was 61 years and body mass index was 24.5 kg/m^2. Seventy-eight percent of subjects were male, 78% had

Table 1 Patient baseline characteristics

Characteristics	Patients (n = 32)*
Age, mean (SD), y	60.8 ± 9.1
Male	25 (78.1%)
Body mass index, mean (SD)†	24.5 ± 2.7
History of hypertension	25 (78.1%)
History of diabetes mellitus	10 (31.3%)
History of coronary heart disease	3 (9.4%)
History of cerebrovascular disease	10 (31.3%)
Current smoking	3 (9.4%)
Concomitant medications	
Aspirin	10 (31.3%)
Antihypertensive	25 (78.1%)
Hypoglycemic agents	10 (31.3%)

*Data are expressed as number (%) unless otherwise specified.
†Calculated as weight (in kilograms) divided by the squared height (in meters).

hypertension, 31% were diabetics, 9% had coronary artery disease and 31% had history of cerebrovascular disease.

Changes in lipid levels under rosuvastatin therapy

Rosuvastatin 5–20 mg/day was initiated at the study entry and dosage adjustment was made at 4 weeks to achieve LDL-C levels < 80 mg/dl. The mean dose was 11 mg/day during the remaining of the study. Lipid levels during the 2 years of rosuvastatin therapy were presented in Table 2. At 3 months, LDL-C levels were significantly reduced by 47% (125.2 ± 24.4 mg/dl vs. 66.7 ± 17.3 mg/dl, $p < 0.001$). HDL-C levels were increased by 4% (49.2 ± 14.7 mg/dl vs. 51.2 ± 11.8 mg/dl, $p = 0.084$). Triglycerides were lowered by 27% (142.3 ± 67.1 mg/dl vs. 103.3 ± 41.6 mg/dl, $p < 0.001$).

Effects of rosuvastatin on plaque lipid content

At 3 months, LRNC volume was significantly decreased by 7.9 mm^3, a reduction of 7.3% (111.5 ± 104.2 mm^3 vs. 103.6 ± 95.8 mm^3, $p = 0.044$). % LRNC was significantly decreased from 18.9% ± 11.9% to 17.9% ± 11.5% ($p = 0.02$) as shown in Table 3.

The time course of plaque LRNC reduction over 24 months is illustrated in Figure 2 and described in Table 3. Following the initial significant reduction at 3 months, LRNC volume continued to decrease moderately at 12 and 24 months. However, there were no statistically significant differences when LRNC at 12 months compared to that at 3 months, and at 24 months vs. at 12 months. The decrease in % LRNC displayed the same trend.

Among the 32 subjects who completed the study, 68.8% showed any decrease in LRNC volume and 62.5% had any decrease in % LRNC. Figure 3 shows a representative MRI of plaque lipid core regression over 2 years. However, there was no subject demonstrated a completed depletion of plaque lipid content over the 24 months. There were 31.2% of subjects showed no change or increase in LRNC.

Furthermore, magnitude of LRNC decrease over 24 months was significantly correlated with the LRNC volume at baseline ($r = -0.53$, $p = 0.002$) as shown in Figure 4.

Effects of rosuvastatin on carotid plaque burden

As shown in Table 3, during the 2 years of rosuvastatin therapy, PWV and the total wall volume slightly decreased, and lumen volume slightly increased. However, none of these changes reached statistical significance.

Nevertheless, the decrease in total wall volume was statistically correlated with reduction in LRNC at 3 ($r = 0.42$, $p = 0.039$), 12 ($r = 0.44$, $p = 0.027$) and 24 months ($r = 0.45$, $p = 0.024$). The decrease in PWV over 24 months was statistically associated with reduction in LRNC ($r = 0.40$, $p = 0.005$).

Discussion

It is well documented that major determinants of plaque rupture are cellular and lipid composition and associated inflammation [1,2] while specific plaque features associated with propensity for disruption include higher lipid [2,13,14] and macrophage content [2,15-17]. These high-risk plaque features have been pursued as therapeutic targets and measurable marker for plaque stabilization [18,19].

In addition to animal studies showed statin therapy let to plaque lipid depletion from the existing plaque [20,21], in a case–control study of patients randomized to 3 months of pravastatin treatment or placebo prior to carotid endarterectomy, Crisby et al. provided histological evidence of plaque lipid content reduction with therapy [22]. The present study demonstrated that carotid plaque lipid content (LRNC volume and % LRNC) measured by MRI decreased significantly at 3 months with moderate-dose rosuvastatin (11 mg/day) lowering LDL-C levels by 47% in a group of lipid treatment naïve subjects. Our study provides *in-vivo* verification of rapid plaque lipid depletion. Furthermore, taken together with a recent published study [23] showing that intensified statin therapy (atorvastatin 80 mg) was associated with rapid reduction in vascular inflammations determined by fluorodeoxyglucose-positron emission tomography, these findings may indicate evidence of an early on-set of plaque stabilization via a rapid reduction in arterial inflammation and a rapid plaque lipid depletion with statin therapy.

After a rapid and statistically significant plaque lipid depletion seen at 3 months in our study, carotid plaque lipid content continued to decrease moderately and no subject achieved completed plaque lipid depletion over 24 months of therapy. However, Carotid Plaque Composition by MRI during Lipid-lowering (CPC) study [9] showed a statistically significant reduction in plaque lipid

Table 2 Lipid levels during the 24-month therapy

	Baseline	3 Months	12 Months	24 Months
Total cholesterol (mg/dl)	200.8 ± 29.8	135.8 ± 24.7*	135.1 ± 36.0*	139.8 ± 24.4*
LDL-cholesterol (mg/dl)	125.2 ± 24.4	66.7 ± 17.3*	65.5 ± 17.0*	69.8 ± 16.6*
HDL-cholesterol (mg/dl)	49.2 ± 14.7	51.2 ± 11.8	52.9 ± 14.2†	53.8 ± 14.8*
Triglycerides (mg/dl)	142.3 ± 67.1	103.3 ± 41.6*	110.6 ± 50.4†	98.7 ± 48.2*

Data are presented as mean ± SD. *LDL* = low-density lipoprotein; *HDL* = high-density lipoprotein. *$p < 0.001$ when compared to baseline. †$p < 0.05$ when compared to baseline.

Table 3 Changes in LRNC and carotid arterial wall burden

	Baseline	3 Months	12 Months	24 Months
LRNC, mm^3	111.5 ± 104.2	103.6 ± 95.8*	101.7 ± 93.4*	97.7 ± 91.5*
LRNC%	18.9% ± 11.9%	17.9% ± 11.5%*	17.5% ± 11.2%*	16.7% ± 11.3%*
Wall volume, mm^3	533.3 ± 208.9	523.1 ± 196.3	521.0 ± 194.2	528.0 ± 198.9
Lumen volume, mm^3	522.1 ± 246.7	514.0 ± 234.2	512.1 ± 245. 6	537.6 ± 265.0
PWV, %	51.0% ± 8.2%	50.8% ± 8.5%	50.9% ± 9.0%	50.3% ± 8.6%

Data are presented as mean ± SD. Changes over time in plaque measurements were compared to baseline using the paired *t*-test (LRNC, LRNC % and lumen volume were logarithmically transformed to normalize their distributions). *LRNC* = lipid-rich necrotic core; % LRNC = proportion of LRNC relative to the wall area; *PWV* = percent wall volume. *$P < 0.05$ when compared to baseline.

content at 12 and 24 months compared to baseline and 11% lower frequency of subjects with measurable LRNC over 3 years. There are several important differences between the present study and CPC: (1) Chinese treatment naïve subjects vs. Caucasian subjects with lipid treat history < 1 year; (2) lower LDL-C (125 mg/dl vs. 163 mg/dl) and triglycerides (142 mg/dl vs. 202 mg/dl) levels at baseline in our study subjects; (3) higher LRNC volume (111.5 mm^3 vs. 60.4 mm^3) and % LRNC (18.9% vs. 14.2%) in present study; (4) statin alone therapy vs. 2/3 of subjects treated with combination lipid therapy. Saam et al. reported significant differences in LRNC area between Chinese and American patients with symptomatic carotid diseases [24]. A large LRNC at baseline and treatment naïve status in our study subjects may play a partial role in the significant rapid plaque lipid depletion. However, the lower dose of rosuvastatin used in current study might be related to the moderated lipid depletion. Further studies are needed to examine the plaque response to therapy in different ethnic groups, population with different lipid abnormalities and different magnitude of plaque lipid depletion associated with intensity of LDL-C lowering.

The application of MRI in prospective serial studies of human atherosclerosis has become more widespread because it is noninvasive, not involve ionizing radiation, superior to other imaging modalities in discriminating tissue contrast, and highly reproducible [25,26]. Prospective MRI studies of carotid lesions [27-29] offer compelling evidence that high-risk plaque features including a large LRNC, strongly associate with clinical cerebrovascular events in patients with asymptomatic 50%-79% carotid stenosis. The high-risk plaque features are also seen in less severe stenosis. In an MR angiography study of carotid arteries with 0% stenosis, LRNC was present in 67.4% of nonocclusive lesions [30]. Importantly, our study showed that plaques with a larger LRNC are more likely to deplete (r = – 0.53, $p = 0.002$) in response to a moderate-dose of rosuvastatin therapy. These data indicate that plaques with large LRNC are associated with a significantly higher risk of plaque rupture and also more likely to respond to statin

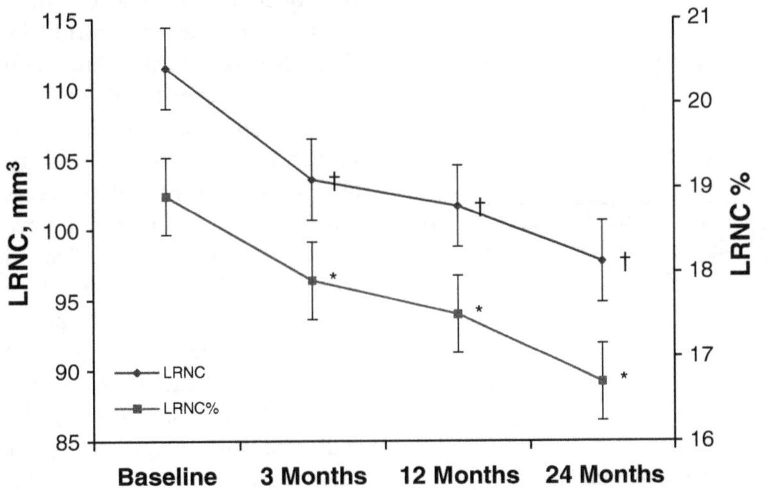

Figure 2 Reduction in LRNC and % LRNC during the 24 months of rosuvastatin therapy. The time course of plaque LRNC reduction over 24 months suggested that LRNC (red rhombuses) significantly decreased by 7.9 mm3, a reduction of 7.3% at 3 months, and continue to decrease moderately at 12 and 24 months. †$p < 0.05$ when compared to baseline. There were no statistically significant differences when LRNC at 12 months compared to that at 3 months, and at 24 months vs. at 12 months. The decrease of % LRNC (green squares) displayed the same trend. *$p < 0.05$ when compared to baseline. Bars around the estimates are standard error bars. LRNC = lipid-rich necrotic core.

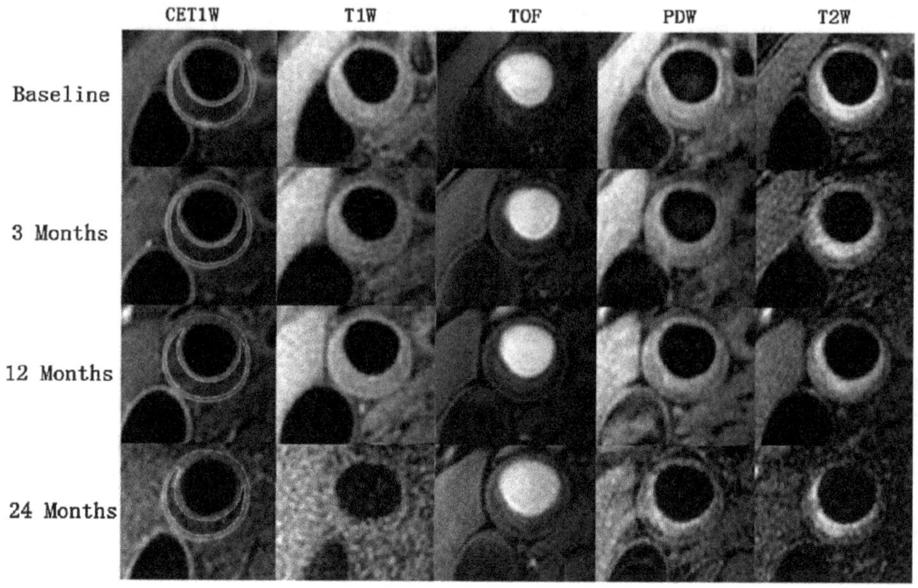

Figure 3 Representative MRIs showing plaque lipid depletion in right common carotid artery over 2 years. The lumen in red, outer wall boundary in blue and lipid content in yellow of the carotid artery were identified and outlined in post-contrast T1W images. LRNC demonstrate isointense on pre-contrast T1W images and TOF, and was detected as non-enhanced areas (relative to surrounding tissues) on CET1W images with the corresponding pre-contrast T1W images used as reference. Regression in LRNC at the same location was found between the baseline, 3 months, 12 months and 24 months MRI scans. MRI = magnetic resonance imaging; LRNC = lipid-rich necrotic core; TOF = time-of-flight; T1W = T1-weighted; T2W = T2-weighted; PDW = proton-density-weighted; CET1W = contrast enhanced T1-weighted.

therapy and suggest a potential mechanism of statin therapy in plaque stabilization leading to a lower risk for future ischemic events. On the other hand, despite a similar LDL-C lowering during the study, 31.2% of subjects showed plaque LRNC no change or increase. The clinical importance of persistent presence of plaque LRNC and other risk features with LDL-C lowering requires to be established in larger prospective clinical trials.

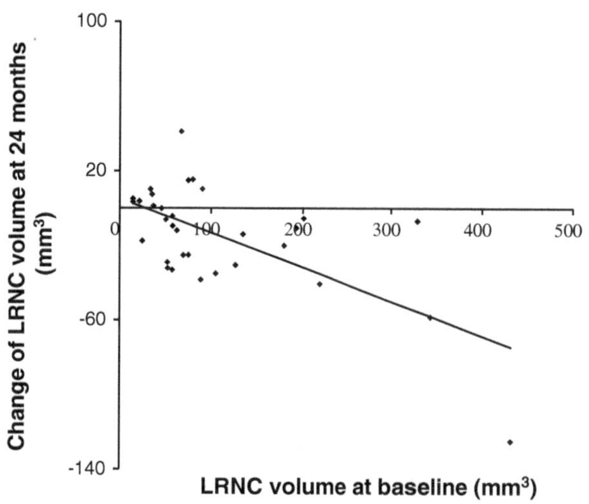

Figure 4 Associations between changes of LRNC volume at 24 months and LRNC volume at baseline. Spearman rank correlation showed that magnitude of LRNC decrease over 24 months was significantly correlated with the LRNC volume at baseline ($r = -0.53$, $p = 0.002$).

Although PWV and total wall volume was decreased and lumen volume was increased non-significantly over two years, these results were consistent with that seen in ORION [8]. Furthermore, the total wall volume reduction was significantly associated with plaque lipid content decrease as indicated in CPC [9]. Considering the natural increase of carotid plaque, the results indicate that rosuvastatin may halt the natural progression of carotid atherosclerotic plaques.

We recognize the limitations of the current study. Firstly, there was no control group since it is not ethically acceptable to study subjects with established carotid atherosclerosis without therapy. Although we performed the MRI analysis by an independent review group blinded to all clinical information, lab results and MRI scan time points, it may reduce the power to detect differences in relevant plaque endpoints. And we cannot exclude the possibility that LRNC may turn into fibrosis in months as a natural process. However, most previous investigations indicated that plaque seemed prone to progress rather than regress without lipid-lowering therapy [31,32], and LRNC was usually regard as one of the important factors leading to plaque increase. Secondly, as subjects were screened to have large plaques in this study, we are unable to discern whether or not the observed changes in LRNC volume and % LRNC occur in population with carotid wall thickness < 3 mm. Finally,due to the rigorous inclusion criteria and image quality requirement,a small number of subjects were enrolled and completed the trial. The degree to which lipid depletion documented by MRI will translate into an improvement in clinical outcomes remains unknown. Thus, larger randomized controlled trials are needed to confirm and further elucidate the effect of rosuvastatin on lipid-core reduction in patients with carotid atherosclerotic plaque in the future.

Conclusions

In summary, the present study demonstrated rapid plaque lipid depletion with a moderate-dose rosuvastatin therapy among treatment naïve subjects with asymptomatic carotid lipid-rich atherosclerotic plaques. These findings may indicate an early on-set of plaque stabilization that could be achieved within the first three months of statin treatment.

Abbreviations

MRI: Magnetic resonance imaging; LDL-C: Low-density lipoprotein cholesterol; HDL-C: High-density lipoprotein cholesterol; TOF: Time-of-flight; PDW: Proton-density-weighted; T2W: T2-weighted; T1W: T1-weighted; LA: Lumen area; WA: Wall area; PWV: Percent wall volume; LRNC: Lipid-rich necrotic core; CET1W: contrast enhanced T1-weighted.

Competing interests

Authors received funding from AstraZeneca to carry out the MR imaging analysis. Other competing interests: none to disclose.

Authors' contributions

PY and LM designed the study and were involved in data analysis and interpretation. RD and JC contributed to data collection and interpretation. PY, XZ and RD wrote the manuscript. All authors were involved in the revision and approved the final manuscript.

Acknowledgments

Thanks to AstraZeneca Pharmaceutical Company for supporting the MR imaging analysis. We thank Professor Geng Li for the language correction.

Funding

This study is partially supported by the grant from the National Nature Science Foundation of China (81270941), the Key National Basic Research Program of China (2012CB517503) and the Key Science and Technology Foundation of China (2012ZX09303004-002) to Dr. Ping Ye.

Author details

[1]Department of Geriatric Cardiology, Chinese PLA General Hospital, No. 28, Fuxing Road, Beijing 100853, China. [2]Department of Radiology, Chinese PLA General Hospital, No. 28, Fuxing Road, Beijing 100853, China. [3]Department of Medicine, Division of Cardiology, University of Washington, Seattle, WA, USA.

References

1. Virmani R, Kolodgie FD, Burke AP, Farb A, Schwartz SM: **Lessons from sudden coronary death: a comprehensive morphological classification scheme for atherosclerotic lesions.** *Arterioscler Thromb Vasc Biol* 2000, **20:**1262–1275.
2. Davies MJ, Richardson PD, Woolf N, Katz DR, Mann J: **Risk of thrombosis in human atherosclerotic plaques: role of extracellular lipid, macrophage, and smooth muscle cell content.** *Br Heart J* 1993, **69:**377–381.
3. Cai JM, Hatsukami TS, Ferguson MS, Small R, Polissar NL, Yuan C: **Classification of human carotid atherosclerotic lesions with *in vivo* multicontrast magnetic resonance imaging.** *Circulation* 2002, **106:**1368–1373.
4. Takaya N, Cai J, Ferguson MS, Yarnykh VL, Chu B, Saam T, Polissar NL, Sherwood J, Cury RC, Anders RJ, Broschat KO, Hinton D, Furie KL, Hatsukami TS, Yuan C: **Intra- and interreader reproducibility of magnetic resonance imaging for quantifying the lipid-rich necrotic core is improved with gadolinium contrast enhancement.** *J Magn Reson Imaging* 2006, **24:**203–210.
5. Cai J, Hatsukami TS, Ferguson MS, Kerwin WS, Saam T, Chu B, Takaya N, Polissar NL, Yuan C: ***In vivo* quantitative measurement of intact fibrous cap and lipid rich necrotic core size in atherosclerotic carotid plaque: a comparison of high resolution contrast enhanced MRI and histology.** *Circulation* 2005, **112:**3437–3444.
6. Corti R, Fuster V, Fayad ZA, Worthley SG, Helft G, Smith D, Weinberger J, Wentzel J, Mizsei G, Mercuri M, Badimon JJ: **Lipid lowering by simvastatin induces regression of human atherosclerotic lesions: two years' follow-up by high-resolution noninvasive magnetic resonance imaging.** *Circulation* 2002, **106:**2884–2887.
7. Corti R, Fuster V, Fayad ZA, Worthley SG, Helft G, Chaplin WF, Muntwyler J, Viles-Gonzalez JF, Weinberger J, Smith DA, Mizsei G, Badimon JJ: **Effects of aggressive versus conventional lipid-lowering therapy by simvastatin on human atherosclerotic lesions: a prospective, randomized, double-blind trial with high-resolution magnetic resonance imaging.** *J Am Coll Cardiol* 2005, **46:**106–112.
8. Underhill HR, Yuan C, Zhao XQ, Kraiss LW, Parker DL, Saam T, Chu B, Takaya N, Liu F, Polissar NL, Neradilek B, Raichlen JS, Cain VA, Waterton JC, Hamar W, Hatsukami TS: **Effect of rosuvastatin therapy on carotid plaque morphology and composition in moderately hypercholesterolemic patients: a high-resolution magnetic resonance imaging trial.** *Am Heart J* 2008, **155**(584):e1–e8.
9. Zhao XQ, Dong L, Hatsukami T, Phan BA, Chu B, Moore A, Lane T, Neradilek MB, Polissar N, Monick D, Lee C, Underhill H, Yuan C: **MR imaging of carotid plaque composition during lipid-lowering therapy a prospective assessment of effect and time course.** *JACC Cardiovasc Imaging* 2011, **4:**977–986.
10. Joint committee for developing Chinese guidelines on prevention and treatment of dyslipidemia in adults: **Chinese guidelines on prevention and treatment of dyslipidemia in adults.** *Zhong hua Xin Xue Guan Bing Za Zhi* 2007, **35:**390–419.
11. Kerwin W, Xu D, Liu F, Saam T, Underhill H, Takaya N, Chu B, Hatsukami T, Yuan C: **Magnetic resonance imaging of carotid atherosclerosis: plaque analysis.** *Top Magn Reson Imaging* 2007, **5:**371–378.
12. Saam T, Hatsukami TS, Yarnykh VL, Hayes CE, Underhill H, Chu B, Takaya N, Cai J, Kerwin WS, Xu D, Polissar NL, Neradilek B, Hamar WK, Maki J, Shaw DW, Buck RJ, Wyman B, Yuan C: **Reader and platform reproducibility for quantitative assessment of carotid atherosclerotic plaque using 1.5T Siemens, philips, and general electric scanners.** *J Magn Reson Imaging* 2007, **26:**344–352.
13. Richardson PD, Davies MJ, Born GV: **Influence of plaque configuration and stress distribution on fissuring of coronary atherosclerotic plaques [see comments].** *Lancet* 1989, **2:**941–944.
14. Mann JM, Davies MJ: **Vulnerable plaque. Relation of characteristics to degree of stenosis in human coronary arteries.** *Circulation* 1996, **94:**928–931.
15. Lendon CL, Davies MJ, Born GV, Richardson PD: **Atherosclerotic plaque caps are locally weakened when macrophages density is increased.** *Atherosclerosis* 1991, **87:**87–90.
16. Galis ZS, Sukhova GK, Kranzhofer R, Clark S, Libby P: **Macrophage foam cells from experimental atheroma constitutively produce matrix-degrading proteinases.** *Proc Natl Acad Sci U S A* 1995, **92:**402–406.
17. Moreno PR, Falk E, Palacios IF, Newell JB, Fuster V, Fallon JT: **Macrophage infiltration in acute coronary syndromes. Implications for plaque rupture.** *Circulation* 1994, **90:**775–778.
18. Li AC, Glass CK: **The macrophage foam cell as a target for therapeutic intervention.** *Nat Med* 2002, **8:**1235–1242.
19. Zhao XQ, Kerwin WS: **Utilizing imaging tools in lipidology: examining the potential of MRI for monitoring cholesterol therapy.** *Clin Lipidol* 2012, **7:**329–343.
20. Reis ED, Li J, Fayad ZA, Rong JX, Hansoty D, Aguinaldo JG, Fallon JT, Fisher EA: **Dramatic remodeling of advanced atherosclerotic plaques of the apolipoprotein E-deficient mouse in a novel transplantation model.** *J Vasc Surg* 2001, **34:**541–547.

21. Williams JK, Sukhova GK, Herrington DM, Libby P: **Pravastatin has cholesterol lowering independent effects on the artery wall of atherosclerotic monkeys.** *J Am Coll Cardiol* 1998, **31:**684–691.
22. Crisby M, Nordin-Fredriksson G, Shah PK, Yano J, Zhu J, Nilsson J: **Pravastatin treatment increases collagen content and decreases lipid content, inflammation, metalloproteinases, and cell deathin human carotid plaques: implications for plaque stabilization.** *Circulation* 2001, **103:**926–933.
23. Tawakol A, Fayad ZA, Mogg R, Alon A, Klimas MT, Dansky H, Subramanian SS, Abdelbaky A, Rudd JH, Farkouh ME, Nunes IO, Beals CR, Shankar SS: **Intensification of statin therapy results in a rapid reduction in atherosclerotic inflammation: results of a multi-center FDG-PET/CT Feasibility Study.** *J Am Coll Cardiol* 2013, **62:**909–917.
24. Saam T, Cai JM, Cai YQ, An NY, Kampschulte A, Xu D, Kerwin WS, Takaya N, Polissar NL, Hatsukami TS, Yuan C: **Carotid plaque composition differs between ethno-racial groups: an MRI pilot study comparing mainland Chinese and American Caucasian patients.** *Arterioscler Thromb Vasc Biol* 2005, **25:**611–616.
25. Kerwin WS, Oikawa M, Yuan C, Jarvik G, Hatsukami T: **MR imaging of adventitial vasa vasorum in carotid atherosclerosis.** *Magn Reson Med* 2008, **59:**507–514.
26. Hatsukami TS, Chun Y: **MRI in the early identification and classification of high-risk atherosclerotic carotid plaques.** *Imaging Med* 2010, **2:**63–75.
27. Takaya N, Yuan C, Chu B, Saam T, Underhill H, Cai J, Tran N, Polissar NL, Isaac C, Ferguson MS, Garden GA, Cramer SC, Maravilla KR, Hashimoto B, Hatsukami TS: **Association between carotid plaque characteristics and subsequent ischemic cerebrovascular events: a prospective assessment with MRI-initial results.** *Stroke* 2006, **37:**818–823.
28. Singh N, Moody AR, Gladstone DJ, Leung G, Ravikumar R, Zhan J, Maggisano R: **Moderate carotid artery stenosis: MRI depicted intraplaque hemorrhage predicts risk of cerebrovascular ischemic events in asymptomatic men.** *Radiology* 2009, **252:**502–508.
29. Altaf N, Daniels L, Morgan PS, Auer D, MacSweeney ST, Moody AR, Gladman JR: **Detection of intraplaque hemorrhage by magnetic resonance imaging in symptomatic patients with mild to moderate carotid stenosis predicts recurrent neurological events.** *J Vasc Surg* 2008, **47:**337–342.
30. Dong L, Underhill HR, Yu W, Ota H, Hatsukami TS, Gao TL, Zhang Z, Oikawa M, Zhao X, Yuan C: **Geometric and compositional appearance of atheroma in an angiographically normal carotid artery in patients with atherosclerosis.** *AJNR Am J Neuroradiol* 2010, **31:**311–316.
31. Okazaki S, Yokoyama T, Miyauchi K, Shimada K, Kurata T, Sato H, Daida H: **Early statin treatment in patients with acute coronary syndrome: demonstration of the beneficial effect on atherosclerotic lesions by serial volumetric intravascular ultrasound analysis during half a year after coronary event: the ESTABLISH Study.** *Circulation* 2004, **110:**1061–1068.
32. Nissen SE, Nicholls SJ, Sipahi I, Libby P, Raichlen JS, Ballantyne CM, Davignon J, Erbel R, Fruchart JC, Tardif JC, Schoenhagen P, Crowe T, Cain V, Wolski K, Goormastic M, Tuzcu EM, ASTEROID Investigators: **Effect of very high-intensity statin therapy on regression of coronary atherosclerosis: the ASTEROID trial.** *JAMA* 2006, **295:**1556–1565.

2

Diagnostic accuracy of resting left ventricular akinesia/hypokinesia in predicting abnormal coronary angiography

Mohamed Faisal Lutfi

Abstract

Background: Although several reports demonstrate the efficacy of stress echocardiography in diagnosing coronary artery disease, comparable studies on the competence of the same imaging technique at rest are limited. This study aimed to evaluate whether ventricular akinesia/hypokinesia and left ventricular ejection fraction (LVEF) < 55 % at rest are useful in predicting abnormal coronary angiography.

Methods: This study prospectively enrolled 100 diagnostic coronary catheterization candidates. Any routine echocardiography that the candidates had undergone before diagnostic coronary catheterization was reviewed. Patients were subclassified according to the presence and location of ventricular akinesia/hypokinesia, LVEF, and the results of diagnostic coronary catheterization. LVEF < 55 % was considered below the normal physiological limit. Abnormal coronary angiography was defined as narrowing of half or more of the caliber of at least one major coronary artery.

Results: Abnormal coronary angiography was significantly associated with akinesia/hypokinesia (OR = 4.85, $P = 0.002$) and LVEF < 55 % (OR = 5.75, $P = 0.001$). Screening of akinesia/hypokinesia and LVEF < 55 % as diagnostic tools for abnormal coronary angiography achieved comparable sensitivities (87.2 % vs. 88.9 %), specificities (41.5 vs. 41.8), and diagnostic accuracies (41.5 vs. 41.8). Left ventricular anterior wall akinesia/hypokinesia achieved a higher diagnostic odds ratio (9.7), sensitivity (95 %), and negative predictive value (96.4 %) compared with other types of akinesia/hypokinesia.

Conclusion: The overall diagnostic accuracy of akinesia/hypokinesia and LVEF < 55 % to predict abnormal coronary angiography was poor, probably owing to significant influences of macro- as well as micro-vascular ischemia on left ventricular function.

Keywords: Akinesia/hypokinesia, Coronary artery disease, Coronary angiography, Ejection fraction

Background

Myocardial ischemia is known to depress cardiac contractility [1]. Reduction of left ventricular wall motion (LVWM) and/or ejection fraction (LVEF) usually indicates myocardial ischemia unless proven otherwise [2]. Depressed left ventricular function (LVF) is likely, whether myocardial ischemia is owing to compromised function of large epicardial vessels [3] or the microcirculation of the heart [4, 5]. The presence of clinical features of myocardial ischemia usually indicates coronary artery disease (CAD) [6]. In such patients, failure of the coronary angiography to demonstrate apparent, or induced, narrowing of the large coronary vessels redirects the possible diagnosis towards microvascular ischemia of the myocardium. Cardiac syndrome X (CSX) is commonly used to describe the triad of: typical cardiac chest pain, significant changes in one or more of the cardiac stress test(s), and normal angiography of the epicardial coronary vessels [7, 8].

Cardiac stress tests evaluate the possible ischemic electrocardiography (ECG) changes, depressed LVWM or LVEF while heart activity is increased by exercise or other inotropic factors [9, 10]. Although there are

Correspondence: mohamedfaisallutfi@gmail.com
Department of Physiology, Faculty of Medicine and Health Sciences, Al-Neelain University, Mailbox: 12702, Khartoum 11121, Sudan

several reports on the efficiency of stress echocardiography in the diagnosis of CAD [11, 12], comparable studies on the competence of the same technique at rest are limited [13]. Clinicians in developing countries are usually forced to use resting ECG and echocardiography for the diagnosis and risk stratification of CAD patients, owing to a lack of facilities and poor financial resources. In Sudan, selection of candidates for diagnostic coronary catheterization (DCC) is partly dependent on depressed LVWM and/or LVEF on resting echocardiography. The present study aimed to evaluate ventricular akinesia/hypokinesia and LVEF < 55 % derived from resting echocardiography as screening tests for the detection of abnormal coronary angiography (ACA). This is the first study to evaluate these two measures as screening tools for ACA in Sudan and probably worldwide.

Methods

This study received clearance from the Ethics Review Committee of the Faculty of Medicine, Khartoum University, Sudan. Written informed consent was provided by each volunteer before being enrolled in the study.

This study prospectively enrolled 100 diagnostic coronary catheterization (DCC) candidates in Al-Shaab Cardiac Center, Khartoum, Sudan. Following evaluation of sociodemographic characteristics, past medical history, and clinical examination of each patient, results of routine echocardiography conducted before DCC were reviewed. Patients were subclassified according to the presence and location of ventricular akinesia/hypokinesia, LVEF, and the results of DCC. The endocardial and epicardial motion, as well as thickening of each segment of the LV, were assessed to assign a wall motion score index (WMSI). Normal wall thickening (WMSI = 1) was considered indicative of normokinesia, while decreased (WMSI = 2) and absent (WMSI = 3) wall thickening were considered indicative of hypokinesia and akinesia respectively. Left ventricular anterior (LVAW), septal (LVSW), inferior (LVIW), and lateral (LVLW) walls were assessed for the presence of akinesia/hypokinesia, irrespective of which particular part of the wall was affected. According to the 16-LV segmentation model, LVSW included the basal anteroseptal, basal inferoseptal, mid-anteroseptal, mid-inferoseptal, and apical parts of the interventricular septum; LVAW included the basal, mid, or apical parts of the anterior LV wall; LVIW included the basal, mid, or apical parts of the inferior LV wall; and LVLW included the basal anterolateral, basal inferolateral, mid-anterolateral, mid-inferolateral, and apical parts of the lateral wall. LVEF < 55 % was considered to be below the normal physiological limit [14]. Patients with narrowing of half or more of the caliber of one or more of the major coronary arteries were considered to have ACA [15]. The following formula was used to estimate body mass index (BMI):

$$\mathrm{BMI}\ (\mathrm{Kg/m^2}) = \mathrm{weight}\ (\mathrm{kg})/(\mathrm{height}\ (\mathrm{m^2}).$$

Statistical analysis was performed using OpenEpi software, version 2.3, and Statistical Package for the Social Sciences (SPSS) for Windows, version 16.0 (SPSS Inc., Chicago, IL, USA). Studied variables were described as the mean ± standard deviation. Proportions of the studied groups were expressed as percentages (%) and 95 % confidence intervals (CI). The unpaired *t*-test was used to evaluate differences in the means of the studied variables between patients with normal coronary angiogram (NCA) and ACA. The binary logestic regression was used to evaluate the association between ACA and akinesia/hypokinesia as well as LVEF < 55 %. Sensitivity, specificity, positive predictive value (PPV), negative predictive value (NPV), diagnostic accuracy (DA), likelihood ratio of a positive test (LRP), likelihood ratio of a negative test (LRN), and diagnostic odds ratio (DOR) were calculated to evaluate akinesia/hypokinesia and LVEF < 55 % as screening tests for ACA. $P < 0.05$ was considered significant.

Results

Coronary angiography confirmed CAD in 72 of 100 patients subjected to DCC (72 %, 95 % CI 62.5–79.9 %). Eight of the subjects with NCA were male (28.6 %, 95 % CI 15.3–47.1 %), and 53 of the subjects with ACA were male (73.6 %, 95 % CI 62.4–82.4 %). Characteristics of the studied groups are given in Table 1. Patients with ACA were significantly older (59.58 ± 9.80 years) and had a significantly lower BMI (25.70 ± 3.97 kg/m^2) compared with those with NCA (49.11 ± 8.16 years, 29.58 ± 4.96 kg/m^2; $P < 0.001$). ACA was significantly associated with male sex (OR = 6.97, $P < 0.001$), diabetes mellitus (OR = 3.89, $P = 0.013$), akinesia/hypokinesia (OR = 4.85, $P = 0.002$; Fig. 1), and LVEF < 55 % (OR = 5.75, $P = 0.001$;

Table 1 Characteristics of the studied groups

	Subjects with normal angiography *N* = 28 M (SD)	Subjects with abnormal angiography *N* = 72 M (SD)	P
Age (Years)	49.11 (8.16)	59.58 (9.80)	<0.001
BMI (kg/m2)	29.58 (4.96)	25.70 (3.97)	<0.001
SBP (mmHg)	129.25 (18.83)	129.49 (24.87)	0.963
DBP (mmHg)	77.64 (11.42)	77.94 (13.06)	0.918
LVEF (%)	59.50 (9.77)	52.10 (12.69)	0.003

M mean, *SD* standard deviation, *BMI* body mass index, *SBP* systolic blood pressure, *DBP* diastolic blood pressure, *LVEF* left ventricular ejection fraction

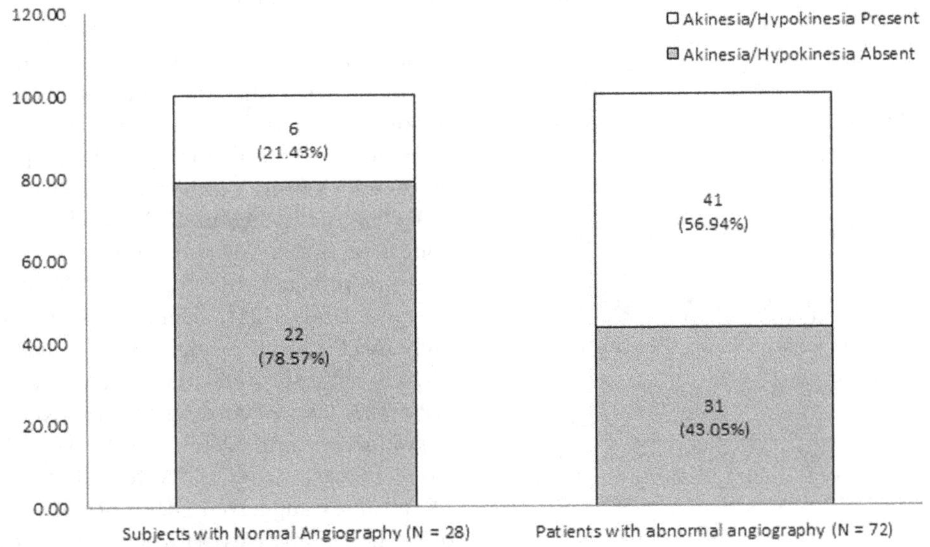

Fig. 1 Distribution of akinesia/hypokinesia among the studied groups

Fig. 2). Evaluation of akinesia/hypokinesia and LVEF < 55 % as screening tests for ACA revealed highly comparable conditional ratios (Table 2). The DORs and sensitivities of akinesia/hypokinesia and LVEF < 55 % as screening tools for diagnosis of CAD were relatively higher than the other conditional ratios (Table 2). LVAW akinesia/hypokinesia achieved the highest DOR (mean 9.7 %; range, 1.2–76.2 %), sensitivity (95 %), and NPV (96.4 %) compared with the other locations (Table 3). Specificities and PPVs were equally poor in all types of akinesia/hypokinesia (Table 3).

Discussion

Presence of LV akinesia/hypokinesia and/or LVEF < 55 % significantly increased the odds of having ACA in patients undergoing DCC. Currently, LVWM and LVEF are important indicators of LVF, and are commonly used to assess severity and prognosis of CAD [2]. In one study, echocardiographic estimates of LVEF were validated using ventriculography measurements of LVEF for comparison; LVWM-derived estimates of ejection fraction faithfully reflected LVEF measured by the standard reference method [16]. Another study by Squeri et al. [3]

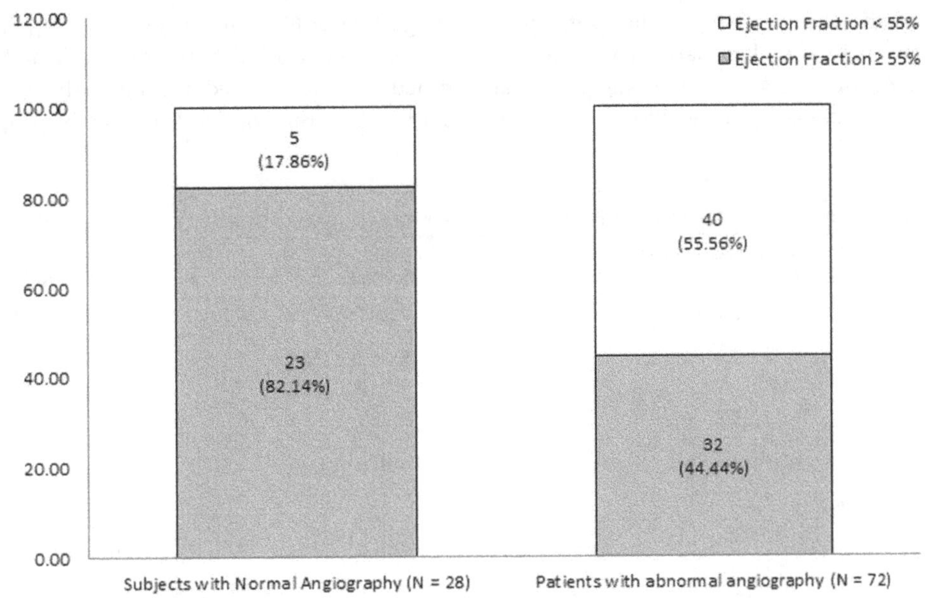

Fig. 2 Distribution of left ventricular ejection fraction values (< or ≥ 55 %) among the studied groups

Table 2 Evaluation of akinesia/hypokinesia and left ventricular ejection fraction < 55 % as screening tests for coronary artery disease

	Akinesia/Hypokinesia	EF < 55 %
	Estimate (95 % CI)	Estimate (95 % CI)
Sensitivity (%)	87.2 (74.8–94.0)	88.9 (76.5–95.2)
Specificity (%)	41.5 (29.2–54.9)	41.8 (29.7–55.0)
PPV (%)	56.9 (45.4–67.7)	55.6 (44.1–66.5)
NPV (%)	78.6 (60.5–89.8)	82.1 (64.4–92.1)
DA (%)	63.0 (53.2–71.8)	63.6 (53.8–72.4)
LRP	1.5 (1.4–1.6)	1.5 (1.4–1.6)
LRN	0.3 (0.2–0.5)	0.3 (0.2–0.4)
DOR	4.8 (1.8–13.4)	5.8 (2.0–16.8)

EF ejection fraction, *CI* confidence intervals, *PPV* positive predictive value, *NPV* negative predictive value, *DA* diagnostic accuracy, *LRP* likelihood ratio of a positive test, *LRN* likelihood ratio of a negative test, *DOR* diagnostic odds ratio

demonstrated the intimate relationship between LVEF and severity of CAD. They assessed stress-induced changes in LVEF (ΔLVEF) in four groups: controls, and patients with single-, two-, and three-vessel disease. The results showed that mean ΔLVEF was negative in patients with three-vessel or left main CAD, indicating that decreased heart contractility followed stress-induced myocardial ischemia [3]. In addition, the ΔLVEF was significantly lower in all other angiographic groups compared with the controls [3]. These previous findings thus reflect the efficiency of LVEF in evaluating the severity of CAD. The present study found that major impairment of LVWM and LVEF increased the odds of having ACA by about five to six times, which gives further support to the findings reported by Squeri et al. [3].

In the present study, the relatively higher sensitivity compared with specificity of akinesia/hypokinesia and LVEF < 55 % as screening tools for ACA suggests that these tests are more efficient in detecting, but not excluding, patients with ACA [17]. The higher NPV relative to PPV suggests a higher proportion of NCA subjects in those with normal LVF compared with the proportion of ACA patients in those with akinesia/hypokinesia and LVEF < 55 % [18]. PPV and NPV are influenced by the disease prevalence [19]; higher prevalence tends to result in increased PPV and decreased NPV [20]. The prevalence of CAD is relatively lower in Sudan compared with developed countries, and is therefore likely to have affected the PPV and NPV assessed in the present study [21]. Hence, LV akinesia/hypokinesia and LVEF < 55 % were also evaluated by LRP and LRN, which showed comparable findings to PPV and NPV [22, 23]. According to the LRP results, akinesia/hypokinesia and LVEF < 55 % was 1.5 times more likely in cases with ACA than those with NCA. The LRN values suggested that normal LVF was 0.3 times more likely in cases with ACA than those with NCA. The wide gap between sensitivity and specificity, as well as between PPV and NPV, indicates poor overall DA of akinesia/hypokinesia and LVEF < 55 % as screening tests for ACA. The variations in the conditional ratios were maintained in different locations of akinesia/hypokinesia when evaluated as screening tests for ACA. LVAW akinesia/hypokinesia achieved the highest DOR, sensitivity, and NPV, and equally poor specificity and PPV, compared with the other locations of akinesia/hypokinesia.

Although it is evident from the current results and previous reports that abnormal LVWM and LVEF are common in CAD patients, the presence of such findings cannot exclude microvascular ischemia. The coexistence of angina and ischemic ECG changes with uneventful DCC in patients with NCA in the current study is highly suggestive of CSX in this group [7, 8]. According to one study, when CSX patients are subjected to exercise, LV function is maintained as long as there is no ST segment shift; worsening of LV function is proportional to the

Table 3 Evaluation of different locations of left ventricular akinesia/hypokinesia in the screening of coronary artery disease

	Anterior wall akinesia/Hypokinesia estimate (95 % CI)	Septal akinesia/Hypokinesia estimate (95 % CI)	Inferior wall akinesia/Hypokinesia estimate (95 % CI)
Sensitivity (%)	95.0 (76.4–99.1)	89.3 (72.8–96.3)	87.0 (67.9–95.5)
Specificity (%)	33.8 (24.4–44.6)	34.7 (24.8–46.2)	32.5 (23.1–43.5)
PPV (%)	26.4 (17.6–37.6)	34.7 (24.8–46.2)	27.8 (18.8–39.1)
NPV (%)	96.4 (82.3–99.4)	89.3 (72.8–96.3)	89.3 (72.8–96.3)
DA (%)	46.0 (36.6–55.7)	50.0 (40.4–59.6)	45.0 (35.6–54.8)
LRP	1.4 (1.4–1.5)	1.4 (1.3–1.4)	1.3 (1.2–1.4)
LRN	0.1 (0.01–1.2)	0.3 (0.1–0.7)	0.4 (0.2–0.9)
DOR	9.7 (1.2–76.2)	4.4 (1.2–16.1)	3.2 (0.9–11.8)

CI confidence intervals, *PPV* positive predictive value, *NPV* negative predictive value, *DA* diagnostic accuracy, *LRP* likelihood ratio of a positive test, *LRN* likelihood ratio of a negative test, *DOR* diagnostic odds ratio

degree of ST segment depression [5]. These findings are further supported by another study that showed decreased myocardial perfusion in 47 % and abnormal wall motion in 35 % of CSX patients following stress testing [4]. The same study concluded that microcirculatory dysfunction of the myocardium in some patients with CSX can result in concordant transient segmental LVWM abnormalities and impaired LVEF [4]. The findings of these previous studies on the pattern of changes in patients with macro- and micro-vascular ischemia explain the poor performance of akinesia/hypokinesia and LVEF < 55 % as screening tools for prediction of ACA.

The current study had some limitations. Although 100 DCC candidates were enrolled, a larger sample size would have enabled more definitive conclusions to be made regarding the diagnostic accuracy of resting LV akinesia/hypokinesia in predicting ACA. In addition, the lack of stress echocardiography testing in Sudan precluded evaluation of LV akinesia/hypokinesia in the studied patients during increased heart activity. Combined evaluation of DCC patients with resting and stress echocardiography tests in the future could offer scientific evidence as to which test has better DA in predicting ACA.

Conclusion

Evaluation of akinesia/hypokinesia and LVEF < 55 % as screening tools for CAD suggests that these tests were more reliable for detection, but not exclusion, of patients with ACA. Overall DA of these measures to discriminate ACA from NCA was poor, probably owing to the comparable influence of macro- and micro-vascular ischemia on LVF.

Abbreviations

ΔLVEF, change in LVEF; ACA, abnormal coronary angiography; BMI, body mass index; CAD, coronary artery disease; CI, confidence intervals; CSX, cardiac syndrome X; DA, diagnostic accuracy; DBP, diastolic blood pressure; DCC, diagnostic coronary catheterization; DOR, diagnostic odds ratio; ECG, electrocardiography; LRN, likelihood ratio of a negative test; LRP, likelihood ratio of a positive test; LVAW, left ventricular anterior wall; LVEF, left ventricular ejection fraction; LVF, left ventricular function; LVIW, left ventricular inferior wall; LVPW, left ventricular posterior wall; LVSW, left ventricular septal wall; LVWM, left ventricular wall motion; M, mean; NCA, normal coronary angiography; NPV, negative predictive value; PPV, positive predictive value; SBP, systolic blood pressure; SD, standard deviation; SPSS, Statistical Package for the Social Sciences

Acknowledgments

I would like to thank patients and medical personnel in Al-Shaab Cardiac Center, Khartoum, Sudan, for their assistance with obtaining the data used in this study.

Funding

None to declare.

Authors' contributions

All work was conducted by MFL (study design, data collection, analysis, interpretation, and draft writing).

Competing interests

The author declares that he has no competing interests.

References

1. Shabana A, El-Menyar A. Myocardial viability: What We Knew and What Is New. Cardiol Res Pract. 2012;2012:607486.
2. Lebeau R, Serri K, Morice MC, Hovasse T, Unterseeh T, Piéchaud JF, Garot J. Assessment of left ventricular ejection fraction using the wall motion score index in cardiac magnetic resonance imaging. Arch Cardiovasc Dis. 2012;105(2):91–8.
3. Squeri A, Gaibazzi N, Reverberi C, Caracciolo MM, Ardissino D, Gherli T. Ejection fraction change and coronary artery disease severity: a vasodilator contrast stress-echocardiography study. J Am Soc Echocardiogr. 2012;25(4):454–9.
4. Demir H, Kahraman G, Isgoren S, Tan YZ, Kilic T, Berk F. Evaluation of post-stress left ventricular dysfunction and its relationship with perfusion abnormalities using gated SPECT in patients with cardiac syndrome X. Nucl Med Commun. 2008;29(3):208–14.
5. Yoshio H, Shimizu M, Kita Y, Ino H, Taki J, Takeda R. Left ventricular functional reverse in patients with syndrome X: evaluation by continuous ventricular function monitoring. J Am Coll Cardiol. 1993;22(5):1465–9.
6. Badar AA, Perez-Moreno AC, Hawkins NM, Jhund PS, Brunton AP, Anand IS, McKelvie RS, Komajda M, Zile MR, Carson PE, Gardner RS, Petrie MC, McMurray JJ. Clinical characteristics and outcomes of patients with coronary artery disease and angina: analysis of the irbesartan in patients with heart failure and preserved systolic function trial. Circ Heart Fail. 2015;8(4):717–24.
7. Douglas PS, Patel MR, Bailey SR, Dai D, Kaltenbach L, Brindis RG, Messenger J, Peterson ED. Hospital variability in the rate of finding obstructive coronary artery disease at elective, diagnostic coronary angiography. J Am Coll Cardiol. 2011;58(8):801–9.
8. Vermeltfoort IA, Raijmakers PG, Riphagen II, Odekerken DA, Kuijper AF, Zwijnenburg A, et al. Definitions and incidence of cardiac syndrome X: review and analysis of clinical data. Clin Res Cardiol. 2010;99(8):475–81.
9. Liu J, Xu Y, Wang J, Zhang B, Liu B, Lü W, Zhi G. Diagnostic value of quantitative low-dose dobutamine stress echocardiography with three-dimensional speckle-tracking for non-ST-elevation acute coronary syndrome. Nan Fang Yi Ke Da Xue Xue Bao. 2015;35(7):947–53.
10. Banerjee A, Newman DR, Van den Bruel A, Heneghan C. Diagnostic accuracy of exercise stress testing for coronary artery disease: a systematic review and meta-analysis of prospective studies. Int J Clin Pract. 2012;66(5):477–92.
11. Health Quality Ontario. Stress echocardiography for the diagnosis of coronary artery disease: an evidence-based analysis. Ontario Health Technol Assess Ser. 2010;10(9):1–61.
12. Peteiro J, Bouzas-Mosquera A. Exercise echocardiography. World J Cardiol. 2010;2(8):223–32.
13. Parato VM, Mehta A, Delfino D, Amabili S, Partemi M, Grossi P, Nardini E. Resting echocardiography for the early detection of acute coronary syndromes in chest pain unit patients. Echocardiography. 2010;27(6):597–602.
14. Ueda T, Kawakami R, Nishida T, Onoue K, Soeda T, Okayama S, Takeda Y, Watanabe M, Kawata H, Uemura S, Saito Y. Left ventricular Ejection Fraction (EF) of 55 % as cutoff for late transition from Heart Failure (HF) with preserved EF to HF with mildly reduced EF. Circ J. 2015;79(10):2209–15.
15. Mohareb MM, Qiu F, Cantor WJ, Kingsbury KJ, Ko DT, Wijeysundera HC. Validation of the appropriate use criteria for coronary angiography: a cohort study. Ann Intern Med. 2015;162(8):549–56.
16. Berning J, Rokkedal Nielsen J, Launbjerg J, Fogh J, Mickley H, Andersen PE. Rapid estimation of left ventricular ejection fraction in acute myocardial infarction by echocardiographic wall motion analysis. Cardiology. 1992;80(3–4):257–66.
17. Parikh R, Mathai A, Parikh S, Chandra Sekhar G, Thomas R. Understanding and using sensitivity, specificity and predictive values. Indian J Ophthalmol. 2008;56(1):45–50.
18. Akobeng AK. Understanding diagnostic tests 1: sensitivity, specificity and predictive values. Acta Paediatr. 2007;96(3):338–41.
19. Stuber KJ. Specificity, sensitivity, and predictive values of clinical tests of the sacroiliac joint: a systematic review of the literature. The Journal of the Canadian Chiropractic Association. 2007;51(1):30–41.
20. Peplow MO, Correa-Prisant M, Stebbins ME, Jones F, Davies P. Sensitivity, specificity, and predictive values of three salmonella rapid detection kits

using fresh and frozen poultry environmental samples versus those of standard plating. Appl Environ Microbiol. 1999;65(3):1055–60.
21. Suliman A. The state of heart disease in Sudan. Cardiovasc J Afr. 2011;22(4):191–6.
22. Spitalnic S. Test properties 2: likelihood ratios, Bayes' formula, and receiver operating characteristic curves. Hosp Physician. 2004;40(10):53–8.
23. Attia J. Diagnostic tests: moving beyond sensitivity and specificity: using likelihood ratios to help interpret diagnostic tests. Aust Prescr. 2003;26(5):111–3.

3

Echocardiographic evaluation of thalassemia intermedia patients in Duhok, Iraq

Ameen Mosa Mohammad

Abstract

Background: Cardiac complications are among the most serious problems of thalassemia intermedia patients. The current study was initiated to address the latter issue through the study of the echocardiographic findings and correlate it with clinical characteristics of thalassemia intermedia patients in Duhok, Kurdistan region, Iraq.

Methods: An echocardiographic assessment of 61beta-thalassemia intermedia cases was performed. It included 30 males and 31 females, with a mean age 19.6 ± 7.5 years. The standard echostudy of two-dimension and M-mode measurements of cardiac chambers were done. The continuous doppler regurgitant jet of tricuspid and pulmonary valves were recorded. Left ventricle diastolic function was assessed by pulsed doppler of mitral valve inflow. To correlate the clinical with echocardiographic findings, patients were divided, according to tricuspid regurgitant velocity, into three groups (<2.5 m/sec, 2.5-2.9 m/sec and ≥3 m/sec).

Results: Tricuspid regurgitant velocity <2.5 m/sec, 2.5-2.9 m/sec and ≥3 m/sec occurred in 42(69%), 11(18%) and 8(13%) respectively. Comparing to other groups patients with tricuspid regurgitant velocity ≥3 m/sec were older and included more males. They had lower hemoglobin levels, but higher ferritin levels. Their age at diagnosis and the age of the initiation of blood transfusion were later. Most of them had significant exertional dyspnea. They also had relatively lower left ventricle ejection fraction values. Right ventricular diameter and right atrial size were larger in the same group. Tricuspid regurgitant velocity as a continuous predictor was associated positively with age, cardiac volumes and pulmonary regurgitation though negatively associated with ejection fraction.

Conclusions: Echo-derived right and left side cardiac complications are not uncommon in thalassemia intermedia patients. Therapeutic trails targeting these complications are indicated, and echocardiographic assessment is necessary to be offered early for thalassemia intermedia.

Keywords: Thalassemia intermedia, Tricuspid velocity jet, Pulmonary hypertension, Iraq

Background

Thalassemia Intermedia (TI) is an inherited hemoglobin disorder that is characterized by a significant genetic and clinical heterogeneity.

Cardiovascular involvement represents a well-known complication and the primary cause of mortality in TI. It is mainly determined by the fact that both ventricles have to maintain a high cardiac output level through a stiff vascular bed. Pulmonary hypertension and steady increase in tricuspid regurgitant jet followed by right heart failure dominates the clinical picture.

The left ventricle has to maintain a high cardiac output in a continuous state of both volume and pressure overload which consequently contributes to left ventricular impairment with time [1-3].

Several factors have been reported to interfere in the pathophysiology of cardiovascular abnormalities in TI. However, the key mechanism is the chronic tissue hypoxia and chronic hemolysis with its consequences [3]. The screening of patients with thalassemia intermedia for evidence of cardiac complications by transthoracic echostudy is a good option for early diagnosis and eventually for future planning of best management of cardiac complications. The purpose of this study is to look for evidence of cardiac involvement by echocardiography

Correspondence: doctoramb@yahoo.com
Department of Medicine, Division of Cardiology, Medical School, Faculty of Medical Sciences, Duhok University, Kurdistan, Iraq

and correlate the echocardiographic findings with clinical characteristics of patients with TI.

Methods

This is a prospective study of 61 beta-thalassemia intermedia patients (out of total 74 registered in Duhok thalassemia center). It included 30 males and 31 females, with a mean age of 19.6(SD7.5) years. All patients were evaluated by history taking and physical examination, laboratory studies, and underwent transthoracic echocardiography between June 2010 and June 2011. Either patients or their relatives provided written informed consent.

Transthoracic echocardiography was performed for all patients by Vivid 3(GE) Echo systems. The standard two-dimension and M-mode measurements of the cardiac chambers including left ventricle ejection fraction (LVEF %) were taken. Cardiac volumes and dimensions were indexed by body surface area. Tricuspid regurgitation was assessed in the apical four chambers, parasternal short axis views, and a minimum of three sequential complexes were recorded. Continuous doppler sampling of the peak regurgitant jet to estimate the right ventricular to right atrial systolic pressure gradient by the modified Bernoulli equation was obtained. To assess the mean pulmonary artery pressure, the pulmonary artery to right ventricular pressure gradient was estimated from the peak pulmonary regurgitant flow velocity (V) in parasternal short axis view by the simplified Bernoulli equation (PG = 4 V2) [4]. Left ventricle diastolic function was assessed by pulsed doppler sampling of mitral valve inflow in four apical chambers view. The peak E and A waves velocities and the E/A ratio of the mitral valve were recorded. All echocardiographic measurements were performed according to American society of echocardiography recommendations [5].

To correlate between the clinical and Echo findings within the studied sample, the patients were divided according to tricuspid regurgitant velocity (TRV) into three groups (TRV < 2.5 m/sec, 2.5-2.9 m/sec and ≥3 m/sec) [6]. Additionally, TRV was taken as a continuous variable to assess its associations with clinical and echocardiographic findings. Data of blood transfusion history were categorized into: regularly transfused (patients transfused at regular intervals every 1–3 months for last year prior to study enrollment) and irregularly transfused (≤ 3 units of blood/ year). Continuous variables were calculated as mean (SD) and categorical variables were presented as counts and percentages. ANOVA and a Fisher's exact tests were used for the comparison of continuous and categorical variables respectively. Scatter plots with line regression were used for the analysis of TRV as a continuous variable with other predictors. P-value < 0.05 was considered significant. The study was approved by the ethical committee at the School of Medicine, Faculty of Medical Sciences, University of Duhok.

Results

Correlations of clinical characteristics to TRV

Since patients have been classified into three groups according to the TRV, 42(69%) had TRV <2.5 m/sec, 8(13%) had ≥ 3 m/sec, the remaining 11(18%) had between these two values. Patients with highest TRV were older. Almost all of them were over 12 years old. Their age at diagnosis and first blood transfusion were later. Majority of them were male with significant exertional dyspnea. Their Hemoglobin level was lower, but ferritin was higher. Most of them were splenectomized. BSA was higher in the same group as shown in Table 1.

Echocardiographic findings in relation to TRV

Higher TRV values were significantly associated with increased cardiac chamber indices. These indices included left ventricle end diastolic diameter (LVEDD), left ventricle end systolic diameter (LVESD), left atrial (LA) diameter, and right ventricle (RV) diameter and right atrial (RA) size. There was a relatively slight decrease in the ejection fraction at the highest levels of jet velocity. There was an increase in the mean of LV wall and septal thickness with higher TRV values, though it did not reach the significant difference. The peak gradients of tricuspid and pulmonary valves were significantly associated with an increasing degree of TRV as shown in Table 2.

Associations of TRV as a continuous variable with other predictors

Scatter plots of TRV with age and echocardiographic predictors showed a significant association with age, LVEDD, LVESD, LA diameter, RV diameter, RA area and PR peak gradient. But there was a negative association with LVEF % as shown in Figures 1, 2, 3, 4, 5, 6, 7 and 8.

Discussion

The main findings of the study are the following: first, both the left and right cardiac chambers, especially the dimensions and volumes, were increased in TI patients with time. Second, patients with higher TRV were presented with advancing age, later age at diagnosis, later onset of initiation of blood transfusion, predominant male gender, lower hemoglobin level, higher ferritin rates, and higher percentage of splenectomised patients. Third, the LVEF % was normal. It was relatively lower for the patients with higher TRV. Three patients had features of congestive heart failure.

Some of TI patients have an exceptional hemodynamic pattern consistent with right ventricular cardiomyopathy and PHT as well as the left ventricular abnormalities that can be a leading cause of cardiopulmonary problems in

Table 1 Clinical characteristics of TI patients in relation to TR jet velocity

Characteristics	Jet velocity <2.5 m/sec 42(69%)	Jet velocity 2.5-2.9 m/sec 11(18%)	Jet velocity ≥ 3.0 m/sec 8(13%)	p-value
Mean Age(year)	14.0(SD11.2)	19.0(SD 5.0)	26(SD 6.30)	0.007
Age ≥ 12 Years	19(45.23%)	8(72.72%)	8(100%)	0.004
Age at Diagnosis(year)	6.40(SD1.74)	8.02(SD1.06)	9.10(SD1.2 0)	<0.001
Sex(male)	16(38%)	8(72%)	6(75%)	0.01
BSA(m^{2})	0.98(SD0.37)	1.40(SD0.25)	1.46(SD0.13)	<0.001
BMI(kg/m^2)	16.95(SD2.91)	18.09(SD2.15)	19.47(SD2.54)	0.05
Exertional dyspnea	4(9.5%)	3(27%)	6(75%)	<0.001
Hemoglobin level(g/dl)	9.10(SD1.2)	8.02(SD1.0)	7.90(SD1.10)	0.003
Ferritin level(ng/ml)	987.5(SD545)	932(SD674)	1650(SD824)	0.01
Age of 1st BT^	7.50(SD5.70)	10.80(SD6.70)	13.7(SD6.20)	0.01
Regular BT^	11(23.8%)	2(9%)	2(12.5%)	0.8
Splenectomized	6(14%)	2(18%)	5(62%)	0.01

^BT = Blood transfusion. Data are presented as count (%) or mean ± SD.

these patients. Frequent monitoring of cardiac function in patients may indicate that those at risk of developing symptomatic cardiac disease. These patients might then become candidates for more intensive therapy including blood transfusion and sustained iron chelation [7,8].

The present study showed that the left ventricular dimensions including (LVEDD and LVESD) in TI were increased with an increase in the TRV. This is in consistence with previous studies by Nouri et al., Aessopos et al. and Vaccari et al. [9,2,10]. The mean of LV septal and posterior wall dimensions during systole and diastole were increased in spite of statistical insignificance. This finding is consistent with those of Aessopos et al. and Nurri et al. studies [2,9]. The larger LV dimensions could be explained by the presence of chronic anemia, which is associated with increased blood volume. The lower capacity of blood to carry an adequate amount of oxygen to peripheral tissues was overcome by higher cardiac output and the venous return was, therefore; increased. This significant volume overload was carried out through the Frank-Starling mechanism [10].

Evaluating LV systolic function, the mean LVEF % in the studied sample was normal. There was a negative association between TRV and LVEF % with correlation coefficient equal to (−0.39). However, comparing LVEF % among subgroups, there was a significant difference

Table 2 Echo findings of TI patients according to TR jet velocity

Echo Findings	Jet velocity <2.5 m/sec 42(69%)	Jet velocity 2.5-2.9 m/sec 11(18%)	Jet velocity ≥3.0 m/sec 8(13%)	p-value
IVSDD(cm/m^2)	0.51(SD0.20)	0.55(SD0.16)	0.56(SD0.13)	0.68
LVEDD(cm/m^2)	2.90(SD0.51)	3.15(SD0.54)	3.40(SD0.40)	0.01
LVPWDD(cm/m^2)	0.52(SD0.14)	0.53(SD0.15)	0.54(SD0.15)	0.92
IVSSD(cm/m^2)	0.75(SD0.20)	0.76(SD0.21)	0.81(SD0.20)	0.74
LVESD(cm/m^2)	1.56(SD0.35)	1.79(SD0.37)	1.91(SD0.40)	0.01
LVPWSD(cm/m^2)	0.57(SD0.15)	0.59(SD0.13)	0.63(SD0.11)	0.54
LVEF (%)	65(SD6.40)	64(SD7.20)	56(SD12.40)	0.01
LA diameter(mm/m^2)	22.53(SD5.0)	25.46(SD5.80)	27.25(SD6.60)	0.01
Transmitralinflow E/A ratio(m/s)	1.70(SD0.61)	1.42(SD0.40)	1.26(SD0.38)	0.07
RV diameter (cm/m^2)	1.24(SD0.62)	1.57(SD0.71)	1.99(SD0.68)	0.01
RA area(cm^2/m^2)	9.11(SD4.20)	12.6(SD3.10)	13.52(SD3.40)	0.003
TAPSE(cm)	2.66(SD1.02)	2.33(SD0.93)	1.8(SD0.40)	0.06
TR peak gradient (mmHg)	21.55(SD10.23)	27.21(SD7.66)	35.44(SD9.1)	0.001
PR peak gradient (mmHg)	10.20(SD4.10)	13.25(SD6.20)	15.01(SD4.41)	0.01

EF: Ejection fraction, IVSDD: Interventricular septum diastolic diameter, LVEDD: Left ventricle end diastolic diameter, LVPWDD: Left ventricle posterior wall diastolic diameter, IVSSD: Interventricular septum systolic diameter, LVESD: Left ventricle end systolic diameter, LVPWSD: Left ventricle posterior wall systolic diameter, LA: Left atrium, RV: Right ventricle, RA: Right atrium, TAPSE: Tricuspid annular plane systolic excursion, TR: Tricuspid regurgitation, PR: Pulmonary regurgitation.

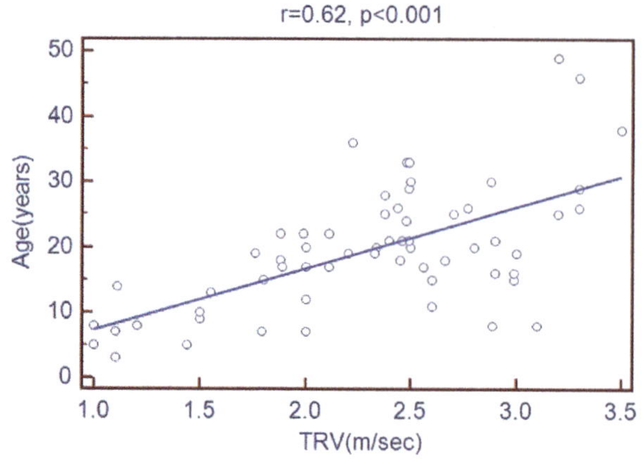

Figure 1 Association of TRV with age of patients.

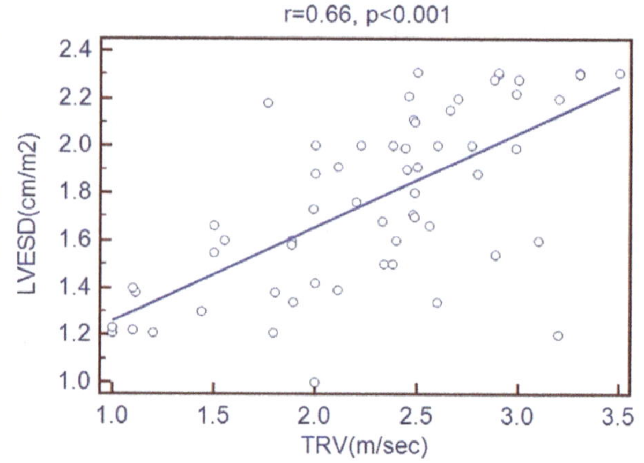

Figure 3 Association of TRV with LVESD.

because of a possible skew caused by a very small highest TRV sample that included three patients with features of congestive heart failure. According to Aessopos et al. [3] the LVEF % was normal in TI. However it was lower than LVEF % of control group with a significant difference ($p < 0.05$) [3]. Noori et al. [11] found significant lower values of LVEF % among TI compared to control group ($p = 0.001$). Vaccari et al. study showed lower LVEF % among TI though insignificant compared to control group [10]. Tissue doppler, a recently introduced method, is known to permit early identification of systolic dysfunction even when left ventricular is still preserved. In this study, however, it was not used [12-14].

Assessing LV diastolic function in TI patients, the mean LA volume and diameter were significantly higher in TI with higher TRV. There was also a progressive increase of the late filling velocity and a relative decrease of the mitral inflow E/A ratio though statistically insignificant. This suggests an increase in LV end diastolic pressure, reflecting an alteration in diastolic property and impairment of LV relaxation, most probably caused by iron deposition which gradually, if not properly managed, leads to restrictive cardiomyopathy [12,15,16]. The left atrial diameter in Aessopos et al. [3] was significantly larger in TI compared to control and the peak late transmitral diastolic velocity was significantly higher in TI. On the other hand the E/A ratio in Vaccari et al. and Noori et al. studies were significantly lower in TI compared to control group [10,11].

Congestive heart failure (CHF) in this study was encountered in 3(4.9%) patients. Yet, the rates of CHF in Aessopos et al. [2] and Aessopos et al. [17] were 2.7% and 5.4% respectively. In TI, the heart is primarily affected by PHT, which is the leading cause of CHF due to subsequent right ventricle dysfunction [18]. The current study showed that there was a decrease in the value of tricuspid annular plane systolic excursion in higher TRV subgroup. However, it did not show a statistical significant difference.

In the present study 8(13%) of cases had TRV ≥ 3.0 m/sec which corresponds to doppler peak systolic tricuspid gradient (PTG) greater than 30 mm Hg and 6(9%) had

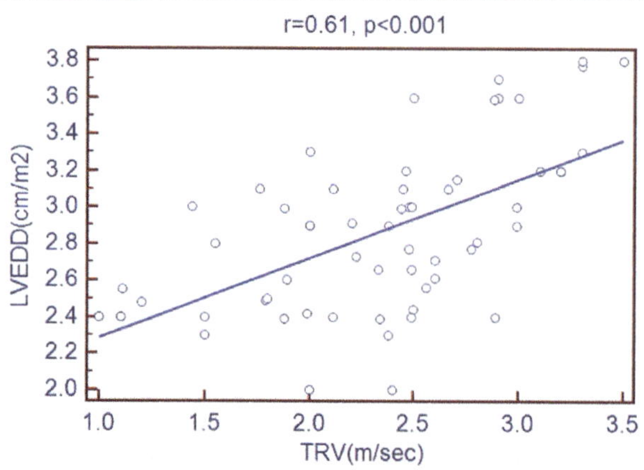

Figure 2 Association of TRV with LVEDD.

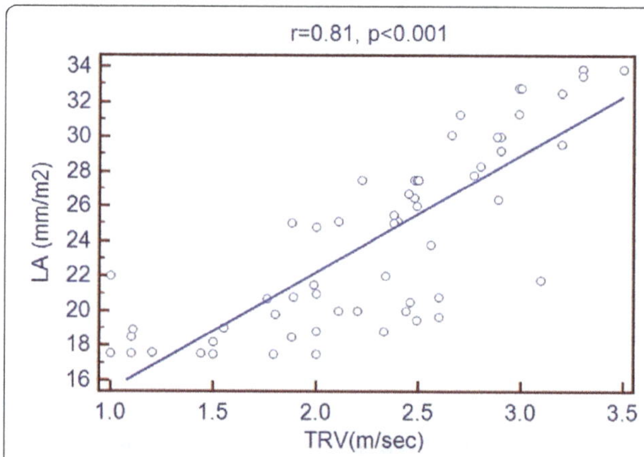

Figure 4 Association of TRV with LA diameter.

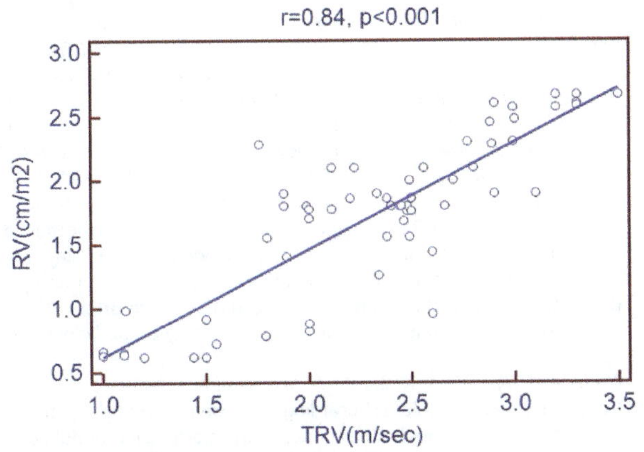

Figure 5 Association of TRV with RV diameter.

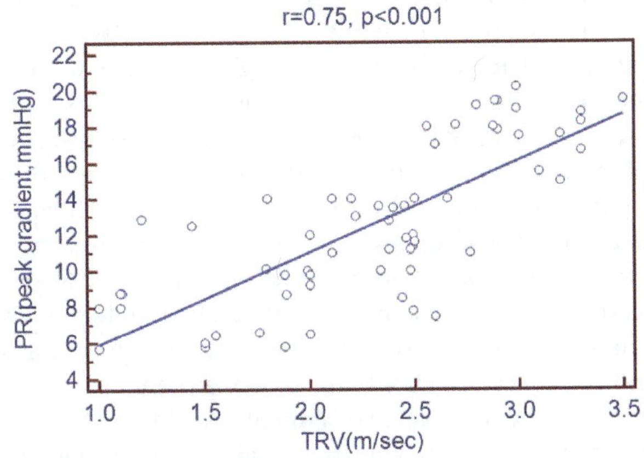

Figure 7 Association of TRV with PR.

TRV > 3.2 m/sec. Despite the lack of cardiac catheterization data the last value was considered to represent the actual cases of PHT in this study relying on diagnostic conclusions of PHT from a recent Italian study [19]. In Aessopos et al. (59.1%) had PTG greater than 30 mmHg and (23%) had PTG > 35 mmHg [17]. The observation that markers of hemolysis are associated with pulmonary hypertension in chronic hemolytic disorders suggests that there is a distinct syndrome of hemolysis-associated pulmonary hypertension. Following the release of hemoglobin into plasma, the plasma hemoglobin can scavenge nitric oxide as well as catalyze the formation of reactive oxygen and nitrogen species, the processes that can lead to acute and chronic pulmonary vasoconstriction [20]. With regard to the TI clinical characteristics, a retrospective analysis showed that splenectomised females with significant anemia, thrombocytosis and elevated ferritin levels, were at greatest risk for developing PHT [21,22].

This study, similar to above analysis, proved that TRV was significantly higher in splenectomised cases, lower hemoglobin, higher ferritin levels, and later onset of blood transfusion. On the contrary, it concluded that higher TRV was associated with male gender. Unsurprisingly, despite of less regular blood transfusion among higher TRV subgroup in the year before this study, relative higher ferritin levels among them was found which was partly attributed to lesser utilization of iron chelation in the same subgroup, the increased risk of progressive ferritn accumulation with advancing age and increased rate of gasrointerstinal iron absorption in TI [23,24].

A recent study demonstrated a significant correlation between iron overload in the liver and pulmonary artery systolic pressure independent of LV filling pressures [25]. Though this study had made no data with regard to iron overload in the liver, a significant association between higher ferritin levels and increase in pulmonary artery systolic pressure and higher jet velocity of tricuspid regurgitation was found. The use of serum ferritin to monitor iron overload is inexpensive and accessible. In TI, serum ferritin assays may underestimate the actual iron load and liver iron concentration (LIC) is more reliable, though invasive [26].

Managing TI patients with cardiac involvement and PHT, regular transfusion and iron chelation therapy is

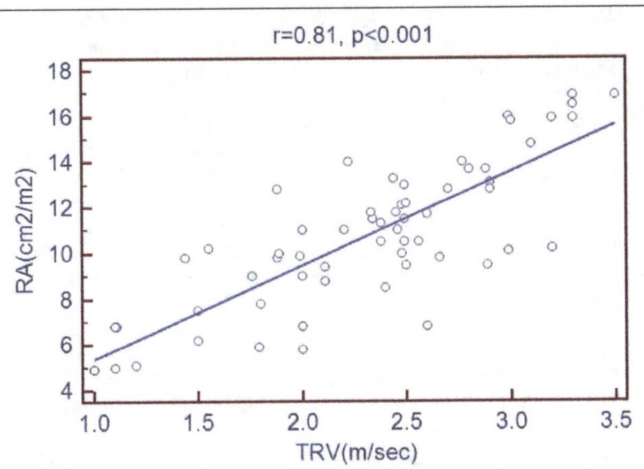

Figure 6 Association of TRV with RA area.

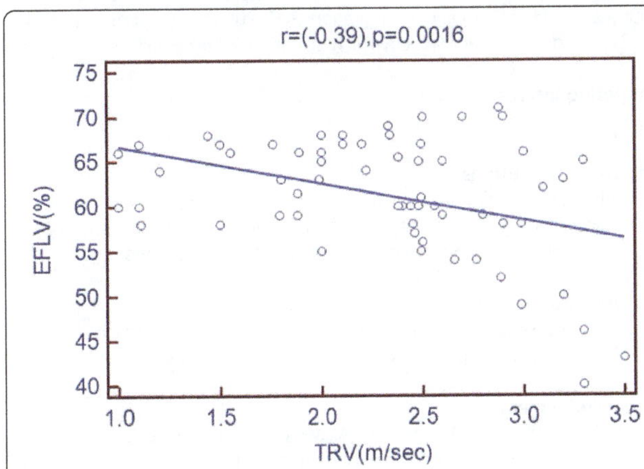

Figure 8 Association of TRV with LVEF %.

indicated even without evidence of cardiac siderosis. This suggests that TI patients may still be at risk for iron related cardiac dysfunction through exposure to non-transferrin bound iron [27,28]. However, only 25% of the studied patients did receive regular blood transfusion, and even among patients with cardiac manifestations only few cases received iron chelation therapy. Sildenafil has been successfully used to treat PHT. However, none of the patients have had received the drug [29]. Hydroxycarbamide may be administered in TI patients in order to minimize, or even obviate, the need for regular transfusions and concomitant iron overload, and eventually minimize the cardiac involvement. Again, only a few cases have been receiving the drug, and with fair outcome and compliance [30].

The main limitations of this study, which is, to my best knowledge, the first attempt conducted in Iraq on echocardiographic evaluation of TI, include reliance on conventional echocardiography. Other diagnostic tools, such as tissue doppler, speckled tracking echocardiography, cardiac catheterization, and cardiac MRI, were not accessible. The studied sample is relatively small to generalize the outcomes, though it resulted in a correlation between accumulative changes in the clinical characteristics and echocardiographic parameters.

Conclusions

Conventional echocardiography for TI cases is a useful tool for preliminary evaluation of cardiac status. It could uncover many cardiac abnormalities that possibly complicate TI. The abnormalities and the underlying pathophysiology could be targeted in the future.

Abbreviations

BT: Blood transfusion; CHF: Congestive heart failure; EF: Ejection fraction; IVSDD: Interventricular septum diastolic diameter; LVEDD: Left ventricle end diastolic diameter; LVPWDD: Left ventricle posterior wall diastolic diameter; IVSSD: Interventricular septum systolic diameter; LVESD: Left ventricle end systolic diameter; LVPWSD: Left ventricle posterior wall systolic diameter; LA: Left atrium; PTG: Peak tricuspid gradient; RV: Right ventricle; RA: Right atrium; TAPSE: Tricuspid annular plane systolic excursion; TR: Tricuspid regurgitation; PR: Pulmonary regurgitation; PHT: Pulmonary hypertension; TRV: Tricuspid regurgitant velocity; TI: Thalassemia intermedia.

Competing interests

The author declares that he has no competing interests.

Authors' contributions

The author declares that he had made substantial contributions to conception and design, acquisition of data, analysis and interpretation of data. He has given final approval of the version to be published.

Authors' information

The author is a senior cardiologist at Duhok heart center and teaches cardiology at Department of Medicine, University of Duhok, Iraqi Kurdistan.

Acknowledgements

I would like to thank Professors Nasir Allawi and Luigi Badano for their revision of the manuscript and valuable notes on it.
Thanks go to the assistant professor Saad Agha for statistical review and Mr. Adress Mosa for linguistic revision.

References

1. Rund D, Rachmilewitz E: **Beta-thalassemia.** *N Engl J Med* 2005, **353:**1135–1146.
2. Aessopos A, Farmakis D, Deftereos S, Tsironi M, Tassiopoulos S, Moyssakis I, Karagiorga M: **Thalassemia heart disease: a comparative evaluation of thalassemia major and thalassemia intermedia.** *Chest* 2005, **127:**1523–1530.
3. Aessopos A, Kati M, Farmakis D: **Heart disease in thalassemia intermedia: a review of the underlying pathophysiology.** *Haematologica* 2007, **92:**658–665.
4. Lang RM, Bierig M, Devereux RB, Flachskampf FA, Foster E, Pellikka PA, Picard MH, Roman MJ, Seward J, Shanewise JS, Solomon SD, Spencer KT, Sutton MS, Stewart WJ: **Recommendations for chamber quantification: a report from the American Society of Echocardiography's Guidelines and Standards Committee and the Chamber Quantification Writing Group, developed in conjunction with the European Association of Echocardiography, a branch of the European Society of Cardiology.** *J Am Soc Echocardiogr* 2005, **18**(12):1440–1463.
5. Masuyama T, Kodama K, Kitabatake A, Sato H, Nanto S, Inoue M: **Continuous-wave Doppler echocardiographic detection of pulmonary regurgitation and its application to noninvasive estimation of pulmonary artery pressure.** *Circulation* 2006, **74**(3):484–492.
6. Gladwin MT, Sachdev V, Jison ML, Shizukuda Y, Plehn JF, Minter K, Brown B, Coles WA, Nichols JS, Ernst I, Hunter LA, Blackwelder WC, Schechter AN, Rodgers GP, Castro O, Ognibene FP: **Pulmonary hypertension as a risk factor for death in patients with sickle cell disease.** *N Engl J Med* 2004, **350:**886–895.
7. Annop L, See O, Sukit Y, Suporn C: **Echocardiographic parameters of right ventricular dysfunction in thalassemic patients.** *Bangkok Medjournal* 2014, **7:**2.
8. Azerkeivan A, Mehravar A, Faranoush M, Vasough P, Ghorbani R, Shahmohamadi A, Ehsani MA, Hedayatiasl AA: **Cardiac involvement in patients with transfusion dependant B-Thalassemia.** *Res J Biol Sci* 2009, **4**(2):195–199.
9. Nouri NM, Naderi M, Rajaie S, Dorgalaleh A, Tabibian SH: **Evaluation of cardiac function in patients with thalassemia intermedia.** *Iran J Pediatr Hematol Oncol* 2013, **3:**1.
10. Vaccari M, Crepaz R, Fortini M, Gamberini MR, Scarcia S, Pitscheider W, Bosi G: **Left ventricular remodeling, systolic function, and diastolic function in young adults with beta-thalassemia intermedia: a Doppler echocardiography study.** *Chest* 2002, **121**(2):506–512.
11. Noori N, Mohamadi M, Keshavarz K, Alavi SM, Mahjoubifard M, Mirmesdagh Y: **Comparison of Right and Left Side Heart Functions in Patients with Thalassemia Major, Patients with Thalassemia Intermedia, and Control Group.** *J Teh Univ Heart Ctr* 2013, **8**(1):35–41.
12. Rodrigues A, Filho FV, Braga JC, Custodio CS, Waib P, Junior AF, Tan DM, Franca ACCV, Okoshi MP, Okoshi K: **Echocardiography in thalassemic patients on blood transfusions and chelation without heart failure.** *Arq Bras Cardiol* 2013, **100**(1):75–81.
13. Yip G, Wang M, Zhang Y, Fung JW, Ho PY, Sanderson JE: **Left ventricular long axis function in diastolic heart failure is reduced in both diastole and systole: time for a redefinition?** *Heart* 2002, **87**(2):121–125.
14. Sanderson JE: **Heart failure with a normal ejection fraction.** *Heart* 2007, **93**(2):155–158.
15. Abhayaratna WP, Seward JB, Appleton CP, Douglas PS, Oh JK, Tajik AJ, Tsang TSM: **Left atrial size: physiologic determinants and clinical applications.** *J Am Coll Cardiol* 2006, **47**(12):2357–2363.
16. Nagueh SF, Appleton CP, Gillebert TC, Marino PN, Oh JK, Smiseth OA, Waggoner AD, Flachskampf FA, Pellikka PA, Evangelista A: **Recommendations for the evaluation of left ventricular diastolic function by echocardiography.** *J Am Soc Echocardiogr* 2009, **22**(2):107–133.
17. Athanasios A, Dimitrios F, Markisia K, Ersi V, Aphrodite L, Antonia H, Jacqueline J, John R, Dimitris L: **Cardiac involvement in thalassemia intermedia: a multicenter study.** *Blood* 2001, **97:**11.
18. Borgna-Pignatti C: **Modern treatment of thalassaemia intermedia.** *Br J Haematol* 2007, **138:**291–304.
19. Derchi G, Galanello R, Bina P, Cappellini MD, Piga A, Lai ME, Quarta A, Casu G, Perrotta S, Pinto V, Musallam KM, Forni GL: **Prevalence and risk factors for pulmonary arterial hypertension in a large group of β-thalassemia patients using right heart catherization: a Webthal(R) study.** *Circulation* 2014, **129**(3):338–345.
20. Reiter CD, Wang X, Tanus-Santos JE, Hogg N, Cannon RO, Schechter AN, Gladwin MT: **Cell-free hemoglobin limits nitric oxide bioavailability in sickle-cell disease.** *Nat Med* 2002, **8:**1383–1389.

21. Atichartakarn V, Likittanasombat K, Chuncharunee S, Chandanamattha P, Worapongpaiboon S, Angchaisuksiri P, Aryurachai K: **Pulmonary arterial hypertension in previously splenectomized patients with beta-thalassemic disorders.** *Int J Hematol* 2003, **78:**139–145.
22. Taher AT, Musallam KM, Cappellini MD: **Thalassemia intermedia: an update.** *Mediterr J Hematol Infect Dis* 2009, **1:**1.
23. Mishra AK, Tiwari A: **Iron overload in beta thalassaemia major and intermedia patients.** *MAEDICA – J Clin Med* 2013, **8**(4):328–332.
24. Gardenghi S, Marongiu MF, Ramos P, Guy E, Breda L, Chadburn A, Liu Y, Amariglio N, Rechavi G, Rachmilewitz EA, Breuer W, Cabantchik ZI, Wrighting DM, Andrews NC, de Sousa M, Giardina PJ, Grady RW, Rivella S: **Ineffective erythropoiesis in beta-thalassemia is characterized by increased iron absorption mediated by down-regulation of hepcidin and up-regulation of ferroportin.** *Blood* 2007, **109:**5027–5035.
25. Isma'eel H, Chafic AH, Rassi FE, Inati A, Koussa S, Daher R, Gharzuddin W, Alam S, Taher AT: **Relation between iron-overload indices, cardiac echo-Doppler, and biochemical markers in thalassemia intermedia.** *Am J Cardiol* 2008, **102:**363–367.
26. Taher AT, Viprakasit V, Musallam KM, Cappellini MD: **Treating Iron overload in patients with non-transfusion-dependent thalassemia.** *Am J Hematol* 2013, **88:**409–415.
27. Musallam KM, Taher AT, Rachmilewitz EA: **Beta-Thalassemia intermedia: a clinical perspective.** *Cold Spring Harb Perspect Med* 2012, **2:**a 013482.
28. Taher AT, Musallam KM, Wood JC, Cappellini MD: **Magnetic resonance evaluation of hepatic andmyocardial iron deposition in transfusion-independent thalassemia intermedia compared to regularly transfused thalassemia major patients.** *Am J Hematol* 2010, **85:**288–290.
29. Derchi G, Forni GL, Formisano F, Cappellini MD, Galanello R, D'Ascola G, Bina P, Magnano C, Lamagna M: **Efficacy and safety of sildenafil in the treatment of severe pulmonary hypertension in patients with hemoglobinopathies.** *Haematologica* 2005, **90:**452–458.
30. Karimi M, Darzi H, Yavarian M: **Hematologic and clinical responses of thalassemia intermedia patients to hydroxyurea during 6 years of therapy in Iran.** *J Pediatr Hematol Oncol* 2005, **27:**380–385.

4

Left atrial appendage morphology, echocardiographic characterization, procedural data and in-hospital outcome of patients receiving left atrial appendage occlusion device implantation

Christian Fastner[1*], Michael Behnes[1], Benjamin Sartorius[1], Mustafa Yildiz[2], Kambis Mashayekhi[3], Ibrahim El-Battrawy[1], Ralf Lehmann[1], Stefan Baumann[1], Tobias Becher[1], Martin Borggrefe[1] and Ibrahim Akin[1]

Abstract

Background: Implantation of left atrial appendage (LAA) occlusion devices was shown to be a feasible and effective alternative to oral anticoagulation in patients with non-valvular atrial fibrillation. However, only few data about in-hospital and peri-procedural data are currently available. This study aims to report about echocardiographic, procedural and in-hospital data of patients receiving LAA occlusion devices.

Methods: This single-center, prospective and observational study includes consecutively patients being eligible for percutaneous implantation of LAA occlusion devices (either Watchman™ or Amplatzer™ Cardiac Plug 2). Data on pre- and peri-procedural transesophageal echocardiography (TEE), implantation and procedure related in-hospital complications were collected. The primary efficacy outcome measure was a successful device implantation without relevant peri-device leaks (i.e., < 5 mm).

Results: In total, 37 patients were included, 22 receiving the Watchman™ and 15 ACP 2 device. Baseline characteristics did not differ significantly in both patient groups. The primary efficacy outcome measure was reached in 91.9 % of patients (90.9 % for the Watchman™, 93.3 % for the ACP 2 group). One device embolization (Watchman™ group) with successful retrieval occurred (2.7 % of patients). No thromboembolism or device thrombosis were present. The majority of bleedings was caused by access site bleedings (88.3 % of all bleedings), consisting mostly of mild hematomas corresponding to a BARC type 1 bleeding (80.0 % of all access-site complications). One patient died due to septic shock (non-procedure related).

Conclusions: In daily real-life practice, percutaneous treatment with LAA occlusion devices appears to be an effective and safe.

Keywords: Left atrial appendage occlusion device implantation, Echocardiography, Procedural data, In-hospital outcome

* Correspondence: christian.fastner@umm.de
[1]First Department of Medicine, University Medical Center Mannheim, University of Heidelberg, DZHK (German Center for Cardiovascular Research), Mannheim, Germany
Full list of author information is available at the end of the article

Background

Atrial fibrillation (AF) represents the most common cardiac arrhythmia with a current age-dependent prevalence of 1–2 % in the Western population, while being assumed to rise significantly within the next couple of years [1]. Cerebral ischemic stroke represents the most important fatal complication of AF deteriorating the prognosis of each individual patient. In the presence of AF, the risk of stroke increases about 5-times [2], being accompanied by a stroke-related mortality rate of about 20 % [3, 4] and a high percentage of patients remaining disabled. The so called CHA_2DS_2-VASc score assesses the patient's individual annual stroke risk and allows a specific risk-adapted anticoagulant treatment [5].

Oral anticoagulation (OAC) with vitamin K antagonists or with new direct oral anticoagulants (DOACs) prevents effectively thromboembolic events in patients with at least one risk factor [6]. In contrast, major bleedings-particularly cerebral bleedings-still represent a most crucial complication of OAC, despite the fact that DOACs were shown to reduce the occurrence of intracranial hemorrhage [7]. The individual bleeding risk as assessed by the HAS-BLED score [5], contraindications against OAC and the patient's preference to deny OAC, need to be considered before initiating OAC. In daily clinical practice, half of patients with an increased risk for thromboembolic complications and without any contraindication against OAC does not receive this treatment [8].

The percutaneous implantation of left atrial appendage (LAA) occlusion devices such as the Watchman™ device (Boston Scientific, Natick, MA) and the Amplatzer™ Cardiac Plug (ACP) replaced by the Amplatzer™ Amulet™ (also known as ACP 2, both St. Jude Medical, St. Paul, MN) was evaluated as an effective alternative to OAC in patients with non-valvular AF and concomitant high bleeding risk or in patients being unwilling to take lifelong OAC. The non-inferiority to warfarin therapy in patients being eligible for OAC was proven in the PROTECT-AF trial for the Watchman™ device [9]. Here, warfarin was prescribed for at least 45 days after successful device implantation. In subsequent studies dual antiplatelet therapy (DAPT) for at least 6 months after implantation was shown to be safe in patients with contraindications for OAC [10]. With regard to the ACP device, a non-inferiority study has not yet been investigated. However, DAPT was shown to be safe and effective for this device [11]. First clinical experience with the ACP 2 did not show significant differences compared to the original ACP with regard to peri- and post-procedural complications [12].

Although the implantation of LAA occlusion devices is well established, there is still a great lack of in-hospital and peri-procedural data addressing the safety and efficacy of these devices [12–19]. Specifically, peri-procedural data have been shown to vary tremendously between individual centers. Today, an increase of and peri-procedural safety has developed compared to early implantation periods [13, 14, 20]. Therefore, this study aims to comparatively evaluate in-hospital single-center registry data of patients scheduled for LAA occlusion device implantation (i.e., Watchman™ versus ACP 2).

Methods

Enrollment

The present study is a single-center, prospective, observational, descriptional and non-randomized registry including consecutively 37 patients with all three types of non-valvular AF, a CHA_2DS_2-VASc score ≥ 2 and, therefore, indication for OAC. Patient enrollment started in June 2014. Further inclusion criteria were age ≥ 18 years, any relative or absolute contraindication for standard OAC - i.e., major bleeding with tendency to recidivity, HAS-BLED score ≥ 3 and neurological symptoms during treatment with OAC or intolerance to OAC. Written informed consent was obtained from all study patients. Patients were excluded if at least one of the following criteria were evident: single episode of AF or treatable reason for AF, catheter ablation of AF within 30 days prior to or after potential LAA occluder implantation, electrical cardioversion within 30 days after potential occluder implantation, congestive heart failure corresponding to functional class NYHA IV, myocardial infarction within the last 3 months, atrial septum defect or interventional/surgical occlusion of ASD, mechanical heart valve, status after heart transplant, symptomatic carotid artery stenosis, transient ischemic attack (TIA) or stroke within last 30 days, intracerebral bleeding within the last 3 months, acute infection, existing or planned pregnancy, existing thrombus. The study was carried out according to the principles of the declaration of Helsinki and was approved by the medical ethics committee II of the Faculty of Medicine Mannheim, University of Heidelberg, Germany.

Procedure

An electrocardiogram (ECG), standard blood analyses and transesophageal echocardiography (TEE) were performed for pre-procedural planning. LAA occlusion device implantation was performed by experienced interventional cardiologists (≥50 LAA closure device implantations each prior to the study). Patients were treated with conscious sedation using intravenous 2,6-di(propan-2-yl)phenol and midazolam. One arterial access sheath (5 French, F) for arterial blood pressure monitoring and one venous access sheath for interventional device implantation were used. Transseptal puncture was performed with a SL1 sheath and BRK1 Brockenbrough needle (St. Jude Medical, St. Paul, MN). Prior transseptal puncture heparin was administered to achieve an active clotting time of at least 250 s. A stiff guide wire (Cook Medical, Bloomington, IN) was placed in the left upper pulmonary vein (LUPV) and the transseptal sheath was removed and replaced by the Watchman™ (14 F), respectively ACP 2 (12 or 14 F) delivery sheath. Device allocation algorithm was performed according to latest consensus recommendations [21]. All patients underwent pre-procedural 2D/3D TEE to assess initially the anatomy, size and absence of thrombus or sludge on all recommended TEE views. Accordingly, peri-procedural imaging was based on fluoroscopy and 2D/3D TEE imaging in order to re-assess prior findings of the LAA and to decide which device size was appropriate in the individual patient. Fluoroscopy was performed using a 5 F pigtail catheter to visualize the LAA in at least 2 standard angulations (RAO 30°/10° cranial, RAO 30°/10° caudal). Regarding TEE, the following parameters of the LAA were assessed for appropriate sizing, as recommended for both devices [21]: LAA ostium, landing zone, angle of the LAA, depth of the LAA, differentiation of main lobes versus smaller side lobes. The device size was chosen at least 20 % larger than the measured diameters at the landing zone [22]. Post-implantation the compression of the devices was measured by 2D TEE and a device compression of at least 10 % was defined as valuable, next to lacking of relevant peri-device leaks (>5 mm), and no compression or attachment of neighboring structures, such as the circumflex coronary artery, mitral annulus or pulmonary veins. A tug test was performed repetitively before final liberation of the device as recommended. Access site was closed with an Angio-Seal™ Evolution™ (St. Jude Medical, St. Paul, MN) for the arterial access and with two ProGlide™ (Abbott Vascular, Santa Clara, CA) for the venous access and followed by a pressure band for 6 hours.

Post-procedural measures

In accordance with our institutional protocol, acetylsalicylic acid (ASA) 100 mg/d was administered lifelong, clopidogrel for at least 6 months commencing the day of implantation with a loading dose of 250 mg, respectively 600 mg, if not taken before. The day after the procedure, a transthoracic echocardiogram (TTE) and a chest X-ray were performed to rule out device dislodgement and pericardial effusion, an ECG was performed to rule out a new bundle branch block (BBB) or atrioventricular (AV) block and repetitive thorough clinical examinations were carried out to rule out other clinical disorders.

Outcome measures

The primary efficacy outcome measure of our in-hospital register was defined as technical success with a successful device implantation without relevant peri-device leaks (i.e., < 5 mm). Primary safety outcome measure was defined as the occurrence of bleeding events classified according to the BARC definition [23], pericardial effusion, device embolization, peri-procedural stroke and peri-procedural death. Events resulting in death, aggravated morbidity or prolonged hospitalization being associated with the procedure were defined as complications. Any events not being associated with the procedure were termed adverse events.

Statistics

Statistical analyses were performed with SPSS Statistics (IBM, Armonk, NY). Descriptive statistics are given as medians (25th and 75th percentiles) or as total numbers with group-related percentages. Normal distribution of data was tested with the Kolmogorov-Smirnov test. In case of normal distribution, the *t*-test was applied to compare scaled data. Scaled variables not normally distributed were compared using the Mann-Whitney *U* test. Categorical variables were compared using the chi-squared test. Level of significance was set at $p < 0.05$ (two-tailed).

Results

Baseline characteristics

Baseline demographic and clinical characteristics of the study population including indications for implantation of LAA occlusion devices and risk-stratification according to CHA_2DS_2-VASc and HAS-BLED scores are shown in Table 1. Of 37 patients, 22 patients received the Watchman™ and 15 patients received the ACP 2 device. The most common indication was a prior history of bleedings (78.4 %) under treatment with OAC. 51.4 % of all patients were not treated with OAC, whereas patients with OAC were mostly treated with DOAC (66.7 %). Table 2 shows two-dimensional (2D) and functional echocardiographic measurements. As assessed by angiography, the majority of patients revealed a chicken-wing shaped LAA (67.6 %).

Procedural data

Procedural data related to the implantation of LAA occlusion devices are summarized in Table 3. The primary efficacy outcome measure in the Watchman™ group was 90.9 %, whereas it was 93.3 % in the ACP 2 group (p = 0.791). Only the Watchman™ device device could not be implanted in two patients (9.1 %) either due to an anatomical mismatch or due to an incomplete occlusion of the LAA landing zone. In contrast, the ACP 2 device was implanted in all patients with one patient with incomplete ostial occlusion (6.7 %). More than one transseptal puncture was needed only in only one patient (2.7 %) due to a transseptal retrieval of an intra-atrial embolized Watchman™ occluder during the procedure.

Table 1 Baseline characteristics of the study collective

	Watchman	ACP 2	All	*p* Value
Patients, n (%)	22 (59.5)	15 (40.5)	37 (100)	-
Male, n (%)	16 (72.7)	9 (60)	25 (67.6)	0.417
Age, y (IQR)	77 (70.75–81)	80 (76–83)	79 (71.5–81.5)	0.213
Height, cm (IQR)	170 (167.75–177)	170 (165–172)	170 (167–175)	0.090
Weight, kg (IQR)	80.5 (67.5–90)	83.5 (69.75–93.25)	81.5 (69.25–90)	0.531
Reason for not taking OAC, n (%)				
- GI bleeding	8 (36.4)	8 (53.8)	16 (43.2)	0.306
- ICB	4 (18.2)	2 (13.3)	6 (16.2)	0.694
- Muscle bleeding	2 (9.1)	0 (0)	2 (5.4)	0.230
- Other bleeding localization	2 (9.1)	3 (20)	5 (13.5)	0.341
- Refusal	3 (13.6)	0 (0)	3 (8.1)	0.136
- Other causes	3 (13.6)	2 (13.3)	5 (13.5)	1.000
AF type, n (%)				
- Paroxysmal	12 (54.5)	7 (46.7)	19 (51.4)	0.638
- Persistent	2 (9.1)	3 (20)	5 (13.5)	0.341
- Permanent	8 (36.4)	5 (33.3)	13 (35.1)	0.850
Heart rhythm at hospitalization, n (%)				
- SR	6 (27.3)	6 (40)	12 (32.4)	0.225
- AF	12 (54.5)	9 (60)	21 (56.8)	0.742
- PM	2 (9.1)	0 (0)	2 (5.4)	0.230
- unsp.	2 (9.1)	0 (0)	2 (5.4)	0.230
Prior PVI, n (%)	2 (9.1)	1 (6.7)	3 (8.1)	0.791
Hypertension, n (%)	21 (95.5)	15 (100)	36 (97.3)	0.403
Diabetes mellitus, n (%)	6 (27.3)	6 (40)	12 (32.4)	0.417
TIA, n (%)	4 (18.2)	0 (0)	4 (10.8)	0.080
Stroke, n (%)	1 (4.5)	2 (13.3)	3 (8.11)	0.336
Coronary artery disease, n (%)	13 (59.1)	8 (53.3)	21 (56.8)	0.729
Peripheral vascular disease, n (%)	3 (13.6)	1 (6.7)	4 (10.8)	0.503
Renal failure, n (%)	8 (36.4)	5 (33.3)	13 (35.1)	0.850
- GFR (IQR)	70 (43.5–70)	70 (41–70)	70 (42–70)	0.636
Liver failure, n (%)	3 (13.6)	1 (6.7)	4 (10.8)	0.503
Prior bleeding, n (%)	16 (72.7)	13 (86.7)	29 (78.4)	0.312
Labile INR, n (%)	2 (9.1)	1 (6.7)	3 (8.1)	0.791
CHA_2DS_2-VASc score (IQR)	4 (3–5)	5 (3–5)	5 (3–5)	0.292
HAS-BLED score (IQR)	4 (3–5)	4 (3–4)	4 (3–5)	0.538
Baseline OAC, n (%)				
- None	10 (45.5)	9 (60)	19 (51.4)	0.385
- Warfarin	3 (13.6)	3 (20)	6 (16.2)	0.606
- Rivaroxaban	6 (27.3)	2 (13.3)	8 (21.6)	0.312
- Dabigatran	1 (4.5)	1 (6.7)	2 (5.4)	0.779
- Apixaban	2 (9.1)	0 (0)	2 (5.4)	0.230
Cardiac device, n (%)				
- PM	4 (18.2)	3 (20)	7 (18.9)	0.890
- ICD	1 (4.5)	2 (13.3)	3 (8.1)	0.336

Values are given as medians (25th and 75th percentiles) or total numbers (percentage). *AF* atrial fibrillation, *GFR* glomerular filtration rate, *GI* gastrointestinal, *ICB* intracerebral bleeding, *ICD* implantable cardioverter defibrillator, *INR* international normalized ratio, *OAC* oral anticoagulation, *PM* pacemaker, *PVI* pulmonary vein isolation, *SR* sinus rhythm, *TIA* transient ischemic attack, *unsp.* unspecified

Table 2 Baseline echocardiographic data

	Watchman	ACP 2	All	*p* Value
LV function, n (%)				
- Normal	14 (63.6)[a]	14 (93.3)[a]	28 (75.5)	0.039
- Mild impairment	6 (27.3)[a]	0 (0)[a]	6 (16.2)	0.027
- Moderate impairment	1 (4.5)	0 (0)	1 (2.7)	0.403
- Severe impairment	1 (4.5)	1 (6.7)	2 (5.4)	0.779
LVEDD, mm (IQR)	49 (44–54.25)	45.5 (40–49.5)	46.5 (42.25–53.75)	0.096
Aortic valve, n (%)				
- Stenosis	2 (9.1)	2 (13.3)	4 (10.8)	0.638
- Regurgitation	10 (45.5)	3 (20)	13 (35.1)	0.111
Pulmonary valve, n (%)				
- Stenosis	0 (0)	0 (0)	0 (0)	-
- Regurgitation	0 (0)	1 (6.7)	1 (2.7)	0.220
Mitral valve, n (%)				
- Stenosis	2 (9.1)	1 (6.7)	3 (8.1)	0.791
- Regurgitation	14 (63.6)	11 (73.3)	25 (67.6)	0.536
Tricuspid valve, n (%)				
- Stenosis	0 (0)	0 (0)	0 (0)	-
- Regurgitation	12 (54.5)	10 (66.7)	22 (59.5)	0.461
Aortic bulb diameter, mm (IQR)	31 (29–35.25)	31 (27.75–35.25)	31 (29–35)	0.737
LAA (IQR)				
- Diameter, mm	48.5 (44.25–55)	40 (40–47.5)	46 (42.5–53)	0.193
- Plane, cm^2	23 (18.5–28.25)	23 (14.5–28.75)	23 (17–28.5)	0.802
- Volume, ml	83.5 (66–101,75)	58.5 (46.75–99.5)	74.5 (57.5–101.75)	0.329
- Depth, mm	34 (27–38.75)	35 (27.5–40.75)	35 (28–40)	0.262
LAA ostial diameter, mm (IQR)				
- 0°	18 (16–23)	20 (13.5–22)	18 (16–22)	0.797
- 45°	18 (16.25–21.75)	19 (14–21)	18 (16–21)	0.727
- 90°	18 (16.75–20.25)	20 (14.75–21)	18.5 (16–21)	0.754
- 135°	20 (16.5–22.5)	21 (17.25–22)	20 (17.25–22)	0.569
Landing zone, mm (IQR)	17 (13.5–21.5)	16 (13.5–19.5)	16 (13.75–20.5)	0.556

Values are given as medians (25th and 75th percentiles) or total numbers (percentage). *LAA* left atrial appendage, *LV* left ventricular, *LVEDD* left ventricular end-diastolic dimension. [a]Indicating significant difference

Pericardial effusion and subsequent intermittent circulatory failure with rapid hemodynamic stabilization without the need for cardiopulmonary resuscitation occurred in one patient of the Watchman™ group (2.7 %). All these results showed no statistically significant difference between the Watchman™ and the ACP 2 group.

In-hospital outcome and peri-procedural safety events

Table 4 shows all relevant data related to in-hospital outcome and peri-procedural safety events. None of the patients died due to the implantation of LAA occlusion devices. However, one patient with a preexisting highly reduced left ventricular function (ejection fraction 28 %) died from an acute heart failure linked to a severe urosepis 20 days after the implantation (i.e., adverse event). In another patient with non-ST elevation myocardial infarction (NSTEMI) and percutaneous coronary intervention (PCI) with stent implantation known clopidogrel non-response, DAPT with ASA and ticagrelor instead of clopidogrel was continued as an individual treatment attempt.

Severe conduction blocks, such as BBB or AV blocks, did not occur. Access site complications, such as groin bruise and bleedings at the access sites represented 75.0 % of all complications. Most of them were mild, corresponding to a BARC type 1 bleeding (76.5 % of all bleeding complications) and only 1 case (2.7 % of all patients) needed transfusion without the need for

Table 3 Procedural data

	Watchman	ACP 2	All	*p* Value
Success rate, n (%)	21 (95.5)	15 (100)	36 (97.3)	0.403
Complete ostial occlusion (i.e., gap < 5 mm), n (%)	20 (90.9)	14 (93.3)	34 (91.9)	0.791
Positioning attempts, n (IQR)	2.5 (1.75–3)	2 (1.5–5)	2 (2–3)	0.555
Changes of device size, n (IQR)	1 (1–1)	1 (1–2)	1 (1–1)	0.169
Final device size, mm (IQR)	24 (21–27)	25 (22–30)	24 (22–27)	-
Duration, min. (IQR)	122.5 (75–136.25)	100 (80–110)	110 (76–135)	0.069
Fluoroscopy time, min. (IQR)	11.7 (7.4–16.8)	12.7 (9.5–17.7)	12.4 (8.5–16.9)	0.244
Reference dose, Gy*cm2 (IQR)	80.5 (45.75–103.25)	62 (52–89)	64 (49–96)	0.842
Amount of contrast agent, ml (IQR)	165 (130–202.25)	140 (110–180)	157 (110–195)	0.833
LAA configuration, n (%)				
- Chicken-wing	14 (63.6)	11 (73.3)	25 (67.6)	0.536
- Windsock	3 (13.6)	1 (6.7)	4 (10.8)	0.503
- Broccoli	4 (18.2)	3 (20)	7 (18.9)	0.890
- Tub	1 (4.5)	0 (0)	1 (2.7)	0.403
Number of lobi, n (%)				
- 1	4 (18.2)	3 (20)	7 (18.9)	0.890
- 2	13 (59.1)	10 (66.7)	23 (62.2)	0.641
- 3	1 (4.5)	0 (0)	1 (2.7)	0.403
- Multi	4 (18.2)	2 (13.3)	6 (16.2)	0.694
Days on ICU/IMC, n (IQR)	1 (1–1)	1 (1–1)	1 (1–1)	0.327
Post-procedural days in hospital, n (IQR)	3 (2.25–4)	4 (2.75–5.25)	4 (2.75–5)	0.341

Values are given as medians (25th and 75th percentiles) or total numbers (percentage). *ICU* intensive care unit, *IMC* intermediate care unit

vascular surgery. The patient with a pericardial effusion (3 mm) in the Watchman™ group could be treated conservatively. Notably, neither peri-procedural nor in-hospital transient ischemic attack, stroke or device thrombosis occurred. Patients could have been discharged with a median of 4 days after the intervention. None of the surviving patients developed persistent neurological or heart-failure related disability.

Discussion

AF is one of the main causes leading to ischemic stroke and persistent neurological disability. In almost 25 % of patients developing an ischemic stroke AF can be documented by ECG recording [3]. Therefore effective prevention of cerebral embolization represents the most important aspect for an optimal treatment of patients with AF. Besides the established vitamin K antagonists such as warfarin, innovative DOACs emerged as reliable treatment alternatives. In a current meta-analysis these drugs were shown to reduce significantly the risk of major cerebral bleedings and hemorrhagic stroke when compared to warfarin [7, 24]. Specific subsets of patients of patients are prone to develop severe bleedings as a consequence of OAC, for instance patients with malignoma, major gastrointestinal bleedings and geriatric patients with an increasing risk to fall in everyday life. Accordingly, most of the patients within the presented study revealed a history of severe bleedings leading to the decision to implant an LAA occlusion device. These patients revealed an increased median HAS-BLED score of 4 points and still revealed an increasing risk of developing stroke, as indicated by an increased median CHA_2DS_2-VASc score of 5 points corresponding to an estimated annual risk of thromboembolic stroke of about 6.7 % [4].

Relative contraindications against the use of OAC have been reported in about 20 % of patients with AF [25, 26]. Even patients without any contraindication against OAC are often not treated by the optimal antithrombotic drug regimes [27, 28]. Within the present study, half of the study patients were not anticoagulated previously due to relevant contraindications. In these patients exclusion of the LAA has become the therapy of choice in order to prevent fatal thromboembolic events apart from OAC [9, 29, 30]. Since we only enclosed patients with a high bleeding risk (a median HAS-BLED score of 4 points indicates "high risk" [6]) or refusal for OAC and, therefore, relative or absolute contraindication for OAC, DAPT with ASA and clopidogrel following implantation procedure was thought to be appropriate for

Table 4 Peri-procedural complications and safety events

	Watchman	ACP 2	All	*p* Value
Overall complications, n (%)	11 (50)	9 (60.0)	20 (54.1)	0.549
Major complications, n (%)	3 (13.6)	0 (0)	3 (8.1)	0.136
Device embolization, n (%)	1 (4.5)	0 (0)	1 (2.7)	0.403
Circulatory failure, n (%)	2 (9.1)	0 (0)	2 (5.4)	0.230
- With CPR	1 (4.5)	0 (0)	1 (2.7)	0.403
- Without CPR	1 (4.5)	0 (0)	1 (2.7)	0.403
Bleeding complications, n (%)	8 (36.4)	9 (60.0)	17 (48.6)	0.157
- Groin bruise	4 (18.2)	5 (33.3)	9 (24.3)	0.292
- Groin bleeding	3 (13.6)	3 (20.0)	6 (16.2)	0.606
- Pericardial effusion	1 (4.5)	0 (0)	1 (2.7)	0.403
- Other (dental)	0 (0)	1 (6.7)	1 (2.7)	0.220
Access-site bleedings, n (%)	7 (31.9)	8 (53.3)	15 (40.5)	0.191
- Venous access	0 (0.0)	1 (6.7)	1 (2.7)	0.220
- Arterial access	4 (18.2)	2 (13.3)	6 (16.2)	0.694
- Both access-sites	3 (13.6)	5 (33.3)	8 (21.6)	0.153
BARC score, each n (%)				
- Type 1	7 (31.8)	6 (40.0)	13 (35.1)	0.609
- Type 2	1 (4.5)	2 (13.3)	3 (8.1)	0.336
- Type 3a	0 (0.0)	1 (6.7)	1 (2.7)	0.220
- Type 3b	0 (0.0)	0 (0.0)	0 (0.0)	-
- Type 3c	0 (0.0)	0 (0.0)	0 (0.0)	-
- Type 4	-	-	-	-
- Type 5a	0 (0.0)	0 (0.0)	0 (0.0)	-
- Type 5b	0 (0.0)	0 (0.0)	0 (0.0)	-

Values are given as total numbers (percentage). *BARC score* Bleeding Academic Research Consortium score, *CPR* cardiopulmonary resuscitation

these patients. The duration of DAPT lasted 6 months as previously been shown to be an effective and safe antithrombotic treatment [10].

Success rates of 95.5–100 %, respectively, were comparable to prior studies using the Watchman™ device [9, 10] or were even higher for the ACP 2 [12, 14]. Since complete coverage of the LAA ostium is crucial for preventing from embolization from the LAA, this was defined as a primary efficacy outcome measure, which was also beyond 90 % for both devices.

The documented high efficacy appears to be associated with a careful and appropriate selection of device sizes according to the pre- and peri-procedural measurements of LAA dimensions being assessed by a multi-modal imaging approach with angiography and TEE imaging [14, 22] allowed a safe and accurate peri-procedural guiding for an optimal positioning and adaption. Diameters of the LAA ostium, landing zone, angulation, deepness and volume appeared most similar in recommended angulations (0, 45, 90 and 135°) with a tendency for larger orifice diameters being measured at 135° of angulation [31]. The median size of the devices was about 40 % larger than the median landing as assessed by TEE, surpassing the 20 % range of recommended oversizing [22].

One patient revealed a flat tub-shaped LAA morphology, which made implantation of both devices impossible, whereas all other typical LAA morphologies were able to be accessed by LAA occlusion devices. Even the relatively frequent occurrence of the chicken-wing morphology, described as often being a challenging morphology for transcatheter occlusion device implantation [32], was not seen to decrease the high success rates of both devices. Time of fluoroscopy was comparable to prior studies [18, 19] and did not differ significantly between both groups despite the fact that decision making algorithm in our study regarding accurate measurements of the LAA and selection of the adequate device size was based on peri-procedural 2D TEE in combination with angiography. 3D TEE has been described as an additional imaging technique for optimal visualization of cardiac anatomy during percutaneous cardiac interventions [22, 33]. However, efficacy data evaluating TEE (either 2D or 3D) versus sole or combined angiography during implantation of LAA occlusion devices are not available at present. Since the procedures were performed by experienced interventional cardiologists, well practiced in LAA closure device implantation, we could not find a certain learning curve neither concerning procedural time nor related to peri-procedural complications [34].

Major peri-procedural complications were rare (8.1 %) and did not reveal persistent disability. At 40.5 %, groin hematomas and groin bleedings occurred more frequently compared to recently published data [10, 18, 20]. However, the majority of access site bleedings were minor hematomas (80.0 % of all access-site complications corresponded to a BARC type 1 bleeding). The majority of patients suffering from access-site complications was affected by combined arterial and venous access-site bleedings (21.6 % of all patients). As must be expected, the arterial access-site was the second most common bleeding site (16.2 % of all patients). Since an arterial access during LAA closure device implantation procedure is not mandatory [35], a certain number of access-site bleedings may be avoidable if this access way would be abandoned. Notably, the arterial access allows a safer performance [35] at the expense of some additional mild hematomas. Only one patient was in need of blood transfusion, whereas vascular surgery was never needed. With respect to major complications, one case of circulatory failure was linked to a post-procedural detected pericardial effusion (3 mm), which could be treated conservatively. Early device thrombosis followed by TIA or stroke did not occur in our population suggesting that DAPT initiated by a loading dose might be effective to prevent thromboembolism at the intraluminal device site prior to neo-endothelialization. One patient with intra-procedural device dislodgement in the left atrium (Watchman™ group) which could be successfully retrieved by a veno-venous double lasso interventional technique.

Limitations of the study

This study is based on observational registry data concerning a relative small real-life patient population and was not intended to reliable calculate significant differences between both device types. Comparison results of both devices are for informative reasons only. The aim was to demonstrate essential peri-interventional efficacy and safety data concerning LAA occlusion device implantation in general. A subsequent enlarged set of this registry data might be able to evaluate further differences between both devices.

As this observational study focused on the peri-procedural time, the follow-up period was limited to the discharge from hospital.

The application of any of the two devices was not randomly assessed and was based on the operator's discretion being mainly based on LAA anatomic considerations. In contrast, this more individualized and clinically driven decision algorithm might have strongly influenced the high achievement of primary efficacy outcome measure, which realistically reflects clinical and interventional practice in experienced centers.

Conclusions

Transcatheter implantation of LAA occlusion devices appears to be a feasible and safe percutaneous cardiac intervention with a rare occurrence of major complications and a high success rate in a real-life patient population.

Competing interests

The authors declare that they have no competing interests.

Authors' contributions

CF conceived the study, participated in its design and coordination, participated in data analysis and interpretation and helped to draft and revise the manuscript for important intellectual content. MBe conceived the study, participated in its design and coordination, participated in data analysis and interpretation and helped to draft and revise the manuscript for important intellectual content. BS participated in the study design and coordination, data acquisition and analysis and helped to draft the manuscript for important intellectual content. MY participated in the study design and coordination, as well as data analysis and revised the manuscript. KM participated in the study design and coordination, as well as data analysis and revised the manuscript. IE-B participated in the study design and coordination, participated in data analysis and interpretation and helped to draft and revise the manuscript for important intellectual content. RL participated in the study design and coordination, as well as data analysis and revised the manuscript. SB participated in the study design and coordination, as well as data analysis and revised the manuscript. TB participated in the study design and coordination, as well as data analysis and revised the manuscript. MBo participated in the study design and coordination, as well as data acquisition and revised the manuscript for important intellectual content. IA conceived the study, participated in its design and coordination, participated in data analysis and interpretation and helped to draft and revise the manuscript for important intellectual content. All authors read and approved the final manuscript.

Author details

[1]First Department of Medicine, University Medical Center Mannheim, University of Heidelberg, DZHK (German Center for Cardiovascular Research), Mannheim, Germany. [2]Department of Cardiology, Istanbul University Cardiology Institute, Istanbul, Turkey. [3]Internal Medicine Clinic II, Helios Vogtland Klinikum Plauen, Academic Teaching Hospital of Leipzig University, Leipzig, Germany.

References

1. Go AS, Hylek EM, Phillips KA, Chang Y, Henault LE, Selby JV, et al. Prevalence of diagnosed atrial fibrillation in adults: national implications for rhythm management and stroke prevention: the AnTicoagulation and Risk Factors in Atrial Fibrillation (ATRIA) Study. JAMA. 2001;285(18):2370–5.
2. Gage BF, Waterman AD, Shannon W, Boechler M, Rich MW, Radford MJ. Validation of clinical classification schemes for predicting stroke: results from the National Registry of Atrial Fibrillation. JAMA. 2001;285(22):2864–70.
3. Marini C, De Santis F, Sacco S, Russo T, Olivieri L, Totaro R, et al. Contribution of atrial fibrillation to incidence and outcome of ischemic stroke: results from a population-based study. Stroke. 2005;36(6):1115–9.
4. European Heart Rhythm Association, European Association for Cardio-Thoracic Surgery, Camm AJ, Kirchhof P, Lip GY, Schotten U, et al. Guidelines for the management of atrial fibrillation: the Task Force for the Management of Atrial Fibrillation of the European Society of Cardiology (ESC). Eur Heart J. 2010;31:2369–429.
5. Lane DA, Lip GY. Use of the CHA(2)DS(2)-VASc and HAS-BLED scores to aid decision making for thromboprophylaxis in nonvalvular atrial fibrillation. Circulation. 2012;126(7):860–5.
6. Camm AJ, Lip GY, De Caterina R, Savelieva I, Atar D, Hohnloser SH, et al. Guidelines ESCCfP: 2012 focused update of the ESC Guidelines for the management of atrial fibrillation: an update of the 2010 ESC Guidelines for the management of atrial fibrillation. Developed with the special contribution of the European Heart Rhythm Association. Eur Heart J. 2012; 33(21):2719–47.
7. Ruff CT, Giugliano RP, Braunwald E, Hoffman EB, Deenadayalu N, Ezekowitz MD, et al. Comparison of the efficacy and safety of new oral anticoagulants with warfarin in patients with atrial fibrillation: a meta-analysis of randomised trials. Lancet. 2014;383(9921):955–62.
8. Waldo AL, Becker RC, Tapson VF, Colgan KJ, Committee NS. Hospitalized patients with atrial fibrillation and a high risk of stroke are not being provided with adequate anticoagulation. J Am Coll Cardiol. 2005;46(9):1729–36.
9. Holmes DR, Reddy VY, Turi ZG, Doshi SK, Sievert H, Buchbinder M, et al. Percutaneous closure of the left atrial appendage versus warfarin therapy for prevention of stroke in patients with atrial fibrillation: a randomised non-inferiority trial. Lancet. 2009;374(9689):534–42.
10. Reddy VY, Mobius-Winkler S, Miller MA, Neuzil P, Schuler G, Wiebe J, et al. Left atrial appendage closure with the Watchman device in patients with a contraindication for oral anticoagulation: the ASAP study (ASA Plavix feasibility study with watchman left atrial appendage closure technology). J Am Coll Cardiol. 2013;61(25):2551–6.
11. Urena M, Rodes-Cabau J, Freixa X, Saw J, Webb JG, Freeman M, et al. Percutaneous left atrial appendage closure with the AMPLATZER cardiac plug device in patients with nonvalvular atrial fibrillation and contraindications to anticoagulation therapy. J Am Coll Cardiol. 2013;62(2):96–102.
12. Gloekler S, Shakir S, Doblies J, Khattab AA, Praz F, Guerios E, et al. Early results of first versus second generation Amplatzer occluders for left atrial appendage closure in patients with atrial fibrillation. Clin Res Cardiol. 2015.
13. Pison L, Potpara TS, Chen J, Larsen TB, Bongiorni MG, Blomstrom-Lundqvist C. Scientific Initiative Committee EHRA: Left atrial appendage closure-indications, techniques, and outcomes: results of the European Heart Rhythm Association Survey. Europace. 2015;17(4):642–6.
14. Freixa X, Abualsaud A, Chan J, Nosair M, Tzikas A, Garceau P, et al. Left atrial

appendage occlusion: initial experience with the Amplatzer Amulet. Int J Cardiol. 2014;174(3):492–6.
15. Meerkin D, Butnaru A, Dratva D, Bertrand OF, Tzivoni D. Early safety of the Amplatzer Cardiac Plug for left atrial appendage occlusion. Int J Cardiol. 2013;168(4):3920–5.
16. Streb W, Szymala M, Kukulski T, Nowak J, Lekston A, Sokal A, et al. Percutaneous closure of the left atrial appendage using the Amplatzer Cardiac Plug in patients with atrial fibrillation: evaluation of safety and feasibility. Kardiol Pol. 2013;71(1):8–16.
17. Lam YY, Yip GW, Yu CM, Chan WW, Cheng BC, Yan BP, et al. Left atrial appendage closure with AMPLATZER cardiac plug for stroke prevention in atrial fibrillation: initial Asia-Pacific experience. Catheter Cardiovasc Interv. 2012;79(5):794–800.
18. Chun KR, Bordignon S, Urban V, Perrotta L, Dugo D, Furnkranz A, et al. Left atrial appendage closure followed by 6 weeks of antithrombotic therapy: a prospective single-center experience. Heart Rhythm. 2013;10(12):1792–9.
19. Gafoor S, Franke J, Bertog S, Boehm P, Heuer L, Gonzaga M, et al. Left atrial appendage occlusion in octogenarians: short-term and 1-year follow-up. Catheter Cardiovasc Interv. 2014;83(5):805–10.
20. Reddy VY, Holmes D, Doshi SK, Neuzil P, Kar S. Safety of percutaneous left atrial appendage closure: results from the Watchman Left Atrial Appendage System for Embolic Protection in Patients with AF (PROTECT AF) clinical trial and the Continued Access Registry. Circulation. 2011;123(4):417–24.
21. Meier B, Blaauw Y, Khattab AA, Lewalter T, Sievert H, Tondo C, et al. EHRA/EAPCI expert consensus statement on catheter-based left atrial appendage occlusion. EuroIntervention. 2015;10(9):1109–25.
22. Wunderlich NC, Beigel R, Swaans MJ, Ho SY, Siegel RJ. Percutaneous Interventions for left atrial appendage exclusion: options, assessment, and imaging Using 2D and 3D Echocardiography. JACC Cardiovasc Imaging. 2015;8(4):472–88.
23. Mehran R, Rao SV, Bhatt DL, Gibson CM, Caixeta A, Eikelboom J, et al. Standardized bleeding definitions for cardiovascular clinical trials: a consensus report from the Bleeding Academic Research Consortium. Circulation. 2011; 123(23):2736–47.
24. Greenspon AJ. A review of oral anticoagulants in patients with atrial fibrillation. Postgrad Med. 2012;124(6):7–16.
25. O'Brien EC, Holmes DN, Ansell JE, Allen LA, Hylek E, Kowey PR, et al. Physician practices regarding contraindications to oral anticoagulation in atrial fibrillation: findings from the Outcomes Registry for Better Informed Treatment of Atrial Fibrillation (ORBIT-AF) registry. Am Heart J. 2014;167(4):601–9. e601.
26. Bradley BC, Perdue KS, Tisdel KA, Gilligan DM. Frequency of anticoagulation for atrial fibrillation and reasons for its non-use at a Veterans Affairs medical center. Am J Cardiol. 2000;85(5):568–72.
27. Jorge E, Pereira FS, Baptista R, Monteiro P, Santos L, Fonseca I, et al. Anticoagulation in elderly patients with atrial fibrillation: from the guidelines to the daily medical practice. Acta Med Port. 2011;24 Suppl 2:293–300.
28. Diez-Manglano J, Gomes-Martin J, Al-Cheikh-Felices P, Perez SI, Diez-Angulo R, Clemente-Sarasa C. Adherence to guidelines and mortality in atrial fibrillation. Int J Cardiol. 2014;176(2):430–6.
29. Madden JL. Resection of the left auricular appendix; a prophylaxis for recurrent arterial emboli. JAMA. 1949;140(9):769–72.
30. Bayard YL, Omran H, Neuzil P, Thuesen L, Pichler M, Rowland E, et al. PLAATO (Percutaneous Left Atrial Appendage Transcatheter Occlusion) for prevention of cardioembolic stroke in non-anticoagulation eligible atrial fibrillation patients: results from the European PLAATO study. EuroIntervention. 2010;6(2):220–6.
31. Chan SK, Kannam JP, Douglas PS, Manning WJ. Multiplane transesophageal echocardiographic assessment of left atrial appendage anatomy and function. Am J Cardiol. 1995;76(7):528–30.
32. Freixa X, Tzikas A, Basmadjian A, Garceau P, Ibrahim R. The chicken-wing morphology: an anatomical challenge for left atrial appendage occlusion. J Interv Cardiol. 2013;26(5):509–14.
33. Kretzschmar D, Lauten A, Goebel B, Doenst T, Poerner TC, Ferrari M, et al. Optimal prosthesis sizing in transcatheter aortic valve implantation by exclusive use of three-dimensional transoesophageal echocardiography. Clin Physiol Funct Imaging. 2014.
34. Cruz-Gonzalez I, Perez-Rivera A, Lopez-Jimenez R, Rodriguez-Collado J, Martin-Moreiras J, Cascon M, et al. Significance of the learning curve in left atrial appendage occlusion with two different devices. Catheter Cardiovasc Interv. 2014;83(4):642–6.
35. Mobius-Winkler S, Majunke N, Sandri M, Mangner N, Linke A, Stone GW, et al. Percutaneous left atrial appendage closure: Technical aspects and prevention of periprocedural complications with the watchman device. World J Cardiol. 2015;7(2):65–75.

5

Required temporal resolution for accurate thoracic aortic pulse wave velocity measurements by phase-contrast magnetic resonance imaging and comparison with clinical standard applanation tonometry

Karolina Dorniak[1], Einar Heiberg[2,3], Marcin Hellmann[1], Dorota Rawicz-Zegrzda[1], Maria Wesierska[1], Rafal Galaska[4], Agnieszka Sabisz[5], Edyta Szurowska[5], Maria Dudziak[1] and Erik Hedström[2,6*]

Abstract

Background: Pulse wave velocity (PWV) is a biomarker for arterial stiffness, clinically assessed by applanation tonometry (AT). Increased use of phase-contrast cardiac magnetic resonance (CMR) imaging allows for PWV assessment with minor routine protocol additions. The aims were to investigate the acquired temporal resolution needed for accurate and precise measurements of CMR-PWV, and develop a tool for CMR-PWV measurements.

Methods: Computer phantoms were generated for PWV = 2–20 m/s based on human CMR-PWV data. The PWV measurements were performed in 13 healthy young subjects and 13 patients at risk for cardiovascular disease. The CMR-PWV was measured by through-plane phase-contrast CMR in the ascending aorta and at the diaphragm level. Centre-line aortic distance was determined between flow planes. The AT-PWV was assessed within 2 h after CMR. Three observers (CMR experience: 15, 4, and <1 year) determined CMR-PWV. The developed tool was based on the flow-curve foot transit time for PWV quantification.

Results: Computer phantoms showed bias 0.27 ± 0.32 m/s for a temporal resolution of at least 30 ms. Intraobserver variability for CMR-PWV were: 0 ± 0.03 m/s (15 years), -0.04 ± 0.33 m/s (4 years), and -0.02 ± 0.30 m/s (<1 year). Interobserver variability for CMR-PWV was below 0.02 ± 0.38 m/s. The AT-PWV overestimated CMR-PWV by 1.1 ± 0.7 m/s in healthy young subjects and 1.6 ± 2.7 m/s in patients.

Conclusions: An acquired temporal resolution of at least 30 ms should be used to obtain accurate and precise thoracic aortic phase-contrast CMR-PWV. A new freely available research tool was used to measure PWV in healthy young subjects and in patients, showing low intra- and interobserver variability also for less experienced CMR observers.

Keywords: Aorta, Pulse wave velocity, Temporal resolution, Magnetic resonance imaging, Phase contrast, Applanation tonometry

* Correspondence: erik.hedstrom@med.lu.se
[2]Lund University, Skane University Hospital, Department of Clinical Sciences Lund, Clinical Physiology, Lund, Sweden
[6]Lund University, Skane University Hospital, Department of Clinical Sciences Lund, Diagnostic Radiology, Lund, Sweden
Full list of author information is available at the end of the article

Background

Aortic stiffness is related to progressive structural changes of the aortic wall with normal aging, [1] but also dependent on cardiovascular disease (CVD) risk factors such as hypertension independent of end-stage renal disease, glucose intolerance, diabetes, and obesity [2, 3]. Pulse wave velocity (PWV) can be used as a biomarker for aortic stiffness, and can predict CVD outcome beyond traditional risk factors [4]. Further, as arterial stiffness occurs earlier than luminal changes, [5] PWV has a potential as an early marker for atherosclerosis. The PWV is defined as the distance between two measurement planes divided by the difference in time between pulse waves at these measurement planes.

Cardiac magnetic resonance (CMR) imaging is increasingly used for cardiovascular assessment, and minor adjustments to a routine CMR protocol yields data for PWV. The CMR-PWV has been previously validated [6, 7] and is thus an attractive option for assessment of aortic stiffness, giving prognostic information at low extra cost.

Applanation tonometry (AT) is another method for assessing PWV, and this method is both generally available and well used in clinical routine as it is easy to apply [8]. The AT measures PWV on a more global arterial scale compared with CMR, between carotid and femoral arteries, whereas CMR usually is applied regionally in the aortic arch or thoracic aorta [9, 10]. The CMR-PWV measurements can however also be performed in a global fashion similar to AT-PWV covering the abdominal aorta or iliac arteries [1, 11]. Depending on the extent of aorta included in CMR-PWV measurements, the CMR-PWV values could be expected to not be interchangeable with AT-PWV, particularly important in follow-up studies.

All PWV methods are susceptible to sampling errors, CMR-PWV particularly so related to noise and temporal resolution, whereas the main limitation for AT-PWV is the estimated distance between flow curve measurement points. With the increasing availability of CMR, the paucity of available software to assess CMR-PWV is also viewed as a major limitation to the wider use of CMR-PWV [12].

The aims of this study were therefore to 1) investigate the acquired temporal resolution needed for accurate measurements of CMR-PWV; and 2) to provide a tool for CMR-PWV measurements and use this to compare CMR-PWV with the clinical standard AT-PWV, by experienced and less experienced CMR observers.

Methods

Study populations and protocol

The local Ethics Committee approved the study and all subjects provided written informed consent.

First, a set of simplistic computer phantoms was created in order to derive the adequate temporal resolution for accurate and precise quantification of CMR-PWV. The following acquisitions of CMR flow data in humans were performed using an acquired temporal resolution above this cut-off.

Irrespective of the PWV measurement method applied, the PWV tend to be lower and less dispersed in younger healthy individuals and higher and more scattered in older subjects, and also increase with presence of cardiovascular disease (CVD) risk factors. Therefore, PWV was obtained by both CMR and AT in younger healthy subjects and in older patients with CVD risk factors.

Healthy subjects ($n = 13$, median age 26 years, range 18 – 43 years, 5 women) were included in whom CMR was performed as part of routine workup due to positive family history or clinical findings raising suspicion of one of the following genetic/familial disorders: arrhythmogenic right ventricular cardiomyopathy, left ventricular non-compaction, Marfan syndrome or hypertrophic cardiomyopathy. In all included subjects the CMR results and other clinical examinations including genetic testing where appropriate were normal. The CMR was considered normal if all volumes, LV mass and thickness and regional and global function were within age and gender reference limits, and valvular pathology including regurgitation/stenosis was not present.

Consecutive patients ($n = 13$, median age 61 years, range 52 – 72 years, 7 women) were included with variable CVD risk profile including dyslipidaemia, hypertension, and history of coronary artery disease. Exclusion criteria were any acute cardiovascular condition such as myocarditis, acute coronary syndrome or overt heart failure within 3 months prior to inclusion, complex congenital heart disease, known familial or genetic cardiomyopathy or aortic stenosis or regurgitation.

Applanation tonometry was used as a clinical standard for comparison, and performed within 2 h after the CMR examination. The brachial arterial blood pressure was also measured in the supine position with a sphygmomanometer in all patients, in conjunction with AT.

Computer phantoms

The velocity profiles and typical aortic centre-line distance between flow measurement planes were extracted from normal subject data with a heart rate of 60 beats per minute and 40 time frames, corresponding to a true temporal resolution of 25 ms. The velocity profiles were up-sampled with cubic interpolation to 10 000 time frames over a cardiac cycle, corresponding to a time resolution of 0.1 ms. Given a known PWV and the distance between flow measurement planes the temporal shift between flow curves was calculated. A set of such fixed temporal shifts was introduced to correspond to known PWV in the range of 2–20 m/s (in 10 steps of 2 m/s). After adding the temporal shift, the velocity profiles were down-sampled to between 20–40 time frames (21 steps per cardiac cycle), resulting in temporal resolutions of 25–50 ms. In the upsample/downsample process the highest temporal resolution thus was kept below the originally collected data based on 40 time frames, i.e. 25 ms. To ensure a mathematically correct down-sampling process optimal anti-aliasing filters were applied. The maximal percentage error between calculated PWV and true PWV was determined for each computer phantom by testing each combination of number of time frames and PWV. In total 210 (10 × 21) phantoms were evaluated. The determination of the cut-off for number of time frames to be used for adequate temporal resolution was based on visual inspection of identity plots and the quantitative bias between calculated and true PWV.

CMR imaging

Patients were imaged in the supine position using either a 1.5 T MR scanner (Siemens Aera, Erlangen, Germany) with an 18-element phased array cardiac coil ($n = 14$) or a 3 T MR scanner (Philips Achieva 3.0 T TX, Eindhoven, the Netherlands) with a 32-channel InVivo cardiac coil ($n = 12$). Oblique sagittal slices covering the thoracic aorta (producing the so-called 'candy-cane view') and 1 phase-contrast image for aortic flow measurements at the level of the diaphragm were added to the routine protocol, which already included a phase-contrast flow acquisition in the ascending aorta. The oblique sagittal slices were acquired either with a HASTE (half fourier single shot turbo spin echo) or a 3D turbo spin-echo sequence. For quantitative flow measurements, a 2D phase-contrast gradient recalled echo (GRE) sequence with retrospective ECG-gating was used. Adequate velocity encoding (Venc) values were selected using a Venc-scout and set to between 150–250 cm/s for through plane flow quantification. Typical parameters for the quantitative flow phase-contrast GRE sequence were TR/TE = 20/3 ms, flip angle = 10/20°, 1.3 × 1.3 × 8 mm^3. Fifty (Siemens) or 40 (Philips) velocity-encoded images were acquired per cardiac cycle, as determined after the computer phantom experiment. The typical segment size was approximately 20 ms for both scanners, ranging from 15 – 27.5 ms. The acquisition matrix in the phase encoding direction was adapted if necessary to meet a segment size < 30 ms.

CMR image analysis

A new module for PWV was introduced in the software Segment (http://www.medviso.com) [13]. Aortic pulse wave travel distance was measured manually along the centre-line of the aorta in the oblique sagittal aorta images, between the acquired flow measurement planes in the ascending aorta and at the level of the diaphragm. For quantitative flow curves, automatic vessel segmentation was performed with manual corrections where needed. Delineations were performed in magnitude images and guided by phase-contrast images where appropriate.

The flow curves from the ascending aorta and the aorta at the level of the diaphragm were superimposed and intersecting tangents between upslope and baseline were determined. The time-to-foot (TTF) approach was applied as this has been shown to be reliable for CMR-PWV [9]. In short, a regression line was fitted to the maximum upslope of each of the two flow curves representative of the ascending aorta and the aorta at the level of the diaphragm. The points at which these upslope tangents intersected the baseline tangents were labelled as the respective intersection points (Fig. 1). Prior to the upslope tangent fitting a Gaussian smoothing kernel was applied to the flow curves, corresponding to sigma = 0.62 ms (for a heart rate of 60 beats per minute; i.e. sigma value 0.025). The amount of smoothing was determined by visual inspection of the flow curves, and can be changed manually as needed. The time delay (Δt) between the intersection points was used as input for calculation of the CMR-PWV. The CMR-PWV was thus calculated by dividing the measured aortic centre-line distance between the ascending aorta and diaphragm level phase-encoded velocity flow planes by the Δt between the 2 flow curves.

Due to concomitant or Eddy current background phase errors a baseline shift of the flow curves may be seen [14]. Built-in Eddy current compensation may solve this, but is also vendor-dependent. Therefore the PWV module also includes an option to adjust the individual flow curves to correct for this, both automatically and manually. The automatic method calculated the baseline as the mean flow rate during 62.5–87.5 % of the cardiac cycle. As this automatic correction may fail in cases with significant aortic regurgitation, a manual method for baseline correction was also implemented. Neither the manual nor the automatic method was however applied in the current study, as baseline shift was not seen.

Three observers blinded to other patient information and each other's results performed independent CMR analyses. The observers had different experience in CMR (15 years, 4 years and less than 1 year). All observers also repeated their measurements more than 10 days later. The CMR-PWV data presented, except for comparisons between observers, are based on measurements by the most experienced observer.

Applanation tonometry

Carotid-femoral PWV was measured noninvasively by AT according to recommended clinical standards [15]. Even though considered clinical standard today, as it is widely available, it is important to note that AT is not a gold standard. In the current study it is thus used as a comparison between non-invasive tools. Carotid and femoral pulse wave recordings were performed in supine

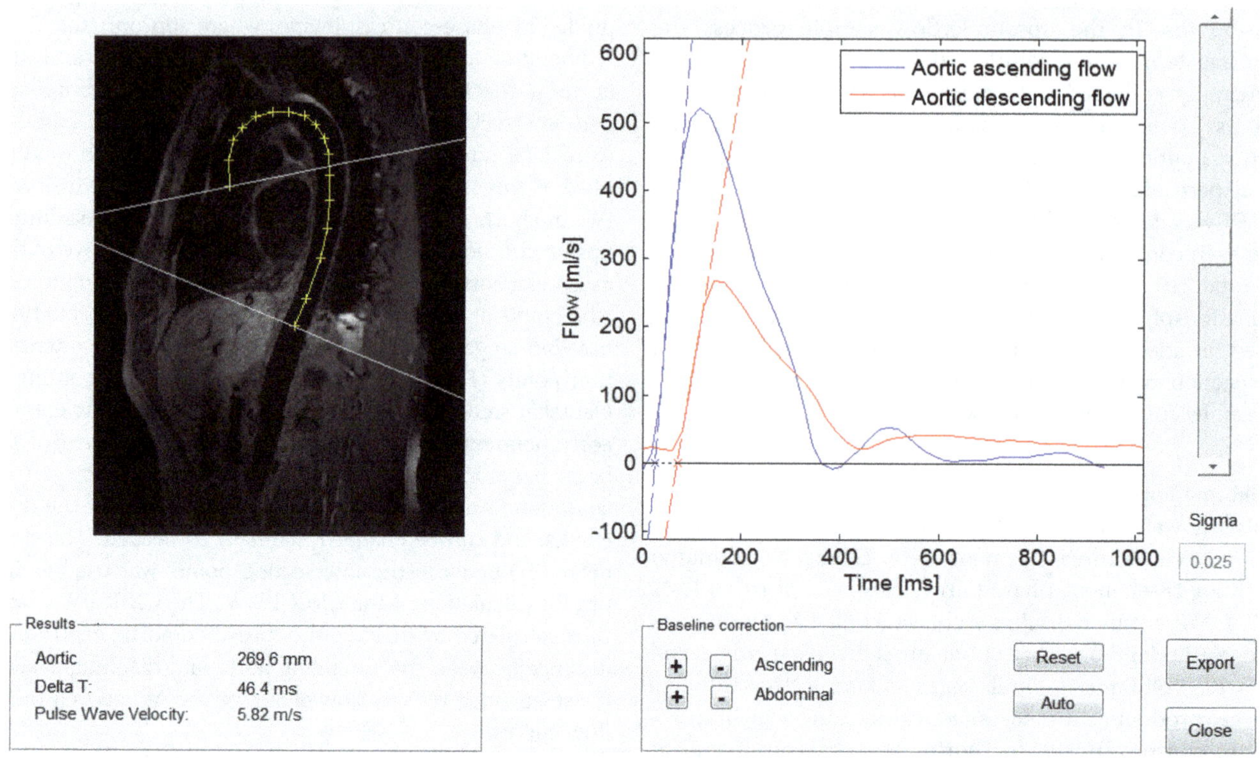

Fig. 1 The graphical user interface for pulse wave velocity assessment. The oblique sagittal image of the aorta (left) shows the perpendicular flow measurement planes (white lines) in the ascending aorta and at the level of the diaphragm. The centre-line aortic distance between flow planes are shown as a yellow line with cross marks. The graph (right) shows the flow curves and respective upslope tangents with their baseline intersection points giving the time delay between flow curves (Δt; dashed part of the baseline tangent)

subjects after 15 min of rest. Measurements were performed on the right common carotid artery [C] and the right femoral artery [F] using the widely available SphygmoCor device (AtCor Medical, Australia). Intravessel distance between measurement points was defined by approximation from body surface tape measurements and calculated as suprasternal notch to [F] - suprasternal notch to [C] [16].

The AT-PWV was calculated using commercial software (SphygmoCor Cardiovascular Management Suite; AtCor Medical, Australia) based on pulse transit time and the approximate intravessel distance between the two measurement points.

Statistical analysis

Data were expressed as median (range) or mean ± SD. Statistical analyses were performed using Prism 6 (GraphPad Software, La Jolla, CA, USA). The observer variability was determined as bias ± SD and agreement was calculated according to Bland-Altman with 95 % limits of agreement. The Student's two-tailed t-test was applied for testing of statistically significant differences in normally distributed data, whereas Fisher's exact test was performed on categorical data, with $p < 0.05$ considered statistically significant.

Results

Demographic and clinical characteristics are summarised in Table 1.

Computer phantoms

The results of the computer phantoms are summarised in Table 2 and Fig. 2. The PWV error seems to increase with increasing number of time frames. The reason for this is that inadequate time resolution (number of time frames) generates smoothing, which prevents calculation of correct slopes and thus leads to incorrect PWV. For each true PWV there is a certain number of time frames where the error is maximal, and thereafter the error again decreases with increasing number of time frames. From 35 time frames per cardiac cycle, a plateau in the error of the PWV estimation is visible, corresponding to a required time resolution of at least 30 ms to accurately quantify PWV over a range of 2 – 20 m/s using phase-contrast CMR. The temporal resolution of at least 30 ms yielded a bias of 0.27 ± 0.32 m/s between calculated and true PWV in the computer phantoms. All human CMR flow data were thus acquired using a temporal resolution of at least 30 ms; i.e. set above 35 time frames also considering the individual cardiac frequency.

Table 1 Demographic and clinical characteristics of the study population

	Healthy young	Patients	p
Number of subjects	13	13	
Male/Female	8/5	6/7	0.70
Age (years)	26 (18 – 43)	61 (52 – 72)	<0.0001
BMI (kg/m^2)	20 (17 – 24)	27 (22 – 35)	<0.0001
Systolic blood pressure (mmHg)	120 (100 – 140)	130 (110 – 160)	0.02
Diastolic blood pressure (mmHg)	80 (55 – 80)	80 (60 – 90)	0.17
History of smoking[a]	0	6	0.01
History of CAD	0	4	0.10
Statins	0	13	<0.0001
Antihypertensive drugs[b]	0	12	<0.0001
Diabetes[c]	0	2	0.48

[a]No current smoker. [b]8 patients with ACE inhibitors, of which 1 with added diuretics, 1 with added calcium channel blockers, and 1 with added beta adrenolytics. Four patients with AT receptor blockers, of which 1 with added beta adrenolytics, 1 with added beta adrenolytics and diuretics, and 1 with added beta adrenolytics, diuretics and alpha adrenolytics. [c]All patients without insulin dependent diabetes

For the Gaussian smoothing sigma value, a 50 % reduction in sigma from 0.68 ms to 0.34 ms resulted in a PWV change of -0.02 ± 0.12 m/s, indicating low impact on standard flow data. In images with a lower signal-to-noise ratio, however, a change in sigma may render more adequate fitting data.

Table 2 The PWV median errors for different number of time frames/temporal resolution based on 210 computer phantoms

Time frames	Temporal resolution [ms]	Median error [m/s]	Median error [%]
20	50.0	2.36	21.3
21	47.6	1.51	17.2
22	45.5	0.72	10.4
23	43.5	0.16	9.1
24	41.7	-0.02	6.5
25	40.0	-0.39	4.4
26	38.5	-1.61	10.8
27	37.0	-2.74	18.1
28	35.7	-2.39	21.3
29	34.5	-1.83	16.2
30	33.3	-1.29	11.4
31	32.3	-0.76	6.7
32	31.3	-0.42	5.1
33	30.3	-0.20	2.6
34	29.4	-0.11	1.3
35	28.6	0.10	0.9
36	27.8	0.48	3.6
37	27.0	0.46	4.1
38	26.3	0.30	3.0
39	25.6	0.23	2.4
40	25.0	0.17	1.8

Errors are expressed as median errors for all velocities in the range of 2–20 m/s

CMR

The CMR-PWV was feasible to perform in all subjects. As good signal-to-noise ratio was seen in all cases in the current study, sigma was not manually altered and thus sigma = 0.025 was used for all CMR-PWV analyses.

The CMR-PWV was statistically significantly higher in patients compared with younger healthy subjects ($p < 0.0001$; Table 3). Intraobserver variability for CMR-PWV for the 3 observers was 0 ± 0.03 m/s (15 years), -0.04 ± 0.33 m/s (4 years), and -0.02 ± 0.30 m/s (<1 year), respectively. The PWV interobserver variability between the 2 less experienced observers and the more experienced observer was for 4 vs. 15 years -0.01 ± 0.32 m/s and for <1 vs. 15 years 0.01 ± 0.30 m/s, and between the 2 less experienced observers PWV interobserver variability was 0.02 ± 0.38 m/s (Fig. 3). The observer variability can be related to aortic distance measurements between flow planes and flow measurements. Intraobserver variability for the aortic centre-line distance between flow planes was 0.2 ± 1.2 mm (15 years), -0.1 ± 4.8 mm (4 years), and -1.0 ± 5.9 mm (<1 year), respectively, with an average distance between flow planes of 250 ± 30 mm. Interobserver variability for aortic centre-line distance between flow planes, comparing the 2 less experienced observers and the more experienced observer, was for 4 vs. 15 years -1.2 ± 4.8 mm and for <1 vs. 15 years -1.9 ± 4.7 mm. Intraobserver variability for flow measurements, calculated as the time difference Δt between flow curves was 0 ± 0.1 ms (15 years), 0.3 ± 1.7 ms (4 years) and 0.3 ± 2.5 ms (<1 year), respectively. Corresponding interobserver variability was for 4 vs. 15 years -0.2 ± 1.4 ms and for <1 vs. 15 years -0.3 ± 3.3 ms. Interobserver variability did not differ between 1.5 T and 3 T (all $p >$ 0.12).

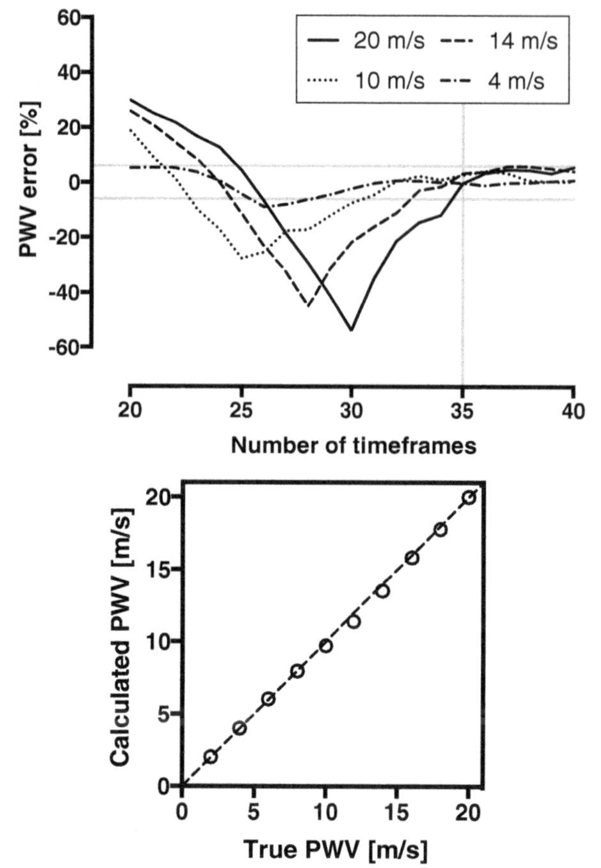

Fig. 2 Median percentage PWV errors for number of time-frame samples for flow data from 210 computer phantoms. For clarity, 4 cases representative of different PWV are shown. All computer phantoms were however used for cut-off calculations. A plateau in the median PWV error is found from 35 time frames per cardiac cycle, corresponding to a temporal resolution of at least 30 ms at a heart rate of 60 beats per minute (top). The grey vertical line represents the cut-off 35 time frames, and the grey horizontal lines indicate the maximum PWV errors (±6 %) above the cut-off 35 time frames. The median error for 35 time frames was 0.27 ± 0.32 m/s between calculated and true PWV in phantoms, and is visualised in the identity plot (bottom). The dashed line indicates line of identity

Applanation tonometry

The AT-PWV values were, as for CMR-PWV, statistically significantly higher in patients than in younger healthy subjects ($p < 0.0001$; Table 3).

The AT-PWV was statistically significantly higher than CMR-PWV for healthy young subjects (5.6 ± 0.7 vs. 4.5 ± 0.8; $p < 0.0001$). For patients a similar trend was found, however not statistically significant (9.0 ± 2.2 vs. 7.8 ± 2.2; $p = 0.07$) (Table 3; Fig. 4).

Table 3 PWV by AT and CMR

	AT-PWV (m/s)	CMR-PWV (m/s)	*p* (between methods)
Healthy young	5.6 ± 0.7	4.5 ± 0.8	<0.0001
Patients	9.0 ± 2.2	7.8 ± 2.2	0.07
p (between groups)	<0.0001	<0.0001	

The bias and variability between AT-PWV and CMR-PWV were similar at 1.5 T and 3 T (1.5 T: 1.1 ± 2.4 m/s; 3 T: 1.6 ± 1.3 m/s; $p = 0.56$).

Discussion

This study shows that an acquired temporal resolution of at least 30 ms is necessary to obtain accurate and precise quantitative flow data for CMR-PWV over the range 2–20 m/s, representative of PWV in the human aorta. Further, a new freely available tool for research was developed and used to measure CMR-PWV in healthy young subjects and in patients, showing low intra- and interobserver variability also for less experienced CMR observers.

The current study showed lower PWV in the younger healthy cohort compared with older patients at risk for CVD, as expected [1, 8]. The current study also showed slightly higher PWV for the healthy young cohort compared with data from an equivalent age group in a recent study including PWV in only the aortic arch (4 m/s), [10] but lower than a study also including parts of the abdominal aorta (5.6 m/s) [17]. This difference may be explained by that measurements for PWV are related to the elastic properties of the vessels, which vary along the arterial tree, with more elastic proximal segments and stiffer distal segments. In an invasive human study, pulse wave velocity increased from 5 m/s in the ascending aorta to 6 m/s in the abdominal aorta, and up to 9 m/s in the iliac and femoral arteries [18]. A recent CMR-PWV study however showed a different order of PWV, with highest PWV in the aortic arch (8–9 m/s), lower PWV in the iliofemoral segment (7–8 m/s), and lowest PWV in the thoracoabdominal segment (5–7 m/s) [11]. This difference is not explained and age groups are similar. Other CMR-PWV studies however also show approximately 4–6 m/s in the aortic arch, [1, 10] or approximately 6 m/s in the thoracic segment, [17] both comparable with the original invasive measurements by Latham et al. [18].

The CMR-PWV was determined with low intraobserver variability in the current study using the TTF approach, which has been previously shown to have high reproducibility [7, 9]. Further, also the less experienced CMR observers in the current study showed low interobserver variability versus the more experienced observer. A previous study showed similar interobserver variability between experienced observers (-0.1 ± 0.3 m/s), [9] which together with the current study indicates that CMR-PWV can be precisely performed also with less CMR experience.

The AT-PWV overestimated CMR-PWV by 1.1 ± 0.7 m/s in young healthy subjects and 1.6 ± 2.7 m/s in the older patients. This is a similar trend compared with previously published data where the corresponding reported

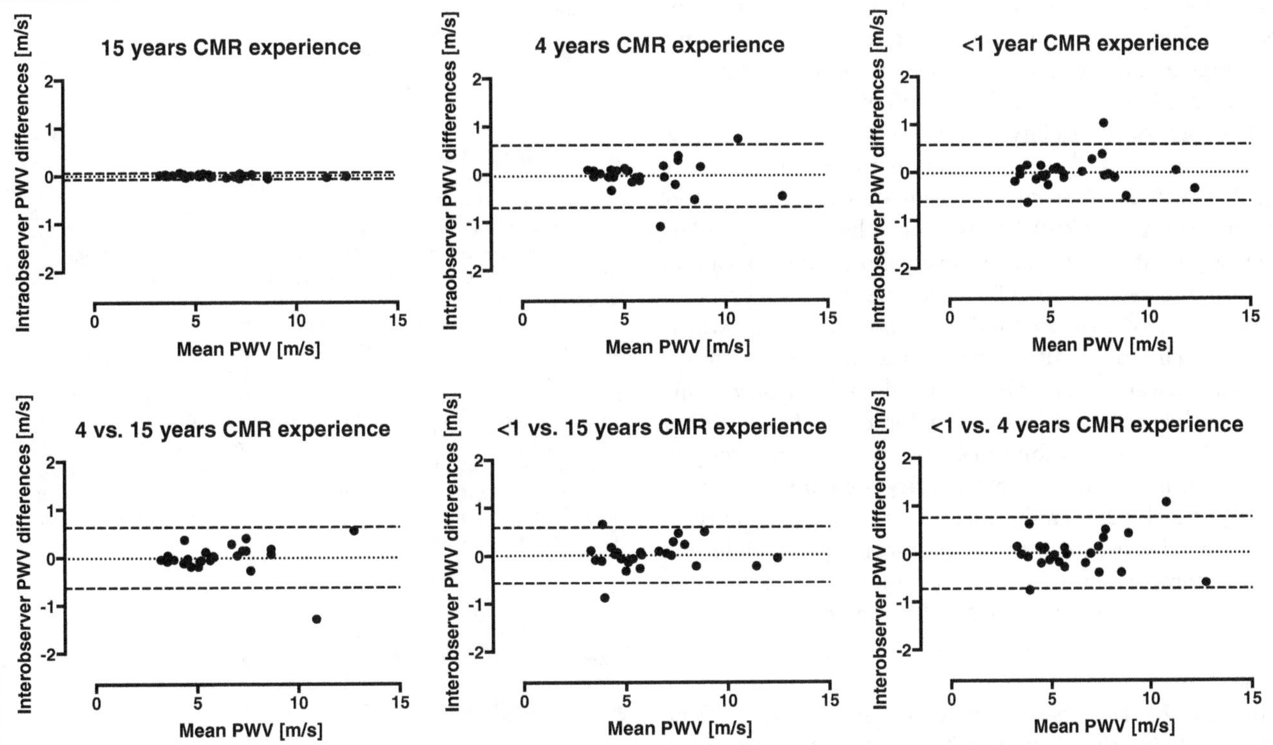

Fig. 3 Bland-Altman plots showing intra- (top) and interobserver (bottom) CMR-PWV variability. Intraobserver variability for CMR-PWV was low for all 3 observers, 0 ± 0.03 m/s (15 years; left), -0.04 ± 0.33 m/s (4 years; middle), and -0.02 ± 0.30 m/s (<1 year; right), respectively. The interobserver variability was also generally low, for 4 vs. 15 years -0.01 ± 0.32 m/s (left), <1 vs. 15 years 0.01 ± 0.30 m/s (middle), and <1 vs. 4 years 0.02 ± 0.38 m/s (right). Dotted lines indicate mean differences and dashed lines represent 95 % limits of agreement

differences were 0.43 m/s and 0.64 m/s [17]. Thus, PWV values are not interchangeable between AT and CMR. In AT-based measurements, age-related elongation or increased tortuosity of the aorta in disease may play a role, as this cannot be accounted for using standard surface tape estimates. Pure age-related elongation of the ascending aorta is considered to be of minor importance for AT-PWV, as this part of aorta is not included in distance measurements for calculation of AT-PWV [19]. When AT-PWV values are compared with CMR-PWV however also the ascending aorta is of importance but even more so the increased tortuosity of the abdominal aorta, which has impact on the vessel distance, not being accurate by surface tape estimates. In CMR-PWV accurate aortic centre-line distance measurements can be acquired in all cases, either by adequate angulation of a stack of oblique sagittal images covering the aorta, which can be combined into a 3D slab

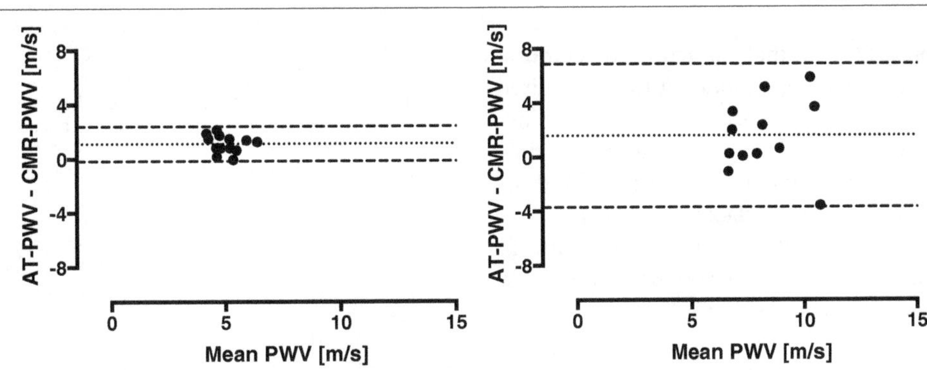

Fig. 4 Bland-Altman plots showing AT-PWV vs. CMR-PWV. The AT-PWV overestimated CMR-PWV by 1.1 ± 0.7 m/s in younger healthy subjects (left) and by 1.6 ± 2.7 m/s in patients (right). Dotted lines indicate mean differences and dashed lines represent 95 % limits of agreement. Also note the PWV differences between younger healthy subjects and older patients where PWV is lower and less dispersed in healthy young subjects

for proper distance measurements in software such as the one used in the current study, or directly assessed using 3D angiography techniques applying curved multiplanar reconstruction, with or without contrast agent.

The lack of availability of CMR-PWV software is currently viewed as a major limitation to the wider use of CMR-PWV [12]. The current study developed a new tool for measuring CMR-PWV, showing values corresponding to previous studies in comparable cohorts, and also a corresponding relation to AT-PWV. The 2D through-plane phase-contrast MRI method was chosen, as it is widely used in clinical CMR routine. This, together with the straightforward TTF method used in post-processing makes this approach attractive for clinical use. Other CMR-based PWV techniques are available, but are both more advanced and less elementary for clinical application [20, 21]. Further, the method applied in the current study has been shown to be the most reproducible in a recent comparison between transit time, cross-correlation and flow-area methods for CMR-PWV assessment [9].

Limitations

The time of day, association with meals, sleep, caffeine and smoking may all impact PWV [15]. All these were corrected for in the current study except for the exact time of day the examination was performed. The differences related to time of day are however small and all subjects underwent AT within 2 h after CMR so potential changes are not considered to have impact on results. The distribution between 1.5 T and 3 T was not randomised but rather resulted from centre logistics. It is however unlikely that randomisation would significantly alter the results. The current study did not use invasive haemodynamics as a gold standard but rather compared two non-invasive methods, which may be considered a limitation. Invasive measures were however not necessary to show the readiness of PWV-CMR imaging and low variability using the proposed tool.

Conclusions

Computer phantoms showed that an acquired temporal resolution of at least 30 ms (corresponding to 35 acquired time frames at a heart rate of 60 beats per minute) is necessary to obtain accurate and precise quantitative flow data for CMR-PWV over the range 2–20 m/s in the thoracic aorta. A new tool, freely available for research, was used to measure PWV in healthy young subjects and in patients showing low intra- and interobserver variability also for less experienced CMR observers.

Abbreviations

AT: applanation tonometry; CVD: cardiovascular disease; CMR: cardiac magnetic resonance; ECG: electrocardiogram; GRE: gradient recalled echo; HASTE: half fourier single shot turbo spin echo; PWV: pulse wave velocity; TTF: time-to-foot; Venc: velocity encoding.

Funding

Funding was received from: Swedish Research Council (621-2012-4944), Swedish Heart and Lung Foundation, Region of Skane, Skane University Hospital in Lund, and Medical University of Gdansk (ST-98).

Authors' contributions

KD made substantial contributions to conception and design, acquired and analysed data, and drafted the manuscript. EiH made substantial contributions to conception and design, acquired and analysed data, and revised the manuscript for important intellectual content. MH made substantial contributions to conception and design, acquired and analysed data, and revised the manuscript for important intellectual content. DRZ acquired and analysed data, and revised the manuscript for important intellectual content. MW, RG and AS acquired data, and revised the manuscript for important intellectual content. ES made substantial contributions to conception and design, acquired data, and revised the manuscript for important intellectual content. MD made substantial contributions to conception and design, and revised the manuscript for important intellectual content. ErH made substantial contributions to conception and design, analysed and interpreted data, and drafted the manuscript. All authors read and approved the final manuscript and agreed to be accountable for all aspects of the work.

Competing interests

The authors declare having no competing interests, with the following exception. Dr. Einar Heiberg founded the company Medviso AB, Lund, Sweden, and is the major shareholder of said company, selling the FDA-approved software version of Segment for commercial use.

Author details

[1]Department of Noninvasive Cardiac Diagnostics, Medical University of Gdansk, Gdansk, Poland. [2]Lund University, Skane University Hospital, Department of Clinical Sciences Lund, Clinical Physiology, Lund, Sweden. [3]Department of Biomedical Engineering, Faculty of Engineering, Lund University, Lund, Sweden. [4]1st Department of Cardiology, Medical University of Gdansk, Gdansk, Poland. [5]2nd Department of Radiology, Medical University of Gdansk, Gdansk, Poland. [6]Lund University, Skane University Hospital, Department of Clinical Sciences Lund, Diagnostic Radiology, Lund, Sweden.

References

1. Rogers WJ, Hu YL, Coast D, Vido DA, Kramer CM, Pyeritz RE, Reichek N. Age-associated changes in regional aortic pulse wave velocity. J Am Coll Cardiol. 2001;38:1123–9.
2. Cruickshank K, Riste L, Anderson SG, Wright JS, Dunn G, Gosling RG. Aortic pulse-wave velocity and its relationship to mortality in diabetes and glucose intolerance: an integrated index of vascular function? Circulation. 2002;106:2085–90.
3. Safar ME, Henry O, Meaume S. Aortic pulse wave velocity: an independent marker of cardiovascular risk. Am J Geriatr Cardiol. 2002;11:295–8.
4. Willum Hansen T, Staessen JA, Torp-Pedersen C, Rasmussen S, Thijs L, Ibsen H, Jeppesen J. Prognostic value of aortic pulse wave velocity as index of arterial stiffness in the general population. Circulation. 2006;113:664–70.
5. Glagov S, Weisenberg E, Zarins CK, Stankunavicius R, Kolettis GJ. Compensatory enlargement of human atherosclerotic coronary arteries. N Engl J Med. 1987;316:1371–5.
6. Bolster BD, Atalar E, Hardy CJ, McVeigh ER. Accuracy of arterial pulse-wave velocity measurement using MR. J Magn Reson Imaging. 1998;8:878–88.
7. Grotenhuis HB, Westenberg JJM, Steendijk P, van der Geest RJ, Ottenkamp J, Bax JJ, Jukema JW, de Roos A. Validation and reproducibility of aortic pulse wave velocity as assessed with velocity-encoded MRI. J Magn Reson Imaging. 2009;30:521–6.
8. The Reference Values for Arterial Stiffness' Collaboration. Determinants of pulse wave velocity in healthy people and in the presence of cardiovascular risk factors: "establishing normal and reference values". Eur Heart J. 2010;31:2338–50.
9. Ibrahim E-SH, Johnson KR, Miller AB, Shaffer JM, White RD. Measuring aortic

pulse wave velocity using high-field cardiovascular magnetic resonance: comparison of techniques. J Cardiovasc Magn Reson. 2010;12:26.
10. Voges I, Jerosch-Herold M, Hedderich JR, Pardun E, Hart C, Gabbert DD, Hansen JH, Petko C, Kramer H-H, Rickers C. Normal values of aortic dimensions, distensibility, and pulse wave velocity in children and young adults: a cross-sectional study. J Cardiovasc Magn Reson. 2012;14:1–1.
11. Langham MC. Effects of age and smoking on endothelial function assessed by quantitative cardiovascular magnetic resonance in the peripheral and central vasculature. 2015. p. 1–14.
12. Wentland AL, Grist TM, Wieben O. Review of MRI-based measurements of pulse wave velocity: a biomarker of arterial stiffness. Cardiovasc Diagn Ther. 2014;4:193–206.
13. Heiberg E, Sjögren J, Ugander M, Carlsson M, Engblom H, Arheden H. Design and validation of Segment–freely available software for cardiovascular image analysis. BMC Med Imaging. 2010;10:1.
14. Bernstein MA, Zhou XJ, Polzin JA, King KF, Ganin A, Pelc NJ, Glover GH. Concomitant gradient terms in phase contrast MR: analysis and correction. Magn Reson Med. 1998;39:300–8.
15. Van Bortel LM, Duprez D, Starmans-Kool MJ, Safar ME, Giannattasio C, Cockcroft J, Kaiser DR, Thuillez C. Clinical applications of arterial stiffness, Task Force III: recommendations for user procedures. Am J Hypertens. 2002; 15:445–52.
16. Vermeersch SJ, Rietzschel ER, De Buyzere ML, Van Bortel LM, Gillebert TC, Verdonck PR, Laurent S, Segers P, Boutouyrie P. Distance measurements for the assessment of carotid to femoral pulse wave velocity. J Hypertens. 2009; 27:2377–85.
17. Suever JD, Oshinski J, Rojas-Campos E, Huneycutt D, Cardarelli F, Stillman AE, Raggi P. Reproducibility of pulse wave velocity measurements with phase contrast magnetic resonance and applanation tonometry. Int J Cardiovasc Imaging. 2012;28:1141–6.
18. Latham RD, Westerhof N, Sipkema P, Rubal BJ, Reuderink P, Murgo JP. Regional wave travel and reflections along the human aorta: a study with six simultaneous micromanometric pressures. Circulation. 1985;72:1257–69.
19. Sugawara J, Hayashi K, Yokoi T, Tanaka H. Age-associated elongation of the ascending aorta in adults. JACC Cardiovasc Imaging. 2008;1:739–48.
20. Hardy CJ, Bolster BD, McVeigh ER, Adams WJ, Zerhouni EA. A one-dimensional velocity technique for NMR measurement of aortic distensibility. Magn Reson Med. 1994;31:513–20.
21. Wentland AL, Wieben O, François CJ, Boncyk C, Munoz Del Rio A, Johnson KM, Grist TM, Frydrychowicz A. Aortic pulse wave velocity measurements with undersampled 4D flow-sensitive MRI: comparison with 2D and algorithm determination. J Magn Reson Imaging. 2012;37:853–9.

6

Assessment of coronary artery intimal thickening in patients with a previous diagnosis of Kawasaki disease by using high resolution transthoracic echocardiography

Valentina Giacchi*, Pietro Sciacca, Ileana Stella, Martina Filippelli, Patrizia Barone, Mario La Rosa and Salvatore Leonardi

Abstract

Background: Kawasaki disease (KD) is a generalized systemic vasculitis of unknown etiology involving medium and small size blood vessels, particularly the coronary arteries. In these vessels a progressive stenosis may result from active remodeling with an intimal proliferation and neoangiogenesis. The aim of our study was to assess, by using high-resolution transthoracic 2D Echocardiography, if subjects with a previous diagnosis of Kawasaki disease after several years show a coronary intimal thickening, suggestive of a persistent cardiovascular risk.

Methods: We assessed measurement of thickening, inner diameter and outer diameter of coronary arteries using 2D Echocardiography (Philips E 33 with multy-frequency S8-3 and S12-4 probes) and examining the proximal portion of left main coronary artery just above the aortic valve with parasternal short axis view.

Results: We found a significant intimal thickening in patients with previous Kawasaki disease compared to healthy controls. In particular, we noticed that also subjects not suffering from coronary impairment in acute phase have higher values of thickening than healthy controls, and this wall thickening may confer a higher cardiovascular risk.

Conclusions: Therefore we concluded that the assessment of coronary artery thickening by high-resolution transthoracic 2D Echocardiography may become an essential instrument to evaluate late cardiovascular risk in subjects with a diagnosis of Kawasaki disease in childhood.

Keywords: Kawasaki disease, High resolution transthoracic echocardiography, Cardiovascular risk, Coronary intimal thickening

Background

Kawasaki disease (KD) is a systemic vasculitis affecting infants and young children [1,2] which may potentially involve heart [3], small and medium-size arteries, and can lead to the formation of aneurysms, especially in the coronary arteries [4,5].

During the acute phase of the disease, mortality peaks from 15 to 45 days after the onset of fever, usually due to cardiac sequelae such as arrhythmia and myocardial infarction (MI) [5,6]. It has been noticed that sudden death from myocardial infarction may also occur after many years in individuals who had previously developed coronary artery aneurysms (CAA) and stenosis, and it seems today that several cases of fatal and nonfatal MIs in young adults have been attributed to "missed" KD diagnosis in childhood [5].

Regarding the pathogenesis of vascular damage, it is well-known that in Kawasaki disease an arterial active remodeling occurs due to intimal proliferation and neoangiogenesis; the intima, rich in smooth muscle cells, and fibrous layers, appears markedly thickened with linearly-arranged microvessels [6].

It has lately been noticed that the high resolution transthoracic echocardiography is able to detect intimal

* Correspondence: valentina.giacchi@yahoo.it
Pediatric Pneumo-Allergology and Cystic Fibrosis Department, Pediatric Cardiology Clinic, AOU "Policlinico-Vittorio Emanuele", University of Catania, Catania, Italy

thickening in the wall of left main and left anterior descending (LAD) coronary arteries in adults with subclinical atherosclerosis [7,8]. We hypothesized that this technique, applied to the study of proximal left main coronary artery, could be useful in monitoring the follow-up of KD after the acute phase.

The aim of the present study was to assess coronary artery intimal thickening by using high resolution transthoracic 2D Echocardiography in patients with a previous diagnosis of Kawasaki disease several years after the acute event.

Methods

We conducted an observational cross-sectional case–control double-blind study on 31 patients with a previous diagnosis of KD who had been hospitalized in childhood since January 1990 to December 2000 in our Pediatric Department of the University of Catania, Italy.

Every patient if of age, or at least one parent or legal guardian if underage, gave their written informed consent before the patient's inclusion in the study. The study was conducted in accordance with the Helsinki Declaration, and the study protocol was approved by the (local) Ethics Committee of the Medical University of Catania.

Five patients were omitted from the study as they were current smokers. In the same way we recruited 26 voluntary healthy subjects among students of school and University to be used as controls.

The main features of the 26 patients at the moment of diagnosis are reported in Table 1.

The diagnosis of Kawasaki disease was performed according to the criteria of the American Heart Association (AHA) Committee on Rheumatic fever, Endocarditis and Kawasaki disease [9,10]: a typical form of Kawasaki disease was detected in 14 patients (53.3%), an incomplete form in 9 (34.6%) and an atypical form in 3 (11.5%).

Every patient was assigned to corresponding risk class: 20 (76.9%) to the first risk class, 3 (11.5%) to the second, 2 (7.7%) to the third and 1 (3.9%) to the fourth. All patients belonging to third and fourth risk classes were affected by typical form, whereas patients of first and second classes presented typical, atypical or incomplete form.

According to the guidelines at the time of diagnosis, 20/26 (76.9%) had been on both acetylsalicylic acid and intravenous immunoglobulin (IVIG) therapy, (400–500 mg/Kg/day for 4–5 consecutive days or 1–2 g/Kg in a single dose), 3/26 (11.5%) only on acetylsalicylic acid therapy, 2/26 (7.7%) only on IVIG therapy, whereas in a single case (3.9%) the parents refused therapy.

At present, the age ranges from 4 to 27, with an average of 13.3 ± 7.4 and a time from the beginning of the illness ranging from 3 to 22 years.

We performed Electrocardiogram and 2D Echocardiography in all patients.

The laboratory and cardiologic data were compared with those of the 26 healthy subjects of the same age.

The same experienced echocardiographer, unaware of whether he was dealing with a case or a control, assessed measurement of thickening, inner diameter and outer diameter of coronary arteries using 2D Echocardiography (Philips E 33 with multy-frequency S8-3 and S12-4 probes, using the setting scheduled by the echo machine) and examining the proximal portion of left main coronary artery just above the aortic valve with parasternal short axis view. Echocardiographic recordings of four separate cardiac cycles were captured by zoom image. Optimal gain setting was adjusted for maximal delineating the outer edge from the inner edge of the line representing the vascular wall. The thicker walled vascular structure was identified as multiple linear echoes which branched off just above from the aortic valve and was measured edge to edge at diastolic period.

Statistical analysis

We calculated means, standard deviation, standard error (SE) and Median for all variables. We adjusted values of coronary thickening for BSA (Body Surface Area) and performed t-student and Mann–Whitney test to compare these values between cases and controls.

P value < 0.05 was considered statistically significant.

Results

We have not found any significant difference in subjective and laboratory parameters between patients and healthy controls Table 2. Both cases and controls presented

Table 1 Features of 26 patients at diagnosis

Gender	Clinical form	ECG	Cardiac manifestations	Risk class	Therapy	Age at diagnosis
M:18 (69.2%)	T: 14 (53.8%)	N: 12 (46.2%)	NCI: 14 (54%)	I: 20 (76.9%)	ASA + IVIG 20 (76.9%)	< 6 ms: 2 (7.7%)
F:8 (30.8%)	I: 9 (34.6%)	SST: 9 (34.6%)	TAC: 3 (11.5%)	II: 3 (11.5%)	ASA 3 (11.5%)	6 ms- 5 ys: 21 (80.8%)
	A: 3 (11.5%)	PRBBB: 3 (11.5%)	PAC: 3 (11.5%)	III: 2 (7.7%)	IVIG 2 (7.7%)	> 5 ys:3 (11.5%)
		NSDVR: 2 (7.7%)	PE: 3 (11.5%)	IV: 1 (3.9%)	No therapy 1 (3.9%)	
			MR: 3 (11.5%)			

Abbreviations: M male, *F* female, *T* Typical, *I* Incomplete, *A* Atypical, *N* normal, *SST* slight sinus tachycardia, *PRBBB* partial right bundle branch block, *NSDVR* non-specific disorders of ventricular repolarization, *NCI* no cardiac impairment, *TAC* transient anomalies of coronaries, *PAC* persistent anomalies of coronaries, *PE* pericardial effusion, *MR* mitral regurgitation.

normal values of cholesterol, Body Mass Index (BMI), blood pressure and nobody was alcohol drinker or had any other risk factor for atherosclerotic disease.

The Electrocardiogram did not show any signs of ischemia in either cases and controls.

The 2D Echocardiographic assessment of systolic and diastolic function showed normal values in both patients and healthy controls.

We confirmed persistent anomalies of coronary arteries already described at diagnosis in two of the patients (one patient with a giant aneurism of left coronary artery and another one with two aneurisms in the left and right coronary arteries respectively), both with previous diagnosis of typical KD, assigned to 3 and 4 risk class respectively.

Regarding intimal thickness, we detected significant higher thickening values adjusted for BSA in cases than healthy controls (5.3 mm ± 4.4, Median 3.7, SE 0.8, versus 2.7 mm ± 1.2, Median 2.6, SE 0.2, p <0.01) Table 3.

Assessing the main values of thickening adjusted for BSA in the different risk classes, we found values equal to 4.5 mm ± 3.7, Median 3.4, SE 0.8 in the risk class 1 and, assembling patients belonging to risk classes 2-3-4, we detected values equal to 7.9 mm ± 5.8, Median 6.0, SE 2.4 in the risk class 2-3-4 group. We noticed significant difference in thickening values between controls and patients belonging to risk class 1 and in controls and patients belonging to risk class 2-3-4 group ($p < 0.05$) but not between patients belonging to risk class 1 and patients belonging to risk class 2-3-4 group (p = ns) Table 4.

Discussion

Our study might provide new data in the long-term follow-up of Kawasaki disease since our patients showed a significant thickening of coronary intimal wall not related to the severity of the Kawasaki disease during the acute phase. Coronary intimal alteration could indirectly mean a higher cardiovascular risk.

Table 2 Subjective and laboratory parameters in cases and healthy controls

Variables	*Cases*	*Controls*	P value
Age (years)	13.3 ± 7,4	12.6 ± 7,4	ns
Male	69%	73%	ns
Female	31%	27%	ns
BMI	20.4 ± 3.9	20.6 ± 2.8	ns
BSA (m^2)	1.33 ± 0.44	1.36 ± 0.40	ns
Total cholesterol (mg/dl)	177 ± 22	170 ± 36	ns
Triglycerides (mg/dl)	61 ± 29	65 ± 24	ns
Low density lipoprotein (mg/dl)	110 ± 19	110 ± 18	ns
C-reactive protein > 0,10 (mg/dl)	11.5%	7.7%	ns
Platelets (x10^3)/mmc	309 ± 93	359 ± 114	ns
Systolic blood pressure (mmHg)	110 ± 14.4	108 ± 12	ns
Diastolic blood pressure (mmHg)	64 ± 9.8	63 ± 11	ns

Table 3 Thickening and thickening adjusted for BSA in cases and healthy controls

Parameter	Cases	Controls	P Value
Thickening (mm)	3.5 ± 2.2	1.9 ± 0.6	**< 0.01**
Thickening adjusted for BSA (mm)	5.3 ± 4.4	2.7 ± 1.2	**< 0.01**

It has been noticed that in coronary atherosclerosis, a diffuse disease process that rarely spares the proximal coronary arteries, a severe intimal thickening may be assessed as a site of localized stenosis. Accurate baseline measurements of the luminal and external diameters and wall thickness of proximal and mid LAD coronary artery have proved to be obtainable by using the high resolution transthoracic echocardiography techniques [11,12].

We successfully applied the same method to the proximal left main coronary artery: by using high resolution transthoracic probes we detected in morphology of proximal left main coronary artery structural features not so far different from atherosclerosis-induced positive remodeling, already showed in other coronary vascular territories of patients with confirmed significant luminal coronary artery disease [13].

In fact studies prior to IVIG therapy showed that a potential mechanism of coronary artery occlusion in long-term KD could be represented by the progression of the thickening of intimal layer and particularly, but not only, in the aneurysm inlet or outlet which is often associated to calcification [14,15]. This, with any combination of thrombus formation [16] might lead to acute myocardial infarction in young adults with sequelae of KD after several years [17].

Afterwards, Takahashi et al. histologically examined twenty-four arteries of six autopsy cases of patients older than 15 years with coronary arterial lesions caused by arteritis in childhood and detected in both patients without aneurysms and those with manifest recanalized lumens after thrombotic occlusion of the aneurysms "new intimal thickening" in addition to the preexisting intimal thickening caused by arteritis in the acute phase of KD. They

Table 4 Thickening and thickening adjusted for BSA in controls, patients belonging to risk class 1 and patients belonging to risk class 2-3-4 group

Category	Thickening (mm)	Thickening adjusted for BSA (mm)
A (Controls)	1.9 ± 0.6	2.7 ± 1.2
B (Risk class 1)	3.0 ± 1.7	4.5 ± 3.7
C (Risk class 2-3-4)	5.3 ± 3.1	7.9 ± 5.8

Thickening: A versus B: $p < 0.01$; A versus C:$p < 0.01$; B versus C: NS;
Thickening adjusted for BSA: A versus B: $p < 0.05$; A versus C:$p < 0.05$; B versus C: NS.

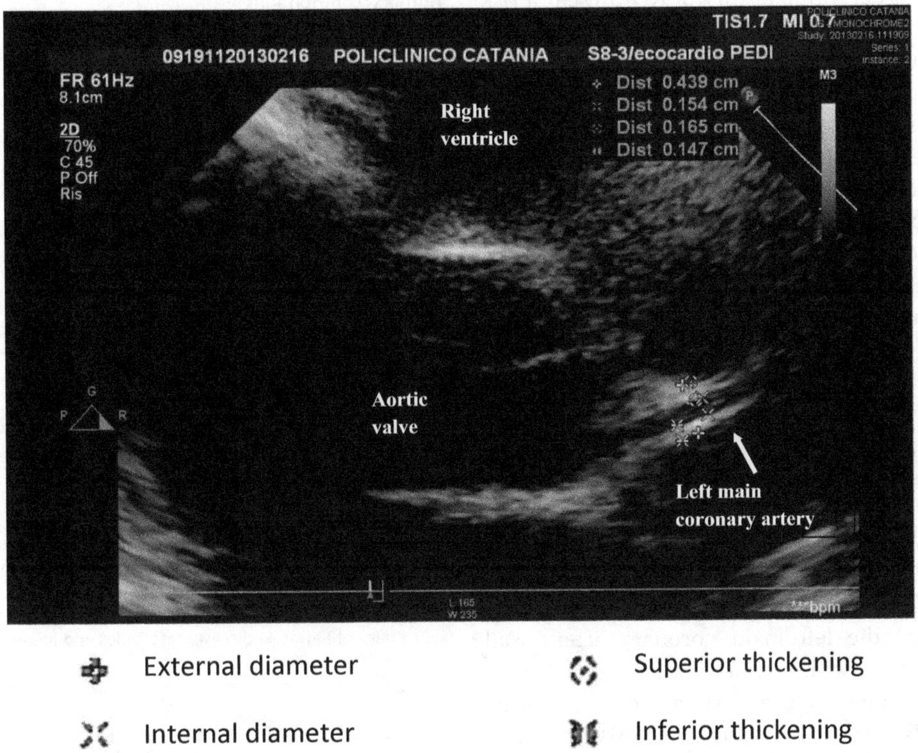

Figure 1 Abnormal left coronary artery. Legend: External diameter; Internal diameter; Superior thickening; Inferior thickening.

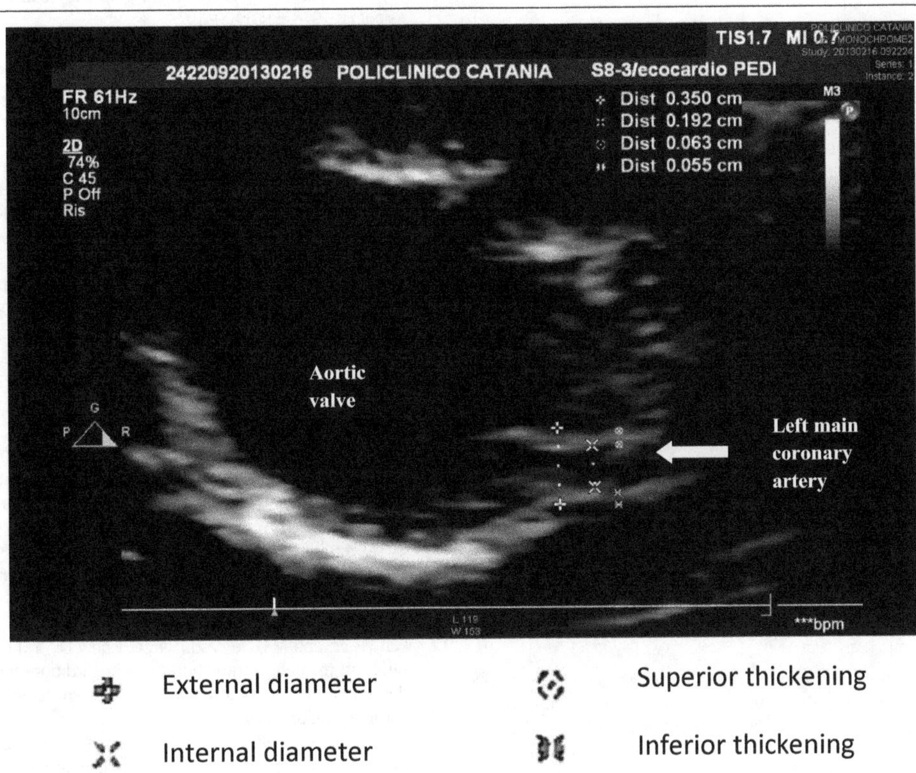

Figure 2 Normal left coronary artery. Legend: External diameter; Internal diameter; Superior thickening; Inferior thickening.

concluded that subjects with a history of KD present a risk factor for atherosclerosis later in life [18].

Iemura et al. found various degrees of intimal thickening but normal media on intravascular ultrasound imaging of the sites of regressed aneurysms. These intravascular ultrasound findings were similar to those in arteriosclerosis [19].

Intimal thickening, detectable in proximal left main coronary artery, occurs as a result of augmented vascular smooth muscle cell proliferation, in addition to increased vascular smooth muscle cell migration, extracellular matrix synthesis and phenotypic change [20,21].

It has recently been proposed that the Wnt/β-catenin pathway, involved in the regulation of embryogenesis and development, but also in cell proliferation, differentiation, polarity, migration, and invasion [22], plays a role in vascular smooth muscle cell proliferation and thereby intimal thickening [23-29].

Therefore, the risk for later KD complications suggests the necessity of a long-term follow-up of KD patients beyond childhood years.

We showed that the left main coronary artery wall thickness of subjects with previous Kawasaki disease were significantly larger (Figure 1) than those of healthy subjects (Figure 2) such as indicating atherosclerotic disease. The inner diameters, instead, were normal in both controls and cases, also in those with previous transient aneurysms suggesting, as an explanation, the phenomenon of positive remodeling.

Conclusion

Our study shows the high sensibility of high resolution transthoracic 2D Echocardiography to the detection of minimal alterations in coronary wall due to intimal thickening in patients with previous Kawasaki disease, also if studied several years after acute phase. In our experience, all patients with a previous diagnosis of Kawasaki disease, independently from the risk class, present a significant thickening of coronary arteries if compared to healthy controls. We state that this may result in premature atherosclerotic cardiovascular disease and therefore the measurement of coronary intimal thickening by high-resolution transthoracic 2D Echocardiography should be added to the follow-up protocol of Kawasaki disease because of its uninvasiveness and reproducibility.

Further investigation is obviously requested to confirm our data. We suggest that this be studied in a larger, multi-institutional study.

Abbreviations

KD: Kawasaki disease; MI: Myocardial infarction; CAA: Coronary artery aneurysms; LAD: Left anterior descending; IVIG: Intravenous immunoglobulin; SE: Standard error; BSA: Body Surface Area; BMI: Body Mass Index.

Competing interests

The authors declare that they have no competing interests.

Authors' contributions

VG carried out the collection and assembly of data, the analysis and interpretation of data, the draft of the manuscript. PS conceived of the study and participated in the design and coordination, helped to draft the manuscript and gave the final approvation. IS participated in the collection, assembly, analysis and interpretation of data, MF and PB participated in collection and assembling of data. MLR participated in the critical revision of the manuscript. SL performed the critical revision of the manuscript and gave the final approval. All authors read and approved the final manuscript.

Acknowledgement

We acknowledge the excellent technical assistance of Nicola Bonanno of the Department of Pediatrics of the University of Catania, Italy. We also acknowledge our secretary Concetta Scuderi for her collaboration in collecting data. All authors report no conflicts of interest to disclose.

References

1. Kawasaki T: **Acute febrile mucocutaneous syndrome with lymphoid involvement with specific desquamation of the fingers and toes in children.** *Arerugi* 1967, **16**:178–222.
2. Takeuchi M, Oda Y, Suzuki I: **Maculopapular rash in the convalescent phase of Kawasaki disease: case series and literature review.** *Eur J Pediatr* 2013, **172**:405–407.
3. Coustasse A, Larry J, Lee D: **Can Kawasaki disease be managed?** *Perm J Spring* 2012, **16**(2):70–72.
4. Yokouchi Y, Oharaseki T, Harada M, Ihara F, Naoe S, Takahashi K: **Histopathological study of lymph node lesions in the acute phase of Kawasaki disease.** *Histopathology* 2013, **62**:387–396.
5. Burns JC, Shike H, Gordon JB, Malhotra A, Shoenwetter M, Kawasaki T: **Sequelae of Kawasaki disease in adolescents and young adults.** *J Am Coll Cardiol* 1996, **28**(1):253–257.
6. Fujiwara H, Hamashima Y: **Pathology of the heart in Kawasaki disease.** *Pediatrics* 1978, **61**(1):100–107.
7. Choi YS, Youn HJ, Park CS, Oh YS, Chung WS, Kim JH: **High echogenic thickening of proximal coronary artery predicts the far advanced coronary atherosclerosis.** *Echocardiography* 2009, **26**(2):133–139. doi:10.1111/j.1540-8175.2008.00766.x. Epub 2008 Nov 1.
8. Gradus-Pizlo I, Feigenbaum H: **Imaging of the left anterior descending coronary artery by high-frequency transthoracic and epicardial echocardiography.** *Am J Cardiol* 2002, **90**(10C):28L–31L.
9. Newburger JW, Takahashi M, Gerber MA, Gewitz MH, Tani LY, Burns JC, Shulman ST, Bolger AF, Ferrieri P, Baltimore RS, Wilson WR, Baddour LM, Levison ME, Pallasch TJ, Falace DA, Taubert KA, Committee on Rheumatic Fever, Endocarditis, and Kawasaki Disease; Council on Cardiovascular Disease in the Young; American Heart Association: **Diagnosis, treatment, and long-term management of Kawasaki disease: a statement for health professionals from the Committee on Rheumatic Fever, Endocarditis, and Kawasaki Disease, Council on Cardiovascular Disease in the Young, American Heart Association.** *Pediatrics* 2004, **114**(6):1708–1733. Erratum in: Pediatrics 2005 Apr;115(4):1118.
10. Council on Cardiovascular Disease in the Young, Committee on Rheumatic Fever, Endocarditis, and Kawasaki Disease, American Heart Association: **Diagnostic guidelines for Kawasaki disease.** *Circulation* 2001, **103**(2):335–336.
11. Gradus-Pizlo I, Sawada SG, Wright D, Segar DS, Feigenbaum H: **Detection of subclinical coronary atherosclerosis using two- dimensional, high-resolution transthoracic echocardiography.** *J Am Coll Cardiol* 2001, **37**:1422–1429.
12. Perry R, Joseph MX, De Pasquale CG, Chew DP, Yiu D, Aylward PE, Mangoni AA: **High resolution transthoracic echocardiography of the left anterior descending coronary artery: a novel non-invasive assessment of coronary vasoreactivity.** *J Am Soc Echocardiography* 2008, **21**(2):134–138.
13. Perry R, De Pasquale CG, Chew DP, Brown L, Aylward PE, Joseph MX: **Changes in left anterior descending coronary artery wall thickness detected by high resolution transthoracic echocardiography.** *Am J Cardiol* 2008, **101**(7):937–940.

14. Japanese Circulation Society Joint Research Group: **Guidelines for diagnosis and management of cardiovascular sequelae in Kawasaki disease.** *Pediatr Int* 2005, **47**:711–732.
15. Sasaguri Y, Kato H: **Regression of aneurysm in Kawasaki disease: a pathological study.** *J Pediatr* 1982, **100**:225–231.
16. Galassi AR, Tomasello SD, Crea F, Costanzo L, Campisano MB, Marza' F, Tamburino C: **Transient impairment of vasomotion function after successful chronic total occlusion recanalization.** *J Am Coll Cardiol* 2012, **59**:711–718.
17. Kato H, Inoue O, Ichinose E, Akagi T, Sato N: **Intracoronary urokinase in Kawasaki disease: treatment and prevention of myocardial infarction.** *Acta Paediatr Jpn* 1991, **33**:27–35.
18. Takahashi K, Oharaseki T, Naoe S: **Pathological study of postcoronary arteritis in adolescents and young adults: with reference to the relationship between sequelae of Kawasaki disease and atherosclerosis.** *Pediatr Cardiol* 2001, **22**(2):138–142.
19. Iemura M, Ishii M, Sugimura T, Akagi T, Kato H: **Long term consequences of regressed coronary aneurysms after Kawasaki disease: vascular wall morphology and function.** *Heart* 2000, **83**(3):307–311.
20. Tsaousi A, Williams H, Lyon CA, Taylor V, Swain A, Johnson JL, George SJ: **Wnt4/β-catenin signaling induces VSMC proliferation and is associated with intimal thickening.** *Circ Res* 2011, **108**(4):427–436.
21. Owens GK: **Regulation of differentiation of vascular smooth muscle cells.** *Physiol Rev* 1995, **75**:487–517.
22. Chien AJ, Conrad WH, Moon RT: **A Wnt survival guide: from flies to human disease.** *J Invest Dermatol* 2009, **129**:1614–1627.
23. Uglow EB, Slater S, Sala-Newby GB, Aguilera-Garcia CM, Angelini GD, Newby AC, George SJ: **Dismantling of cadherin-mediated cell-cell contacts modulates smooth muscle proliferation.** *Circ Res* 2003, **92**:1314–1321.
24. Slater SC, Koutsouki E, Jackson CL, Bush RC, Angelini GD, Newby AC, George SJ: **R-cadherin:_-catenin complex and its association with vascular smooth muscle cell proliferation.** *Arterioscler Thromb Vasc Biol* 2004, **24**:1204–1210.
25. Quasnichka H, Slater S, Beeching C, Boehm M, Sala-Newby G, George S: **Regulation of smooth muscle cell proliferation by _-catenin/TCF signaling involves modulation of cyclin D1 and p21 expression.** *Circ Res* 2006, **99**:1329–1337.
26. Wang X, Xiao Y, Mou Y, Zhao Y, Blankesteijn M, Hall JL: **A role for the _-catenin/T-cell factor signaling cascade in vascular remodeling.** *Circ Res* 2002, **90**:340–347.
27. Wang X, Adhikari N, Li Q, Hall JL: **The LDL receptor related protein LRP6 regulates proliferation and survival through the Wnt cascade in vascular smooth muscle cells.** *Am J Physiol Heart Circ Physiol* 2004, **287**:H2376–H2383.
28. Mao C, Malek T-BO, Pueyo ME, Steg PG, Soubrier F: **Differentitial expression of rat frizzled-related *frzb-1* and frizzled receptor *fz1* and *fz2* genes in the rat aorta after balloon injury.** *Arterioscler Thromb Vasc Biol* 2000, **20**:43–51.
29. Ezan J, Leroux L, Barandon L, Dufourcq P, Jaspard B, Moreau C, Allieres C, Daret D, Couffinhal T, Duplaa C: **FrzA/sFRP-1, a secreted antagonist of the Wnt-Frizzled pathway, controls vascular cell proliferation in vitro and in vivo.** *Cardiovasc Res* 2004, **63**:731–738.

7

Evaluation of the left and right ventricular systolic and diastolic function in asthmatic children

Esra Akyüz Özkan[1*] and Hashem E. Khosroshahi[2]

Abstract

Background: Asthma is the most common cause of respiratory disorders among children. We aimed to investigate left (LV) and right (RV) ventricular function in asthmatic children as detected by conventional and tissue Doppler echocardiography.

Methods: Fifty pediatric patients with asthma and forty healthy children were studied. Pulmonary function tests, electrocardiography and echocardiographic examinations were performed on all children.

Results: Rate-corrected velocity of circumferential fiber shortening (VCFc) ($p = 0.044$), the ratio between heights of early and late diastolic flow velocity peaks (E/A) ($p = 0.019$) and LV end-systolic wall stress (ESWSm) was lower ($p = 0.003$), RV stroke volume (SV) ($p = 0.002$), LV SV ($p = 0.001$), tricuspid annular plane systolic excursion (TAPSE) ($p = 0.034$), tricuspid annular peak velocity during systole (S') ($p = 0.022$), tricuspid and mitral early diastolic velocities (E') ($p = 0.012$, $p = 0.003$ respectively) were lower in asthmatic children than controls. The mitral valve ejection time (ET) was high in asthmatic group ($p = 0.027$).
FEV1 was positively correlated with isovolumetric relaxation time (IVRT) ($p = 0.018$) ($r = 0.382$) and mitral ET ($p = 0.018$) ($r = 0.381$). PEF was negatively correlated with the RV work index ($p = 0.032$) ($r = -0.348$) and LV work index ($p = 0.005$) ($r = -0.457$).

Conclusion: Although cardiac systolic function was found to be impaired in asthmatic patients, contrary to the literature, diastolic dysfunction was not observed in these patients, even by tissue Doppler imaging, and this finding may be attributed to using inhaled corticosteroid

Keywords: Asthma, Children, Echocardiography, Tissue Doppler imaging, Ventricular function

Background

Asthma is a chronic inflammatory disease of the airways which is related to airway obstruction, hyperresponsiveness and characterized recurrent wheezing, coughing and breathlessness [1]. Bronchial asthma affects many organs including the heart. There are many explanations for the occurrence of cardiac dysfunction in asthmatic children [2–4]. It is suggested that chronic hypoxia may cause pulmonary arterial hypertension, which causes RV hypertrophy and/or dilatation [2]. It is also suggested that recurrent hypoxemia and the release of various mediators and cytokines in bronchial asthma may cause chronic inflammation, which could induce pulmonary vasoconstriction [3, 4]. Other hypotheses concluded that the exaggerated respiratory efforts may raise intrathoracic pressure that increases RV afterload and consequently pulmonary hypertension with RV hypertrophy and/or dilatation. As a result, pulmonary hypertension occurs and leads to RV hypertrophy and/or dilatation [3–5]. As a result of chronic pressure overload, the RV hypertrophies and dilates and leads to both systolic and diastolic dysfunction [5]. The level of RV diastolic dysfunction depends on the degree of RV hypertrophy and total pulmonary resistance. Interaction between the RV and LV related to increased LV afterload and decreased LV preload, and thus LV dysfunction [6]. There are important limitations to determining RV

* Correspondence: esra.akyuz@mynet.com
[1]Department of Pediatrics, Bozok University Medical Faculty, Yozgat, Turkey
Full list of author information is available at the end of the article

function by conventional echocardiography [7]. The unavailability of the RV at the back the sternum leads to poor image quality. Also, locating the endocardial boundary of the anterior wall is a problem owing to the thicker trabeculations compared with the LV. Furthermore, the RV cavity has a more complex geometry than the LV, and RV performance depends on extrinsic conditions, such as afterload, preload, and LV performance.

Our study aimed to investigate ventricular diastolic and systolic functions, LV wall stresses and circumferential fiber shortening by using tissue Doppler imaging (TDI) and conventional echocardiography in asthmatic children, using regular inhaled corticosteroid, without any cardiovascular symptoms.

Methods

We studied 50 pediatric patients (35 male and 15 female), selected randomly from those with bronchial asthma, and 40 healthy subjects. Inclusion criteria include all patients meeting the criteria for bronchial asthma [1]. Exclusion criteria were patients with comorbid diseases, such as upper or lower respiratory infection, allergic rhinitis, gastroesophageal reflux, obesity, chronic cardiovascular or pulmonary diseases and acute asthma attack during the last 4 weeks.

The control group was chosen from healthy individuals. The ethics committee of the institution approved the study and informed consent forms signed by the parents were obtained. All the children included in the study were subjected to full history taking. Complete physical examinations were performed by the same physician. Body height and weight, blood pressure (BP) and heart rate of all children were recorded. The patients and the controls who were >6 years underwent pulmonary function tests using spirometry forced expiratory volume in 1 s (FEV1), forced vital capacity (FVC), the ratio of FEV1 to FVC, and peak expiratory flow (PEF), which were all documented.

All asthmatic patients involved in this study were moderately asthmatic and received inhaled corticosteroid treatment for different periods of time and doses.

An electrocardiogram was simultaneously recorded for all patients. Transthoracic echocardiography was performed by a single experienced pediatric cardiologist, blinded to the subjects, and the following parameters were monitored: LV end-diastolic pressures (LVEDPs), LV mass (LVM, g) according to the formula of Devereux [8], stroke volume (SV), ejection fraction (EF, %), fractional shortening (FS, %), ratio between heights of early and late diastolic flow velocity peaks (E/A ratio) for both mitral and tricuspid valves, deceleration time (DT, ms), LV meridional end-systolic wall stress (ESWSm, g/cm^2), Midwall Shortening Fraction (SFmid), heart rate corrected circumferential fiber shortening (VCFc), midwall VCFc, myocardial fiber stress (MFS, g/cm^2), RV and LV work index (RVWI, LVWI respectively), LV and RV relative wall thickness (LVRWT, RVRWT, mm) mitral and tricuspid annular plane systolic excursion (MAPSE, TAPSE), RV Pre-ejection Period/RV ejection time (RVPEP/RVET), RV Pre-ejection period/RV acceleration time (RPEP/AT), and Acceleration time/Pulmonary artery ejection time (AT/PAET).

The following parameters were monitored by TDI: annular peak velocity during late diastole (A') annular peak velocity during early diastole (E'), isovolumetric relaxation time (IVRT), isovolumetric contraction time (IVCT), myocardial performance index (MPI), annular peak velocity during systole (S'), ejection time (ET), time velocity integral for aortic valve (Aort VTI), time velocity integral for pulmonary artery (PA VTI), mitral valve myocardial acceleration during isovolumic contraction (IVMA-MV), tricuspid valve myocardial acceleration during isovolumic contraction (IVMA-TV), and pulmonary artery myocardial acceleration during isovolumic contraction (IVMA-PA).

EF, SV, LVOT and AoVTI were calculated as described in previous studies [9].

LV fractional shortening (FS) was calculated as LVVD-LVDS/LVDD [10].

Mitral and tricuspid filling velocities were recorded from the apical four-chamber view with the pulse-wave Doppler during diastole. E/A and DT were used as both ventricular diastolic function parameters. The ratios of E to A were calculated for mitral and tricuspid valves [11].

The Doppler-derived myocardial performance index (MPI) for LV and RV, combining systolic and diastolic time intervals, were calculated IVCT+ IVRT/ET [12].

VCFc (circ/s) = (SF x (1500/heart rate)$^{0.5}$/LV ET)

Midwall VCFc was calculated as = 0.0007xMFS + 0.65

ESWSm was calculated by the method of Grossman et al [12] and MFS according to the formula recommended by Regen [13].

SFmid = $[(\text{LVED} + h_d/2 + s_d/2) - \text{LVES} - \textit{mwst}]/(\text{LVED} + h_d/2 + s_d/2)$

Where the *mwst* calculared as = $[(\text{LVED} + (h_d + s_d)/2)^3 - \text{LVED}^3 + \text{LVES}^3)^{0,333} - \text{LVES}]$

h_d : left ventricular end-diastolic posterior wall thickness

s_d: end-diastolic septal thickness

LVES stands for LV end systolic dimension and LVED stands for LV end diastolic dimension.

LVEDP = 21.6 (Q-M1/A2-OS) + 1.1, OS: opening snap of the mitral valve, A2: aortic component of the second heart sound, Q: Q wave on the ECG, M1: mitral component of the first heart sound [14].

RV and LV function were also evaluated using TDI: Peak systolic (S') and early and late diastolic velocities (E' and A') were measured from the apical four-chamber view with the pulsed-wave Doppler sample volume placed at the tricuspid and mitral annulus.

Cardiac time intervals comprising RV included IVCT from the end of the tricuspid flow to the beginning of the pulmonary flow, IVRT from the end of the pulmonary flow to the beginning of the tricuspid flow, and ET from the beginning to the end of the pulmonary flow were also measured.

Statistical analysis

The statistical analyses were performed by the Statistical Package for Social Sciences (SPSS). Kolmogorov–Smirnov and Shapiro Wilk tests were used to assess normality of distribution.

Parametric variables were compared using the Student's *t* test for normally distributed data and the Mann Whitney *u* test for not normally distributed data. Bivariate associations of the variables were assessed using Pearson's correlation coefficients. Variables were expressed as mean ± SD and *p* value <0.05 was considered to indicate statistical significance.

Results

The current study enrolled 50 patients (35 boys and 15 girls) with a mean age of 10.56 ± 3.03 years who had diagnosis of bronchial asthma. The characteristics of the children and healthy subjects are shown in Table 1. The spirometry findings are summarized in Table 2.

LV and RV echocardiographic findings are listed in Tables 3 and 4. The rate-corrected velocity of circumferential fiber shortening (VCFc) ($p = 0.044$), E/A ratio ($p = 0.019$), ESWSm was lower ($p = 0.003$), RSV ($p = 0.002$), LSV ($p = 0.001$), tricuspid annular peak velocity during systole (S') ($p = 0.022$), TAPSE ($p = 0.034$) and tricuspid and mitral E' ($p = 0.012$, $p = 0.003$ respectively) were lower in asthmatic children than control subjects. Mitral valve ET was higher in the asthmatic group ($p = 0.027$). Distribution of ESWSm between groups is showed in Fig. 1. TDI parameters are listed in Table 5.

Table 1 Comparison (mean ± SD) of clinical characteristics

Variable	asthmatic children $n = 50$	Healthy control $n = 40$	p value
Age (years)	10.56 ± 3.03	12.08 ± 3.21	0.250[a]
Male/female	35/15	17/23	0.314[c]
Body height (cm)	142.8 ± 12.2	144.5 ± 12.4	0.120[b]
Body weight (kg)	28.6 ± 12.5	28.6 ± 12.5	0.480[b]
Heart rate (bpm)	84.68 ± 14.93	86.42 ± 10.87	0.537[a]
Systolic BP (mmHg)	104.74 ± 8.94	103.78 ± 9.47	0.345[b]
Diastolic BP (mmHg)	64.02 ± 5.88	61.38 ± 9.63	0.175[b]

[a] Student's t test, [b] Man-Whitney u test, [c] Chi-square test

Table 2 Comparison (mean ± SD) of spirometry findings

Variable	asthmatic children $n = 50$	Healthy controls $n = 40$	p value[a]
PEF	90.02 ± 9.7	92.7 ± 8.9	0.320
FEV1	82.8 ± 12.2	92.2 ± 9.3	**0.002***
FVC	92.1 ± 8.5	95.2 ± 11.4	0.123
FEV1/FVC	89.6 ± 9.7	96.2 ± 10.5	**0.012***

[a] Student's *t* test

*Correlation is significant at the 0.05 level

We performed pulmonary function tests on patient and control groups and correlated FEV1, FVC, FEV1/FVC and PEF with cardiac parameters. There were no differences between the asthmatic and control group. In correlation analysis, FEV1 was positively correlated with IVRT ($p = 0.018$) ($r = 0.382$) and ET-MV ($p = 0.018$) ($r = 0.381$). PEF was negatively correlated with RVWI ($p = 0.032$), ($r = -0.348$) and LVWI ($p = 0.005$), ($r = -0.457$).

Discussion

Asthma is the most common cause of respiratory disability in children [3]. We aimed to investigate both ventricular

Table 3 Comparison (mean ± SD) of left ventricular echocardiographic findings

Variable	Asthmatic children 50 (M/F = 35/15)	Healthy controls 40 (M/F = 17/23)	p value
LSV (ml)	40.75 ± 14.26	50.99 ± 13.08	0.001[a]
LVWT (cm)	0,40 ± 0,087	0,38 ± 0,055	0,172[a]
LV-EF (%)	0.66 ± 0.1	0.63 ± 0.07	0.182[a]
DT (msn)	184.79 ± 53.98	192.50 ± 45.60	0.465[a]
LV-FS (%)	0.36 ± 0.08	0.34 ± 0.05	0.185[a]
LVM (gr)	67.03 ± 22.89	69 ± 18.26	0.440[b]
E/A	1.78 ± 0.27	1.93 ± 0.32	0.019[a]
L-sist (ms)	340.34 ± 42.89	346.83 ± 28.01	0.485[b]
MAPSE (cm)	1.09 ± 0.18	1.07 ± 0.17	0.672[b]
LVEDP (mmHg)	26.45 ± 5.11	26.96 ± 4.63	0.451[b]
LVWI (gm-m/m^2)	35.61 ± 9.41	33.32 ± 7.24	0.387[b]
WSM (g/cm^2)	1114.18 ± 595.42	1356.16 ± 562.54	0.053[a]
ESWSm (g/cm^2)	172.5 ± 58.05	209.22 ± 55.53	0.003[a]
VCFc (circ/s)	0.0051005 ± 0.00	0,0057375 ± 0.00	0.044[b]
Sfmid (%)	-0.36 ± 0.10	-0.38 ± 0.07	0.257[b]
Fiber stress (g/cm^2)	36.55 ± 9.32	39.74 ± 11.61	0.160[b]
Midwall VCFc (circ/s)	0.67 ± 0.01	0.68 ± 0.01	0.160[b]

LSV Left ventricle stroke volume, *LVWT* Left ventricular wall thickness, *EF* Ejection fraction, *DT* Deceleration time, *LV_FS* Left ventricle fractional shortening, *LVM* Left ventricular mass, *A* Peak velocity during late diastole, *E* Peak velocity during early diastole, *L-sist T* Left Systolic Time (Contraction time), *MAPSE* Mitral annular plane systolic excursion; *LVEDP* Left Ventricle end-diastolic Pressure, *LVWI* Left ventricular work index; *WSM* Meridional LV wall stress, *ESWSm* Meridional end-systolic wall stress, *VCFc* Rate-corrected velocity of circumferential fiber shortening

[a] Student's *t* test, [b] Mann-Whitney *u* test

Table 4 Comparison (mean ± SD) of right ventricular echocardiographic findings

Variable	asthmatic children 50 (M/F = 35/15)	Healthy controls 40 (M/F = 17/23)	*p* value
RSV (ml)	50.01 ± 18.26	64.70 ± 23.66	0.002[b]
RVWT (cm)	0,47 ± 0,11	0,47 ± 0,10	0.980[a]
RV-EF (%)	0.73 ± 0.15	0.71 ± 0.13	0.385[b]
DT (msn)	198.19 ± 62.73	189.87 ± 46.76	0.490[b]
RV-FS (%)	0.42 ± 0.12	0.39 ± 0.10	0.372[a]
E/A	1.72 ± 0.26	1.80 ± 0.33	0.243[a]
R-sist (ms)	362.78 ± 32.74	362.72 ± 28.90	0.807[b]
TAPSE (cm)	2.02 ± 0.20	2.15 ± 0.32	0.034[b]
RV WI (gm-m/m^2)	4.24 ± 1.20	4.57 ± 1.68	0.572[b]
RVPEP/RVET (ms)	0.19 ± 0.04	0.19 ± 0.03	0.767[b]
RPEP/AT (ms)	0.50 ± 0.13	0.51 ± 0.11	0.679[b]
AT/PAET (ms)	0.39 ± 0.06	0.38 ± 0.05	0.372[b]

RSV Right ventricle stroke volume, *RVWT* Right ventricular wall thickness, *RV-EF* Right ventricle ejection fraction; *RV-FS* Right ventricle fractional shortening, *A* Peak velocity during late diastole, *E* Peak velocity during early diastole, *DT* Deceleration Time, *R-sist T* Right ventricle systolic time (contraction time), *TAPSE* Tricuspid annular plane systolic excursion, *RVWI* Right ventricular work index, *RVPEP/RVET* Right Ventricle Pre-Ejection Period/Right ventricle Ejection Time, *RPEP/AT* Right ventricle Pre-Ejection Period/Right ventricle Acceleration Time, *AT/PAET* Acceleration time/Pulmonary artery Ejection Time
[a] student's *t* test, [b] Mann-Whitney *u* test

function in children with bronchial asthma as detected by conventional echocardiography and TDI.

Our results confirms the results reported by Shedeed et al [15] and Mahmoud et al [16] who found no statistically significant differences between asthmatic children and controls regarding heart rate and systolic and diastolic BP.

According to some studies right ventricular (RV) systolic and diastolic dysfunction were detected, even in mild cases, by echocardiography. On the other hand, left ventricular (LV) dysfunction usually presents itself in severe asthmatic cases which may be reversible in acute conditions [17, 18].

Some studies showed that there were no differences in echocardiographic findings regarding the ventricular function with the exception of RV wall thickness [15, 19]. We couldn't find any differences between the two groups regarding RVWT and LVWT.

IVMA, MPI, EF, FS, TAPSE, MAPSE, SV, VCFc and ESWSm values of both ventricles were evaluated to assess ventricular systolic function. IVMA, MPI, EF, FS and MAPSE were similar in both groups. TAPSE was lower in asthmatic patients.

IVMA is a measurement of ventricular contractile function that is unaffected by preload and afterload changes in a physiological range [20]. In this study we couldn't show any differences between IVMA values in either group.

The SV of both the RV and LV were lower in asthmatic children than in the controls in our study. Hedlin et al

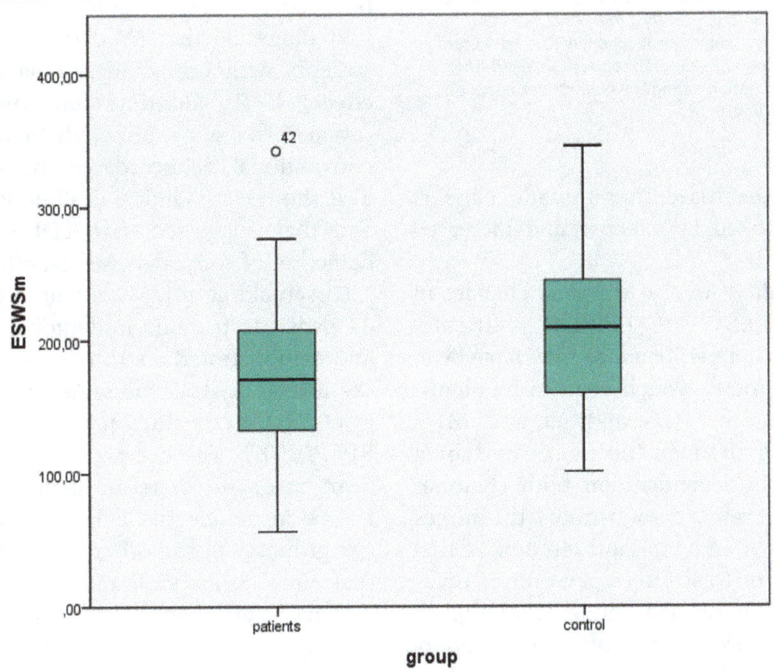

Fig. 1 Distribution of LV meridional end-systolic wall stress (ESWSm) between groups

Table 5 TDI findings (mean ± SD) of the patients and control group

Variable	asthmatic children 50 (M/F = 35/15)	Healthy controls 40 (M/F = 17/23)	*p* value
Mitral annulus			
E'(m/sn)	0.17 ± 0.03	0.19 ± 0.03	0.003[a]
A'(m/sn)	0.08 ± 0.02	0.12 ± 0.21	0.635[b]
S'(m/sn)	0.072 ± 0.022	0.077 ± 0.013	0.147[a]
Aort-VTI (cm)	21.96 ± 3.91	22.48 ± 3.60	0.514[a]
IVCT (ms)	65.89 ± 11.57	69.05 ± 15.08	0.533[a]
IVRT (ms)	64.13 ± 8.87	64.05 ± 8.48	0.880[b]
ET-MV (ms)	265.53 ± 40.58	245.80 ± 30.90	0.027[b]
IVMA-MV (m/s^2)	0.07 ± 0.03	0.08 ± 0.04	0.575[b]
Mitral-MPI (ms)	0.50 ± 0.09	0.54 ± 0.10	0.089[b]
Tricuspid annulus			
E' (m/sn)	0.17 ± 0.02	0.18 ± 0.02	0.012[b]
A'(m/sn)	0.11 ± 0.04	0.12 ± 0.03	0.968[b]
S'(m/sn)	0,08 ± 0,022	0,10 ± 0,028	0.022[a]
PA-VTI (cm)	21.87 ± 2.73	22.39 ± 2.80	0.377[a]
IVCT (ms)	66.63 ± 10.87	66.40 ± 13.07	0.517[b]
IVRT (ms)	65.74 ± 9.77	64.35 ± 8.26	0.436[b]
ET-TV (ms)	253.79 ± 36.58	241.10 ± 30.01	0.118[b]
IVMA-TV(m/s^2)	0.09 ± 0.04	0.08 ± 0.04	0.955[b]
IVMA-PA(m/s^2)	0.10 ± 0.17	0.08 ± 0.031	0.557[a]
Tricuspit MPI (ms)	0.53 ± 0.08	0.56 ± 0.09	0.070[a]

A' Annular peak velocity during late diastole, *E'* Annular peak velocity during early diastole; *IVRT* Izovolumetric relaxation time, *IVCT* Izovolumetric contraction time, *MPI* Myocardial performance index, *S'* Annular peak velocity during systole, *ET* Ejection time, *Aort VTI* Time velocity integral for aortic valve, *PA VTI* Time velocity integral for pulmonary artery, *IVMA-MV* Mitral valve myocardial acceleration during izovolumetric contraction, *IVMA-TV* Tricuspid valve myocardial acceleration during izovolumetric contraction, *IVMA-PA* Pulmonery artery myocardial acceleration during izovolumetric contraction
[a] student's *t* test, [b] Mann-Whitney *u* test

[21] reported that SV decreased in asthmatic patients whose asthma was provoked by exercise and increased with inhale salbutamol.

To assess LV contractility, we also analyzed changes in LV VCFc and afterload (ESWSm) [12]. The ventricular contractility and myocardial performance may have been affected by chamber geometry, which need to be identified by measuring ESWSm, VCFc-midwall and MFS. ESWSm was accepted as afterload (no more shortening point). ESWSm, which is dependent on both chamber shape and mass/volume ratio, demonstrates the forces opposing predominantly meridional and circumferential planes. This is an index of total forces per unit of myocardium, and therefore may cause an underestimation in true afterload. MFS, as representative of myofiber afterload, is a more accurate index of afterload in hypertrophied or dilated LV [22]. In the current study, ESWSm and VCFc were low, while MFS was similar in the asthmatic group. SFmid as a systolic ejection index of deeper layers of myocardium provides more physiologically appropriate measurements of LV in wall thickness and conditions like LV concentric hypertrophy and provides information to assess the myocardial performance [22]. In this study, SFmid was similar in both groups. As an indication of compromised LV contractility, LV ESWSm was significantly lower in asthmatic patients.

To evaluate ventricular diastolic function we used mitral and tricuspid E/A, E', A', DT, IVRT and IVCT by using conventional echocardiography and TDI. There are some studies which reported RV and LV diastolic dysfunction in patients with moderate to severe asthma [2, 23, 24]. In contrast with these studies, we turned away from the diagnosis of diastolic dysfunction in asthmatic patients because both mitral and tricuspid E/A values were >1 without any sign of pseudo-normal E/A values.

Mitral and tricuspid annulus early diastolic velocities were different by TDI. Mitral E', tricuspid E' and S' were lower in the asthmatic group. There were no significant differences among the IVCT, IVRT and DT in either the mitral or tricuspid annulus. These findings showed that there was no diastolic dysfunction among our asthmatic children even by TDI. This result may due to use of inhaled corticosteroids. Shedeed [15] reported that E', A', and S' were significantly lower, and E'/A', IVRT, and IVCT significantly greater in asthmatic children as detected by TDI. Zeybek et al [18] showed that lateral annular velocities of tricuspid and IVRT were different between asthmatic children and controls. Abdalla et al [25] suggested that LV diastolic function is impaired in patients with bronchial asthma despite there being no effect on RV diastolic function. Ozdemir et al [19] revealed the same, although there was no difference by conventional echocardiography in asthmatic children. TDI showed subclinical dysfunction of the right ventricle and they suggested that TDI was useful in the early detection of some detrimental effects of asthmatic cases.

Hirschfeld et al [26] measured the RPEP and RVET in 64 pediatric patients undergoing cardiac catheterization and demonstrated a strong correlation between pulmonary artery diastolic pressure and the ratio RPEP/RVET ($r = 0.72$). In one study it has been suggested that normal RPEP/RVET was not significantly influenced by age or heart rate, and therefore could be used as an index of RV performance throughout a wide range of pediatric age groups. On the other hand, the same study revealed that the RPEP/RVET ratio correlated with mean pulmonary artery pressure and was associated with pulmonary vascular resistance [27]. The current study failed to demonstrate any differences regarding the RVPEP/RVET ratio between the groups.

We performed pulmonary function tests in both groups. FEV1 was positively correlated with IVRT and ET-MV. PEF was negatively correlated with RVWI and LVWI. Ozdemir et al [19] reported that PEF was negatively correlated with tricuspid E'/A', while Sheeded et al [15] demonstrated a negative correlation between PEF and IVRT.

Inhaled corticosteroids exert a strong anti-inflammatory effect on airways; they represent the most effective agents for long-term asthma control [28]. Some studies showed that inhaled corticosteroids have protective effects on cardiac function in asthmatic patients [29]. In the current study, all the children were using inhaled corticosteroids with a different period of time and doses and this study showed that, even with this protective effect, myocardial function can be impaired in asthmatic children.

In our previous study on asthmatic children who use inhaled corticosteroid, arterial stiffness were decreased, distensibility and strain were increased [30]. We suggested that using inhaled corticosteroids could have provided certain protective effects in asthmatic children. A proposed mechanism that may explain the decrease in arterial stiffness involves nitric oxide synthesis and vasodilatation [31].

Conclusion

Asthma affects ventricular contractility in children. Although cardiac systolic function was found to be impaired in asthmatic patients, contrary to the literature diastolic dysfunction didn't observed in these patients even by tissue Doppler imaging, may be due to using inhaled corticosteroid. This was one of the most comprehensive studies among asthmatic patients. Further studies with larger sample sizes or without using corticosteroid treatment warranted to better elucidate the cardiac function in asthmatic children.

Abbreviations

A, Peak velocity during late diastole; A', Annular peak velocity during late diastole; Aort VTI, Time velocity integral for aortic valve; AT/PAET, Acceleration time/Pulmonary artery Ejection Time; BP, Blood pressure; DT, Deceleration time; E, Peak velocity during early diastole; E', Annular peak velocity during early diastole; EF, Ejection fraction; ESWSm, Meridional end-systolic wall stress; ET, Ejection time; FEV1, Forced expiratory volume in 1 s; FVC, Forced vital capacity; IVCT, Izovolumetric contraction time; IVMA-MV, Mitral valve myocardial acceleration during izovolumetric contraction; IVMA-PA, Pulmonery artery myocardial acceleration during izovolumetric contraction; IVMA-TV, Tricuspid valve myocardial acceleration during izovolumetric contraction; IVRT, Izovolumetric relaxation time; L-sist T, Left Systolic Time (Contraction time); LSV, Left ventricle stroke Volume; LVEDP, Left Ventricle end-diastolic Pressure; LV-FS, Left ventricle fractional shortening; LVM, Left ventricular mass; LVWI, Left ventricular work index; LVWT, Left ventricular wall thickness; MAPSE, Mitral annular plane systolic excursion; MFS, Myocardial fiber stress; MPI, Myocardial performance index; PA VTI, Time velocity integral for pulmonary artery; PEF, Peak expiratory flow; RPEP/AT, Right ventricle Pre-Ejection Period/Right ventricle Acceleration Time; R-sist T, Right ventricle systolic time (contraction time); RSV, Right ventricle stroke volume; RV-EF, Right ventricle ejection fraction; RV-FS, Right ventricle fractional shortening; RVPEP/RVET, Right ventricle Pre-Ejection Period/Right ventricle Ejection Time; RVWI, Right ventricular work index; RVWT, Right ventricular wall thickness; S', Annular peak velocity during systole; TAPSE, Tricuspid annular plane systolic excursion; TDI, Tissue Doppler imaging; VCFc, Rate-corrected velocity of circumferential fiber shortening; WSM, Meridional LV wall stress.

Acknowledgements
None.

Funding
This research received no grant from any funding agency in the public, commercial or not-for-profit sectors.

Authors' contributions

EAO: designed, drafted and wrote the manuscript, performed the statistical analysis, collected the data. HEK: have made substantial contributions to conception and design, performed echocardiography and collected the data. All authors read and approved the final manuscript.

Competing interests

The authors declare that they have no competing interests.

Author details
[1]Department of Pediatrics, Bozok University Medical Faculty, Yozgat, Turkey. [2]Department of Pediatric Cardiology, Bozok University Medical Faculty, Yozgat, Turkey.

References

1. Global Strategy for Asthma Management and Prevention, Global Initiative for Asthma (GINA) (2015) Available at: http://ginasthma.org/.
2. Bardsley P, Evely R, Howard P. Hypoxic cor pulmonale: a review. Herz. 1986; 11:155–1568.
3. Davenport PW, Cruz M, Stecenko AA, Kifle Y. Respiratory-related evoked potentials in children with life-threatening asthma. Am J Respir Crit Care Med. 2000;161:1830–5.
4. Massoud MN, el-Nawawy AA, el-Nazar SY, Abdel-Rahman GM. Tumour necrosis factor-alpha concentration in severely asthmatic children. East Mediterr Health J. 2000;6:432–6.
5. Han MK, McLaughlin VV, Criner GJ, Martinez FJ. Pulmonary diseases and the heart. Circulation. 2007;116:2992–3005.
6. Healy F, Hanna BD, Zinman R. Clinical practice. The impact of lung disease on the heart and cardiac disease on the lungs. Eur J Pediatr. 2010;169:1–6.
7. Oldershaw P, Bishop A. The difficulties of assessing right ventricular function. Br Heart J. 1995;74:99–100.
8. Devereux RB, Alonso DR, Lutas EM, Gottlieb GJ, Campo E, Sachs I, Reichek N. Echocardiographic assessment of left ventricular hypertrophy: comparison to necropsy findings. Am J Cardiol. 1986;57:450–8.
9. Khosroshahi HE, Ozkan EA, Kilic M. Arterial and left ventricular end-systolic elastance in normal children. Eur Rev Med Pharmacol Sci. 2014;18:3260–6.
10. Lang RM, Bierig M, Devereux RB Flachskampf FA, Foster E, Pellikka PA, Chamber Quantification Writing Group; American Society of Echocardiography's Guidelines and Standards Committee; European Association of Echocardiography, et al. Recommendations for chamber quantification: a report from the American Society of Echocardiography's Guidelines and Standards Committee and the Chamber Quantification Writing Group, developed in conjunction with the European Association of Echocardiography, a branch of the European Society of Cardiology. J Am Soc Echocardiogr. 2005;18:1440–63.
11. Correale M, Totaro A, Ieva R, Brunetti ND, Di Biase M. Time intervals and myocardial performance index by tissue Doppler imaging. Intern Emerg Med. 2011;6:393–402.

12. Grossman W, Jones D, McLaurin LP. Wall stress and patterns of hypertrophy in the human left ventricle. J Clin Invest. 1975;56:56–64.
13. Regen DM. Calculation of left ventricular wall stress. Circ Res. 1990;67:245–52.
14. Palomo AR, Quinones MA, Waggoner AD, Kumpuris AG, Miller RR. Echo-phonocardiographic determination of left atrial and left ventricular filling pressures with and without mitral stenosis. Circulation. 1980;61: 1043–7.
15. Shedeed SA. Right ventricular function in children with bronchial asthma: a tissue Doppler echocardiographic study. Pediatr Cardiol. 2010;31:1008–15.
16. Mahmoud MMK, Mohamed EA, Tarek AR. Doppler echocardiographic evaluation of ventricular function in patients with bronchial asthma. Alex J Pediatr. 2005;19:7–11.
17. Peng SM, Sun P, Zeng J, Deng XM. Cardiac function of children with bronchial asthma. Zhongguo Dang Dai Er Ke Za Zhi. 2006;8:388–90.
18. Zeybek C, Yalcin Y, Erdem A, Polat TB, Aktuglu-Zeybek AC, Bayoglu V, Akdeniz C, Celebi A. Tissue Doppler echocardiographic assessment of cardiac function in children with bronchial asthma. Pediatr Int. 2007;49:911–7.
19. Ozdemir O, Ceylan Y, Razi CH, Ceylan O, Andiran N. Assessment of ventricular functions by tissue Doppler echocardiography in children with asthma. Pediatr Cardiol. 2013;34:553–9.
20. Vogel M, Schmidt MR, Kristiansen SB, Cheung M, White PA, Sorensen K, Redington AN. Validation of myocardial acceleration during isovolumic contraction as a novel noninvasive index of right ventricular contractility: comparison with ventricular pressure-volume relations in an animal model. Circulation. 2002;105:1693–9.
21. Hedlin G, Freyschuss U. Cardiac output and blood pressure in asthmatic children before and during induced asthma. Acta Paediatr Scand. 1984;73: 441–7.
22. Allen DH, Dr scoll DJ, Shaddy ER, Feltes FT. Echocardiography, in: Moss abd Adams' Heart Disease in infants, Children and Adolescents. Wlaters Kluwer/ Lippincott, Williams & Wilkins; 2008, pp. 128-31.
23. Chicherina EN, Shipitsyna W. The cardiovascular system in patients with bronchial asthma of varying severity. Probl Tuberk Bolezn Legk. 2003;8:25–8.
24. Uyan AP, Uyan C, Ozyurek H. Assessment of right ventricular diastolic filling parameters by Doppler echocardiography. Pediatr Int. 2003;45:263–7.
25. Mohamed E. Abdalla, Hamdy Abd El Azeem. Echocardiographic evaluation of ventricular function in young adults with bronchial asthma. Egypt J Chest Dis Tuberc 2013; 62: 27-31.
26. Hirschfeld S, Meyer R, Schwartz DC, Kofhagen J, Kaplan S. The echocardiographic assessment of pulmonary artery pressure and pulmonary vascular resistance. Circulation. 1975;52:642–50.
27. Riggs T, Hirschfeld S, Borkat G, Knoke J, Liebman J. Assessment of the pulmonary vascular bed by echocardiographic right ventricular systolic time intervals. Circulation. 1978;57:939–47.
28. Statement by the British Thoracic Society, the British Paediatric Association, the Research Unit of the Royal College of Physicians of London, the King's Fund Centre, the National Asthma Campaign, the Royal College of General Practitioners, the General Practitioners in Asthma Group, the British Association of Accident and Emergency Medicine and the British Paediatric Respiratory Group. Guidelines on the management of asthma. Thorax. 1993;48:S1–24.
29. Suissa S, Assimes T, Brassard P, Ernst P. Inhaled corticosteroid use in asthma and the prevention of myocardial infarction. Am J Med. 2003;115:377–81.
30. Akyüz Özkan E, Serin Hİ, Khosroshahi HE, Kılıç M, Ekim M, Beysel P, Geçit UA, Domur E. Arterial Stiffness, Distensibility, and Strain in Asthmatic Children. Med Sci Monit. 2016;22:251–7.
31. Dawes M, Chowienczyk PJ, Ritter JM. Effects of inhibition of the L-arginine/ nitric oxide pathway on vasodilation caused by beta-adrenergic agonists in human forearm. Circulation. 1997;95:2293–7.

8

Measurement of pulse wave velocity in normal ageing: comparison of Vicorder and magnetic resonance phase contrast imaging

Jehill D. Parikh[1], Kieren G. Hollingsworth[1], Vijay Kunadian[1,3], Andrew Blamire[1] and Guy A. MacGowan[2,3*]

Abstract

Background: Pulse wave velocity is an important measure of cardiovascular risk, and can be measured by several different techniques. We compared age-related changes in pulse wave velocity derived from carotid and femoral artery waveforms using the Vicorder device and descending thoracic aorta time velocity curves using phase contrast magnetic resonance imaging (MRI) in a group of normal healthy volunteers, without cardiovascular disease, aged between 20 and 79 years.

Methods: Eighty subjects underwent same-day measurements of Vicorder and MRI pulse wave velocity measurements.

Results: Both Vicorder and MRI-based pulse wave velocity measurements were significantly increased with age ($R = 0.59$ and 0.57 respectively, both $P < 0.0001$). Vicorder and MRI pulse wave velocities were also significantly related to each other ($R = 0.27$, $P < 0.05$), and Bland Altman plots showed that on average Vicorder measurements were 1.6 m/s greater than MRI. In 5 % of cases, agreement between the values of the two techniques were above and below 2 standard deviations, and these were at higher levels of pulse wave velocities. Multiple linear stepwise regression analysis confirmed highly significant relationships of both techniques to age (both $P < 0.0001$), and MRI was also significantly related to heart rate ($P = 0.006$) but Vicorder was not.

Conclusions: Both Vicorder and MRI perform similarly in detecting age-related changes in pulse wave velocity. Thus, the choice of using one or the other will depend on other aspects of the investigation, such as the need for portability favouring Vicorder, or need for additional cardiovascular imaging favouring MRI.

Keywords: Pulse wave velocity, Vicorder, Phase contrast magnetic resonance imaging, Ageing

Background

Arterial stiffness is an important determinant of cardiovascular risk, and measurement of pulse wave velocity is the most accepted measure of arterial stiffness [1–3]. This can be non-invasively measured by Doppler [4] or high fidelity pressure measuring devices to measure pulse wave velocity [5]. A quite different approach is to use phase contrast magnetic resonance imaging (MRI), measuring velocity in two or more slices of the thoracic aorta from flow waveforms [6, 7]. These inherently different techniques have distinct advantages and disadvantages. Measurements from pressure waveform techniques are relatively easily done, do not require extensive training, are quick, and can be brought to the patient. A disadvantage of the pressure techniques is that the measurement of carotid to femoral length is an external anatomical surface measure along the course of the major blood vessels and so is prone to error [8]. MRI requires significant expertise, highly trained staff, and can only be done at specialised centres. Nevertheless, the measurement of length along

* Correspondence: guy.macgowan@nuth.nhs.uk
[2]Institute of Genetic Medicine, Newcastle University, Newcastle upon Tyne, UK
[3]Cardiothoracic Centre, Freeman Hospital, Newcastle upon Tyne, UK
Full list of author information is available at the end of the article

the aorta between the two slices where flow is measured is very accurate. Furthermore, MR imaging can be used to measure several aspects of cardiac and vascular function – so if these are already being acquired using MRI, the addition of MRI to measure vascular stiffness is relatively straightforward with advanced 4D phase contrast MRI [9].

The Vicorder device (Skidmore Medical, UK) is an inflatable cuff-based device that simultaneously measures the upstroke of carotid and femoral pulsations to calculate pulse wave velocity. It has shown good reproducibility [10] even when used by subjects with limited experience in using the device [11], and compares well with invasive measures of central blood pressure [12], and with measures of pulse wave velocity from the SphygmoCor device [10]. The purpose of this study was to compare measurements of pulse wave velocity using MRI and the Vicorder device in a population of normal subjects, without cardiovascular disease, but a wide range of ages.

Methods

Subjects

This study was performed as part of a larger project of ageing effects on cardiovascular function in normal subjects without a cardiovascular diagnosis, hypertension diabetes, or renal disease requiring dialysis (Cardiac Energetics and Function in Normal Human Ageing, ClinicalTrials.Gov identifier NCT01504828). Exclusion criteria were as above and also known claustrophobia. To get a consistent spread of ages we recruited subjects stratified by age ranges from 20 to 79 years. These and other general data are shown in Table 1. Informed consent was obtained for all patients, and this study was approved by a UK National Health Service Research Ethics Committee (NRES Committee North East - Newcastle & North Tyneside 1, reference number 12/NE/0057). All subjects had measurements of pulse wave velocity by the Vicorder device and Phase Contrast MRI on the same day within 2 h.

Vicorder pulse wave velocity and other haemodynamic measurements

The Vicorder measurements were performed by trained research nurses. Patients (non fasting) were laid on an a couch in a quiet clinic room, with the head raised to approximately 30^0, so that the skin and muscles over the carotid were relaxed though not too tense. Pulse wave velocity was measured by a cuff placed over the right carotid and the right thigh. The length between the carotid and femoral arteries was done by measuring the length between the suprasternal notch and the mid-point of the thigh cuff (Table 2). Measurements were taken until pressure waveforms over the carotid and thigh area were clear and reproducible. At a later date the lead investigator reviewed all tracings and if necessary selected only those data with clear pressure waveform upstrokes. Additional measurements with the Vicorder device were performed with a cuff placed on the right upper arm. These included oscillatory blood pressure measurement and using a global transfer function, central aortic pressures [13] and augmentation and augmentation index. Interobserver measurements of pulse wave velocity with these methods ($N = 32$) were 7.8 ± 1.6 and 7.6 ± 1.6 m/s with mean difference of 0.2 ± 0.8 m/s (linear regression $r = 0.89$), and intra-observer measurements ($N = 3$) of 6.1 ± 1.0 and 6.1 ± 0.9 m/s with mean difference of 0.03 ± 0.25 m/s.

Phase contrast MRI

Phase contrast MRI acquisitions were specifically designed to acquire time-velocity curves at two slices locations (aortic arch and descending aorta approximately 10 cm apart) to estimate transit time (ΔT) as shown in Fig. 1. Subjects were scanned using a Philips Achieva 3 Tesla scanner and a six channel cardiac coil was employed for signal reception. Phase contrast MRI data was acquired by

Table 1 Patient characteristics by age groups

	Age groups (years):					
	20–29	30–39	40–49	50–59	60–69	70–79
N	15	14	14	14	12	11
Gender (male)	5	7	6	6	8	6
Height	172 ± 8.1	174 ± 9.1	176 ± 12.5	174 ± 8.5	171 ± 9.1	164 ± 11.4
Weight	77 ± 16.6	75 ± 12.8	78 ± 9.9	77 ± 17.1	74 ± 18.1	70 ± 16.5
Glucose	4.8 ± 0.4	4.8 ± 0.5	4.9 ± 0.3	5.0 ± 0.5	5.3 ± 0.6	4.9 ± 0.5
Cholesterol	4.6 ± 0.9	4.2 ± 0.6	4.8 ± 0.9	4.9 ± 0.7	4.8 ± 0.7	5.1 ± 1.0
Triglycerides	0.9 ± 0.5	0.8 ± 0.3	0.9 ± 0.4	0.9 ± 0.7	0.9 ± 0.4	1.0 ± 0.3
HDL	1.5 ± 0.4	1.7 ± 0.3	1.5 ± 0.5	1.8 ± 0.6	1.7 ± 0.5	1.6 ± 0.3
LDL	2.7 ± 0.8	2.3 ± 0.6	2.9 ± 0.7	2.7 ± 0.8	2.7 ± 0.6	3.0 ± 0.8

Height (cm), weight (kg), all lipids and glucose measured in mmol/L
HDL high density lipoprotein, *LDL* low density lipoprotein

Table 2 Pulse wave velocities and the arterial length measured by age group

	Age groups (years):					
	20–29	30–39	40–49	50–59	60–69	70–79
Vicorder PWV	6.7 ± 0.9	6.9 ± 1.0	7.5 ± 1.2	8.0 ± 1.7	8.1 ± 1.2	9.5 ± 1.4
MRI PWV	4.5 ± 1.5	5.1 ± 0.8	6.5 ± 1.7	6.2 ± 1.6	6.8 ± 2.1	7.9 ± 1.5
Vicorder Length	63 ± 6	65 ± 6	64 ± 6	68 ± 7	67 ± 7	65 ± 9
MRI Length	10 ± 1	10 ± 2	10 ± 1	9.9 ± 8	10 ± 1	10 ± 2

PWV pulse wave velocity, m/sec, and lengths: cm

experienced radiographers using a high temporal resolution sequence (repetition time / echo time / flip angle / number of excitations / slice thickness = 5 ms/2.9 ms/10^0/ 1/8 mm, SENSE factor 2, field of view 300 mm × 225 mm, reconstructed voxel size 1.17 mm^2, velocity encoding = 150 m/s, 44 phases, breath hold duration ~19 s) at both slice locations which were the aortic arch (AAo) and the descending (DAo) aorta (Fig. 1). Additional scout images were acquired to facilitate positioning of the phase contrast MR acquisitions and to ensure that the slices were positioned perpendicular to aorta at both locations. Q-flow analysis package (Philips, Viewform) was employed to extract time-velocity curves as shown in Fig. 1 and to estimate precise distance (ΔX) between the two slice locations. The time-velocity curves were then used to determine transit time (ΔT) and compute MR pulse wave velocity = ΔX/ΔT using an in house Matlab based program. A reproducibility analysis of this technique was performed in seven normal volunteers, repeating scans at two sessions, and within each session performing the scanning twice. For session one the values were 4.9 ± 1.6 and 4.5 ± 1.6 m/s (mean difference 0.4 ± 0.9) and session two 5.5 ± 1.6 and 5.2 ± 1.2 m/s (mean difference 0.3 ± 0.7).

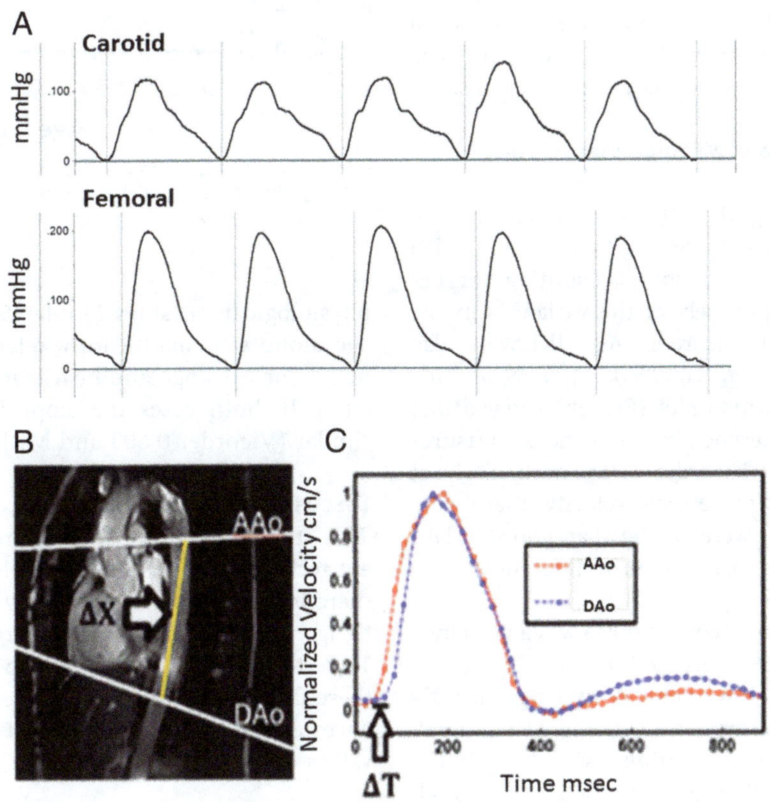

Fig. 1 Illustration of Vicorder and phase contrast MRI techniques. In panel **a**, examples of simultaneous Vicorder carotid and femoral arterial waveforms are shown. Panel **b** shows the two slices of thoracic aorta (AAo – aortic arch, and DAo descending aorta) between which distance is measured (ΔX), and in panel **c** phase contrast MRI flow images showing ΔT which is the time delay between of the initial upstroke in flow between the two slices

Data and statistical analysis

Data are expressed as mean ± standard deviation. Univariate associations of both Vicorder and MRI were tested with Pearson's correlation, and multiple linear stepwise regression models to test the role of multiple parameters incorporating all the parameters from the Univariate analysis. Stepwise criteria were: Probability-of-F-to-enter < = 0.050, Probability-of-F-to-remove > = 0.100). SPSS version 21 was used for all statistics. $P < 0.05$ was considered significant.

Results

Ninety nine patients were recruited to the main research study (between 16 and 18 subjects for each age decile from 20 to 79 years). Nine patients were excluded from this study because the Vicorder data was not adequate, usually because the carotid waveform was unclear. Six of these patients were over 50 years. Ten patients were excluded due to issues with the MR imaging. Three patients could not tolerate the MR scanning due to claustrophobia so were withdrawn. Six patients had very short transit times measured in the thoracic aorta (> 2 standard deviations from the mean). Review of these individual cases revealed that there were difficulties in positioning slices perpendicular to the aorta, particularly in those with more curved aortic arches. Five out of seven of these subjects were above 60 years of age. The remaining 80 subjects are the subject of this analysis.

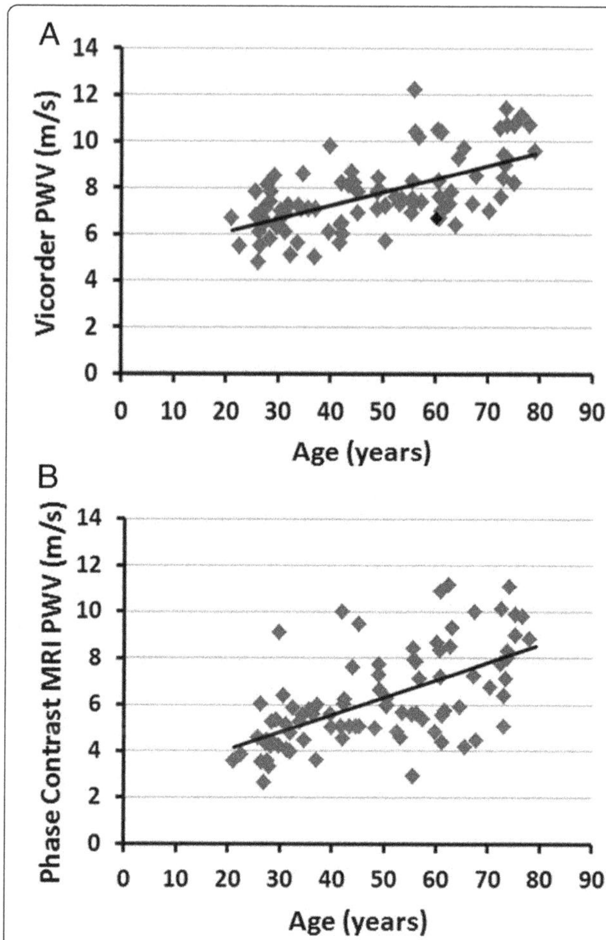

Fig. 2 Relationship of Vicorder to age (**a**) ($y = 0.055x + 5.033$, $R^2 = 0.353$, $R = 0.594$, $P < 0.0001$) and phase contrast MRI to age (**b**) ($y = 0.067x + 2.859$, $R^2 = 0.327$, $R = 0.572$, $P < 0.0001$). PWV: pulse wave velocity

Comparison of Vicorder and MRI measures of pulse wave velocity

Both techniques were significantly and similarly related to age (Table 2 and Fig. 2, Vicorder $R = 0.594$, and MRI $R = 0.572$), with R^2 values in both accounting for between 35 and 33 % respectively of the variances in the model (both $P < 0.0001$). Vicorder and MRI were also significantly correlated (Fig. 3a, $R = 0.271$, 7 % of variance, $P < 0.05$). Bland Altman plot (Fig. 3b) showed that in general the mean difference between the 2 measures was 1.6 m/s greater for Vicorder. Also, particularly at higher measurements of pulse wave velocity, there were four individual cases that were greater than two standard deviations greater or less than the mean difference.

Correlates of both measurements of pulse wave velocity

Hemodynamic data are presented by age group in Table 3. Vicorder pulse wave velocity was significantly related to all these hemodynamic variables. In general, the extent of significant correlations with these measurements were less with the MRI (Table 4), though there were highly significant correlations with aortic pulse pressure, augmentation and augmentation index. Multivariate analysis was performed separately for both techniques to compare how they related to other physiological variables (Tables 5 and 6). For Vicorder, age alone was significantly related to pulse wave velocity. For MRI age and heart rate were significantly related. In both cases the slope (Beta) against age was similar (Vicorder 0.603 and MRI 0.632).

Discussion

This study shows that when comparing two very different techniques for measuring pulse wave velocity that a) there is a very similar and highly significant relationship to age, b) there is a similar failure rate of approximately 10 % to obtain usable data in both techniques, c) that these failures and higher variances from the mean differences are greater in older subjects and those with higher values of pulse wave velocity.

Two different techniques

The Vicorder and MRI are fundamentally two different techniques. The Vicorder measurements rely on pressure waveforms whereas MRI is based on flow. The other

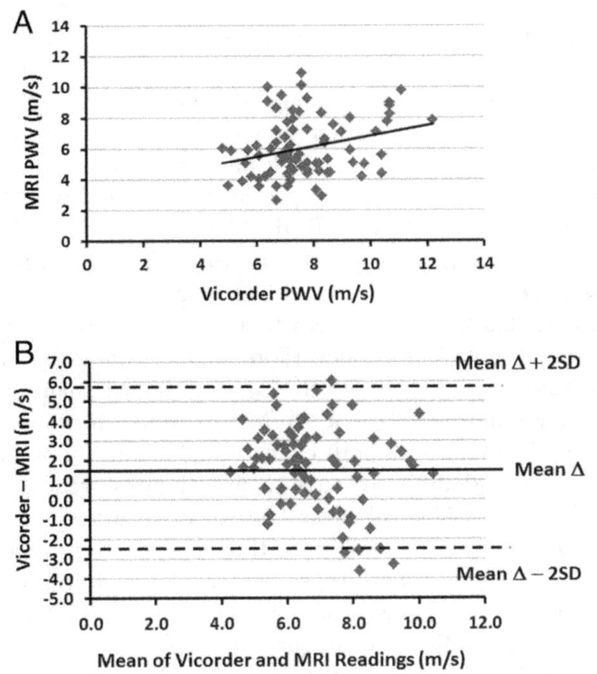

Fig. 3 Relationship of Vicorder to phase contrast MRI (**a**) ($y = 0.345x + 3.45$, $R^2 = 0.073$, $R = 0.271$ $P < 0.05$), and Bland Altman plot of the two techniques (**b**). On average Vicorder values are 1.6 m/s greater than MRI values. PWV: pulse wave velocity, and SD: standard deviation

major difference is the region from which the pulse wave velocity is measured. The MRI is measured in a relatively small segment (10 cm) in the descending aorta, whereas the Vicorder measurements go from the carotid to femoral artery. This can explain why the Vicorder measurements are on average 1.6 m/s greater than the MRI as the peripheral arteries are stiffer than the aorta [14, 15]. The measurement of length with MRI is accurate, though with the Vicorder an anatomical external surface measure along the length of the major blood vessels is used, which is a potential source of error. Despite these differences it is reassuring that both are closely and similarly related to age.

Table 4 Univariate correlations

	Vicorder PWV	P =	MRI PWV	P =
Height	−0.042	0.363	−0.054	0.325
Weight	0.053	0.328	−0.044	0.354
Heart Rate	0.253	0.015	−0.213	0.035
Systolic Pressure	0.392	0.000	0.162	0.085
Diastolic Pressure	0.284	0.007	0.026	0.414
Mean Arterial Pressure	0.371	0.001	0.098	0.204
Pulse Pressure	0.286	0.007	0.224	0.028
Aortic Systolic Pressure	0.466	0.000	0.251	0.016
Aortic Pulse Pressure	0.389	0.000	0.347	0.001
Augmentation	0.358	0.001	0.419	0.000
Augmentation Index	0.290	0.006	0.377	0.000

Comparisons with other studies

Vicorder pulse wave velocity has been assessed comprehensively in healthy subjects by Müller and colleagues [16]. In comparison with the present study, they obtained mean values of pulse wave velocity for 20–29 year olds of 5.8 ± 0.7 m/s and for 40–49 years of 7.1 ± 0.9 m/s which is slightly lower than our data particularly at the younger age (6.7 ± 0.9 and 7.5 ± 1.2 m/s respectively, Table 2). A likely explanation for this difference is in the measurement of the carotid-femoral length. Müller et al. have used the length from the suprasternal notch to the top of the femoral cuff, whereas we have taken the measurement to the middle of the cuff. Thus, our longer length will record higher pulse wave velocities. We have done this as the centre of the cuff has been shown to be where the pressure measurement is actually recorded [10]. Rogers et al [7] have looked at phase contrast MRI to measure pulse wave velocity in different regions of the aorta. Their values obtained from the proximal

Table 3 Vicorder haemodynamic data

	Age groups (years):					
	20–29	30–39	40–49	50–59	60–69	70–79
Heart Rate	64 ± 14	63 ± 14	61 ± 7	64 ± 9	59 ± 9	69 ± 14
Systolic Pressure	121 ± 11	128 ± 11	123 ± 8	124 ± 8	123 ± 12	136 ± 11
Diastolic Pressure	65 ± 7	73 ± 7	67 ± 6	68 ± 10	67 ± 9	73 ± 6
Mean Pressure	88 ± 9	95 ± 9	90 ± 7	93 ± 8	91 ± 10	100 ± 8
Pulse Pressure	60 ± 6	55 ± 5	56 ± 5	56 ± 8	55 ± 6	64 ± 9
Ao Systolic Pressure	115 ± 10	121 ± 9	120 ± 7	122 ± 8	120 ± 12	134 ± 12
Ao Pulse Pressure	50 ± 5	49 ± 5	53 ± 4	53 ± 8	53 ± 6	61 ± 9
Augmentation	6.9 ± 3.5	7.0 ± 4.3	11.2 ± 3.6	11.9 ± 3.9	13.4 ± 3.8	16.5 ± 4.4
Augmentation Index	13.7 ± 6.9	13.9 ± 8.0	21.4 ± 6.3	21.9 ± 5.0	25.5 ± 6.6	27.0 ± 6.4

Heart rate (beats per minute), all other pressures measured in mmHg, and augmentation index is a percentage
Ao aortic

Table 5 Multivariate Linear Regression Analysis

Vicorder PWV as dependent variable:	Beta	SE	P =
Age	0.603	0.009	0.000

Model $R^2 = 0.363$, $F = 40.5$, ANOVA $P < 0.0001$
SE standard error

descending aorta which is a similar area as used in our study are comparable to our study, though values particularly in the older age groups are lower. However, this study was in a smaller cohort of patients and significant variability is seen in the older subjects. For instance, in the 20–29 year old Rogers et al. obtained a pulse wave velocity of approximately 5 m/s (compared to 4.5 ± 1.5 m/s in the present study), and for 60–69 years old approximately 9 m/s compared to 6.8 ± 2.1 m/s in the present study. In a larger study of 162 normal subjects Hickson and colleagues [17] have compared the SphygmaCor and Vicorder devices and phase contrast MRI. Their values of phase contrast MRI pulse wave velocity in the descending thoracic aorta are very similar to the current study. They did however show a closer relationship of Vicorder pulse wave velocity measurements to phase contrast MRI measurements than in the current study ($r = 0.64$ vs $r = 0.27$ in current study). This higher level of correlation may be due to the larger number of subjects studied and the measurement of pulse wave velocity along the whole length of the descending aorta by phase contrast MRI. Nevertheless Bland Altman plots show a similar pattern to the current study with higher overall mean values for Vicorder, and individual points outside two standard deviations particularly at higher levels of pulse wave velocity. Thus, the values of both Vicorder and MRI pulse wave velocity obtained in this study match very closely to published data.

Clinical significance

There are two issues of particular clinical significance with these data. Firstly, measurement of pulse wave velocity is recommended in the 2013 European Society of Cardiology/European Society of Hypertension guidelines for assessment of cardiovascular risk [18], though there are continuing issues regarding clinical application that have been recently highlighted [19]. The issue that is most relevant to this study is that there are a myriad of devices that can measure pulse wave velocity and that these are not necessarily interchangeable. In that regard, our data is very important comparing these two techniques. In particular, as MR imaging becomes more widely adapted in clinical cardiovascular diagnostics, how this performs compared to other techniques is very important. The second issue of clinical significance is that with both techniques there were approximately 10 % of cases in which data was not obtainable or usable. This was more prevalent in older subjects. One of the advantages with the Vicorder system is that it is easy to use, and so in this study all examinations were performed by research nursing staff. However, despite this there are cases where the carotid waveform is simply not clear enough to identify the upstroke and therefore not usable, and this appears higher than previously reported [11]. For the MRI scanning there were similarly issues with both claustrophobia and tolerating the scan, and also poor data quality which is predominantly in the older subjects. The scans were performed by experienced radiographers, though there were issues with obtaining scans perpendicular to the descending aorta in older subjects as a result of increased aortic curvature. As these techniques move from a purely research domain to clinical tools, these data are important to understand how these techniques perform. Our data suggests that assessing pulse wave velocity in older subjects requires careful attention to these technical issues to avoid loss of potentially important data, and more information is required to determine how other techniques perform in these older subjects.

Table 6 Multivariate Linear Regression Analysis

MRI PWV as dependent variable	Beta	SE	P =
Age	0.632	0.010	0.000
Heart Rate	−0.256	0.014	0.006

Model $R^2 = 0.442$, $F = 27.7$, ANOVA $P < 0.0001$
SE standard error

Limitations

These data are in normal subjects, so in subjects with cardiovascular disease with increased vascular stiffness the relationships described may be altered, and also there may be additional issues with acquiring high quality data. Gender differences have been described with measures of vascular stiffness [20], but this study was not statistically powered to detect gender differences. There are other methods to measure pulse wave velocity with MRI. For instance, other areas of the aorta can be assessed using phase contrast MRI. Hickson and colleagues [17] have shown that the abdominal aorta has slightly higher rates of age-related increases in pulse wave velocity relative to the descending thoracic aorta. Other phase contrast techniques include determination of flow-area [21], and cross-correlation methods [22] (where flow is determined at several points along the descending aorta). Ibrahim et al. [23] have shown that the transit time (as used in this study) and cross-correlation methods resulted in more reproducible measurements compared to the flow-area method. Our MRI reproducibility studies have more variation than the data published by Ibrahim et al. explained by their much larger study number. A dependency of heart rate on augmentation index has been reported for the SphygmoCor device

[24]. As there is no published data on this issue with the Vicorder device, we have not normalised data to heart rate.

Conclusions

Both the Vicorder device and phase contrast MRI measurements of pulse wave velocity are similarly and strongly related to age. The decision on whether to use one or the other in studies of vascular ageing will thus be related to other factors – such as the portability and ease of use of the Vicorder device, or need for additional cardiovascular MR imaging.

Abbreviations

MRI: magnetic resonance imaging; AAo: arch of aorta; DAo: descending aorta; HDL: high density lipoprotein; LDL: low density lipoprotein; PWV: pulse wave velocity; Ao: aortic; SE: standard error.

Competing interests

The authors declare that they have no competing interests.

Authors' contributions

JP: performed and analysed MR data, KH and AB designed and oversaw MR techniques, VK assisted with Vicorder data, GMG all aspects of study. All authors have read and approved final manuscript.

Acknowledgments

This study was funded by British Heart Foundation Clinical Leave Research Fellowship to Dr MacGowan (FS/11/89/29162).

Author details

[1]Institute of Cellular Medicine, Newcastle University, Newcastle upon Tyne, UK. [2]Institute of Genetic Medicine, Newcastle University, Newcastle upon Tyne, UK. [3]Cardiothoracic Centre, Freeman Hospital, Newcastle upon Tyne, UK.

References

1. Laurent S, Cockcroft J, Van Bortel L, Boutouyrie P, Giannattasio C, Hayoz D, et al. Expert consensus document on arterial stiffness: methodological issues and clinical applications. Eur Heart J. 2006;27:2588–605.
2. Lin F, Zhu P, Huang F, Li Q, Yuan Y, Gao Z, et al. Aortic stiffness is associated with the central retinal arteriolar equivalent and retinal vascular fractal dimension in a population along the southeastern coast of China. Hypertens Res. 2015;38:342–8.
3. Seidlerová J, Filipovský J, Mayer O, Wohlfahrt P, Cífková R. Positive effects of antihypertensive treatment on aortic stiffness in the general population. Hypertens Res. 2014;37:64–8.
4. Avolio AP, Chen SG, Wang RP, Zhang CL, Li MF, et al. Effects of aging on changing arterial compliance and left ventricular load in a northern Chinese urban community. Circulation. 1983;68:50–8.
5. Ring M, Eriksson MJ, Zierath JR, Caidahl K. Arterial stiffness estimation in healthy subjects: a validation of oscillometric (Arteriograph) and tonometric (SphygmoCor) techniques. Hypertens Res. 2014;37:999–1007.
6. Groenink M, de Roos A, Mulder BJ, Spaan JA, van der Wall EE. Changes in aortic distensibility and pulse wave velocity assessed with magnetic resonance imaging following beta-blocker therapy in the Marfan syndrome. Am J Cardiol. 1998;82:203–8.
7. Rogers WJ, Hu YL, Coast D, Vido DA, Kramer CM, Pyeritz RE, et al. Age-associated changes in regional aortic pulse wave velocity. J Am Coll Cardiol. 2001;38:1123–9.
8. Bossuyt J, Van De Velde S, Azermai M, Vermeersch SJ, De Backer TL, Devos DG, et al. Noninvasive assessment of carotid-femoral pulse wave velocity: the influence of body side and body contours. J Hypertens. 2013;31:946–51.
9. Markl M, Draney MT, Hope MD, Levin JM, Chan FP, Alley MT, et al. Time-resolved 3-dimensional velocity mapping in the thoracic aorta: visualization of 3-directional blood flow patterns in healthy volunteers and patients. J Comput Assist Tomogr. 2004;28:459–68.
10. Hickson SS, Butlin M, Broad J, Avolio AP, Wilkinson IB, McEniery CM. Validity and repeatability of the Vicorder apparatus: a comparison with the SphygmoCor device. Hypertens Res. 2009;32:1079–85.
11. McGreevy C, Barry M, Bennett K, Williams D. Repeatability of the measurement of aortic pulse wave velocity (aPWV) in the clinical assessment of arterial stiffness in community-dwelling older patients using the Vicorder® device. Scand J Clin Lab Invest. 2013;73:269–73.
12. Pucci G, Cheriyan J, Hubsch A, Hickson SS, Gajendragadkar PR, Watson T, et al. Evaluation of the Vicorder, a novel cuff-based device for the noninvasive estimation of central blood pressure. J Hypertens. 2013;31:77–85.
13. O'Rourke MF. Influence of ventricular ejection on the relationship between central aortic and brachial pressure pulse in man. Cardiovasc Res. 1970;4:291–300.
14. Latham RD, Westerhof N, Sipkema P, Rubal BJ, Reuderink P, Murgo JP. Regional wave travel and reflections along the human aorta: a study with six simultaneous micromanometric pressures. Circulation. 1985;72:1257–69.
15. McDonald DA. Regional pulse-wave velocity in the arterial tree. J Appl Physiol. 1968;24:73–8.
16. Müller J, Oberhoffer R, Barta C, Hulpke-Wette M, Hager A. Oscillometric carotid to femoral pulse wave velocity estimated with the Vicorder device. J Clin Hypertens (Greenwich). 2013;15:176–9.
17. Hickson SS, Butlin M, Graves M, Taviani V, Avolio AP, McEniery CM, et al. The relationship of age with regional aortic stiffness and diameter. JACC Cardiovasc Imaging. 2010;3:1247–55.
18. Mancia G, Fagard R, Narkiewicz K, Redón J, Zanchetti A, Böhm M, et al. 2013 ESH/ESC guidelines for the management of arterial hypertension: the task force for the management of arterial hypertension of the European Society of Hypertension (ESH) and of the European Society of Cardiology (ESC). J Hypertens. 2013;31:1281–357.
19. Wilkinson IB, Cockcroft JR, McEniery CM. Aortic stiffness as a cardiovascular risk predictor. BMJ. 2015;351:h3764.
20. Coutinho T, Borlaug BA, Pellikka PA, Turner ST, Kullo IJ. Sex differences in arterial stiffness and ventricular-arterial interactions. J Am Coll Cardiol. 2013;61: 96–103.
21. Vulliemoz S, Stergiopulos N, Meuli R. Estimation of local aortic elastic properties with MRI. Magn Reson Med. 2002;47:649–54.
22. Fielden SW, Fornwalt BK, Jerosch-Herold M, Eisner RL, Stillman AE, Oshinski JN. A new method for the determination of aortic pulse wave velocity using cross-correlation on 2D PCMR velocity data. J Magn Reson Imaging. 2008;27:1382–7.
23. Ibrahim e-SH, Johnson KR, Miller AB, Shaffer JM, White RD. Measuring aortic pulse wave velocity using high-field cardiovascular magnetic resonance: comparison of techniques. J Cardiovasc Magn Reson. 2010;12:26.
24. Wilkinson IB, MacCallum H, Flint L, Cockcroft JR, Newby DE, Webb DJ. The influence of heart rate on augmentation index and central arterial pressure in humans. J Physiol. 2000;525:263–70.

9

A unique association of arrhythmogenic right ventricular dysplasia and acute myocarditis, as assessed by cardiac MRI

Andrea Ponsiglione*, Marta Puglia, Carmine Morisco,
Luigi Barbuto, Antonio Rapacciuolo, Mario Santoro, Letizia Spinelli, Bruno Trimarco, Alberto Cuocolo
and Massimo Imbriaco

Abstract

Background: Arrhythmogenic right ventricular dysplasia (ARVD), is a genetic disorder of the heart, which mainly involves the right ventricle. It is characterized by hypokinetic areas at the free wall of the right ventricle (RV) or both ventricles, where myocardium is replaced by fibrous or fatty tissue. ARVD is an important cause of ventricular arrhythmias in children and young adults. Although the transmission of the disease is based on hereditary, in young adults it may not show any symptoms. The main differential diagnoses with other frequent etiological causes of sudden arrhythmia are: idiopathic outflow tract ventricular tachycardia of the RV, myocarditis, dilated cardiomyopathy and sarcoidosis.

Case presentation: We describe an unusual case of a 44-year-old woman who was hospitalized for ventricular tachycardia, deep asthenia and dyspnoea with no previous history of cardiac disease. The patient had a ten-year history of palpitations, which started immediately after her last pregnancy. She was diagnosed with both acute/subacute viral myocarditis and arrhythmogenic right ventricular dysplasia, based on established clinical and cardiac MRI criteria. After the diagnosis the patient received an automatic implantable cardioverter defibrillator. Currently, she is on clinical follow-up with no apparent further complications.

Conclusion: Analyzing this rare case, we have shown the link between myocarditis and arrhythmogenic right ventricular dysplasia, and how important is to perform a cardiac MRI, in the context of acute myocarditis and ventricular arrhythmia.

Keywords: Myocarditis, Cardiac, Magnetic resonance imaging, Right ventricle, Case report

Background

Arrhythmogenic right ventricular dysplasia (ARVD), is a genetic disorder of the heart, that mainly involves the right ventricle [1, 2]. It is characterized by hypokinetic areas at the free wall of the right ventricle (RV) or both ventricles, where myocardium is replaced by fibrous or fatty tissue. ARVD is an important cause of ventricular arrhythmias in children and young adults. Although the transmission of the disease is based on hereditary, in young adults it may not show any symptoms. The main differential diagnoses with other frequent etiological causes of sudden arrhythmia are: idiopathic outflow tract ventricular tachycardia of the RV, myocarditis [3], dilated cardiomyopathy and sarcoidosis. We hereby describe a rare case of a patient with both acute viral myocarditis and ARVD, as assessed by echocardiography and cardiac MR (CMR).

Case presentation

The patient is a 44 year-old woman with a ten-year history of palpitations, who started immediately after her last pregnancy. She wasn't an active smoker and had a family history

* Correspondence: andreaponsiglione@hotmail.it
Department of Advanced Biomedical Sciences, University "Federico II", Via Pansini, 5, 80123 Naples, Italy

of cardiac disease (her father died at the age of 49 years-old for myocardial infarction). The patient was admitted to the emergency department for palpitations, deep asthenia and dyspnoea appearing suddenly when she was at home, under resting conditions. The patient was not febrile and did not show any episodes of chest pain or syncope. At physical examination, the patient revealed no symptoms of right heart failure. ECG performed at her admission showed a ventricular tachycardia (VT) with heart rate of 192 bpm (Fig. 1). Initially the VT was treated by intravenous bolus of lidocaine. For the resistance of the VT to lidocaine, was injected an intravenous bolus of amiodarone and adenosine. In response to the combined antiarrhythmic treatment, the patient had a drop of systemic blood pressure (80/50 mmHg), developed bradycardia (junctional rhythm at 38 bpm) associated with dizziness. For this reason she was moved to the coronary care unit (CCU). Here she was treated with temporary endocardial pacing and hydration therapy. Within 24 h the patient restored the sinus rhythm and normal blood pressure. ECG recorded in sinus rhythm, showed frequent polymorphic ectopic ventricular beats associated with negative T waves in right precordial leads. On admission in CCU the blood tests revealed an elevated troponin level (23 ng/mL, normal value: <5 ng/mL ng/mL) and an elevated CK-MB level (1240 IU/L, normal value < 120 IU/L). The inflammation markers were also elevated with a C-reactive protein (CRP) of 30,5 mg/L (normal value: < 8 mg/L) and 21.000/mL white blood cells (normal value: 4000-10000/mL). Her plasma electrolyte levels were normal.

Echocardiography showed a normal geometry of the left ventricle, with a slightly reduced systolic function (EF: 51%), a normal diastolic pattern and mild tricuspid regurgitation; the right ventricle was dilated with evidence of hypokinesia of the apical segment and severely reduced systolic function (TAPSE: 16 mm), hinting the diagnosis of ARVD. CMR was performed using a superconducting system 1.5 T MR (Gyroscan Intera, Philips Medical System, Best, The Netherlands) with a maximum gradient capability of 30 MT/m and maximum slow rate of 150 MT/Ms. MR acquisition was triggered by ECG and included a T1-weighted (T1W) sequence and cine-MR images in the short-axis, and vertical long-axis and horizontal long-axis planes for displaying cardiac contraction. Short time inversion recovery (STIR) T2-weighted (T2W) sequence was obtained to suppress fatty tissue signal. Finally, three-dimensional (3D) T1-delayed enhancement sequences, were acquired at 10, 15 and 20 min, after the intravenous injection of Gd-DTPA at a dose of 0.1 mmol/kg. CMR revealed findings that were consistent with the major criteria of arrhythmogenic right ventricular dysplasia: dilated right ventricle with high end-diastolic volume (EDV) normalized for body surface area (BSA) (116 mL/m2); right ventricular dysfunction with ejection fraction (RVEF) of 18% and regional wall motion abnormalities (diffuse hypokinesia, free wall iper-trabeculation, dyskinesia and mid-RV free wall pseudo-aneurysm) (Fig. 2a and b). On CMR there was a slightly reduced global left ventricular systolic function (EF: 50%) with normal morpho-

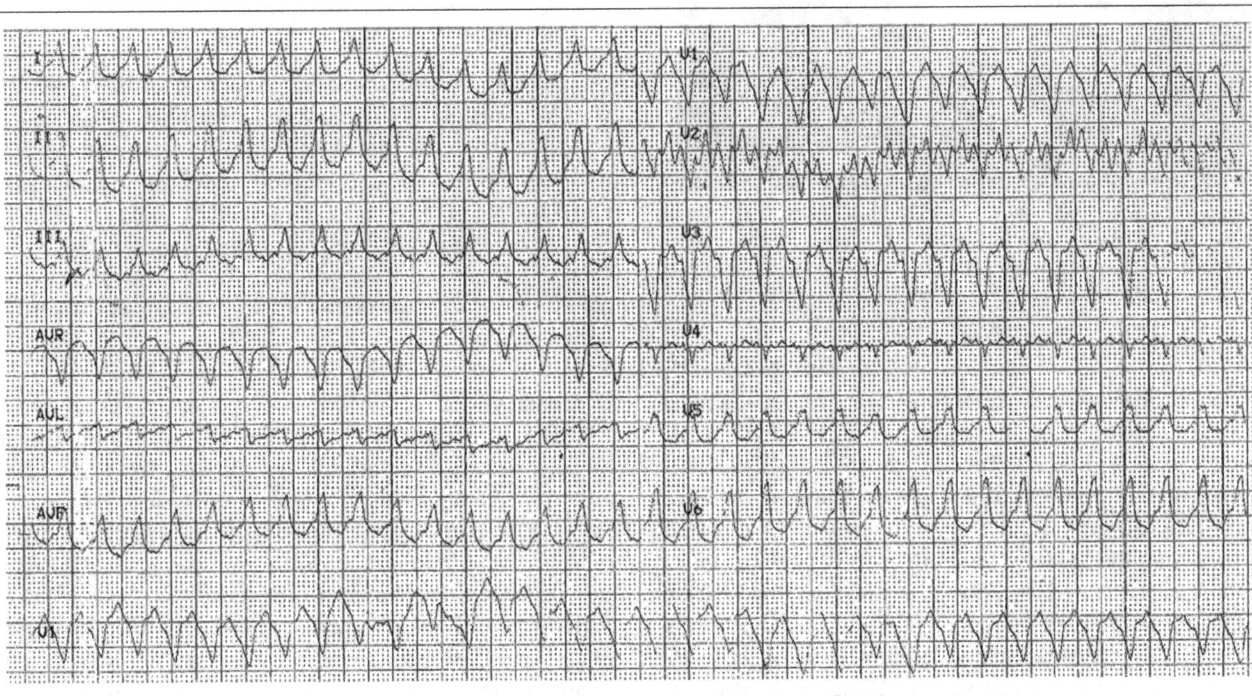

Fig. 1 ECG performed on patient admission, showing a ventricular tachycardia with heart rate of 192 bpm

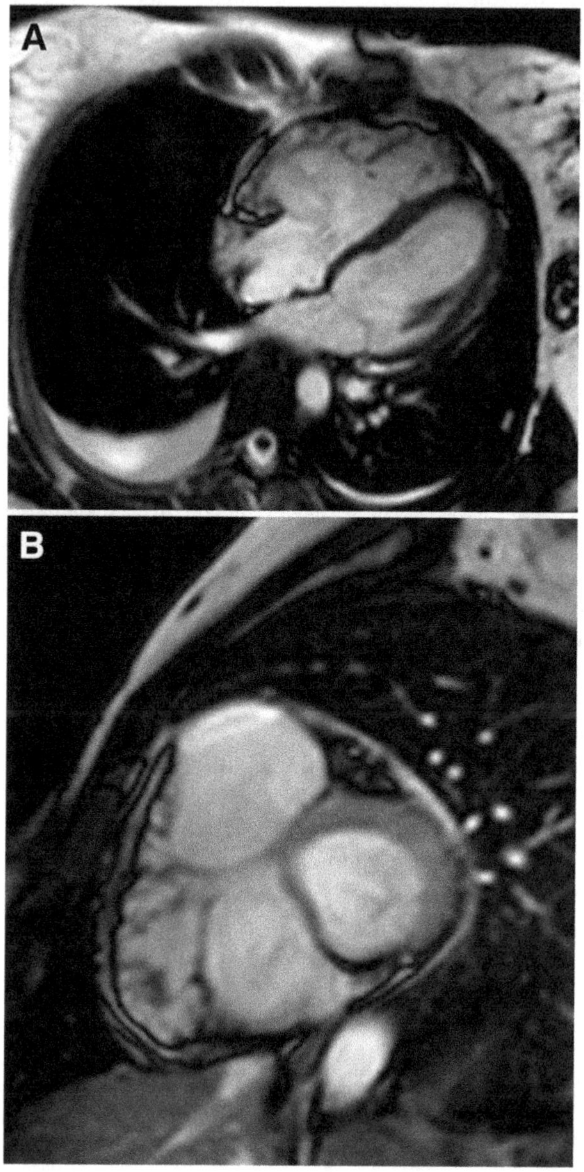

Fig. 2 Horizontal long axis (**a**) and short axis (**b**) balanced FFE images showing a dilated right ventricle, with diffuse free wall iper-trabeculation and dyskinesia, and mid-RV free wall pseudo-aneurysm. Bilateral pleural effusion is also present; more conspicuous on the right side

volumetry of the left ventricle. CMR also revealed the following findings that were consistent with a diagnosis of acute/subacute viral myocarditis: diffuse edema of the right ventricular free wall on STIR images (Fig. 3a and b), associated with sub-epicardial late gadolinium enhancement (Fig. 4a and b) of the same region. Overall, the patient met the criteria for both ARVD and acute/sub acute viral myocarditis. After the diagnosis the patient received an automatic implantable cardioverter defibrillator (AICD) and a beta-blocker (Sotalol) was prescribed at discharge. There was no recurrent VT up to the 4-month follow-up. At 6-month follow-up, the patient complained

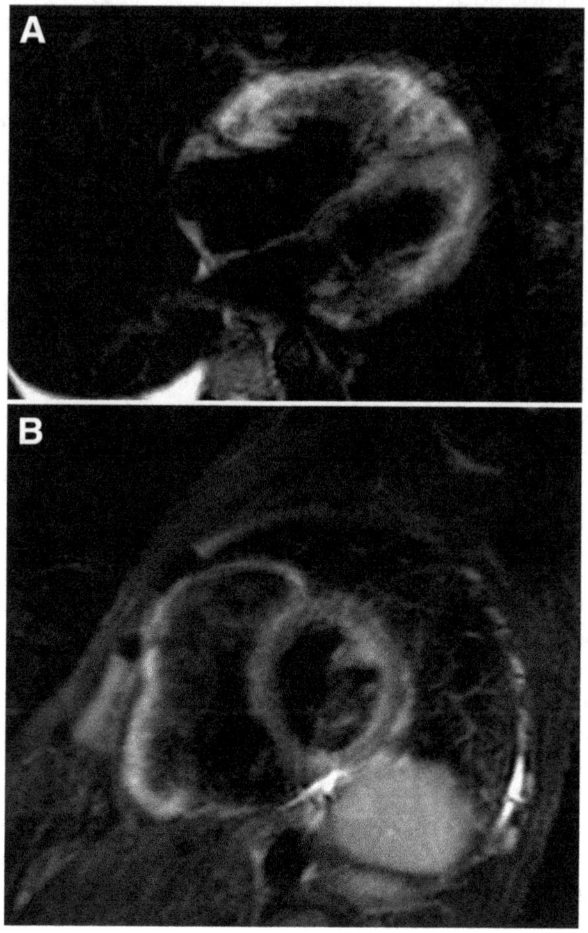

Fig. 3 Horizontal long axis (**a**) and short axis (**b**) STIR-T2W images showing a diffuse edema of the right ventricular free wall

for palpitation and dizziness. AICD recordings demonstrated 5 sustained VT episodes with appropriate device intervention in all the cases. Transthoracic echocardiography demonstrated a preserved systolic function of the left ventricle (EF: 59%) and a dilated and hypokinetic RV, owing a severely reduced systolic function (TAPSE = 14 mm, fractional change area of 30%). Currently, the patient is on clinical follow-up with no apparent further complications.

Discussion

ARVD is predominantly a genetically determined heart muscle disorder, pathologically characterized by fibro-fatty replacement of the right ventricular myocardium [1, 2]. This pathology predisposes to ventricular arrhythmias and sudden cardiac death and it can be divided in three progressive phases: in the early "concealed phase" patients are often asymptomatic; in the overt "electrical phase" patients present with symptomatic arrhythmias; finally, in the diffuse disease patients may present with right, left or biventricular heart failure with associated

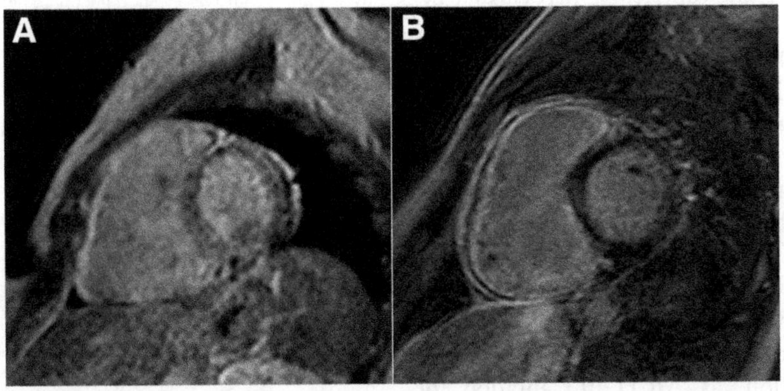

Fig. 4 Early (**a**) and delayed (**b**) dynamic contrast enhanced 3D short axis images, showing abnormal contrast enhancement of the dilated right ventricular free wall

ventricular arrhythmias. Current Task Force Criteria for ARVD diagnosis include, repolarization or depolarization abnormalities on electrocardiography (ECG), presence of ventricular arrhythmias, morphological and functional changes, in addition to histopathology, family history, and genetic findings [2]. Our patient fulfilled the major criteria set by the Task Force [2, 3]: repolarization abnormalities (inverted T waves in right precordial leads in the absence of complete right bundle-branch block), sustained ventricular tachycardia of left bundle-branch morphology with superior axis, RV EDV to BSA $\geq$ 100 mL/m^2 and RVEF $\leq$ 40%, as assessed by echocardiography and CMR. In addition, the patient fulfilled two of the Lake-Louise criteria for CMR in acute myocarditis [4]. Infact, CMR showed the presence of myocardial edema on STIR-T2W sequences and sub-epicardial necrosis on post-contrast T1W sequences; therefore, these imaging findings added to troponin I and CK-MB release and an elevation of CRP and white blood cells, strongly suggested an acute myocarditis. Several studies have demonstrated that myocarditis may affect the RV, causing structural abnormalities, including microaneurysms, as well as the arrhythmic manifestations that are typical of ARVD. Some cardiotropic viruses (enterovirus or adenovirus), detected in patients with sporadic ARVD, were considered to have a potential role for the disease; in fact the activation of inflammatory mediators, determined by the myocardial infection, could damage the cardiac adherents junctions and the T-tubule system, resulting in ventricular irritability and/or ion channel disruption and consequent ARVD symptomatology [5]. However, this hypothesis is controversial, because the inflammation could be a secondary event; infact, an already diseased myocardium could have an increased susceptibility to viral infection with resulting myocardial inflammation [6]. Therefore, the precise relationship between ARVD and acute myocarditis is not yet determined [7].

In a previous manuscript, Mavrogeni et al. described the case of a patient with Naxos disease, a recessively inherited arrhythmogenic cardiomyopathy (ACM), characterized by woolly hair and palmo-plantar keratoderma [8]. This patient was asymptomatic and presented with chest pain and increased troponin I. A deletion in plakoglobin (cell adhesion protein) gene (Pk2157del2TG) was identified as the cause of Naxos disease [9]; therefore, it has been proposed that a defect in proteins involved in cell–cell adhesion, particularly under mechanical stress conditions, could result in cell death and progressive myocardial fibro-fatty replacement [10]. Moreover, myocardial inflammatory infiltrates, frequently detected in patients with ARVD, have been assumed as a reaction to cell death rather than a consequence of an infective process [11]. As described in recent papers, the reactive nature of myocarditis in ARVD has been supported by the massive inflammatory cell infiltrates found after acute myocardial necrosis in early stages of disease in desmoglein-2 transgenic animal model [12]. In particular, Kant et al. have shown the etiologic role of a deletion of the adhesive extracellular domain of the desmosomal cadherin in mice with an arrhythmogenic right ventricular cardiomyopathy like phenotype, with ventricular dilation and fibrosis. Disturbed sarcomer structure, multiple autophagic vacuoles and swollen mitochondria are typical findings of this cardiomyopathy, inducing cardiomyocyte death, aseptic inflammation and fibrotic replacement, with consequent impairment of the cardiac function [13].

It must be underlined that in our case the patient started to suffer of palpitations and fatigue for light efforts after giving birth her third child in 2009. Therefore, it is reasonable to raise the hypothesis that pregnancy, the hormonal changes and/or inflammatory stress occurring during pregnancy may unmask ARVD. Due to the rarity of cases, the relation between the two events is not yet established. Furthermore, idiopathic right ventricular outflow tract ventricular tachycardia, right ventricular myocardial infarction, dilated cardiomyopathy, myocarditis, pulmonary hypertension, atrial and ventricular septal defects are possible differential diagnoses including a dilated right ventricle. Moreover, sarcoidosis with cardiac involvement can mimic ARVC, making the differential diagnosis very challenging. Uhl's disease, an unusual cardiac disorder with almost complete absence of right ventricular myocardium, should also be considered as differential diagnosis [14]. ARVD and myocarditis have often different prognosis and treatment; in fact, the former is a complex and progressive entity that requires major clinical intervention, as AICD implantation, or heart transplantation, while the latter is often a self-limited pathology responding to a conservative approach.

To the best of our knowledge, only one case has been published in the English literature showing in a 23 years old man this rare linkage between ARVD and acute myocarditis, based on echocardiography and CMR findings [15]. In agreement with this article, in our case and according to the current international task force consensus statement for ARVD [16] the patient underwent an AICD implantation and is currently in clinical follow up, with no further complications.

In the case presented, CMR allowed the correct identification of the two different clinical entities; in addition, the enhancement pattern as shown on delayed CMR images, may also serve as a map for the exact location of ablation or an endomyocardial biopsy [17].

Conclusions

This case shows the rare association between acute myocarditis and ARVD, highlighting the importance of a complete RV assessment through a CMR study in the context of ventricular arrhythmia. CMR is the most accurate and reproducible technique for assessing the morphology and segmental wall motion of the RV; in addition, it can evaluate the presence of myocardial inflammation with specific STIR-T2W sequences and myocardial fibrosis or necrosis with post-contrast T1W sequences, leading the physician to the correct final diagnosis and to the most appropriate management of patients presenting with ventricular arrhythmias.

Abbreviations

3D: Three-dimensional; ACM: Arrhythmogenic cardiomyopathy; AICD: Automatic implantable cardioverter defibrillator; ARVD: Arrhythmogenic right ventricular dysplasia; BSA: Body surface area; CCU: Coronary care unit; CMR: Cardiac MR; CRP: C-reactive protein; ECG: Electrocardiography; EDV: End-diastolic volume; RV: Right ventricle; RVEF: Right ventricular ejection fraction; STIR: Short time inversion recovery; T1W: T1-weighted; T2W: T2-weighted; VT: Ventricular tachycardia

Acknowledgements

Gennaro Fraia and Fabio Garbino (Technologists) for their contribution in making this study possible.

Funding

Not applicable.

Authors' contributions

MI, MP, AP, AC and BT: Study design and conception, Cardiac MR interpretation and manuscript preparation; CM, MS, LS and AR: acquisition of data, coronary care unit, drafting the manuscript; LB, MP, AP and MI: acquisition of cardiac MR data and interpretation of images. AC and BT: manuscript critical revision. All authors read and approved the final manuscript.

Authors' information

All authors belong to the Department of Advanced Biomedical Sciences, University *"Federico II"*, Via Pansini 5, 80123, Naples, Italy.

Competing interests

Not applicable.

References

1. Basso C, Corrado D, Marcus FI, Nava A, Thiene G. Arrhythmogenic right ventricular cardiomyopathy. Lancet. 2009;373:1289–300.
2. Marcus FI, McKenna WJ, Sherrill D, Basso C, Bauce B, Bluemke DA, et al. Diagnosis of arrhythmogenic right ventricular cardiomyopathy/dysplasia: proposed modification of the Task Force Criteria. Eur Heart J. 2010;31:806–14.
3. Marcus FI, McKenna WJ, Sherrill D, Basso C, Bauce B, Bluemke DA, et al. Diagnosis of arrhythmogenic right ventricular cardiomyopathy/dysplasia: proposed modification of the Task Force Criteria. Circulation. 2010;121:1533–41.
4. Friedrich MG, Sechtem U, Schulz-Menger J, Holmvang G, Alakija P, Cooper LT, et al. International Consensus Group on Cardiovascular Magnetic Resonance in Myocarditis. Cardiovascular magnetic resonance in myocarditis: A JACC White Paper. J Am Coll Cardiol. 2009;53:1475–87.
5. Bowles NE, Ni J, Marcus F, Towbin JA. The detection of cardiotropic viruses in the myocardium of patients with arrhythmogenic right ventricular dysplasia/cardiomyopathy. J Am Coll Cardiol. 2002;39:892–5.
6. Chimenti C, Pieroni M, Maseri A, Frustaci A. Histologic findings in patients with clinical and instrumental diagnosis of sporadic arrhythmogenic right ventricular dysplasia. J Am Coll Cardiol. 2004;43:2305–13.
7. Jordan AN, Lyne J, De Silva R, Wong T. Myocarditic appearance of arrhythmogenic right ventricular cardiomyopathy. Circulation. 2010;122:e556–7.
8. Mavrogeni S, Protonotarios N, Tsatsopoulou A, Papachristou P, Sfendouraki E, Papadopoulos G. Naxos disease evolution mimicking acute myocarditis: The role of cardiovascular magnetic resonance imaging. Int J Cardiol. 2013; 166(1):e14–5. doi:10.1016/j.ijcard.2012.12.078.
9. McKoy G, Protonotarios N, Crosby A, Tsatsopoulou A, Anastasakis A, Coonar A, et al. Identification of a deletion in plakoglobin in arrhythmogenic right ventricular cardiomyopathy with palmoplantar keratoderma and woolly hair (Naxos disease). Lancet. 2000;355:2119–24.
10. Asimaki A, Tandri H, Huang H, Halushka MK, Gautam S, Basso C, et al. A new diagnostic test for arrhythmogenic right ventricular cardiomyopathy. N Engl J Med. 2009;360:1075–84.
11. Basso C, Thiene G, Corrado D, Angelini A, Nava A, Valente M. Arrhythmogenic right ventricular cardiomyopathy. Dysplasia, dystrophy, or myocarditis? Circulation. 1996;94:983–91.
12. Pilichou K, Remme CA, Basso C, Campian ME, Rizzo S, Barnett P, et al. Myocyte necrosis underlies progressive myocardial dystrophy in mouse dsg2-related arrhythmogenic right ventricular cardiomyopathy. J Exp Med. 2009;206:1787–802.

13. Kant S, Krull P, Eisner S, Leube RE, Krusche CA. Histological and ultrastructural abnormalities in murine desmoglein 2-mutant hearts. Cell Tissue Res. 2012;348:249–59. doi:10.1007/s00441-011-1322-3.
14. Haugaa KH, Haland TF, Leren IS, Saberniak J, Edvardsen T. Arrhythmogenic right ventricular cardiomyopathy, clinical manifestations, and diagnosis. Europace. 2015. doi:10.1093/europace/euv340.
15. Huttin O, Frikha Z, Brembilla-Perrot B, Sellal JM, Mandry D, Aliot E, et al. Acute myocarditis presenting with ventricular arrhythmias: the role of CMR in the differential diagnosis of ARVD. Intern Med. 2013;52:1915–8.
16. Corrado D, Wichter T, Link MS, Hauer R, Marchlinski F, Anastasakis A. Treatment of arrhythmogenic right ventricular cardiomyopathy/dysplasia: an international task force consensus statement. Eur Heart J. 2015;36:3227–37.
17. Tavano A, Maurel B, Gaubert JY, Varoquaux A, Cassagneau P, Vidal V, et al. MR imaging of arrhythmogenic right ventricular dysplasia: What the radiologist needs to know. Diagn Interv Imaging. 2015;96:449–60.

10

Electrocardiographic features of disease progression in arrhythmogenic right ventricular cardiomyopathy/dysplasia

Ardan M Saguner[1], Sabrina Ganahl[1], Andrea Kraus[2], Samuel H Baldinger[3], Deniz Akdis[1], Arhan R Saguner[1], Thomas Wolber[1,4], Laurent M Haegeli[1], Jan Steffel[1], Nazmi Krasniqi[1], Thomas F Lüscher[1,4], Felix C Tanner[1,4], Corinna Brunckhorst[1] and Firat Duru[1,4*]

Abstract

Background: Arrhythmogenic right ventricular cardiomyopathy/dysplasia (ARVC/D) is considered a progressive cardiomyopathy. However, data on the clinical features of disease progression are limited. The aim of this study was to assess 12-lead surface electrocardiographic (ECG) changes during long-term follow-up, and to compare these findings with echocardiographic data in our large cohort of patients with ARVC/D.

Methods: Baseline and follow-up ECGs of 111 patients from three tertiary care centers in Switzerland were systematically analyzed with digital calipers by two blinded observers, and correlated with findings from transthoracic echocardiography.

Results: The median follow-up was 4 years (IQR 1.9–9.2 years). ECG progression was significant for epsilon waves (baseline 14% vs. follow-up 31%, $p = 0.01$) and QRS duration (111 ms vs. 114 ms, $p = 0.04$). Six patients with repolarization abnormalities according to the 2010 Task Force Criteria at baseline did not display these criteria at follow-up, whereas in all patients with epsilon waves at baseline these depolarization abnormalities also remained at follow-up. T wave inversions in inferior leads were common (36% of patients at baseline), and were significantly associated with major repolarization abnormalities ($p = 0.02$), extensive echocardiographic right ventricular involvement ($p = 0.04$), T wave inversions in lateral precordial leads ($p = 0.05$), and definite ARVC/D ($p = 0.05$).

Conclusions: Our data supports the concept that ARVC/D is generally progressive, which can be detected by 12-lead surface ECG. Repolarization abnormalities may disappear during the course of the disease. Furthermore, the presence of T wave inversions in inferior leads is common in ARVC/D.

Keywords: Arrhythmogenic Right Ventricular, Cardiomyopathy, Dysplasia, Electrocardiography, T wave inversion

Background

Arrhythmogenic right ventricular cardiomyopathy/dysplasia (ARVC/D) is an inherited heart muscle disorder characterized by fibro-fatty infiltration of the right ventricle (RV) [1,2]. The disease is a common cause of sudden cardiac death among young adults and athletes [3-5]. ARVC/D can manifest with multiple facets ranging from primarily ventricular tachyarrhythmia to biventricular heart failure that may eventually lead to heart transplantation or cardiac death [6,7].

The diagnosis of ARVC/D according to the 2010 Task Force Criteria (TFC) is based on six categories with major and minor criteria in each. These categories comprise: 1. Global or regional dysfunction and structural alteration of the RV visualized by echocardiography, cardiac magnetic resonance tomography, or RV angiography 2. Tissue characterization of the RV free wall by endomyocardial biopsy 3. 12-lead surface electrocardiographic (ECG) repolarization abnormalities 4. ECG depolarization abnormalities 5. Ventricular tachyarrhythmias 6. Family history/genetic testing. The diagnosis is possible if 2 minor criteria

* Correspondence: firat.duru@usz.ch
[1]Department of Cardiology, University Heart Center Zurich, Rämistrasse 100, CH-8091 Zurich, Switzerland
[4]Center for Integrative Human Physiology, University Zurich, Zurich, Switzerland
Full list of author information is available at the end of the article

or 1 major criterion are present. It is borderline if 1 major and 1 minor or 3 minor criteria are present, and it is definite if 2 major or 1 major plus 2 minor or 4 minor criteria are present [6,7].

Recent data suggests that diagnostic features of ARVC/D such as epsilon waves and T wave inversions (TWI) may disappear on serial ECG evaluations during follow-up [8], although ARVC/D is generally considered an irreversible and progressive cardiomyopathy [9-11]. TWI in inferior leads have recently been proposed as valuable diagnostic and prognostic markers in this entity, but have not been incorporated in the TFC [12,13]. Whereas TWI in V1- V2 or in V4, V5, or V6 are a minor criterion for ARVC/D, epsilon waves constitute a major criterion owing to the fact that epsilon waves are rather specific for ARVC/D. Precordial TWI are more sensitive, but lack specificity as they are often present in other diseases such as ischemic or congenital heart disease. Moreover, precordial TWI in V1-V3 and inferior lead TWI can be observed in a minority of healthy probands [14]. Since data on clinical features of disease progression are limited, and correlations between inferior lead TWI and other diagnostic parameters have not been well defined in ARVC/D, the aim of this study was to identify associations between inferior lead TWI, other ECG variables, and echocardiographic findings, and to assess ECG changes during long-term follow-up in a large cohort of patients with ARVC/D [14-16].

Methods

Study population

The study population included 111 patients from three tertiary-care centers in Switzerland with a definite (n = 80), borderline (n = 19), and possible (n = 12, all first degree family members of patients with confirmed ARVC/D) diagnosis of ARVC/D according to the 2010 TFC, who had an ECG recorded between February 1987 and March 2013 [7]. This baseline ECG was the first available ECG. Clinical information regarding demographics and symptoms were obtained from hospital records at the time of the baseline ECG. Coronary ischemia was ruled out in the presence of precordial TWI. If patients with precordial TWI presented with typical angina, or were >35 years old and presented with ventricular tachycardia or arrhythmogenic syncope, coronary angiography was performed to rule out significant coronary artery disease. In all other patients noninvasive tests such as cardiac MRI, myocardial perfusion scintigraphy, stress TTE or treadmill stress testing were performed to rule out coronary ischemia. This study was approved by the Ethics Committee of the Canton of Zurich and the Ethics Committee of the Canton of Bern, Switzerland, and has been performed in accordance with the ethical standards laid down in the 1964 Declaration of Helsinki and its later amendments. Patients gave written informed consent for prospective inclusion in this study.

Definitions of 12-lead surface ECG and transthoracic echocardiography parameters

ECG and transthoracic echocardiography (TTE) definitions and criteria used in this study are presented in Table 1.

ECG analysis

ECGs were recorded at rest (25 mm/s, 10 mm/mV amplitude) with standard lead positions, digitized with a high-resolution scanner, and analyzed with a digital caliper (Iconico; screen caliper version 4.0; www.iconico.com) [15]. To increase the accuracy of measurements, all ECGs were enlarged four times. ECG intervals were measured in two consecutive sinus beats in each lead; the mean value of the two beats was used. If the difference between the two beats was >10 ms, then the mean of three beats was taken. Each ECG was independently analyzed by two blinded experienced readers. Differences in the interpretation of the ECG parameters were adjudicated by a third cardiologist, and a final conclusion was made by consensus. ECG variables were measured as previously described [13].

Transthoracic Echocardiography

Conventional M-mode, 2-D, and color Doppler echocardiography was performed in 111 patients at the time of the baseline ECG by experienced cardiologists according to guidelines [16,17]. Left ventricular (LV) involvement was diagnosed when regional wall motion abnormalities or a reduced ejection fraction (EF <50% by Simpson's biplane method) were present, and other causes were excluded [18]. Some ECG data from 90 patients and TTE data from 70 patients used in this study has been previously reported by our group [11,13]. While we focused on predictors of adverse outcome in these previous studies, the current study investigates ECG changes during long-term follow-up, and their associations with TTE findings. Thus, data on follow-up ECGs have not been previously reported by our group.

Statistical analysis

Continuous variables are presented as mean ± SD or median (with interquartile ranges, IQR), and were compared using a two-sided t-test or Mann–Whitney U-test, as appropriate. Categorical variables are reported as frequency (percentage) and compared between groups by Fisher's exact test or χ^2 –test of independence, as appropriate. Logistic univariate regression analysis was used to correlate between TWI in inferior leads as the response, and number of precordial leads with TWI as the explanatory variable. For comparison of ECG data between baseline and follow-up, we used the Wilcoxon signed-rank test for continuous variables, and Mc Nemar's test for categorical variables. A two-sided

Table 1 Definitions of electrocardiographic and echocardiographic parameters used in this study

Variables	Definitions
Epsilon wave (major depolarization criterion)	Distinct waves of small amplitude that occupy the ST segment in right precordial leads (V1-V3) and are distinct from the QRS complex
Terminal activation duration (minor depolarization criterion)	Longest value in V1 through V3 from the nadir of the S wave to the end of all depolarization
T wave inversion	Any T wave negativity
Inferior leads T wave inversion	Inverted T waves in 2 out of 3 inferior leads (II, III, and aVF)
Major repolarization criteria	Inverted T waves in right precordial leads (V1, V2, and V3) or beyond in individuals >14 years of age (in the absence of complete right bundle branch block)
Minor repolarization criteria	- Inverted T waves in leads V1 and V2 in individuals >14 years of age (in the absence of complete right bundle branch block) or in V4, V5, or V6
	- Inverted T waves in leads V1, V2, V3, and V4 in individuals >14 years of age in the presence of complete right bundle branch block
Complete right bundle branch block	QRSd ≥120 ms and:
	A1: R′ or r′ in V1 or V2
	A2: S duration > R duration in I and V6
	A3: S duration >40 ms in I and V6
	A4: R peak time >50 ms in V1 or V2
	a: A1 + A2
	b: A1+ A3
	c: A4+ (A2 or A3)
Incomplete right bundle branch block	QRS <120 ms and R peak time in V1 or V2 > 50 ms
QRS notching	Additional deflections/notches at the beginning of the QRS, on top of the R-wave, or in the nadir of the S-wave in the absence of bundle branch block
Left ventricular involvement	Echocardiographic documentation of LV wall motion abnormalities or a reduced ejection fraction (<50%) in the absence of other causes
Right ventricular regional wall motion abnormalities	Echocardiographic documentation of regional right ventricular akinesia/dyskinesia

p-value of ≤0.05 was considered significant. Statistical analysis was performed using R programming language (R Development Core Team, 2009) and GraphPad Prism 5 (GraphPad Software Inc., La Jolla, CA, USA).

Results

Baseline characteristics

Patient baseline characteristics are summarized in Table 2. A baseline ECG was available in 111 patients. TTE at the time of the baseline ECG was performed in all 111 patients. Ninety-eight patients were index patients, and 13 were family members. Sixty-four (58%) patients had an implantable cardioverter-defibrillator. ECG did not display abnormal findings in 14 patients (13%). Epsilon-waves were most frequently observed in V1 (14%). Epsilon-like waves in any lateral precordial lead (V4, V5, or V6) were present in a minority of patients (5%), with one patient displaying these potentials in V2 through V6. Complete right bundle branch block (RBBB) was observed in 14 (13%), incomplete RBBB in 3 (3%), complete left bundle branch block in 2 (2%), left anterior fascicular block in 7 (6%), and unspecific QRS notching in 29 (26%) patients. On echocardiography, regional wall motion abnormalities were most commonly observed in the RV subtricuspid region (n = 66; 60%).

12-lead ECG changes during follow-up

A follow-up ECG was available in 77 patients. In the remaining 34 patients, a follow-up ECG was not obtained due to short follow-up periods (n = 14) or loss of follow-up/heart transplantation/death (n = 20). The median time between baseline and follow-up ECG was 4 years (IQR 1.9-9.2 , range 0.3–21.8 , mean 5.6 years). The follow-up ECG was considered normal in 9 patients (12%). On average, ECG findings were progressive during follow-up, although individual disease course showed some variations. This progression was statistically significant for major depolarization criteria, which was

Table 2 Baseline characteristics

Patient characteristic	All patients (n = 111)
Male, n (%)	71 (64%)
Age at baseline ECG (years)	43 (30–56)
Systolic blood pressure (mmHg)	120 ± 19
Diastolic blood pressure (mmHg)	76 ± 9
Heart rate (bpm)	65 (57–74)
Body mass index (kg/m^2)	24.3 ± 3.2
Medication	
Amiodarone, n (%)	17 (15%)
Beta-blocker, n (%)	47 (42%)
Sotalol, n (%)	13 (12%)
12-lead surface ECG	
Epsilon waves in V1, V2, or V3	21 (19%)
Minor ECG depolarization criteria (2010 TFC)	25 (23%)
Terminal activation duration (ms)	52 (43–64)
Major ECG repolarization criteria (2010 TFC)	37 (33%)
Minor ECG repolarization criteria (2010 TFC)	21 (19%)
TWI in inferior leads	38 (34%)
TWI in V4, V5, or V6	43 (39%)
Number of leads with TWI	4.5 ± 2.5
Number of precordial leads with TWI	2.6 ± 1.9
QRS duration (ms)	111 (100–116)
Corrected QT duration (ms)	444 (426–480)
Transthoracic echocardiography	
Patients with RV regional wall motion abnormalities	85 (77%)
1 RV region involved	25 (23%)
≥2 RV regions involved	56 (50%)
Patients with LV involvement	15 (14%)

Abbreviations: *ARVC/D* Arrhythmogenic right ventricular cardiomyopathy/dysplasia, *LV* left ventricular, *RV* right ventricular, *TFC* 2010 Revised ARVC/D Task Force Criteria, *TWI* T wave inversions.
Values are means ± standard deviation, medians with interquartile ranges and numbers (percentages).

Table 3 ECG variables in 77 patients, in whom a baseline and follow-up 12-lead surface ECG was available

ECG variable	Baseline ECG	Follow-up ECG	p-value
Epsilon waves in V1, V2, or V3	11 (14%)	24 (31%)	0.01
Late potentials in inferior leads	6 (8%)	9 (12%)	0.45
Minor ECG depolarization criterion	21 (27%)	19 (25%)	0.56
Terminal activation duration (ms)	50 (44–64)	50 (45–60)	0.47
Major ECG repolarization criterion	29 (38%)	28 (36%)	0.58
Minor ECG repolarization criterion	14 (18%)	18 (23%)	0.55
T wave inversions in inferior leads	28 (36%)	31 (40%)	0.65
T wave inversions in V4, V5, or V6	33 (43%)	40 (52%)	0.25
Number of leads with T wave inversions	4 (2-6)	5 (2–7)	0.18
Number of precordial leads with T wave inversions	2 (1–4)	3 (1–5)	0.1
QRS duration (ms)	111 (100–125)	114 (100–128)	0.04
QT duration (ms)	431 (399–435)	420 (400–441)	0.57

Values are means ± standard deviation, medians with interquartile ranges and numbers (percentages).

particularly attributed to an increase in patients with epsilon waves in V2 at follow-up, and an increase in the maximum QRS duration (Table 3). More patients had TWI in the precordial leads at follow-up. Out of 8 patients without any precordial TWI at baseline, 4 (50%) later displayed precordial TWI. An illustrative diagram of electrocardiographic de- and repolarization abnormalities at baseline and their changes during follow-up is shown in Figure 1. Three patients with minor repolarization criteria at baseline did not have any repolarization criteria at follow-up. Four patients with major repolarization criteria at baseline had minor repolarization criteria in the absence of complete RBBB at follow-up (Figure 2), whereas two patients with major repolarization criteria displayed minor repolarization criteria in the presence of complete RBBB at follow-up. Repolarization criteria were completely absent in three patients, who had major repolarization criteria at baseline (Figure 3).

From the patients without epsilon waves at baseline, 19% had these abnormalities at follow-up. In all patients displaying epsilon waves at baseline these potentials also remained at follow-up. In one patient, follow-up ECG revealed a dynamic Brugada-like ECG pattern (Figure 4). Epsilon-like waves in V4, V5 or V6 were present in a higher proportion of patients at follow-up compared to baseline (9%). Median terminal activation duration (TAD) at follow-up was similar compared to baseline. An increase in the number of precordial leads with TWI was particularly attributed to new TWI in leads V4 and V5 at follow-up compared to baseline (49% vs. 36% for V4, and 38% vs. 26% for V5, respectively). At follow-up, complete RBBB was observed in 12 (16%), incomplete RBBB in 2 (3%), complete left bundle branch block in 2 (3%), left anterior fascicular block in 5 (6%), and unspecific QRS notching in 23 (30%) patients. The maximum corrected QT interval did not significantly differ between baseline and follow-up.

Transthoracic echocardiographic findings at follow-up

TTE data was available in all 77 patients at the time of the follow-up ECG. Echocardiographic data also indicated disease progression, and correlated with the ECG findings.

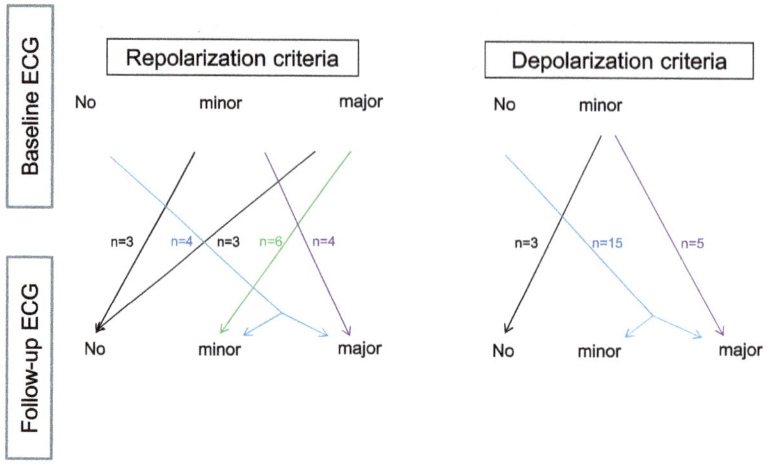

Figure 1 Illustrative diagram of changes in depolarization and repolarization criteria during follow-up in patients with ARVC/D. Patients not presented in this figure remained in the same category of depolarization and repolarization criteria at baseline and follow-up.

Accordingly, LV involvement was present in 20 patients at follow-up (26% vs. 14% at baseline, p = 0.04). At follow-up, 15 (19%) patients remained with only one RV region involved, whereas 48 patients (62%) had ≥2 RV regions involved (p = 0.14 compared to baseline).

Association between ECG and TTE findings

TWI in inferior leads were significantly associated with major repolarization criteria (p = 0.02), extensive RV involvement (p = 0.04), the presence of TWI in either lateral precordial lead (V4, V5 or V6; p = 0.05), and the

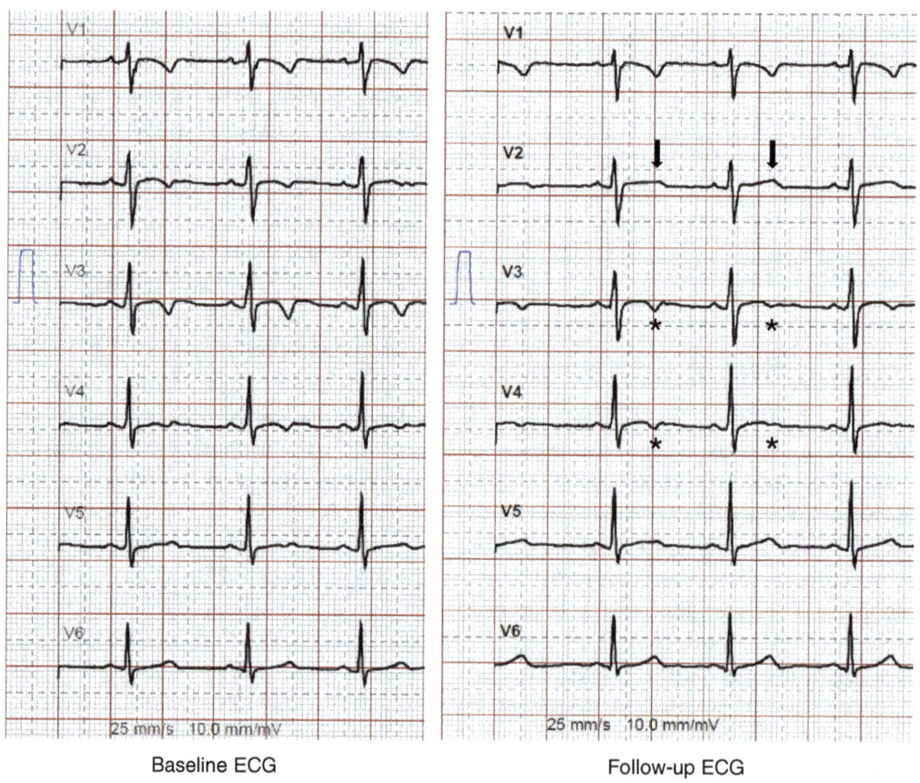

Figure 2 Representative 12-lead surface ECG (25 mm/s, 10 mm/mV) from a patient with ARVC/D displaying major repolarization 2010 task force criteria at baseline (left panel), and minor repolarization criteria (in the absence of complete RBBB) at follow-up due to normalization of T waves in lead V2 (black arrows, right panel). This variation may have been caused by slightly different fixation of V2, although R/S transition occurs in V3 in both ECGs. Also note the beat-to-beat variation of T wave morphology in leads V3 and V4 (asterisks).

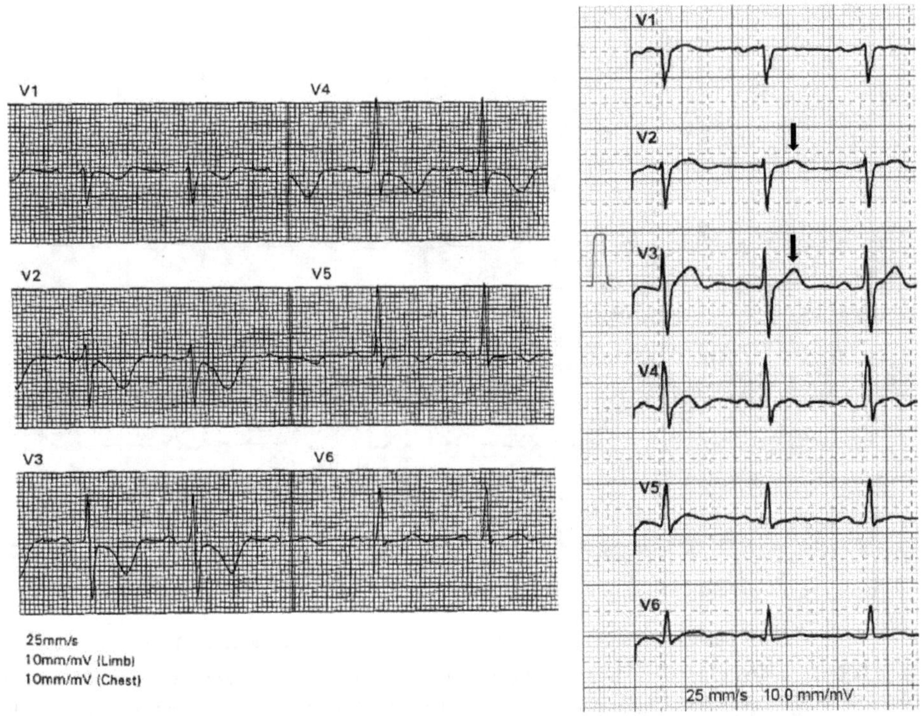

Figure 3 Representative 12-lead surface ECG (25 mm/s, 10 mm/mV) from a patient with ARVC/D and dynamic repolarization abnormalities, presumably T wave memory. The left panel shows major repolarization abnormalities according to the 2010 task force criteria at baseline, but no repolarization criteria at follow-up with normalization of T waves in leads V1-V5 (right panel, black arrows). This patient suffered from sustained ventricular tachycardia from the RV outflow tract, and imaging revealed akinesia of the RVOT corresponding to scar visualized by electroanatomical voltage mapping.

presence of definite ARVC/D (p = 0.05), whereas the presence of echocardiographic LV involvement (p = 0.11) did not reach statistical significance. Regional wall motion abnormalities of the subtricuspid region were not significantly associated with TWI in inferior leads (p = 0.16). Univariate logistic regression revealed a highly significant incremental association between the absolute number of precordial leads with TWI and TWI in inferior leads (odds ratio 1.45, 95% confidence interval 1.16 - 1.83, p = 0.001).

Discussion

This observational study constitutes the largest series investigating ECG changes during long-term follow-up in patients with ARVC/D, and has three main findings: First, our study supports the concept that ARVC/D is generally progressive in nature, and that surface 12-lead ECG is able to detect disease progression. Second, precordial T wave inversions may disappear during the disease course, whereas epsilon waves persist; and third, the presence of TWI in inferior leads is common.

Previous studies - disease progression

Except for one study [19], four previous studies have suggested that ECG changes are generally progressive in patients with ARVC/D. Yet, the extent and speed of disease progression shows some individual variability that may be based on genetic and environmental factors [9-11,20-22].

Previous studies – dynamic ECG changes

Recent data suggests that electrocardiographic diagnostic features of ARVC/D such as epsilon waves and TWI may be dynamic and transient [8], which may potentially impede appropriate diagnosis of ARVC/D at certain time points during the disease course, particularly at early stages.

Our findings

This study focused on patients with less advanced disease in comparison to previous studies analyzing data from patients with more advanced forms of ARVC/D, and underscores that disease progression can be visualized by consecutive ECG tracings, although the disease

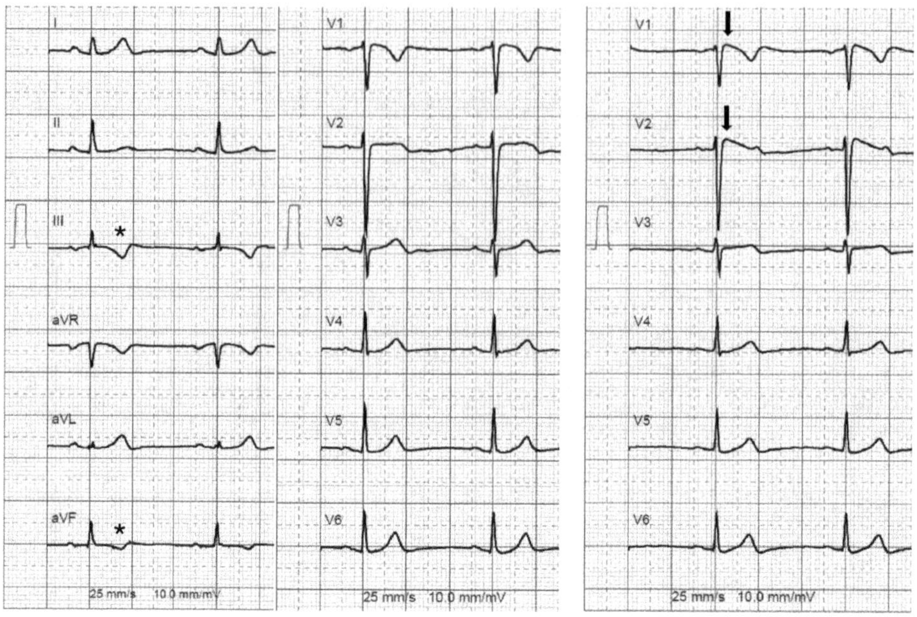

Figure 4 12-lead surface ECG (25 mm/s, 10 mm/mV) from a patient with ARVC/D and a dynamic Brugada-like ECG pattern (criteria for Brugada Type I ECG not fulfilled). The right panel shows a coved-type Brugada-like ECG in leads V1 and V2 at follow-up (black arrows), which is not visible at baseline (left panel). Also note the T wave inversions in the inferior leads (III and aVF) in the absence of repolarization criteria (asterisks).

course shows some individual variations. Importantly, the percentage of patients with epsilon waves and average QRS duration significantly increased over time, and the increase in the number of precordial leads with TWI showed a tendency towards significance. With regard to TWI, the percentage of patients with precordial TWI beyond V3 and TWI in inferior leads increased, and correlated well with more extensive echocardiographic RV involvement and new onset LV involvement at follow-up. ARVC/D has been recently recognized as a biventricular disease with early LV involvement [23]. With respect to this, repolarization abnormalities beyond V1-V3, but also inferior lead TWI may serve as early ECG markers of biventricular involvement and widespread disease. The fact that depolarization abnormalities appear to better reflect disease progression compared to TWI is not completely clear. It is possible that repolarization abnormalities are not only caused by structural myocardial changes, but may also constitute a physiological variant [14], may vary depending on exercise status of a given patient [24], be caused by prolonged bouts of paroxysmal tachyarrhythmia or frequent ventricular premature contractions, i.e. T wave memory [25], and subtle differences in positioning the precordial electrodes, i.e. ECG reproducibility [26]. Anatomic predisposition, particularly in women, may affect lead positioning, and thus alter the presence and distribution of leads with TWI (Figure 3). Of note, in this study all four patients with major repolarization criteria at baseline, who presented with minor repolarization criteria in the absence of complete RBBB at follow-up, were women [8]. We were also able to document a dynamic Brugada-like ECG pattern in leads V1/V2 in one patient, as previously reported, although the criteria for Brugada Type I ECG were not fulfilled in the absence of J-point elevation ≥2 mm and TWI in V2 [27,28]. Interestingly, this patient was one out of 13, in whom TWI in inferior leads were documented in the absence of major and minor repolarization criteria (34% of patients with TWI in inferior leads). In contrast to the study by Quarta et al. [8], dynamic ECG changes in our study primarily originated from changes in repolarization rather than depolarization abnormalities. Furthermore, as opposed to that previous study, all three patients with major repolarization criteria at baseline and absence of any repolarization criteria at follow-up had advanced forms of ARVC/D, suggesting that dynamic repolarization abnormalities may not only affect early forms of the disease.

Based on our data, depolarization abnormalities seem to be far less prone to reversal, because they probably better reflect myocardial infiltration by fibro-fatty tissue. This interpretation is further supported by our data on QRS duration, which also significantly increased during follow-up. As the proportion of patients with antiarrhythmic medication were not significantly different at baseline and follow-up, and TAD did not change over time, this increase can be attributed to a progression in depolarization abnormalities also affecting early depolarization such as bundle branch block and QRS notching. As such, the percentage of patients with RBBB and QRS notching increased during follow-up.

TWI in inferior leads

The presence of TWI in lateral leads in patients with ARVC/D is well established, and a noninvasive indicator of biventricular involvement and severe RV dilation [29-32]. However, data about TWI in inferior leads in ARVC/D is scarce and their role not completely understood. Whereas most studies support the concept that TWI in inferior leads are a marker of progressive disease with extensive RV involvement and LV involvement [31,32], other studies suggest that such ECG changes could also be associated with isolated wall motion abnormalities of the subtricuspid region. Steriotis et al. have recently reported a considerable prevalence of TWI in inferior leads in ARVC/D, particularly in the presence of severe RV dilation, but did not report on the prevalence of LV involvement in their cohort. Our study confirms these previous findings with more than one third of patients displaying TWI in inferior leads at baseline – far more than depolarization abnormalities in these leads. We further add to the concept that inferior lead TWI in ARVC/D are associated with extensive disease as reflected by a significant association with definite disease status, extensive RV involvement, and TWI in lateral precordial leads, and a tendency towards significance for LV involvement. On the contrary, we did not observe a significant association between inferior lead TWI and isolated regional wall motion abnormalities of the subtricuspid region. TWI in inferior leads could even constitute markers for widespread biventricular disease, especially in the presence of major repolarization abnormalities implying that TWI in inferior leads may have a rather non-benign character. Based on our findings, we believe that ECGs obtained once yearly can serve as an informative, cheap and readily available monitoring tool. In case of progressive ECG findings, further more expensive diagnostic tests such as echocardiography, cardiac MRI or Holter monitoring can be performed, and follow-up strategies can be refined. In the absence of ECG changes and a clinical deterioration during follow-up, in our routine clinical practice we perform TTE every 2 years, and cardiac MRI every 2–5 years to monitor disease progression. Yet, as an isolated diagnostic test ECG may not drive therapy per se, and ECG findings have to be incorporated in the whole clinical picture, especially when arrhythmic episodes are lacking. Accordingly, as a sole diagnostic method, ECG is not sensitive and specific enough to establish the diagnosis of ARVC/D. Therefore, other diagnostic tests including imaging (e.g. cardiac MRI with stress testing), genetic testing, family history and endomyocardial biopsy are necessary and required by the TFC. Since TWI in the precordial leads are not very specific for ARVC/D, e.g. are commonly seen in patients suffering from coronary artery disease immediately after a coronary ischemic episode, and can persist for several weeks thereafter, it is important to exclude coronary ischemia by diagnostic tests such as coronary angiography or cardiac MRI.

Limitations

Due to the observational and partially retrospective nature of this study, echocardiographic data was mainly obtained from previous reports. The duration of individual follow-up and lack of a follow-up ECG in some patients is a limitation that may have led to an underestimation of ECG changes. Variable ECG filtering may have affected the detection of epsilon waves, but not the detection of TWI, which was the main reversible ECG feature found in our cohort. Due to the retrospective study design our ECGs did not include right-sided chest leads (V1R, V2R, V3R, V4R), which could be included in future prospective studies investigating the diagnostic and prognostic utility of ECG in ARVC/D. Baseline and follow-up cardiac MRI were only available in a minority of patients, and thus associations between ECG and MRI findings could not be addressed in this study.

Conclusions

This study supports the concept that ARVC/D is generally progressive, which can be detected by 12-lead surface ECG. Repolarization abnormalities may disappear during the course of the disease. Furthermore, the presence of TWI in inferior leads is common. Our findings support the use of 12-lead surface ECG to monitor disease progression in ARVC/D.

Competing interests

The authors declare that they have no competing interests.

Authors' contributions

AMS: concept/design, data collection and analysis/interpretation/drafting article/statistics/approval of the submitted and final versions. SG: concept/design, data analysis/revising article critically/data collection/approval of the submitted and final versions. AK: concept/design, data analysis/statistics/revising article critically/approval of the submitted and final versions. SHB: data collection/revising article critically/approval of the submitted and final versions. DA: design/ revising article critically/approval of the submitted and final versions. ARS: data collection/revising article critically/approval of the submitted and final versions. TW: interpretation of data, revising article critically/approval of the submitted and final versions. LMH: interpretation of data, revising article critically/approval of the submitted and final versions. JS: interpretation of data, revising article critically/approval of the submitted and final versions. NK: interpretation of data, revising article critically/approval of the submitted and final versions. TFL: funding secured, interpretation of data, revising article critically/approval of the submitted and final versions. FCT: data collection, revising article critically/approval of the submitted and final versions. CB: funding secured, interpretation of data, revising article critically/approval of the submitted and final versions. FD: concept/design, funding secured, data collection and interpretation/drafting article/approval of the submitted and final versions. All authors read and approved the final manuscript.

Acknowledgements
This work is supported by a grant from the Georg and Bertha Schwyzer-Winiker Foundation, Zurich, Switzerland.

Author details
[1]Department of Cardiology, University Heart Center Zurich, Rämistrasse 100, CH-8091 Zurich, Switzerland. [2]Division of Biostatistics, Institute for Social and Preventive Medicine, University Zurich, Zurich, Switzerland. [3]Department of Cardiology, University Hospital Bern, Bern, Switzerland. [4]Center for Integrative Human Physiology, University Zurich, Zurich, Switzerland.

References

1. Herren T, Gerber PA, Duru F. Arrhythmogenic right ventricular cardiomyopathy/dysplasia: a not so rare "disease of the desmosome" with multiple clinical presentations. Clin Res Cardiol. 2009;98:141–58.
2. Azaouagh A, Churzidse S, Konorza T, Erbel R. Arrhythmogenic right ventricular cardiomyopathy/dysplasia: a review and update. Clin Res Cardiol. 2011;100:383–94.
3. Fontaine G, Fontaliran F, Hebert JL, Chemla D, Zenati O, Lecarpentier Y, et al. Arrhythmogenic right ventricular dysplasia. Annu Rev Med. 1999;50:17–35.
4. Basso C, Calabrese F, Corrado D, Thiene G. Postmortem diagnosis in sudden cardiac death victims: macroscopic, microscopic and molecular findings. Cardiovasc Res. 2001;50:290–300.
5. Kim C, Wong J, Wen J, Wang S, Wang C, Spiering S, et al. Studying arrhythmogenic right ventricular dysplasia with patient-specific iPSCs. Nature. 2013;494:105–10.
6. Fontaine GH. The multiple facets of right ventricular cardiomyopathies. Eur Heart J. 2011;32:1049–51.
7. Marcus FI, McKenna WJ, Sherrill D, Basso C, Bauce B, Bluemke DA, et al. Diagnosis of arrhythmogenic right ventricular cardiomyopathy/dysplasia: proposed modification of the Task Force Criteria. Eur Heart J. 2010;31:806–14.
8. Quarta G, Ward D, Tome Esteban MT, Pantazis A, Elliott PM, Volpe M, et al. Dynamic electrocardiographic changes in patients with arrhythmogenic right ventricular cardiomyopathy. Heart. 2010;96:516–22.
9. Jaoude SA, Leclercq JF, Coumel P. Progressive ECG changes in arrhythmogenic right ventricular disease. Evidence for an evolving disease. Eur Heart J. 1996;17:1717–22.
10. Nava A, Folino AF, Bauce B, Turrini P, Buja GF, Daliento L, et al. Signal-averaged electrocardiogram in patients with arrhythmogenic right ventricular cardiomyopathy and ventricular arrhythmias. Eur Heart J. 2000;21:58–65.
11. Saguner AM, Vecchiati A, Baldinger SH, Rueger S, Medeiros-Domingo A, Mueller-Burri AS, et al. Different Prognostic Value of Functional Right Ventricular Parameters in Arrhythmogenic Right Ventricular Cardiomyopathy/Dysplasia. Circ Cardiovasc Imaging. 2014;7(2):230–9.
12. Jain R, Dalal D, Daly A, Tichnell C, James C, Evenson A, et al. Electrocardiographic features of arrhythmogenic right ventricular dysplasia. Circulation. 2009;120:477–87.
13. Saguner AM, Ganahl S, Baldinger SH, Kraus A, Medeiros-Domingo A, Nordbeck S, et al. Usefulness of electrocardiographic parameters for risk prediction in arrhythmogenic right ventricular dysplasia. Am J Cardiol. 2014;113:1728–34.
14. Aro AL, Anttonen O, Tikkanen JT, Junttila MJ, Kerola T, Rissanen HA, et al. Prevalence and prognostic significance of T-wave inversions in right precordial leads of a 12-lead electrocardiogram in the middle-aged subjects. Circulation. 2012;125:2572–7.
15. Roten L, Derval N, Sacher F, Pascale P, Scherr D, Komatsu Y, et al. Heterogeneous response of J-wave syndromes to beta-adrenergic stimulation. Heart Rhythm. 2012;9:1970–6.
16. Lang RM, Bierig M, Devereux RB, Flachskampf FA, Foster E, Pellikka PA, et al. Recommendations for chamber quantification. Eur J Echocardiogr. 2006;7:79–108.
17. Schuler PK, Haegeli LM, Saguner AM, Wolber T, Tanner FC, Jenni R, et al. Predictors of appropriate ICD therapy in patients with arrhythmogenic right ventricular cardiomyopathy: long term experience of a tertiary care center. PLoS One. 2012;7:e39584.
18. Lemola K, Brunckhorst C, Helfenstein U, Oechslin E, Jenni R, Duru F. Predictors of adverse outcome in patients with arrhythmogenic right ventricular dysplasia/cardiomyopathy: long term experience of a tertiary care centre. Heart. 2005;91:1167–72.
19. Metzger JT, de Chillou C, Cheriex E, Rodriguez LM, Smeets JL, Wellens HJ. Value of the 12-lead electrocardiogram in arrhythmogenic right ventricular dysplasia, and absence of correlation with echocardiographic findings. Am J Cardiol. 1993;72:964–7.
20. Xu T, Yang Z, Vatta M, Rampazzo A, Beffagna G, Pilichou K, et al. Compound and digenic heterozygosity contributes to arrhythmogenic right ventricular cardiomyopathy. J Am Coll Cardiol. 2010;55:587–97.
21. James CA, Bhonsale A, Tichnell C, Murray B, Russell SD, Tandri H, et al. Exercise increases age-related penetrance and arrhythmic risk in arrhythmogenic right ventricular dysplasia/cardiomyopathy-associated desmosomal mutation carriers. J Am Coll Cardiol. 2013;62:1290–7.
22. Rigato I, Bauce B, Rampazzo A, Zorzi A, Pilichou K, Mazzotti E, et al. Compound and digenic heterozygosity predicts lifetime arrhythmic outcome and sudden cardiac death in desmosomal gene-related arrhythmogenic right ventricular cardiomyopathy. Circ Cardiovasc Genet. 2013;6:533–42.
23. Saguner AM, Duru F, Brunckhorst CB. Arrhythmogenic right ventricular cardiomyopathy: a challenging disease of the intercalated disc. Circulation. 2013;128:1381–6.
24. Zorzi A, ElMaghawry M, Rigato I, Cardoso Bianchini F, Crespi Ponta G, Michieli P, et al. Exercise-induced normalization of right precordial negative T waves in arrhythmogenic right ventricular cardiomyopathy. Am J Cardiol. 2013;112:411–5.
25. Patberg KW, Shvilkin A, Plotnikov AN, Chandra P, Josephson ME, Rosen MR. Cardiac memory: mechanisms and clinical implications. Heart Rhythm. 2005;2:1376–82.
26. Lehmann MH, Katona AM. Proposed bedside maneuver to facilitate accurate anatomic orientation for correct positioning of ECG precordial leads V1 and V2: a pilot study. J Emerg Med. 2012;43:584–92.
27. Corrado D, Basso C, Buja G, Nava A, Rossi L, Thiene G. Right bundle branch block, right precordial st-segment elevation, and sudden death in young people. Circulation. 2001;103:710–7.
28. Schmidt T, Gerckens U, Ortmeyer D, Bootsveld A, Lampe E, Grube E. [Brugada syndrome or ARVD (arrhythmogenic right ventricular dysplasia) or both? Significance and value of right precordial ECG changes]. Z Kardiol. 2002;91:416–22.
29. Nava A, Canciani B, Buja G, Martini B, Daliento L, Scognamiglio R, et al. Electrovectorcardiographic study of negative T waves on precordial leads in arrhythmogenic right ventricular dysplasia: relationship with right ventricular volumes. J Electrocardiol. 1988;21:239–45.
30. Peters S, Peters H, Thierfelder L. Risk stratification of sudden cardiac death and malignant ventricular arrhythmias in right ventricular dysplasia-cardiomyopathy. Int J Cardiol. 1999;71:243–50.
31. Corrado D, Basso C, Thiene G, McKenna WJ, Davies MJ, Fontaliran F, et al. Spectrum of clinicopathologic manifestations of arrhythmogenic right ventricular cardiomyopathy/dysplasia: a multicenter study. J Am Coll Cardiol. 1997;30:1512–20.
32. Steriotis AK, Bauce B, Daliento L, Rigato I, Mazzotti E, Folino AF, et al. Electrocardiographic pattern in arrhythmogenic right ventricular cardiomyopathy. Am J Cardiol. 2009;103:1302–8.

11

Myocardial fibrosis as the first sign of cardiac involvement in a male patient with Fabry disease: report of a clinical case and discussion on the utility of the magnetic resonance in Fabry pathology

Annalisa Sechi[1*], Gaetano Nucifora[2], Gianluca Piccoli[3], Andrea Dardis[1] and Bruno Bembi[1]

Abstract

Background: Cardiovascular magnetic resonance (CMR) with late gadolinium enhancement (LGE) imaging is increasingly used to assess myocardial involvement in patients with Fabry disease, an X linked lipid storage disorder. However, it is often proposed as an optional tool. A different cardiomyopathic disease progression between male and female patients was hypothesised in previous studies, as in female myocardial fibrosis was found without left ventricular (LV) hypertrophy, while myocardial fibrosis was always detected in association to LV hypertrophy in men.

Case presentation: A male Caucasian patient, 19 years old, diagnosed through a family-based molecular screening, presented with LGE of the LV inferolateral wall evidenced at the CMR, without LV hypertrophy, or other clinical signs of the disease.

Conclusion: This is the first report of cardiac fibrosis as the first sign of organ involvement in a male patient with Fabry disease. This finding stresses the importance of performing CMR with LGE imaging for the initial staging and monitoring of Fabry patients of both genders.

Keywords: Fabry disease, Cardiovascular magnetic resonance, Myocardial fibrosis, Late gadolinium enhancement

Background

Fabry disease is an X linked lysosomal storage disorder, characterised by the deficient activity of the enzyme α-galactosidase A, involved in the catabolism of glycosphingolipids. This enzymatic defect results in the accumulation of globotrialosylceramide within the cells, particularly in cardiomyocytes, kidney, neural and vascular endothelial cells, causing a progressive systemic disease, which can lead to severe cardiac, renal, and cerebrovascular complications [1]. Heterozygous females may become as severely affected as males, although generally at a later age [2]. In males the diagnosis is made by the demonstration of α-gal deficiency in leukocytes and/or by the identification of pathogenic mutations in the α-galactosidase gene (*GLA*, Xq22.1 region). In heterozygous females, the enzymatic activity is not a reliable test, due to random X-chromosome inactivation, rendering DNA sequencing of the *GLA* gene the only reliable test for the diagnosis confirmation in females. Once the GLA mutation is identified, a screening within the family is indicated in order to detect Fabry patients at an early stage [3], when the disease seems to be more responsive to the specific enzyme replacement therapy (ERT) [4,5].

Cardiac involvement in Fabry disease includes arrhythmias, ischemia, and cardiomyopathy and is associated with increased morbidity and mortality in both male and female patients [6]. Left ventricular (LV) hypertrophy is considered the most common cardiologic finding [1]. Studies using cardiovascular magnetic resonance (CMR), demonstrated that myocardial fibrosis, detected with late

* Correspondence: sechi.annalisa@aoud.sanita.fvg.it
[1]Regional Coordinator Centre for Rare Diseases, University Hospital Santa Maria della Misericordia, Udine, Italy
Full list of author information is available at the end of the article

gadolinium enhancement (LGE), is also part of the natural history of Fabry disease [7,8]. A recent cardiovascular imaging research on patients with Fabry disease, showed a different cardiomyopathic involvement between male and female subjects: myocardial fibrosis was always detected in association to LV hypertrophy in men, while in females LGE was found even with normal LV thickness [9].

As far as we know, this is the first report of cardiac fibrosis as the first sign of organ involvement in a male patient with Fabry disease.

Case presentation

A 19 years old boy was diagnosed with Fabry disease through a family-based molecular screening, demonstrating the presence of the R112H mutation in the *GLA* gene. The diagnosis was further confirmed by the assessment of enzymatic α-gal activity in leucocytes, which resulted undetectable. Subsequently, he was admitted for a global screening of disease clinical manifestations although, at the time of diagnosis, he appeared completely asymptomatic. His neurological and general examination, including cardiac auscultation, were unremarkable. Biochemical tests (including 24 h microalbuminuria, proteinuria and creatinine clearance), ophthalmologic assessment, audiometry, pulmonary function tests, brain and kidney magnetic resonance imaging did not show any abnormality.

For the cardiac assessment he underwent first transthoracic echocardiography, 12-lead electrocardiogram, 24-hour Holter recording, and bicycle stress test, all resulting normal. Finally CMR with LGE imaging was performed; cine images (steady-state free precession) confirmed normal biventricular size and systolic function and normal LV wall thickness (Figure 1A-B). No signal alterations were detected on black-blood T1-weighted fast spin-echo imaging and T2-weighted short TI inversion recovery imaging (Figure 1C-E). Conversely, delayed enhancement imaging performed 10 minutes after injection of Gadolium chelate contrast agent showed LGE of the LV inferolateral wall with intramyocardial distribution (Figure 1F-G). Of note, despite the absence of LV wall motion abnormalities, feature-tracking analysis of cine LV mid short-axis slice demonstrated reduced circumferential strain of the mid inferolateral wall (Figure 2).

Considering the male gender and the evidence of a cardiac involvement, ERT treatment with recombinant agalsidase alfa was started and administered intravenously at the standard dosage of 0.2 mg/kg every other week, without side effects. After 12 months of ERT cardiological assessment including ECG, echocardiography and CMR was repeated, showing no changes compared to baseline (Figure 3); in particular LGE of the LV inferolateral wall was still observed and unchanged (Figure 3C-D).

Discussion

To our knowledge this is the first case reported so far, which demonstrates the presence of LGE without LV hypertrophy in a male affected by Fabry disease. Nevertheless, few CMR studies on Fabry patients have been published until now. Indeed, in the international consensus guidelines for Fabry disease, CMR is not included among the recommended exams for the basal evaluation

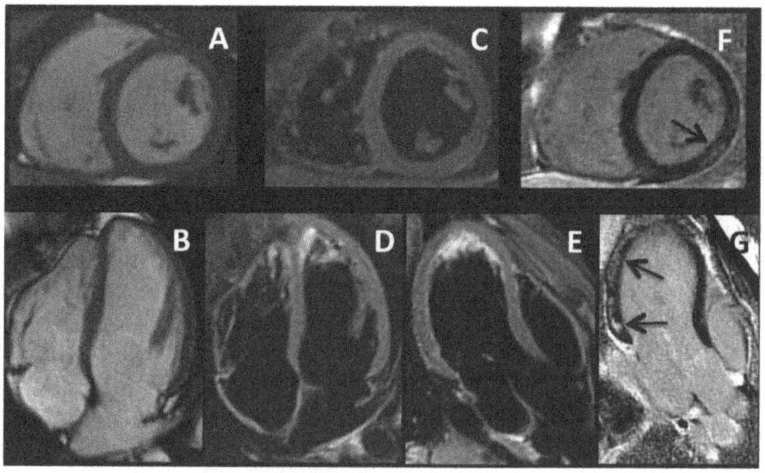

Figure 1 Cine and late gadolinium enhancement (LGE) CMR images of the patient at baseline. Panel **A** and **B**: cine (steady-state free precession sequence) CMR of short-axis **(A)** and 4-chamber **(B)** view showing normal left ventricular wall thickness. Panel **C**, **D** and **E**: T2-weighted short-TI inversion-recovery fast spin-echo image of short-axis **(C)**, 4-chamber **(D)** and 3-chamber **(E)** view showing the absence of myocardial oedema. Panel **F** and **G**: contrast-enhanced inversion recovery gradient echo image of short-axis **(F)** and 3-chamber **(G)** view showing LGE involving the inferolateral wall with intramyocardial distribution (black arrow).

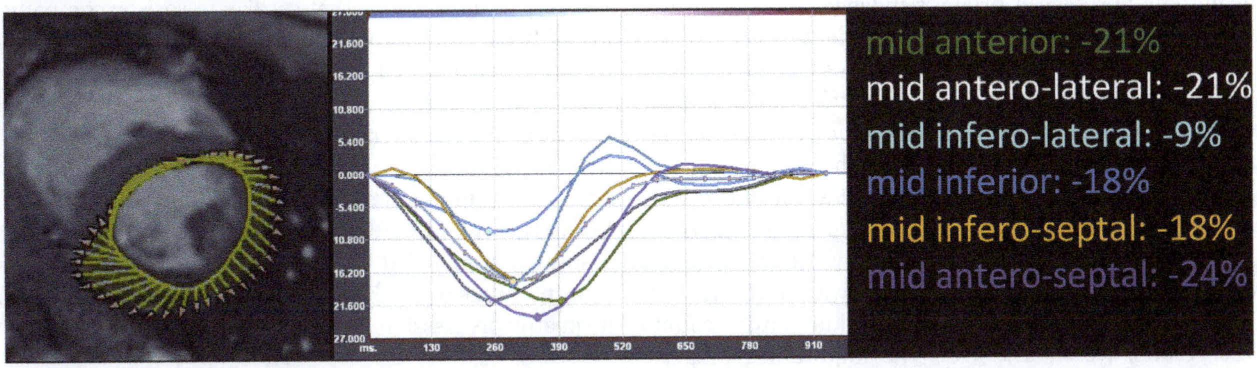

Figure 2 Feature-tracking analysis. 2D Cardiac Performance Analysis Software (TomTec, Munich, Germany) was used to measure LV deformation directly from cine CMR images (left panel). Feature-tracking analysis of cine LV mid short-axis slice demonstrated reduced circumferential strain of the mid infero-lateral wall (pale blue line in the right panel).

and monitoring of cardiac complications and therefore it is not routinely performed [3,10,11].

In 2003 Moon and colleagues first reported CMR findings in 18 male and 8 female patients with Fabry disease, describing LGE in 9/18 males and 4/8 females. In 92% of patients LGE occurred in the basal inferolateral wall, with intramyocardial pattern. Two male patients with severe LV hypertrophy had additional hyperenhancement in other myocardial sites. One female patient with LGE had normal echocardiography [7].

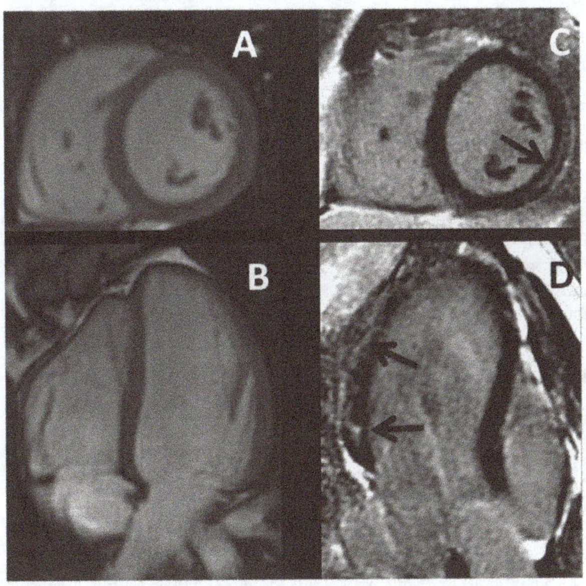

Figure 3 Cine and late gadolinium enhancement (LGE) CMR images of the patient, acquired after 12 months of ERT. Panel **A** and **B**: cine (steady-state free precession sequence) CMR of short-axis **(A)** and 4-chamber **(B)** view showing normal left ventricular wall thickness. Panel **C** and **D**: contrast-enhanced inversion recovery gradient echo image of short-axis **(C)** and 3-chamber **(D)** view showing LGE involving the inferolateral wall with intramyocardial distribution (black arrow), without significant changes from baseline examination (Figure 1).

In 2005 Weidemann and colleagues published a further cardiac imaging study (using echocardiography, strain rate imaging, and CMR) on 39 Fabry patients, finding LGE in 12 of them (2 females and 10 males). The inferolateral wall was confirmed as the typical LGE location. All subjects, of both genders, had also LV hypertrophy associated to LGE. All patients with LGE had severely reduced radial and longitudinal function. One patient with LGE died and histology confirmed fibrotic tissue in the inferolateral wall [8].

Recently, Niemann and colleagues published a large CMR study, including 104 patients (58 females and 46 males) with genetically proven Fabry disease. LGE was detected in 33% (n.19) of females and 48% (n.22) of males. Sixty-eight % of these patients showed LGE in the typical basal lateral location. Interestingly, 10 female patients without LV hypertrophy already presented LGE positive segments, while LGE was not found in male patients with LV thickness < 12 mm. Based on these results, the authors concluded that cardiomyopathy disease progression in Fabry disease differs between male and female patients, only the latter showing fibrosis before hypertrophy [9].

On the contrary, our findings suggest that LGE can be the first sign of cardiomyopathy even in male patients. It is possible that LGE without LV hypertrophy has never been found in males affected by Fabry disease because only few patients have been studied with CMR until now and most of them, being older than the patient reported here (i.e. 46 ± 12 years in the study by Niemann), had already developed both LV hypertrophy and fibrosis at the time of the study. Since the proposed temporal sequence of Fabry cardiomyopathy (increasing wall thickness➔ replacement fibrosis) [8] is not always present even in men, further pathogenetic studies are needed to explain why fibrosis can progress independently from the development of hypertrophy in Fabry patients.

It is worth noting that our case, as well as 11 females already reported [9,7], did not manifest any cardiac symptom and had no wall motion abnormalities at the echocardiography but showed LGE at the CMR, suggesting that conventional assessment is not sufficient to detect subtle cardiac abnormalities. Our patient and 7/10 female with isolated LGE described by Niemann et al were diagnosed by genetic screening within the family after the identification of a proband. Taking into account these results, we should stress the importance to perform CMR to stage and monitor Fabry cardiomyopathy, after diagnosis in both genders, even in apparently asymptomatic patients with a normal echocardiogram. CMR can be also fundamental in the diagnostic process of patients evaluated for cardiomyopathy, as LGE in the midmyocardium of the basal-inferolateral wall seems to be characteristic of Fabry disease [12]. It should be acknowledged that LGE in the midmyocardium of the basal-inferolateral wall can also be observed in other pathologies, including previous myocarditis [13]. In our patient, however, history of symptoms suggestive of remote myocarditis was negative. Moreover, recently, non contrast T1 mapping by CMR has been proposed by Thompson et al. as a tool to distinguish LV hypertrophy do to Fabry disease, from other causes. In fact, septal T1 was found to be lower in Fabry patients compared with healthy controls and patients with similar patterns of LV hypertrophy, probably reflecting glycosphingolipids accumulation. The authors concluded that reduced non-contrast myocardial T1 values are the most sensitive and specific cardiovascular MRI parameter in patients with Fabry disease irrespective of sex and LV morphology and function [14]. Unfortunately this technique is not available at our hospital.

Of note, feature-tracking analysis of cine LV mid short-axis slice demonstrated reduced circumferential strain of myocardial segment presenting LGE, despite the absence of LV wall motion abnormalities; this underlines the utility of myocardial deformation imaging techniques (including speckle-tracking echocardiography, tagged-CMR and feature-tracking CMR) for the identification of subtle changes of myocardial function which cannot be detected with conventional measures such as qualitative wall motion assessment [15].

Cardiac fibrosis is considered a negative prognostic factor towards ERT response in patients who already show LV hypertrophy [16], and an increased amount of LGE (from 0.5 to 7.1%) after 12 months of ERT has been reported [17]. To date, no data are available on the effect of ERT in patients with isolated cardiac fibrosis. Our patient did not show any LGE change after one year of ERT treatment at the CMR assessment. Therefore, it is possible to hypothesise that cardiac fibrosis accompanied by LV hypertrophy would be a sign of a late stage cardiac disease, which rapidly progresses despite ERT. Instead, when cardiac fibrosis appears early in a non-hypertrophic myocardium, it may have a more favourable response to treatment. However, we do not know what would have been the natural course of fibrosis in our patient without ERT. Further CMR studies on large cohorts and long term follow up are needed to assess whether ERT initiated before the onset of LV hypertrophy can prevent the cardiomyopathy progression.

Conclusions

The development of myocardial fibrosis does not necessarily require myocardial hypertrophy in both male and female patients with Fabry disease. CMR should be included in the routing diagnostic assessment and follow-up monitoring of all Fabry patients.

Consent

Written informed consent was obtained from the patient for publication of this Case report and any accompanying images. A copy of the written consent is available for review by the Editor of this journal.

Abbreviations

ERT: Enzyme replacement therapy; LV: Left ventricle; CMR: Cardiovascular magnetic resonance; LGE: Late gadolinium enhancement.

Competing interests

The authors declare that they have no competing interests.

Authors' contributions

AS was the primary physician during patient's first assessment and follow up, conceived the report and drafted the manuscript. GN provided cardiology supervision during scanning, and helped to draft the manuscript. GP assisted in image acquisition and interpretation and helped to draft the manuscript. AD performed the enzymatic and genetic tests and critically reviewed the manuscript. BB provided additional supervision and critically reviewed the manuscript. All authors read and approved the final manuscript.

Acknowledgments

The authors would like to thank all the staff of the Regional Coordinator Centre for Rare Diseases of Udine for their assistance.

Author details

[1]Regional Coordinator Centre for Rare Diseases, University Hospital Santa Maria della Misericordia, Udine, Italy. [2]Cardiothoracic Department, University Hospital Santa Maria della Misericordia, Udine, Italy. [3]Department of Diagnostic Imaging, University Hospital Santa Maria della Misericordia, Udine, Italy.

References

1. Desnick R, Ioannou Y, Eng C: **Alpha-Galactosidase A deficiency: Fabry disease.** In *The Metabolic and Molecular Bases of Inherited Disease.* 8th edition. Edited by Scriver CR BA, Sly WS, Valle D. New York: McGraw-Hill; 2001:3733–3774.
2. Deegan PB, Baehner AF, Barba Romero MA, Hughes DA, Kampmann C, Beck M, European FOS Investigators: **Natural history of Fabry disease in females in the Fabry Outcome Survey.** *J Med Genet* 2006, **43:**347–352.

3. Martins AM, D'Almeida V, Kyosen SO, Takata ET, Delgado AG, Gonçalves AM, Benetti Filho CC, Martini Filho D, Biagini G, Pimentel H, Abensur H, Guimarães HC, Gomes JG, Sobral Neto J, D'Almeida LO, Carvalho LR, Harouche MB, Maldonado MC, Nascimento OJ, Montoril PS, Bastos RV: **Guidelines to diagnosis and monitoring of Fabry disease and review of treatment experiences.** *J Pediatr* 2009, **155**(4 Suppl):S19–S31.
4. Breunig F, Weidemann F, Strotmann J, Knoll A, Wanner C: **Clinical benefit of enzyme replacement therapy in Fabry disease.** *Kidney Int* 2006, **69:**1216–1221.
5. Engelen MA, Brand E, Baumeister TB, Marquardt T, Duning T, Osada N, Schaefer RM, Stypmann J: **Effects of enzyme replacement therapy in adult patients with Fabry disease on cardiac structure and function: a retrospective cohort study of the Fabry Munster Study (FaMuS) data.** *BMJ Open* 2012, **21:**2(6).
6. Mehta A, Clarke JT, Giugliani R, Elliott P, Linhart A, Beck M, Sunder-Plassmann G, FOS Investigators: **Natural course of Fabry disease: changing pattern of causes of death in FOS - Fabry Outcome Survey.** *J Med Genet* 2009, **46:**548–552.
7. Moon JC, Sachdev B, Elkington AG, McKenna WJ, Mehta A, Pennell DJ, Leed PJ, Elliott PM: **Gadolinium enhanced cardiovascular magnetic resonance in Anderson-Fabry disease. Evidence for a disease specific abnormality of the myocardial interstitium.** *Eur Heart J* 2003, **24:**2151–2155.
8. Weidemann F, Breunig F, Beer M, Sandstede J, Störk S, Voelker W, Ertl G, Knoll A, Wanner C, Strotmann JM: **The variation of morphological and functional cardiac manifestation in Fabry disease: potential implications for the time course of the disease.** *Eur Heart J* 2005, **26:**1221–1227.
9. Niemann M, Herrmann S, Hu K, Breunig F, Strotmann J, Beer M, Machann W, Voelker W, Ertl G, Wanner C, Weidemann F: **Differences in Fabry cardiomyopathy between female and male patients: consequences for diagnostic assessment.** *JACC Cardiovasc Imaging* 2011, **4:**592–601.
10. Desnick RJ, Brady R, Barranger J, Collins AJ, Germain DP, Goldman M, Grabowski G, Packman S, Wilcox WR: **Fabry disease, an under-recognized multisystemic disorder: expert recommendations for diagnosis, management, and enzyme replacement therapy.** *Ann Intern Med* 2003, **138:**338–346.
11. Eng CM, Germain DP, Banikazemi M, Warnock DG, Wanner C, Hopkin RJ, Bultas J, Lee P, Sims K, Brodie SE, Pastores GM, Strotmann JM, Wilcox WR: **Fabry disease: guidelines for the evaluation and management of multi-organ system involvement.** *Genet Med* 2006, **8:**539–548.
12. Gange CA, Link MS, Maron MS: **Utility of cardiovascular magnetic resonance in the diagnosis of Anderson-Fabry disease.** *Circulation* 2009, **120:**e96–e97.
13. Nucifora G, Miani D, Di Chiara A, Piccoli G, Artico J, Puppato M, Slavich G, De Biasio M, Gasparini D, Proclemer A: **Infarct-like acute myocarditis: relation between electrocardiographic findings and myocardial damage as assessed by cardiac magnetic resonance imaging.** *Clin Cardiol* 2013, **36:**146–152.
14. Thompson RB, Chow K, Khan A, Chan A, Shanks M, Paterson I, Oudit GY: **T1 mapping with cardiovascular MRI is highly sensitive for fabry disease independent of hypertrophy and sex.** *Circ Cardiovasc Imaging* 2013, **6:**637–645.
15. Sengupta PP, Korinek J, Belohlavek M, Narula J, Vannan MA, Jahangir A, Khandheria BK: **Left ventricular structure and function: basic science for cardiac imaging.** *J Am Coll Cardiol* 2006, **48:**1988–2001.
16. Weidemann F, Niemann M, Breunig F, Herrmann S, Beer M, Störk S, Voelker W, Ertl G, Wanner C, Strotmann J: **Long-term effects of enzyme replacement therapy on fabry cardiomyopathy: evidence for a better outcome with early treatment.** *Circulation* 2009, **119:**524–529.
17. Beer M, Weidemann F, Breunig F, Knoll A, Koeppe S, Machann W, Hahn D, Wanner C, Strotmann J, Sandstede J: **Impact of enzyme replacement therapy on cardiac morphology and function and late enhancement in Fabry's cardiomyopathy.** *Am J Cardiol* 2006, **97:**1515–1518.

12

Severe mitral regurgitation due to mitral leaflet aneurysm diagnosed by three-dimensional transesophageal echocardiography

Takao Konishi[1,3*], Naohiro Funayama[1], Tadashi Yamamoto[1], Daisuke Hotta[1], Kenjiro Kikuchi[1], Katsumi Ohori[2], Hiroshi Nishihara[3] and Shinya Tanaka[3]

Abstract

Background: A small mitral valve aneurysm (MVA) presenting as severe mitral regurgitation (MR) is uncommon.

Case presentation: A 47-year-old man with a history of hypertension complained of exertional chest discomfort.
A transthoracic echocardiogram (TTE) revealed the presence of MR and prolapse of the posterior leaflet. A 6-mm
in diameter MVA, not clearly visualized by TTE, was detected on the posterior leaflet on a three-dimensional (3D) transesophageal echocardiography (TEE). The patient underwent uncomplicated triangular resection of P2 and mitral valve annuloplasty, and was discharged from postoperative rehabilitation, 2 weeks after the operation. Histopathology of the excised leaflet showed myxomatous changes without infective vegetation or signs of rheumatic heart disease.

Conclusions: A small, isolated MVA is a cause of severe MR, which might be overlooked and, therefore, managed belatedly. 3D TEE was helpful in imaging its morphologic details.

Keywords: Mitral leaflet aneurysm, Mitral regurgitation, Three-dimensional transesophageal echocardiography, Case report

Background

Mitral valve aneurysm (MVA), a rare disorder first described by Saphir and Leroy in 1948 [1], is usually a complication of infective endocarditis [2–7]. Other causes of this disorder are rheumatic heart disease, Marfan's syndrome [8], aortic regurgitation and hypertrophic cardiomyopathy. Furthermore, the reports of surgical case have usually described MVA 15 to 30 mm in diameter [5, 7, 9–14]. The complications of MVA includes expansion, perforation and severe valvular regurgitation. An early diagnosis followed by surgical treatment is of critical importance to reduce the rate of these complications. We report a 6-mm in diameter, isolated aneurysm of a mitral leaflet in a man who presented with severe mitral regurgitation (MR).

Case presentation

A 47-year-old man with a 10-year history of hypertension complained of exertional chest discomfort. On physical examination, he was alert, his height and body weight were 168.5 cm and 78 kg, respectively, body temperature 36.3 °C, systemic blood pressure 152/

* Correspondence: takaokonishi0915@gmail.com
[1]Department of Cardiology, Hokkaido Cardiovascular Hospital, 1-30, West 13, South 27, Chuou-ku, Sapporo 064-8622, Japan
[3]Department of Cancer Pathology, Hokkaido University, Graduate School of Medicine, Sapporo, Japan
Full list of author information is available at the end of the article

82 mmHg and heart rate 56 bpm. The percutaneous oxygen saturation on room air was 97%. A III/VI systolic murmur was heard at the apex, radiating to the left axilla, without manifestation of cardiac decompensation. He had no sign of Marfan's syndrome. The laboratory tests revealed a $4.0 \times 10^3/mm^3$ white blood cell count with 66% granulocytes and 27% lymphocytes, a $20.4 \times 10^4/mm^3$ platelet count, 15.7 g/dl haemoglobin concentration, and 0.03 mg/dl C-reactive protein serum concentration. A chest roentgenogram showed a 48% cardiothoracic ratio, and the 12-lead electrocardiogram showed a high QRS voltage in the lateral precordial leads. A transthoracic echocardiogram (TTE) revealed MR with prolapse of the posterior leaflet (Fig. 1a-c) without vegetation or aortic regurgitation. The echocardiographic left atrial and left ventricular (LV) dimensions and LV ejection fraction are shown in Table 1A. A two-dimensional transoesophageal echocardiogram (TEE) showed mitral valve prolapse (Fig. 2a and c) and MR with a significant proximal isovelocity surface area (PISA) (Fig. 2b and d). On three-dimensional (3D) TEE, a 6-mm in diameter aneurysm was present on the posterior mitral valve leaflet, which was not clearly visible on TTE (Fig. 2e and Additional file: Video S1). 3D full-volume colour TEE was also useful for illustrating the spatial relationship between the MVA and the MR jet (Fig. 2f and Additional file: Video S2). A LV angiogram (Fig. 3 and Additional file: Video S3) showed grade 3–4 MR and coronary angiograms showed no significant stenosis. The pressures measured during right heart catheterization are shown in Table 1B. Cardiac index was within normal limits (Table 1B).

The patient underwent open-heart, triangular resection of the P2 segment of the mitral valve and annuloplasty with a 28-mm Séguin ring. Intraoperative inspection confirmed the presence of an aneurysm on the posterior mitral leaflet (Fig. 4a-c). High- and low-power histopathologic microphotographs showed myxomatous degeneration, without active mitral valve endocarditis or inflammatory cellular infiltration of the posterior leaflet (Fig. 5a-c). The postoperative course was uneventful and the chest discomfort resolved during the postoperative rehabilitation program. The patient was discharged from postoperative rehabilitation, 2 weeks after the operation, and has remained free from significant MR over a 2-year follow-up.

Table 1 Transthoracic echocardiographic and right heart catheterisation measurements

A. Transthoracic echocardiogram	
Left ventricular ejection fraction, %	61
Diameters, mm	
Left atrial	47
Left ventricular (end-diastolic)	55
B. Right heart catheterization	
Pressures, mmHg	
Right	
Atrial	10 (1–5)
Ventricular	
End-systolic	36 (15–30)
End-diastolic	4 (1–7)
Pulmonary	
Arterial	
Systolic	35 (15–30)
Diastolic	18 (4–12)
Mean	24 (9–18)
Capillary wedge	18 (4–12)
Cardiac index, $l/min/m^2$	3.2 (2.5–4.0)

Normal values are shown in parentheses

Discussion

This case illustrates the rare characteristics of an isolated, non-infective MVA, which, albeit small, caused severe MR. This observation, to the best of our

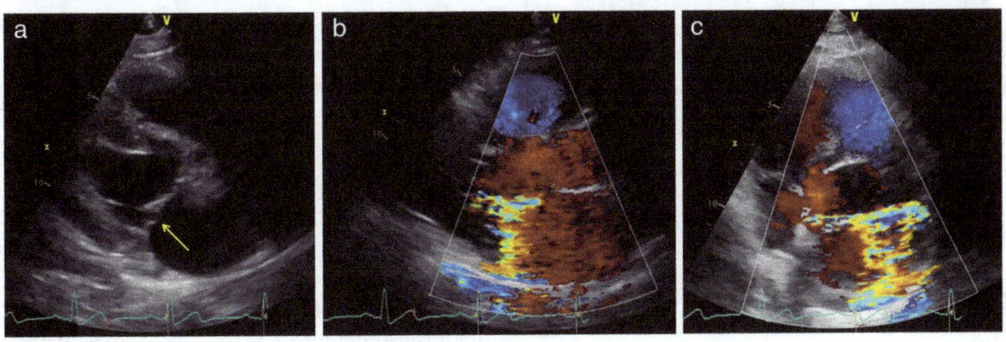

Fig. 1 Transthoracic echocardiogram. **a**, **b** and **c**. Parasternal long **a** and **b** and short **c** axis view of the posterior mitral valve leaflet slightly protruding into the left atrium (*arrow*) with severe eccentric mitral regurgitation

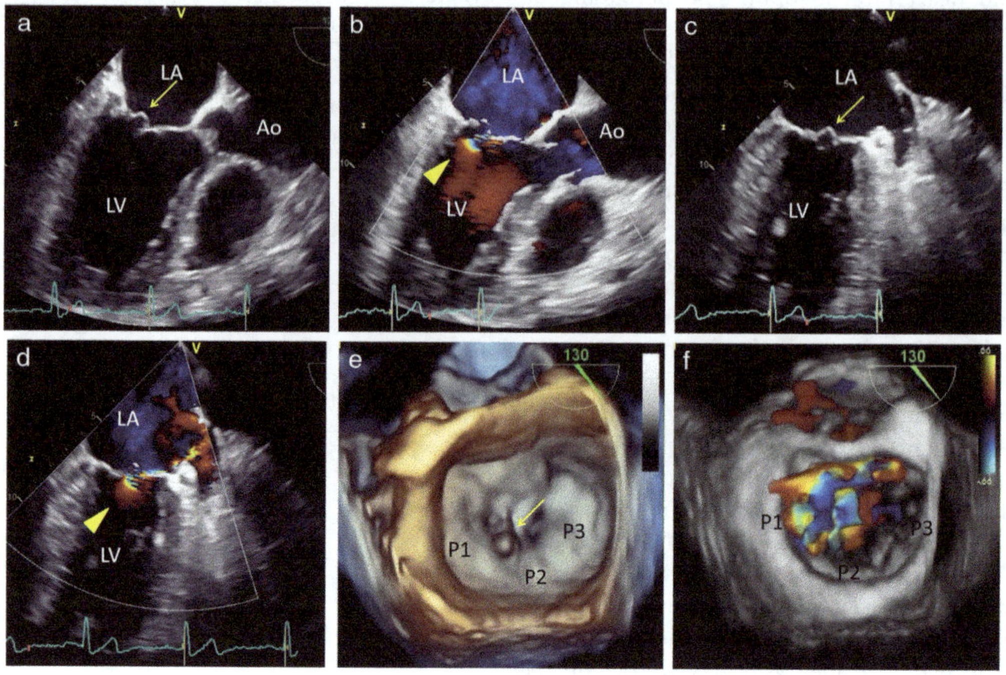

Fig. 2 Transoesophageal echocardiogram. **a** and **c**. Part of the posterior leaflet protrudes into the left atrium at a 129° (**a**) and 63° (**c**) angle in early systole (arrows). LA = left atrium; LV = left ventricle; Ao = Aorta. **b** and **d**. The colour Doppler images shows a considerably large proximal isovelocity surface area (PISA) (arrowheads) and a prominently eccentric mitral regurgitation at a 129° (**b**) and 63° (**d**) angle in end-systole. **e**. Three-dimensional transoesophageal echocardiogram, observed from the left atrium towards the mitral valve annulus, showing the 6-mm in diameter aneurysm on the posterior leaflet (arrow). The aneurysm was located at mid-posterior leaflet (P2) near lateral-posterior leaflet (P1). **f**. Three-dimensional full-volume colour acquisition of the mitral valve illustrating the spatial relationship between the MVA and the MR jet

knowledge, has not been previously reported in the English language medical literature.

A MVA is a discrete bulge of the mitral leaflet toward the left atrium expanding during systole and collapsing during diastole [15]. Its formation is associated with congenital, structural diseases of the connective tissues, including Marfan's syndrome [8], mitral valve prolapse [15], LV outflow tract obstruction, hypertrophic cardiomyopathy [16, 17] and bicuspid or quadricuspid aortic valves [18, 19]. From these predisposing disorders, MVA is formed by acquired factors, such as rheumatic fever, Libman-Sachs endocarditis and, in most cases, infective endocarditis [2, 3, 20–22]. It is usually detected on the anterior leaflet, due to infective endocarditis caused by an aortic regurgitant jet striking the leaflet [9, 21, 22]. In this patient, however, it was on the posterior leaflet, in absence of regurgitant jet. In addition, the histopathology showed myxomatous degeneration without active endocarditis or inflammatory cells in the excised valve specimen (Fig. 5a-c). This supports our hypothesis that, in this patient, the prolonged hypertensive LV pressure overload, besides the congenital structural weakness secondary to myxomatous degeneration, caused the development of an isolated MVA of the posterior mitral leaflet in absence of infection.

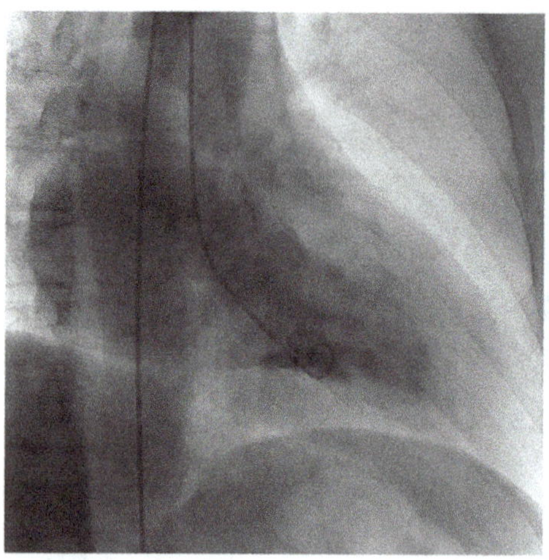

Fig. 3 Left ventriculography. Right anterior oblique, 30° view of grade 3 to 4 mitral regurgitation (Seller's grading)

The diagnosis of a small MVA, as was discovered in this patient, is often challenging, because its 3 dimensions are difficult to detect and identify on TTE. The superior performance of 3-dimensional TEE in clarifying the anatomical details of MVA has been reported [10, 23]. Since they may cause serious complications, such as systemic embolization, leaflet perforation, and recurrent infective

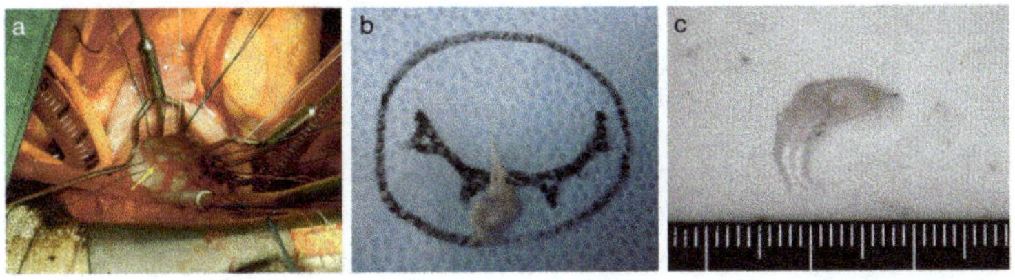

Fig. 4 Intraoperative aspect and histopathology of the posterior mitral valve leaflet. **a**. Intraoperative aspect of the MVA on the posterior mitral leaflet (*arrow*). **b**. The excised MVA was a part of the mid-posterior leaflet (P2). **c**. The excised MVA measured 6 mm in diameter

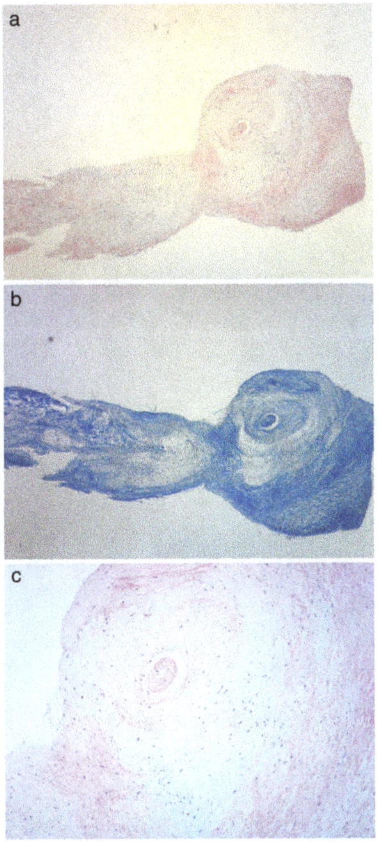

Fig. 5 Histopathology of the mitral valve aneurysm. **a** and **b.** Low-power (X 5 original magnification) microphotograph of the mitral valve aneurysm showing prominent myxomatous changes observed after **a** haematoxylin and eosin, and **b** Masson Trichrome staining. **c**. Low-power (X 10 original magnification) microphotograph showing no infiltration by inflammatory cells or active endocarditis in the posterior mitral leaflet

endocarditis [21, 24, 25], their prompt diagnosis and surgical management is of utmost importance. In this patient, 3-dimensional TEE showed a small MVA, which could not be detected by TTE. This case also highlights the severity of MR caused by a MVA as small as 10 mm in diameter.

Conclusions

Small, isolated MVA causing significant MR are rare and may be neither visible on TTE nor managed in a timely fashion. Regardless of their size, MVA can cause severe MR. 3D TEE is an effective means of detecting their presence.

Abbreviations

3D: Three-dimensional; MR: Mitral regurgitation; MVA: Mitral valve aneurysm; TEE: Transesophageal echocardiography; TTE: Transthoracic echocardiography.

Acknowledgments

We thank Ms. Seiko Oono for her contribution in acquiring the echocardiographic images.

Funding

None.

Authors' contributions

TK drafted the manuscript and prepared the figures. HN and ST analysed the histopathologic preparations. NF, TY, DH, KK and KO contributed to the composition of the manuscript. All authors have read and approved the submission of the final version of the manuscript.

Competing interests

The authors declare that they have no competing interests.

Author details

[1]Department of Cardiology, Hokkaido Cardiovascular Hospital, 1-30, West 13, South 27, Chuou-ku, Sapporo 064-8622, Japan. [2]Department of Cardiovascular Surgery, Hokkaido Cardiovascular Hospital, Sapporo, Japan. [3]Department of Cancer Pathology, Hokkaido University, Graduate School of Medicine, Sapporo, Japan.

References

1. Saphir O, Leroy EP. True aneurysms of the mitral valve in subacute bacterial endocarditis. Am J Pathol. 1948;24(1):83–95.
2. Azevedo O, Ferreira F, Guardado J, Durães C, Quelhas I, Pereira A, et al. Mitral and aortic valve aneurysms secondary to infective endocarditis: impressive images of a rare echocardiographic finding. Eur J Echocardiogr. 2010;11(7):E28.

3. Gao C, Xiao C, Li B. Mitral valve aneurysm with infective endocarditis. Ann Thorac Surg. 2004;78(6):2171–3.
4. Harada M, Hirai H, Inoue T, Sakai H, Lee T, Sugiyama Y, et al. Aortic and mitral valve aneurysms complicated with infective endocarditis: a case report. J Cardiol. 1998;31 Suppl 1:105–13.
5. Hotchi J, Hoshiga M, Okabe T, Nakakoji T, Ishihara T, Katsumata T, et al. Impressive echocardiographic images of a mitral valve aneurysm. Circulation. 2011;123(14):e400–2.
6. Michelena HI, Suri RM, Enriquez-Sarano M, Dearani J. Ruptured mycotic aneurysm of the mitral valve on real-time 3-dimensional transesophageal echocardiography. J Am Coll Cardiol. 2010;56(2):154.
7. Reid CL, Chandraratna AN, Harrison E, Kawanishi DT, Chandrasoma P, Nimalasuriya A, et al. Mitral valve aneurysm: clinical features, echocardiographic-pathologic correlations. J Am Coll Cardiol. 1983;2(3):460–4.
8. Edynak G, Rawson A. Ruptured aneurysm of the mitral valve in a Marfan-like syndrome. Am J Cardiol. 1963;11(5):674–677.
9. Northridge DB, Gnanapragasam JP, Houston AB. Diagnosis of mitral valve aneurysm by transoesophageal echocardiography. Br Heart J. 1991;65(4):227–8.
10. Al-Refai MA, Oueida FM, Lui RC, Al-Saif SM, Al-Omran HM. Impressive echocardiographic images of a rare pathology: Aneurysm of the mitral valve - Report of two cases and review of the literature. J Saudi Heart Assoc. 2012;25(1):47–51.
11. Anzouan-Kacou JB, Kramoh E, Coulibaly I. Perforated aneurysm of the anterior mitral valve. A rare cause of severe mitral regurgitation. Arch Cardiovasc Dis. 2010;103(4):275–6.
12. Subban V, Krishnamurthy V, Mohanraj A, Ajit MS. Posterior mitral leaflet aneurysm - a rare cause of mitral regurgitation. Indian Heart J. 2012;64(4):402–3.
13. Zhang H, Chen H, Sun X, Yang S, Wang C. Repair for mitral valve aneurysm using autologous pericardium: a case of our experience. J Cardiothorac Surg. 2014;9:148.
14. Gajjar TP, Desai NB. True aneurysm of anterior mitral leaflet–a rare entity. J Thorac Cardiovasc Surg. 2012;144(3):e93–5.
15. Ruckel A, Erbel R, Henkel B, Kramer G, Meyer J. Mitral valve aneurysm revealed by cross-sectional echocardiography in a patient with mitral valve prolapse. Int J Cardiol. 1984;6(5):633–7.
16. de Castro S, Adorisio R, Pelliccia A, Papetti F, Fedele F, Pandian NG. Perforated aneurysms of left side valves during active infective endocarditis complicating hypertrophic obstructive cardiomyopathy. Eur J Echocardiogr. 2002;3(2):100–2.
17. Carpenter PM, Atai M, Hoit B. Aneurysm of the mitral valve in a patient with hypertrophic cardiomyopathy. Am J Cardiovasc Pathol. 1988;2(3):273–6.
18. Hori D, Tanaka M, Yamaguchi A, Adachi H, Ino T. Extracardiac aneurysm of the interleaflet triangle above the aortic-mitral curtain due to infective endocarditis of the bicuspid aortic valve. Gen Thorac Cardiovasc Surg. 2008; 56(8):424–6.
19. Unger P, Preumont N, Stoupel E. Images in cardiology. Ruptured sinus of Valsalva aneurysm with right ventricular obstruction, quadricuspid aortic valve, and ventricular septal defect. Heart. 2000;84(4):424.
20. Takayama T, Teramura M, Sakai H, Tamaki S, Okabayashi T, Kawashima T, et al. Perforated mitral valve aneurysm associated with Libman-Sacks endocarditis. Intern Med. 2008;47(18):1605–8.
21. Kharwar RB, Mohanty A, Sharma A, Narain VS, Sethi R. Ruptured anterior mitral leaflet aneurysm in aortic valve infective endocarditis–evaluation by three-dimensional echocardiography. Echocardiography. 2014;31(3):E72–6.
22. Marcos-Alberca P, Rey M, Serrano JM, Fernandez-Rozas I, Navarro F, Contreras A, et al. Aneurysm of the anterior leaflet of the mitral valve secondary to aortic valve endocarditis. J Am Soc Echocardiogr. 2000; 13(11):1050–2.
23. Edwards NC, Smith NL, Steeds RP. Beyond the artery and ventricle - an aneurysm of the mitral valve leaflet. Echocardiography. 2013;30(8):E258–9.
24. Vijay SK, Tiwari BC, Misra M, Dwivedi SK. Incremental value of three-dimensional transthoracic echocardiography in the assessment of ruptured aneurysm of anterior mitral leaflet. Echocardiography. 2014;31(1):E24–6.
25. Lee CH, Tsai LM. Transesophageal echocardiographic recognition of mitral valve aneurysm. J Ultrasound Med. 2005;24(8):1141–4.

13

Diastolic dysfunction in spontaneous type 2 diabetes rhesus monkeys: a study using echocardiography and magnetic resonance imaging

Can Qian[1,2], Li Gong[2], Zunyuan Yang[2], Wei Chen[3], Yushu Chen[3], Ziqian Xu[3], Bing Wu[3], Chungui Tang[4], Fabao Gao[3*] and Wen Zeng[1,2*]

Abstract

Background: Diastolic heart failure is a common and deadly complication of diabetes mellitus, with the development of diabetic cardiomyopathy as one of the key determinants of the disease's complex pathology. The cause of the association is unknown and has no approved therapy strategies as of yet. However significant advances in this area may come from studies on suitable animal models.

Methods: A total of 25 male rhesus monkeys (12-16 years, 9-13 kg) were enrolled. Fifteen of them were diagnosed as spontaneous type 2 diabetes mellitus (T2DM, FPG ≥ 104 mg/dl, HbA1c: 4.7-5.5 %, diabetes duration: 1-4 years). The other 10 monkeys were non-diabetic (ND, FPG < 90 mg/dl). Echocardiography and cardiac magnetic resonance were used for evaluating the cardiac structure and function. One T2DM monkey with impaired diastolic function and another ND monkey were both sacrificed to gain the necessary pathology and protein expression studies displayed here.

Results: Six out of 15 T2DM rhesus monkeys were diagnosed with diastolic dysfunction (DD) by echocardiography. Additionally, no abnormalities were found in the group which we determined as the ND monkeys. The six DD monkeys all showed low e' velocity and decreased e'/a' ratio, among which three of them showing decreased E/A ratio and the other 3 having elevated E/A ratio, this appears to be similar to the impaired relaxation pattern and pseudonormal pattern found in human patients respectively. The EF and FS of monkeys with pseudonormal pattern decreased significantly compared with ND subjects. A CMR study showed that LVID at end systole of 5 DD monkeys is significantly longer than that of 3 ND monkeys. Of great interest, myocardium lesions and mitochondria impairments and increased expression of AGEs and caspase-3 were found in a sacrificed DD subject.

Conclusion: The changes in the imaging and physiological markers of spontaneous T2DM rhesus monkeys are similar to those key markers found in human type 2 diabetes and diastolic dysfunction. This monkey model could help the medical community and us to understand the pathology of this debilitating disease and serve as a beginning to explore important measures to prevent and treat diabetic cardiomyopathy.

* Correspondence: gaofabao@yahoo.com; zengwen10@vip.163.com
[3]Department of Radiology, West China Hospital, Sichuan University, Chengdu, China
[1]Sichuan Industrial Institute of Antibiotics, Chengdu, China
Full list of author information is available at the end of the article

Background

Cardiovascular diseases (CVD) are the leading causes of death and disability among people with diabetes. At least 65 % of people with diabetes die from certain forms of cardiovascular diseases [1]. As a major outcome of diabetes, cardiac failure is the most severe comorbidity [2]. A high prevalence of cardiac failure is seen in individuals with diabetic cardiovascular complications, therefore diabetic cardiomyopathy (DCM) is one of the key determinants in understanding and controlling the dire effects of the onset and progression of diabetes mellitus [3].

DCM has been defined as ventricular dysfunction that occurs in diabetic patients independent of a recognized cause, such as coronary artery disease (CAD) or hypertension [4]. Additionally, DCM is marked by diastolic dysfunction (DD) early on the disease's progression [5–7] that leads to the loss of contractile (systolic) function as time passes by [7–9]. The pathogenesis of this ventricular dysfunction remains unknown, but several hypotheses have been proposed, including autonomic dysfunction, metabolic derangements, abnormalities in ion homeostasis, alteration in structural proteins and the presence of interstitial fibrosis.

Alterations of certain biomarkers have also been reported to play key roles in the development of cardiac dysfunction and are therefore important to monitor. For example, advanced glycosylation end products (AGEs) can covalently crosslink and biochemically modify collagen structures in diabetes induced myocardial stiffness [10]. Another biomarker of interest is caspase-3 activation triggered by ROS generation in hyperglycemia-induced cardiac cell apoptosis in vivo [11]. Monitoring PKA-mediated phosphorylation of cMyBP-C is also helpful as it is linked to the modulation of cardiac contractions [12]. Determinations of these biomarkers contribute to providing the evidence of impairments by monitoring the abnormal effects in different metabolic pathways.

Significant advances in diabetic-related diseases may come from the studies on suitable animal models. Abnormalities in cardiac functionality and structure in diabetic subjects have been demonstrated in a variety of type 1 and type 2 diabetic rodent models [13–18]. In most studies of type 1 diabetes mellitus, diabetes is induced after administration of the pancreatic beta-cell toxin streptozotocin (STZ). Additionally, most studies of type 2 diabetes mellitus have been performed in genetic models demonstrating obesity and insulin resistance such as the Zucker fatty rat or db/db mice, both of which have mutations that impair leptin receptor signaling, or ob/ob mice, which lack leptin [4]. STZ induced and transgenic/gene knock-out diabetic rodent models may have advantages in studying some particular mechanisms. However, as for the complicated pathogenesis of DM, neither the rats nor the mice appear to have similar cardiac dysfunction that stimulates diabetic cardiomyopathy in diabetic humans.

Compared with other animal models, rhesus monkeys (*Macaca mulatta*) are more similar to humans in physiology and to the susceptibility of known metabolic diseases in human patients [19]. Though naturally occurring spontaneous type 2 diabetes has been extensively studied in rhesus [20–22], diabetic cardiovascular complications in rhesus monkeys have not been adequately discerned. In our previous work, a certain number of spontaneous T2DM rhesus monkeys have been screened and found within our colony, and their DM related parameters were demonstrated to be similar to humans [23]. Therefore, to investigate cardiac characteristics of those subjects, T2DM and age matched non-diabetic (ND) rhesus monkeys were enrolled in this study. Multiple complementary image techniques such as M-mode echocardiography, pulsed wave Doppler ultrasound, tissue Doppler imaging and cardiac magnetic resonance (CMR) were used to assess and categorize the DD group. Furthermore, light-scope was utilized to observe the microstructure within major organs to help us visualize the pathology present. Transmission electron microscope (TEM) was also used to observe the myocardium mitochondrial ultrastructure. These images were obtained through the application of immunohistochemical staining to determine and show the cardiac proteins of interest.

Methods

Animals

Fifteen previously screened spontaneous T2DM rhesus monkeys from ages 12 to 16 years, with 1–4 years' duration of diabetes [23] were matched with 10 ND rhesus monkeys of a similar age for testing. The criteria used for the rhesus monkey selections were guided by our previous work [23] along with similar criteria for rhesus monkeys [24, 25]. Monkeys were singly housed in a climate controlled room at 19 °C to 26 °C (66 °F to 79 °F), with a relative humidity of 50 % ± 20 %. The rate of ventilation was 10 times/h and the lighting cycle was 12 (day)/12 (night) hours. Monkeys were continually fed with mild high-calorie diet (containing 18 % protein, 60 % carbohydrates, 14 % water, and 8 % fat) approximately 300 g/day; a daily allotment of apples or vegetable was also provided. Tap water was provided as drinking water ad libitum. The monkeys were maintained in conformity with the requirements of "the National Institutes of Health Guide for the Care and Use of Laboratory Animal" of the United States, and all experimental protocols had been reviewed and approved by the Institutional Animal Care and Use Committee of Sichuan PriMed Group Co., Ltd.

Trial arrangements

There was a 4-week long acclimation period before the initial image study, during which gravimetry and metabolic profiles of all enrolled monkeys were acquired, see Table 1. Fasting plasma glucose (FPG) were determined semi-monthly for four weeks. Hemoglobin A1c (HbA1c), 2 h post-challenge plasma glucose (2hPPG), total cholesterol (TC), triglyceride (TG), low density lipoprotein cholesterol (LDL-c) and high density lipoprotein cholesterol (HDL-c) were determined at the end of the acclimation period. Body weight (BW), crown-rump length (CRL) of all monkeys were measured after the last blood collection to calculate BMI. Blood pressure of all the monkeys were measured before each image examination. Echocardiography were performed on all monkeys in 48 h after the last blood collection. Cardiac magnetic resonance (CMR) were performed sequentially on some of the monkeys. One monkey with moderate diastolic dysfunction, together with one ND monkey was sacrificed for histopathological and protein study. Some of the pathology was detailed by use of transmission electron microscope for observing microstructure and ultrastructure. Immunohistochemistry staining were performed for the protein studies.

Laboratory measurements

FPG, 2hPPG, HbA1c and lipid parameters were measured as we previously performed [23, 26]. Body mass index (BMI) was calculated using body weight divided by the square of CRL. Blood pressures were measured by an intelligent non-invasive blood pressure monitor while the monkeys were seated upon a monkey chair.

Table 1 Gravimetry and metabolic profile of monkeys enrolled for the study showing measurements in the acclimation period

Groups		ND ($n = 10$)	T2DM ($n = 15$)
Age (year)		12-16	12-16
BW (kg)		9.2 ± 1.9	11.3 ± 1.2
BMI		28.8 ± 2.8	38.0 ± 2.8*
Diabetes Duration (year)		0	1-4
FPG (mg/dL)	day 14	82.6 ± 10.3	119.8 ± 12.9*
	day 28	78.6 ± 9.8	113.9 ± 8.6*
2hPPG (mg/dL)		98.1 ± 16.4	137.8 ± 24.5*
HbA1c (%)		4.2 ± 0.4	5.1 ± 0.2*
TC (mg/dL)		131.6 ± 27.1	140.0 ± 17.6
TG (mg/dL)		44.4 ± 22.9	51.0 ± 30.9
LDL-c (mg/dL)		46.4 ± 11.6	53.7 ± 13.5
HDL-c (mg/dL)		61.4 ± 10.8	62.1 ± 11.6
SBP (mmHg)		129 ± 6	154 ± 7*
DBP (mmHg)		114 ± 7	109 ± 19

*$p < 0.05$, compared with ND group

Image examination

Echocardiography: All monkeys were fasted overnight prior to echocardiography examination. Monkeys were sedated by ketamine hydrochloride (Bioniche Teoranta) at a dosage of 10 mg/kg i.m. and the coat of monkey was bilaterally shaved from the cervical part to the navel, and rinsed copiously with water in order that acoustic coupling was obtained using ultrasound gel. Transthoracic echocardiography was performed by using a commercially available ultrasound system (Mindray M7vet) with the same investigator taking the measurements with the monkeys placed in a dorsal decubitus position while in a stable sedation state. All measurements were performed around the midday to avoid the influence of circadian rhythm on the left ventricular diastolic function [27]. All echographic acquisitions were obtained according to the recommendations of the American Society of Echocardiography and digitally stored from at least three consecutive heartbeats for offline analysis.

Pulsed-wave Doppler measurements: Blood flow velocity was recorded at the mitral diastolic inflow at the level of the mitral leaflet tips from the apical 4-chamber view. The following velocities were observed and recorded according to the current standards of the practice of echocardiography: E wave, A wave and E/A ratio. Early filling deceleration time (EDT) and isovolumic relaxation time (IVRT) were measured and averaged from 3 consecutive beats. Pulmonary venous flow (PVF) was recorded from the same acoustic window, placing a sampling volume 1 cm into the right upper pulmonary vein. Peak systolic (S), diastolic (D), and atrial reversal (AR) velocities were measured and averaged from 3 consecutive beats.

Conventional M-mode Doppler ultrasound: Real-time two-dimensional targeted M-mode echocardiograms of the LV minor axis was taken at the papillary muscle level to measure the EF and FS. EF = (EDV-ESV)/EDV. In this study, the values of EDV and ESV were measured by using the Teichholz-corrected formula in standard software included in the ultrasound equipment. EF and FS were calculated automatically by the system when relative cardiac borders were set.

Tissue Doppler imaging: to perform this, the ultrasound equipment was switched into tissue Doppler imaging mode, sample volume was located at the septal side of the mitral annulus from the apical 4-chamber view. Early (e') and late (a') diastolic mitral annulus velocities and the ratio of early to late peak velocities (e'/a') were obtained.

Cardiovascular magnetic resonance

In one week after echocardiography examination, CMR imaging was performed with a 3.0-T whole-body MR system (MAGNETOM Trio, Siemens Medical Solutions, Erlangen, Germany) on four ND monkeys and only five DD monkeys (anesthesia failure happened to one monkey with moderate DD). Intravenous propofol were used for anesthesia induction, and inhalation isoflurane were used for anesthesia maintenance. Data were acquired during end-inspiratory breath holding. After scout images, TrueFISP cine sequence (TE/TR = 11/500 ms; field of view (FOV) = 20 cm x 20 cm, NEX = 2; matrix = 256 x 256; flip angle, 50°; slice thickness = 2 mm; slice gap = 2 mm) with retrospective ECG-gating was used to acquire dynamic cine loops of the LV for function analysis. The LV was imaged in its entirety from the base to the apex in 9–12 short-axis cine images without interslice gaps or overlaps.

Cine function analysis was performed off-line with commercial software (Argus, Siemens Medical Solutions). At the same mid-ventricular level, endocardial and epicardial boundaries were traced semi-automatically during the end-diastolic and end-systolic phases in order to obtain the dimensional parameters: LVIDd, LVIDs, SWTd, SWTs, AWTd, AWTs, PWTd, and PWTs. Left ventricular cine images were analyzed by an experienced radiologist who was blinded to the echocardiographic results.

Light scope and transmission electron microscopy (TEM) observation

Extracted heart, liver, kidney and pancreas of a DD monkey were processed for H & E staining. The ultrastructure of myocardial mitochondria were observed by transmission electron microscope (TEM) as we previously did [28]. Fresh tissues (cardiac muscle) were cut into 1 mm cubes, which were fixed in 3 % glutaraldehyde for 2 h, and then fixed in 1 % osmium tetroxide, with stepwise dehydration in graded acetone, then after being infiltrated and embedded, tissue was polymerized in EPON 812. The semi-thin sections were optically positioned and further sectioned with ultramicrotome into 50–60 nm pieces, which were collected on copper grids, double-stained with uranyl acetate and lead citrate, and then observed under Hitachi H-600IV transmission electron microscope and photographed.

Immunohistochemistry assessment for protein study

Five-micron serial paraffin sections of LV were used to stain for AGEs, caspase-3 and phosphorylated cMyBP-C. Sections were dewaxed in xylene, rehydrated through a graded series of ethanol, washed in distilled water and phosphate-buffered saline (PBS), and then blocked for endogenous peroxidase by incubation with 3 % H_2O_2 in methanol for 15 min. The sections were subjected to antigen retrieval procedure by microwaving in 0.01 M pH 6.0 sodium citrate buffer. Additional washing in PBS was performed before the next 30 min of incubation at 37 °C in 10 % normal goat serum. The sections were incubated overnight at 4 °C with diluted (1:100) primary antibodies. The antibodies used were polyclonal goat anti-rabbit AGEs antibodies, goat anti-rabbit caspase-3 antibody and goat anti-rabbit phosphorylated cMyBP-C antibody (Boster, China). For negative controls, the sections received PBS in place of the primary antibody. After washing in PBS, the sections were exposed to a 1 % biotinylated secondary antibody goat and anti-rabbit IgG (Boster, China) for 1 h at 37 °C. The sections were then incubated with the HRP-streptavidin (Boster, China) for 30 min at 37 °C. To visualize the immunoreaction, the sections were immersed in blue diaminobenzidine hydrochloride (DAB). The reaction was monitored microscopically and stopped by the immersion into distilled water as soon as a brown color staining was clearly visualized.

Statistical analysis

Statistical analysis was performed using SPSS 19.0 software. The data is presented as the mean ± SD unless otherwise specified. Comparison among the two groups of subjects for various parameters was carried out by one-way analysis of variance. When normality and/or equal variance testing conditions were not met, the Kruskal-Wallis rank test and/or the Dunn's test for multiple comparisons were used, respectively. A p value less than 0.05 was considered statistically significant.

Results

Gravimetry and metabolic profile

Hyperglycemia and elevated HbA1c percentage were confirmed in all spontaneous T2DM monkeys enrolled (Table 1). In terms of both of the FPG determinations, T2DM group showed significantly higher FPG level compared with the ND group. All T2DM monkeys enrolled not only met our criteria for T2DM, but also showed relatively stable FPG in the acclimation period. 2hPPG and HbA1c percentage in the T2DM group were also significantly higher than those in ND group (137.8 ± 24.5 *vs* 98.1 ± 16.4 mg/dL for 2hPPG, $p < 0.05$; 5.1 ± 0.2 *vs* 4.2 ± 0.4, %, for HbA1c, $p < 0.05$). Obesity was observed in all T2DM monkeys, whose BMI average body weight was larger than that of ND group (38.0 ± 2.8 *vs* 28.8 ± 2.8, kg/m^2, $p < 0.05$), while there was no significance in body weight (11.3 ± 1.2 *vs* 9.2 ± 1.9, kg). There were no significant differences between groups in their lipid profiles. Average systolic blood pressure of the diabetic monkeys was found to be higher than that of the ND monkeys (154 ± 7.0 *vs* 129 ± 5.6, mmHg, $p < 0.05$).

Echocardiography findings

The monkeys tolerated the anesthesia and procedure without difficulty. There were no post study deaths. Echocardiograms with high definition were acquired from all monkeys, representative echo images were shown in Fig. 1. Six out of 15 T2DM monkeys were found having manifestations that are similar to those of human patients with diastolic dysfunction. These six monkeys all showed low e' velocity and a decreased e'/a' ratio. Among these six monkeys, three showed decreased E/A ratio (below 0.9), which was similar to the echographic characteristics of mild diastolic dysfunction in human patients. While another three monkeys showed increased E/A ratio (above 1.3) accompanying abnormalities of the TDI parameters described above, which were similar to the manifestations of moderate diastolic dysfunction in human patients. Since there are no criteria for diastolic function grading in monkeys, we attempt here to classify all monkeys enrolled into 4 groups: ND, T2DM with preserved DD, mild DD (considered as impaired relaxation) and moderate DD (pseudonormal pattern), for the following analyzes.

In ND (n = 10) and T2DM with preserved diastolic function (n = 9) subjects averaged E/A ratio for both groups were slightly greater than 1 (1.1 ± 0.2 and 1.2 ± 0.2, see Table 2, Fig. 2), while E/A ratio significantly decreased in mild DD group (0.8 ± 0.1, n = 3) but increased in moderate DD group (1.5 ± 0.2, n = 3). Mitral annulus velocity e' were 8.7 ± 0.6 cm/s for the ND group and 9.3 ± 0.9 cm/s for the T2DM with preserved diastolic function group, while e' velocity decreased in DD subjects: 5.7 ± 1.7 cm/s for the mild DD group and 7.7 ± 1.6 cm/s for the moderate DD group. Significance was only found between the T2DM with the preserved diastolic function group and the mild DD group ($p < 0.05$). e'/a' ratio was found to be 1.2 ± 0.3 for the ND group and 1.4 ± 0.3 for the T2DM with preserved diastolic function group, however this parameter decreased below 1 in the DD subjects: 0.7 ± 0.1 for the mild DD group ($p < 0.01$ compared with the T2DM group with preserved diastolic function) and 0.8 ± 0.1 for the moderate DD group ($p < 0.01$ compared with the T2DM with preserved diastolic function group).

The mild DD group had the longest average EDT (See Table 2). Significant difference was found between the mild DD group and the T2DM with preserved LV function group (92 ± 20 *vs* 66 ± 18, ms, $p < 0.05$). However, the difference between mild DD group and the moderate DD group was not significant. As for the IVRT, no significances were found among any of the groups.

As for pulmonary venous flow pattern, monkeys in the ND group and T2DM with preserved LV function group showed similar levels of S, D and AR (See Table 2 and Fig. 3). In normal PVF patterns, values of S/D were around 1. In monkeys with mild DD, we have the highest peak S (61.4 ± 9.0 cm/s) and lowest D (37.1 ± 2.0 cm/s), resulting in the highest S/D ratio in this group. However, peak S decreased but D increased in the group with pseudonormal pattern, which lead to S/D < 1. As for PV AR velocity, though the highest AR waves were seen in the mild DD group, nonetheless,

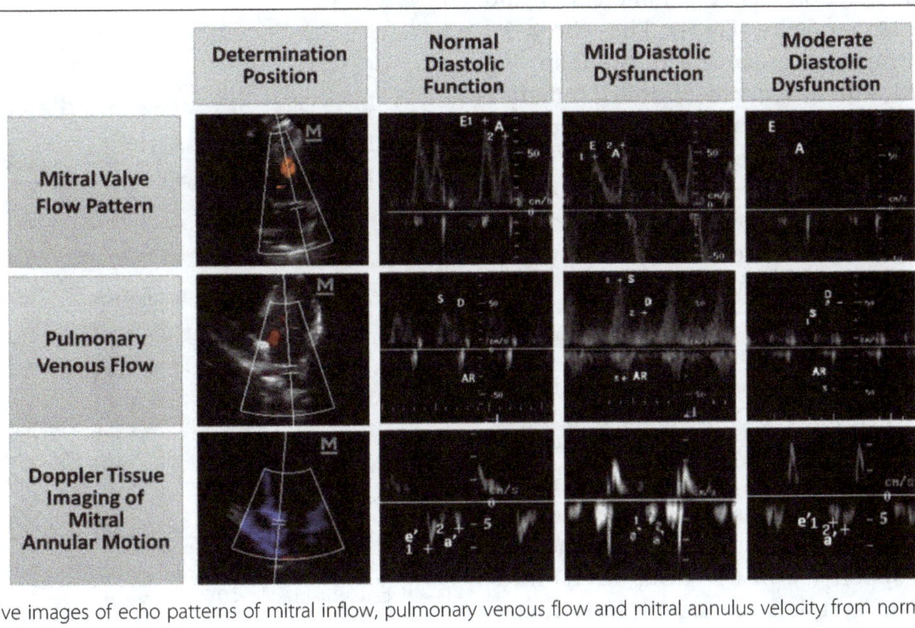

Fig. 1 Representative images of echo patterns of mitral inflow, pulmonary venous flow and mitral annulus velocity from normal to moderate diastolic dysfunction in rhesus monkeys

Table 2 Echocardiographic measurements in 10 ND monkeys and 15 spontaneous T2DM monkeys

parameters	normal (*n* = 10)	T2DM with preserved diastolic function (*n* = 9)	impaired relaxation (*n* = 3)	pseudonormal pattern (*n* = 3)
transmitral flow				
E/A	1.1 ± 0.2	1.2 ± 0.2	0.8 ± 0.1*	1.5 ± 0.2*#
EDT (ms)	70 ± 12	66 ± 18	92 ± 20*	75 ± 10
IVRT (ms)	48 ± 7	51 ± 10	55 ± 16	49 ± 19
pulmonary venous flow				
S(cm/s)	46.8 ± 6.1	48.5 ± 11.0	61.4 ± 9.0*	38.2 ± 2.7#
D(cm/s)	43.8 ± 11.0	45.9 ± 10.8	37.1 ± 2.0	56.9 ± 4.5*#
AR(cm/s)	43.7 ± 11.2	42.1 ± 7.9	54.7 ± 13.1	44.4 ± 2.0
myocardial velocities				
e'(cm/s)	8.7 ± 0.6	9.3 ± 0.9	5.7 ± 1.7*	7.0 ± 0.4
e'/a'	1.2 ± 0.3	1.4 ± 0.3	0.7 ± 0.1*	0.8 ± 0.1*
LA diameters				
LAAD (mm)	16.8 ± 1.0	15.1 ± 1.1	15.1 ± 2.1	15.7 ± 1.8
LATD (mm)	18.4 ± 0.7	17.8 ± 3.4	16.2 ± 2.0	16.8 ± 3.8
LAVD (mm)	21.6 ± 2.1	21.0 ± 2.2	19.3 ± 3.0	22.0 ± 5.9

*$p < 0.05$ compared with the T2DM with preserved diastolic function group
#$p < 0.05$ compared with the impaired relaxation group

the differences among groups were not statistically significant.

M-mode Doppler ultrasound was used for the measurement of left ventricular contractile capacity. Left ventricular systolic function related parameters EF and FS share similar characteristics (Fig. 4). They showed a tendency to decrease in accordance with the following order: ND, T2DM with preserved diastolic function, mild DD and moderate DD. Though there were significant differences between the moderate DD group and ND group (EF: 63.1 ± 7.0 *vs* 76.8 ± 4.9, %, p < 0.05; FS: 28.6 ± 4.5 *vs* 43.0 ± 4.0, %, p < 0.001) for these two parameters, whether they were still within normal physical limits still needs to be further studied.

Cardiac magnetic resonance findings

Left ventricular cine images at the mid-ventricular level were obtained from 5 DD monkeys and 4 ND monkeys who have been through the echocardiographic examination (Fig. 5). LV internal diameter (LVID), anterior, posterior and septum wall thickness (AWT, PWT, SWT) were measured at both end diastole (d) and end systole (s). In DD group, LVID measured at the end of systole were significantly longer

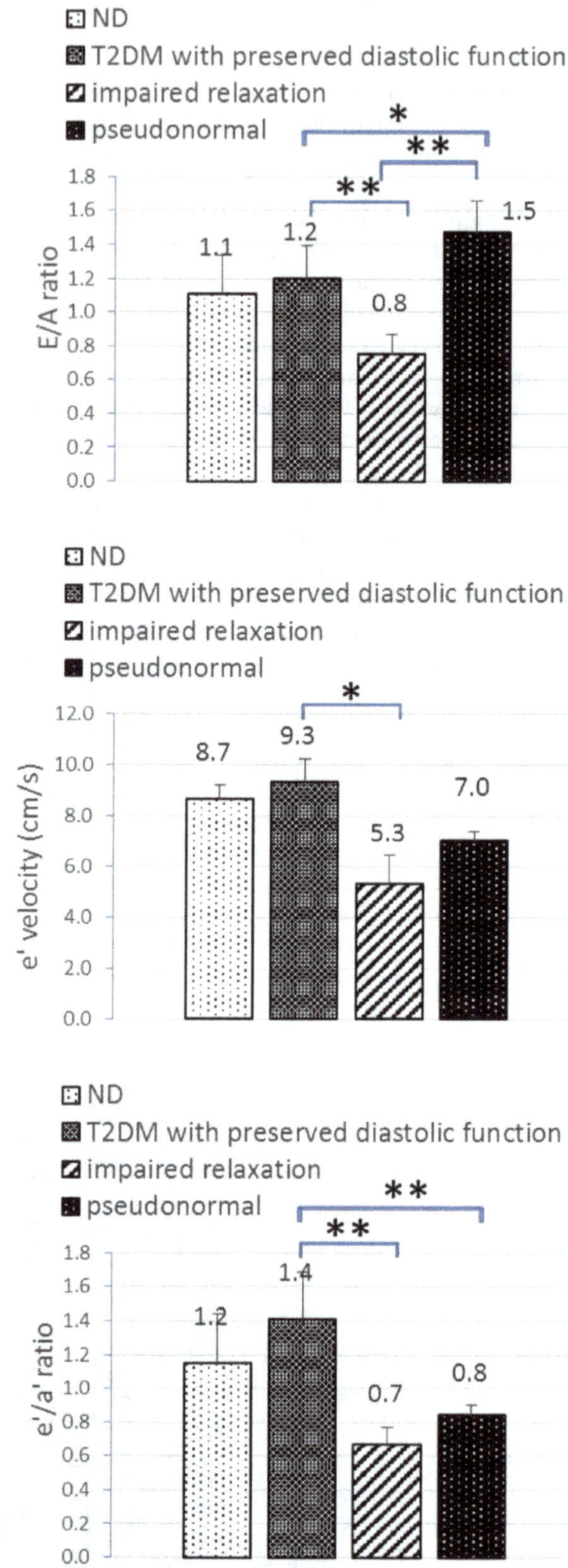

Fig. 2 Diastolic function related parameters measured by echocardiography. *$p < 0.05$, **$p < 0.01$

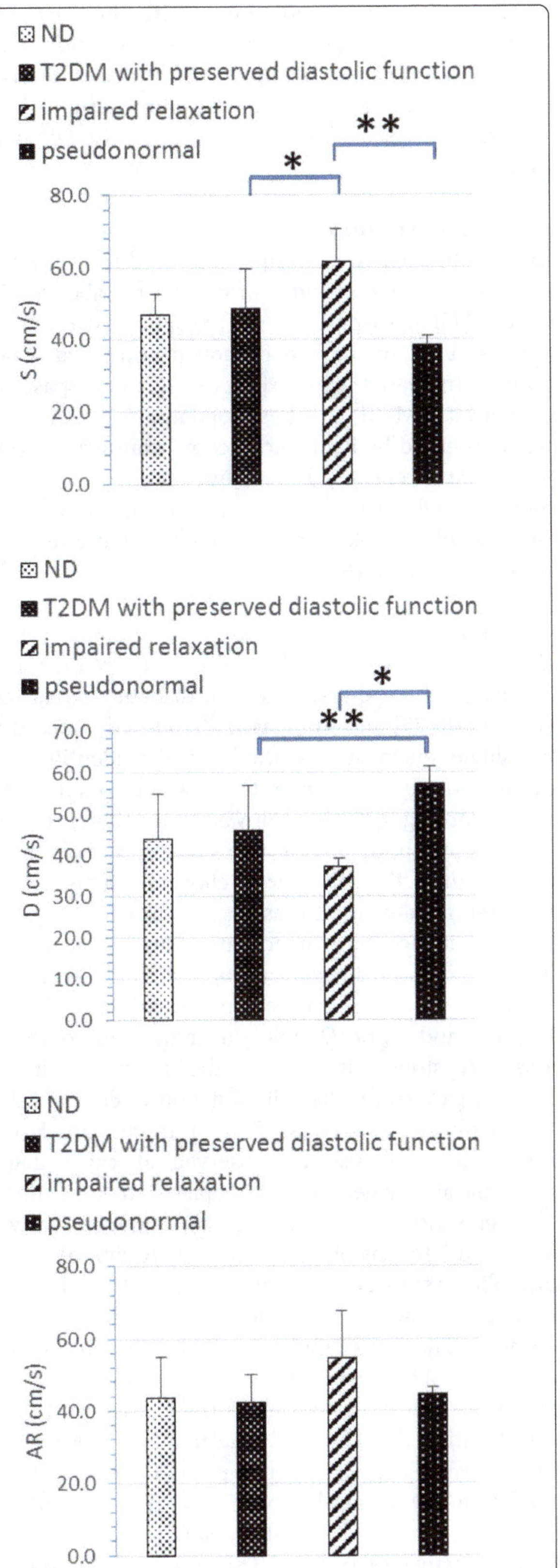

Fig. 3 Pulmonary venous flow parameters measured by echocardiography. $^*p < 0.05$, $^{**}p < 0.01$

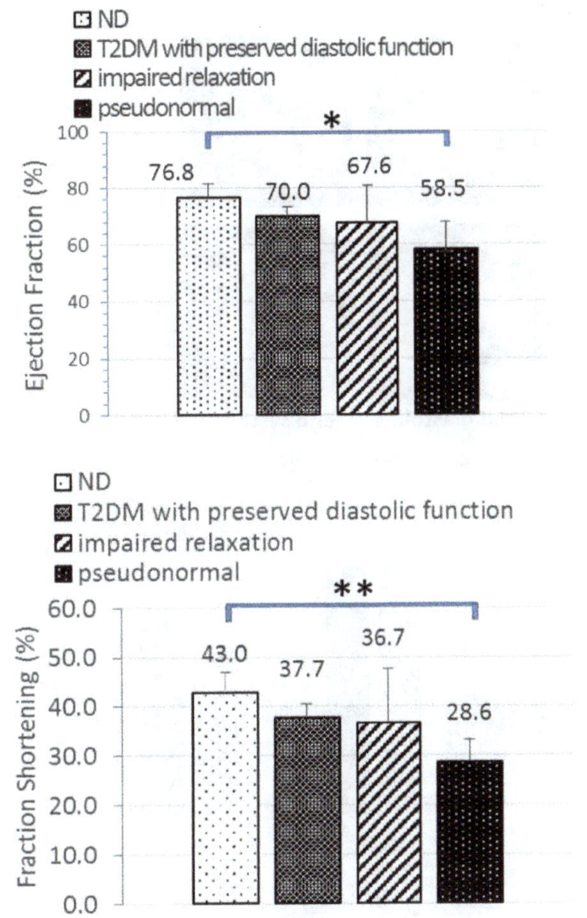

Fig. 4 Systolic function related parameters measured by echocardiography. $^*p < 0.05$

than that of ND (21.8 ± 2.9 *vs* 17.5 ± 0.1, mm, $p < 0.05$). As for LV wall thickness parameters (AWTd, AWTs, PWTs), they all showed a tendency to be thinner in the DD group than those in the ND group but still without statistical significance.

Myocardial microstructure and ultrastructure findings

Pathologic analyses were used to assess the myocardial microstructure of a monkey with moderate LV diastolic dysfunction. H&E staining revealed myocardium swelling with granular degeneration and myocardial atrophy accompanying interstitial expansion (Fig. 6a). At the same time, lesions were found in other major organs: liver, kidney and pancreas (Fig. 6b, c and d). Firstly, cellular atrophy, hepatic sinusoid expansion, multifocal proliferation of the connective tissue and hepatic cords vanishment were found in the section of liver tissue. Secondly, shrinkage of the glomerulus, kidney tubules granular degeneration and sectional tubular epithelial detachment were observed in the

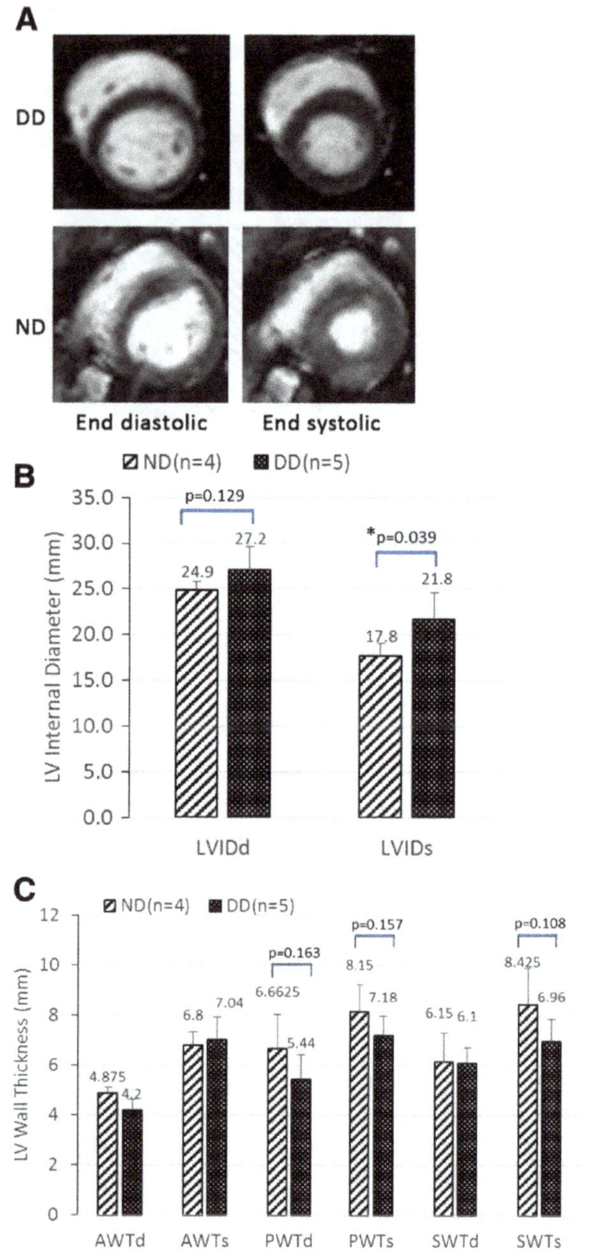

Fig. 5 Cardiac cine-MR results measured from 5 DD monkeys and 4 ND monkeys. **a** End-diastolic (left) and end-systolic (right) cine-MR images in a mid-ventricular slice from a DD (top) and an ND (bottom) monkey. **b** Left ventricular internal dimension measured at both end diastole and end systole. **c** Left ventricular wall thickness measured at both end diastole and end systole

section of kidney tissue. Thirdly, cellular swelling, decreasing cell numbers and cell shrinkage were observed in the section of pancreas tissue. Transmission electron microscopy was used to observe the mitochondrial ultrastructure of the hearts of a ND monkey and a monkey with moderate diastolic dysfunction (Fig. 7a and b). In the myocardial mitochondria of a ND monkey, mitochondria were regularly shaped and arranged between myofilaments with the cristae being clear and undamaged. However mitochondrial swelling and vacuolation, atrophy and rupture of myocardial fibers along with nuclear chromatin migration towards the cell's edge are observed in the DD monkey images.

Cardiac protein study

Immunohistochemical stains were used to assess the expression of different kinds of protein metabolized in the heart. AGEs, caspase-3 and phosphorylated cMyBP-C were stained by blue diaminobenzidine hydrochloride (DAB). Increased expression of AGEs, caspase-3 and decreased cMyBP-C phosphorylation in myocardium were observed by light-microscopic examination (Fig. 8), which were reflected by positive staining of these proteins throughout the field of microscope. However, there were no observable abnormal staining patterns as these in the sections of the ND monkey heart.

Discussion

Echocardiography and CMR have been used for invasive cardiac phenotype assessment in diabetic animal models [15, 17, 18, 29] and humans [7, 8, 30–35]. Since there is no single diagnostic method for the identification of diastolic dysfunction, these tools can be complementary.

Echocardiography is an invasive and inexpensive tool that allows sonographers to evaluate changes in heart structure/function that are echogenic. This technique has been already used to assess the cardiac structure and function in non-human primates [36–39], all for establishing standardized echocardiographic reference values.

Mitral valve blood inflow measured by pulsed-wave Doppler and tissue Doppler imaging were combined to assess diastolic function in the hearts of monkeys. Normal pattern for diastolic function under pulsed-wave Doppler were defined as $E/A > 1$ in human. However, this value may also be observed at early stages of ischemia and hypertrophy. Doppler pattern of impaired LV relaxation, characterized by reduced early and increased late diastolic flow, is an early sign of DD (mild diastolic dysfunction) which shows $E/A < 1$ [40]. More advanced grades, manifested by predominant early diastolic filling and rapid velocity deceleration, known as restrictive filling patterns, cause an increase in filling pressure, lead to an increase in the E-wave, and result in a E/A ratio > 2 [41]. The hinge point of these grades is the intermediary values, the pseudonormal pattern or moderate DD group, has an $E/A > 1$ which results from an increase in the left atrial pressure [41] in the presence of a defective relaxation. The impaired LV relaxation leads to an increase in filling pressures in order to maintain normal cardiac output as a complement of the variables of mitral valve inflow velocity. A combination of

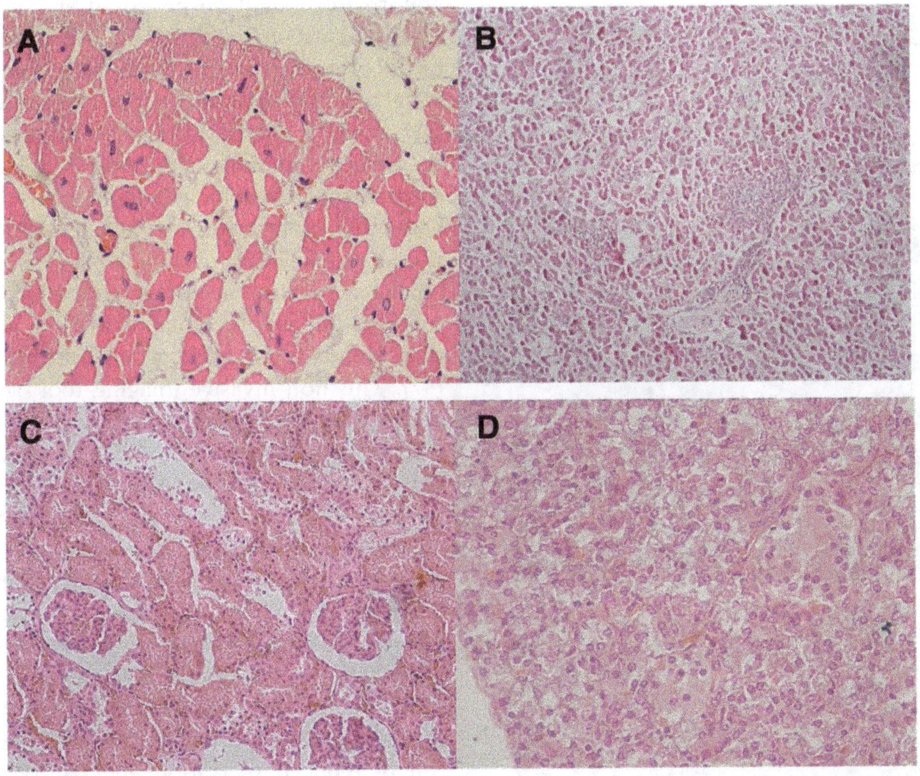

Fig. 6 Myocardial microstructure and ultrastructure pictures observed by light scope and transmission electron microscope. **a**, **b**, **c** and **d** Myocardium, liver, kidney and pancreas pathological image of a DD monkey, respectively

mitral annulus velocity with peak e' velocity < 8.5 cm/s and e'/a' ratio < 1 was used to indicate relaxation abnormality, this mitral annulus velocity pattern could identify the underlying relaxation abnormality with a sensitivity of 88 % and specificity of 67 % [31]. Moreover, mitral annulus motion is less load dependent than conventional mitral inflow variables. This technique appears to be useful for evaluating diastolic function, especially in the detecting of a pseudonormal pattern. In this study, DD diagnosing and grading were referred to as a combination of parameters measured from pulsed-wave Doppler and TDI. Monkeys in ND group and T2DM with preserved diastolic function group showed that E/A > 1, e' velocity < 8 cm/s, e'/a' < 1 and E/e' > 8. Subjects with E/A < 0.9 (impaired relaxation) and E/A > 1.3 (pseudonormal) were considered as mild DD and moderate DD, which were supported by TDI results such as decreased e' velocity and e'/a' < 1. The E/A ratio measured from T2DM monkeys in our trials was found to show a U-shaped prognostic behavior, which were similar to T2DM patients [7, 42].

Impairment of LV relaxation results in prolongation of the IVRT and EDT. In contrast, increasing filling pressure shortens IVRT and reduces EDT [43]. In this study, the mild DD group had the longest average EDT. Significant difference was found between the mild DD group and the T2DM with preserved diastolic function group. Though the difference of EDT between mild DD and the moderate DD groups were not significant, there was a tendency to register a decrease in the moderate DD group. As for the IVRT, no significances were found among groups. Heart rates (HR) of monkeys are usually twice or three times faster than that of the human being. During our echo study, heart rates ranged from 110 to 175 bpm when monkeys were sedated by ketamine. The wide variability of HR can influence the IVRT and EDT in evaluating the LV diastolic function.

Pulmonary venous flow pattern has also been used to distinguish normal from pseudonormal transmitral Doppler filling. Impairment of LV relaxation results in increased systolic (S) pulmonary venous flow, in contrast increasing filling pressure reduces PV systolic flow [43]. It has been reported that PVF indexes also change in a typical U-shaped pattern during the progression from normal to severe DD. In this study, the highest peak S and S/D ratio were seen in the mild DD group, whereas S was reduced in the moderate DD group and resulted in the reversal of S/D ratio (S/D < 1). As for AR velocity, differences between groups were unremarkable, which may be caused by the relative difficulty in obtaining

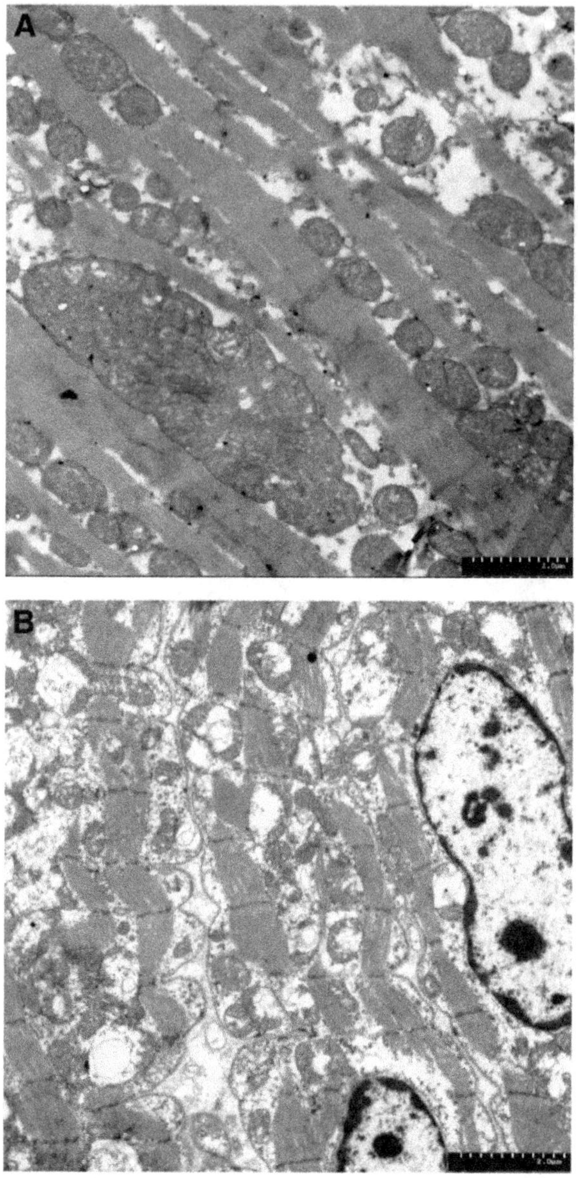

Fig. 7 Myocardium ultrastructure TEM image of an ND monkey and a DD monkey. **a** ND monkey; **b** DD monkey

accurate tracings by the transthoracic approach. Assisted by the TDI indexes, the PVF patterns seen provided more evidence of DD in these monkeys.

Decreased EF and FS were only seen in moderate DD subjects. It is still under debate as to which left ventricular function is impaired earlier in the evolution of diabetic cardiomyopathy. More studies stated that diastolic function is more commonly impaired than systolic and that diastolic dysfunction might be the initial abnormality in patients with the onset of diabetes [5, 7, 9, 42, 44, 45]. However, other researchers have recently shown that systolic strain alterations may exist despite normal diastolic function, which indicates systolic strain abnormality might be proposed as the first indicator of diabetic cardiomyopathy [46]. According to the results of the groupings in this study, significances of EF and FS were only found between the moderate DD group and ND group, indicating that diastolic dysfunction may be the earliest functional alteration in the course of diabetic cardiomyopathy, which lead to contractile abnormality with the progression of DD in spontaneous T2DM rhesus monkeys.

MRI provides accurate, reproducible, noninvasive representations of cardiac structure and function and measurements of regional myocardial wall thickening [47]. This non-invasive imaging tool has been proved to be powerful in evaluating the cardiac morphology of the diabetic rodent models [15, 17] and patients [35]. However, in vivo cine MRI studies on T2DM monkey models are very limited. In the present study, it was observed that T2DM rhesus monkeys with diastolic dysfunction showed significantly dilated LV internal diameter at end systole compared with ND monkeys. Though statistical differences were not seen, average LV internal diameter at end diastole were 12 % higher in DD subjects when compared with the ND group. These cardiac structural changes reflex the adaptive mechanism of reduced relaxation and contractility. As for left ventricular wall and septum thickness, no significant changes were seen between DD subjects and ND monkeys. Similarly, LV dilatation were accompanied by no significant changes in LV wall thickness as observed in diabetes rodents [48–50]. In this study, alterations of systolic function indicators were observed with the progression of DD by echocardiography, which included reductions in EF and FS. Increases in LV inner dimensions were also indicators of reduced contractile ability. Though significant changes were not found in LV wall and septal thickness, the average PWTd, PWTs and SWTs of the DD monkeys were 18.3 %, 11.9 % and 17.4 % all lower values than found in the ND ones. In a study using STZ treated rats [48, 50], it reported there is a gradual decrease in PWT after 8 weeks of diabetes while continuing after 12 weeks of recorded measurements. A relatively small sample number in this study may be a limitation in observing the differences between groups. Moreover, additional longitudinal studies are needed to trace the alteration with the progression of diabetes.

Histological abnormalities of myocardium were reported both in diabetic rodent models and human patients [51–53]. Characteristics of the pathological changes of the myocardium in the T2DM accompanying DD monkeys were consistent with the previous DCM studies. Meanwhile, lesions found in the liver, kidney and pancreas indicates that other diabetes complications also exist in these monkeys. Mitochondrial

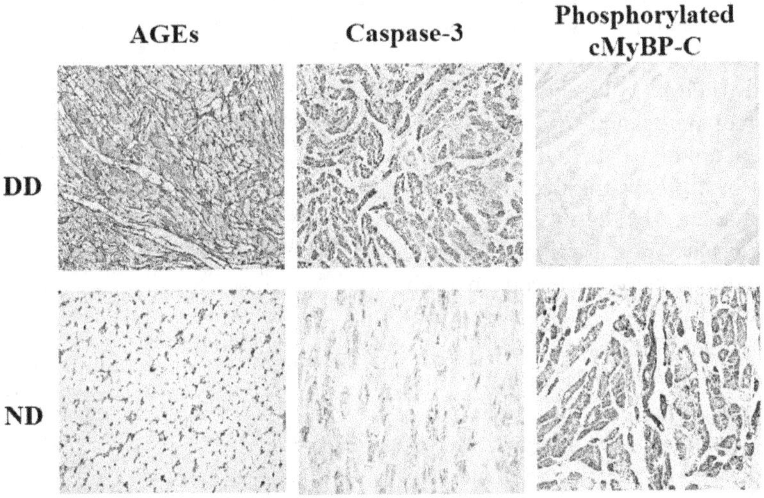

Fig. 8 Immunohistochemistry stain results of AGEs, caspase-3 and cMyBP-C of an ND monkey and a DD monkey respectively

ultrastructure damage were also observed by TEM. Many laboratories have generated data suggesting that diabetic damage is a consequence of elevated production of reactive oxygen species (ROS) found at the mitochondrial respiratory chain during hyperglycemia [54, 55]. More and more laboratory findings support the hypothesis that mitochondrial ROS mediated the diabetes induced cardiac defects. Manifestations of mitochondria in our DCM rhesus monkeys were similar to those in previous rodent studies.

Assisted by immunohistochemistry stain, positive products were observed to be abnormally expressed in the DCM monkey myocardium compared with the ND monkey. The formation of AGEs on extracellular matrix components leads to accelerated increases in collagen cross linking that contributes to the myocardial stiffness in diabetes [10]. Apoptotic cell death occurs in the diabetic myocardium through the mitochondrial cytochrome c-mediated caspase-3 activation pathway, which plays a critical role in cardiac pathogenesis related to hyperglycemia [11]. Basal levels of cMyBP-C phosphorylation may be necessary for maintaining thick-filament orientation, dynamic regulation and contractile mechanics [12]. However, cMyBP-C phosphorylation was significantly decreased during the development of heart failure or pathologic hypertrophy. Phosphorylated cMyBP-C were lightly stained in the myocardium of the DCM monkey, which is indicative of contractile abnormality. Thus, myocardial impairments were observed at molecular level in abnormal organ functioning.

The spontaneously diabetic monkeys are of great importance in both biomedical investigation and for pharmaceutical studies. Literatures and our previous work demonstrated that the clinical manifestations of T2DM monkeys were highly similar to those of human beings. Results show that some if not most of our middle-aged rhesus monkeys were confirmed to have obesity, β-cell impairment, insulin level decline and persistent hyperglycemia verifying the development of spontaneous T2DM. The FPG of healthy monkeys in our monkey model is only approximately 10 %-15 % lower than that of humans. As for DD in monkeys diagnosed by echocardiography, relative parameters exhibit human-like echo patterns with diastolic dysfunction progression, which has not been reported in rodent models. As for other features like MRI parameters, cardiac structure and biomarkers in cardiomyopathy, the monkeys share the same features as reported in human and rodents. Moreover, the development of spontaneous diabetes and its complications is a multifactorial slow progression. Of note, monkeys have a long enough life span that allows both disease progression and thorough longitudinal studies, which may shed light on the origins, pathways and pathogenesis of these pathologic changes. Meanwhile, these monkeys live in a highly controlled and stable environment with their metabolic history well documented. Thus long-term relationships between cardiovascular pathology changes and diabetic status can now be studied without the confounding lifestyle factors encountered in humans.

Limitations of the study

The present study primarily demonstrated diastolic dysfunction and related myocardial impairments in spontaneous T2DM rhesus monkeys. Nevertheless, there are several limitations need to be addressed. Firstly, the echocardiographic parameters we examined in this study were not so sufficient as to allow us to draw a full picture of the dimension and function of the ventricle. It has been reported that EDV, ESV, and V_P obtained by color M-mode Doppler also change with cardiac dysfunction in a diabetic heart. Secondly, CMR can provide more information about cardiomyopathy by using late gadolinium enhancement (LGE), MR tagging and T1 mapping, which we unfortunately failed to obtain in the present study. We are planning to further investigate DCM in rhesus monkeys by CMR in the near future. In consideration of the maintenance of the model, we only sacrificed 2 monkeys for invasive measurements. Luckily, certain myocardial impairments were observed on both microstructure and ultrastructure levels. However, quantified measurements of these biomarkers need to be done on a larger scale for these animals to determine reliability. We are also preparing non-invasive assessments for a better understanding of the mechanisms of these biomarkers and more, hoping to provide evidence for the hypotheses proposed regarding the pathogenesis of DCM.

Conclusions

The present study primarily demonstrated cardiomyopathy in spontaneous T2DM rhesus monkeys. Left ventricular diastolic dysfunction was diagnosed in six out of 15 T2DM monkeys, accompanied with structural abnormalities such as significantly increased LVID at end systole. Systolic related parameters, EF and FS, decreased with DD progression, however significance was found only between the moderate DD group and the ND group. Myocardial microstructure and ultrastructure damages were observed in a DD monkey. Meanwhile, the expression of DCM related proteins altered in a DD monkey. Characteristics of cardiomyopathy in spontaneous T2DM monkeys with DD are similar to those in DCM human patients. We will not only conduct more studies in these subjects for further investigations, but we will also screen for more diseased animals in the future to create a more effective drug testing platform.

Ethics statement

The protocols were approved by the Institutional Animal Care and Use Committee (IACUC) of Sichuan PriMed Bio-Tech Group Co., Ltd.

Abbreviations

E: Peak velocity of mitral blood flow during the rapid ventricular filling (cm/s); A: Peak velocity of mitral blood flow during the atrial contraction (cm/s); e': Peak velocity of mitral annulus during the rapid ventricular filling (cm/s); a': Peak velocity of mitral annulus during the atrial contraction (cm/s); S: Pulmonary venous flow peak systolic velocity (cm/s); D: Pulmonary venous flow diastolic velocity (cm/s); AR: Pulmonary venous flow atrial reversal velocity (cm/s); EDV: End diastolic left ventricular volume (ml); ESV: End systolic left ventricular volume (ml); SV: Stroke volume (ml); FS: Fractional shortening of the left ventricular (%); EF: Ejection fraction (%); SWTd: Septum wall thickness at end diastole (mm); SWTs: Septum wall thickness at end systole (mm); AWTd: Anterior wall thickness at end diastole (mm); AWTs: Anterior wall thickness at end systole (mm); PWTd: Posterior wall thickness at end diastole (mm); PWTs: Posterior wall thickness at end systole (mm); LVIDd: Left ventricular internal dimension at end diastole (mm); LVIDs: Left ventricular internal dimension at end systole (mm); LAAD: Left atrial anterior-posterior diameter (mm); LATD: Left atrial transverse diameter (mm); LAVD: Left atrial vertical diameter (mm)..

Competing interests

Other than the grants listed in the acknowledgement section, the authors declare that they have no other competing interests.

Author's contributions

CQ, WZ and FG were responsible for designing the experiment and overall investigation. CQ, LG and ZY carried out the experiment procedures and monkey maintenance. FG, YC, ZX, BW, CT and WC were responsible for coordinating and performing the echocardiographic and CMR measurements. CQ, ZY and WC were responsible for data collection and image analysis. CQ wrote the manuscript. All authors have given final approval of the version to be published. Each author has participated sufficiently in the work to take public responsibility for appropriate portions of the content.

Author's information

The PriMed group has been studying human disease monkey models for many years. For more information, please visit PriMed website: http://www.scprimed.com/.
The Sichuan University group consists of sonographers and radiologists from the Imaging Center of West China Hospital, Sichuan University. See website: http://www.cd120.com/.

Acknowledgements

This study was supported by the Key Projects in the National Science & Technology Pillar Program during the Twelfth Five-year Plan Period (2012BAI23B08), the State Key Program of National Natural Science Foundation of China (81130027), the National Key Basic Research Program of China (2011CB935800) and the Innovation Fund for Small and Medium-Sized Technology-Based Firms of the China Ministry of Science and Technology (14C26215102969).

Author details

[1]Sichuan Industrial Institute of Antibiotics, Chengdu, China. [2]Sichuan PriMed Shines Bio-Tech Co., Ltd, Chengdu, China. [3]Department of Radiology, West China Hospital, Sichuan University, Chengdu, China. [4]Department of Radiology, Yaan People's Hospital, Yaan, China.

References

1. American Heart Association. Cardiovascular Disease & Diabetes accessed at http://www.heart.org/. 2013.
2. Yancy CW, Jessup M, Bozkurt B, et al. 2013 ACCF/AHA guideline for the management of heart failure: a report of the American College of Cardiology Foundation/American Heart Association Task Force on Practice Guidelines. Journal of the American College of Cardiology. Oct 15 2013;62(16):e147-239.
3. Tziakas DN, Chalikias GK, Kaski JC. Epidemiology of the diabetic heart. Coron Artery Dis. 2005;16 Suppl 1:S3–s10.
4. Boudina S, Abel ED. Diabetic cardiomyopathy revisited. Circulation. 2007;115(25):3213–23.
5. Fang ZY, Prins JB, Marwick TH. Diabetic cardiomyopathy: evidence, mechanisms, and therapeutic implications. Endocr Rev. 2004;25(4):543–67.
6. Hayat SA, Patel B, Khattar RS, Malik RA. Diabetic cardiomyopathy: mechanisms, diagnosis and treatment. Clin Sci. 2004;107(6):539–58.
7. Poirier P, Bogaty P, Garneau C, Marois L, Dumesnil J-G. Diastolic Dysfunction in Normotensive Men with Well-Controlled Type 2 Diabetes: Importance of maneuvers in echocardiographic screening for preclinical diabetic cardiomyopathy. Diabetes Care. 2001;24(1):5–10.
8. Zabalgoitia M, Ismaeil MF, Anderson L, Maklady FA. Prevalence of diastolic dysfunction in normotensive, asymptomatic patients with well-controlled type 2 diabetes mellitus. Am J Cardiol. 2001;87(3):320–3.

9. Raev DC. Which left ventricular function is impaired earlier in the evolution of diabetic cardiomyopathy? An echocardiographic study of young type I diabetic patients. Diabetes Care. 1994;17(7):633–9.
10. Candido R, Forbes JM, Thomas MC, et al. A breaker of advanced glycation end products attenuates diabetes-induced myocardial structural changes. Circ Res. 2003;92(7):785–92.
11. Cai L, Li W, Wang G, Guo L, Jiang Y, Kang YJ. Hyperglycemia-induced apoptosis in mouse myocardium mitochondrial cytochrome c–mediated caspase-3 activation pathway. Diabetes. 2002;51(6):1938–48.
12. Sadayappan S, Gulick J, Osinska H, et al. Cardiac myosin-binding protein-C phosphorylation and cardiac function. Circ Res. 2005;97(11):1156–63.
13. Aasum E, Hafstad AD, Severson DL, Larsen TS. Age-dependent changes in metabolism, contractile function, and ischemic sensitivity in hearts from db/db mice. Diabetes. 2003;52(2):434–41.
14. Rodrigues B, McNeill JH. Cardiac dysfunction in isolated perfused hearts from spontaneously diabetic BB rats. Can J Physiol Pharmacol. 1990;68(4):514–8.
15. Loganathan R, Bilgen M, Al-Hafez B, Alenezy MD, Smirnova IV. Cardiac dysfunction in the diabetic rat: quantitative evaluation using high resolution magnetic resonance imaging. Cardiovasc Diabetol. 2006;5(1):7.
16. Kralik PM, Ye G, Metreveli NS, Shen X, Epstein PN. Cardiomyocyte dysfunction in models of type 1 and type 2 diabetes. Cardiovasc Toxicol. 2005;5(3):285–92.
17. Yu X, Tesiram YA, Towner RA, et al. Early myocardial dysfunction in streptozotocin-induced diabetic mice: a study using in vivo magnetic resonance imaging (MRI). Cardiovasc Diabetol. 2007;6(1):6.
18. Hoit BD, Castro C, Bultron G, Knight S, Matlib MA. Noninvasive evaluation of cardiac dysfunction by echocardiography in streptozotocin-induced diabetic rats. J Card Fail. 1999;5(4):324–33.
19. Gibbs RA, Rogers J, Katze MG, et al. Evolutionary and biomedical insights from the rhesus macaque genome. Science. 2007;316(5822):222–34.
20. Ortmeyer HK, Bodkin N, Hansen BC. Insulin-mediated glycogen synthase activity in muscle of spontaneously insulin-resistant and diabetic rhesus monkeys. Am J Physiol Regul Integr Comp Physiol. 1993;265(3):R552–8.
21. Hansen B, Bodkin N. Beta-cell hyperresponsiveness: earliest event in development of diabetes in monkeys. Am J Physiol Regul Integr Comp Physiol. 1990;259(3):R612–7.
22. Hansen B, Bodkin N. Heterogeneity of insulin responses: phases leading to type 2 (non-insulin-dependent) diabetes mellitus in the rhesus monkey. Diabetologia. 1986;29(10):713–9.
23. Gong L, Zeng W, Yang Z, et al. Comparison of the Clinical Manifestations of Type 2 Diabetes Mellitus Between Rhesus Monkey (Macaca mulatta lasiotis) and Human Being. Pancreas. 2013;42(3):537–42.
24. Hansen BC. Investigation and treatment of type 2 diabetes in nonhuman primates. Methods Mol Biol. 2012;933:177–85.
25. Wagner JD, Kavanagh K, Ward GM, Auerbach BJ, Harwood HJ, Kaplan JR. Old world nonhuman primate models of type 2 diabetes mellitus. ILAR J. 2006;47(3):259–71.
26. Zeng W, Wen X, Gong L, et al. Establishment and ultrasound characteristics of atherosclerosis in rhesus monkey. Biomed Eng Online. 2015;14 Suppl 1:S13.
27. Voutilainen S, Kupari M, Hippelainen M, Karppinen K, Ventila M. Circadian variation of left ventricular diastolic function in healthy people. Heart. 1996;75(1):35–9.
28. Zeng W, Cheng A-c, Chen Z-l, et al. In vivo assessment of mitochondrial toxicity of metacavir in rhesus monkeys after three months of intravenous administration. Acta Pharmacol Sin. 2009;30(12):1666–73.
29. Semeniuk LM, Kryski AJ, Severson DL. Echocardiographic assessment of cardiac function in diabeticdb/db and transgenic db/db-hGLUT4 mice. Am J Physiol Heart Circ Physiol. 2002;283(3):H976–82.
30. Moreo A, Ambrosio G, De Chiara B, et al. Influence of myocardial fibrosis on left ventricular diastolic function noninvasive assessment by cardiac magnetic resonance and echo. Circ Cardiovasc Imaging. 2009;2(6):437–43.
31. Sohn D-W, Chai I-H, Lee D-J, et al. Assessment of mitral annulus velocity by Doppler tissue imaging in the evaluation of left ventricular diastolic function. J Am Coll Cardiol. 1997;30(2):474–80.
32. Paulus WJ, Tschöpe C, Sanderson JE, et al. How to diagnose diastolic heart failure: a consensus statement on the diagnosis of heart failure with normal left ventricular ejection fraction by the Heart Failure and Echocardiography Associations of the European Society of Cardiology. Eur Heart J. 2007;28(20):2539–50.
33. Hirai J, Ueda K, Takegoshi T, Mabuchi H. Effects of metabolic control on ventricular function in type 2 diabetic patients. Intern Med. 1992;31(6):725–30.
34. Boyer JK, Thanigaraj S, Schechtman KB, Pérez JE. Prevalence of ventricular diastolic dysfunction in asymptomatic, normotensive patients with diabetes mellitus. Am J Cardiol. 2004;93(7):870–5.
35. Khan JN, Wilmot EG, Leggate M, et al. Subclinical diastolic dysfunction in young adults with Type 2 diabetes mellitus: a multiparametric contrast-enhanced cardiovascular magnetic resonance pilot study assessing potential mechanisms. European Heart Journal Cardiovascular Imaging. Nov 2014;15(11):1263-1269.
36. Korcarz CE, Padrid PA, Shroff SG, Weinert L, Lang RM. Doppler echocardiographic reference values for healthy rhesus monkeys under ketamine hydrochloride sedation. J Med Primatol. 1997;26(6):287–98.
37. Tang HL, Wang LL, Cheng G, Wang L, Li S. Evaluation of the cardiovascular function of older adult rhesus monkeys by ultrasonography. J Med Primatol. 2008;37(2):101–8.
38. Sleeper MM, Gaughan JM, Gleason CR, Burkett DE. Echocardiographic reference ranges for sedated healthy cynomolgus monkeys (Macaca fascicularis). Am Assoc Lab Anim Sci. 2008;47(1):22.
39. Keenan CM, Vidal JD. Standard morphologic evaluation of the heart in the laboratory dog and monkey. Toxicol Pathol. 2006;34(1):67–74.
40. Maya L, Villarreal FJ. Diagnostic approaches for diabetic cardiomyopathy and myocardial fibrosis. J Mol Cell Cardiol. 2010;48(3):524–9.
41. Danzmann LC, Bodanese LC, Köhler I, Torres MR. Left atrioventricular remodeling in the assessment of the left ventricle diastolic function in patients with heart failure: a review of the currently studied echocardiographic variables. Cardiovasc Ultrasound. 2008;6(1):56.
42. Galderisi M. Diastolic dysfunction and diabetic cardiomyopathy: evaluation by Doppler echocardiography. J Am Coll Cardiol. 2006;48(8):1548–51.
43. Farias CA, Rodriguez L, Garcia MJ, Sun JP, Klein AL, Thomas JD. Assessment of diastolic function by tissue Doppler echocardiography: comparison with standard transmitral and pulmonary venous flow. J Am Soc Echocardiogr. 1999;12(8):609–17.
44. From AM, Scott CG, Chen HH. The Development of Heart Failure in Patients With Diabetes Mellitus and Pre-Clinical Diastolic DysfunctionA Population-Based Study. J Am Coll Cardiol. 2010;55(4):300–5.
45. Bonito P, Moio N, Cavuto L, et al. Early detection of diabetic cardiomyopathy: usefulness of tissue Doppler imaging. Diabet Med. 2005;22(12):1720–5.
46. Ernande L, Bergerot C, Rietzschel ER, et al. Diastolic dysfunction in patients with type 2 diabetes mellitus: is it really the first marker of diabetic cardiomyopathy? J Am Soc Echocardiogr. 2011;24(11):1268–75. e1261.
47. Sechtem U, Pflugfelder P, Higgins CB. Quantification of cardiac function by conventional and cine magnetic resonance imaging. Cardiovasc Intervent Radiol. 1987;10(6):365–73.
48. Mihm MJ, Seifert JL, Coyle CM, Bauer JA. Diabetes related cardiomyopathy time dependent echocardiographic evaluation in an experimental rat model. Life Sci. 2001;69(5):527–42.
49. Joffe II, Travers KE, Perreault-Micale CL, et al. Abnormal cardiac function in the streptozotocin-induced, non–insulin-dependent diabetic rat: Noninvasive assessment with Doppler echocardiography and contribution of the nitric oxide pathway. J Am Coll Cardiol. 1999;34(7):2111–9.
50. Akula A, Kota M, Gopisetty S, et al. Biochemical, histological and echocardiographic changes during experimental cardiomyopathy in STZ-induced diabetic rats. Pharmacol Res. 2003;48(5):429–35.
51. Factor SM, Bhan R, Minase T, Wolinsky H, Sonnenblick EH. Hypertensive-diabetic cardiomyopathy in the rat: an experimental model of human disease. Am J Pathol. 1981;102(2):219.
52. Factor SM, Minase T, Sonnenblick EH. Clinical and morphological features of human hypertensive-diabetic cardiomyopathy. Am Heart J. 1980;99(4):446–58.
53. Kuethe F, Sigusch H, Bornstein S, Hilbig K, Kamvissi V, Figulla H. Apoptosis in patients with dilated cardiomyopathy and diabetes: a feature of diabetic cardiomyopathy? Horm Metab Res. 2007;39(09):672–6.

14

Assessment of left ventricular preload by cardiac magnetic resonance imaging predicts exercise capacity in adult operated tetralogy of Fallot

Jonathan Yap[1], Ju Le Tan[1], Thu Thao Le[1], Fei Gao[1,2], Liang Zhong[1], Reginald Liew[2], Swee Yaw Tan[1,2] and Ru San Tan[1,2*]

Abstract

Background: The optimal timing of pulmonary homograft valve replacement (PVR) is uncertain. Cardiopulmonary exercise testing (CPET) and cardiac magnetic resonance (CMR) are often used to guide the clinical decision for PVR in operated tetralogy of Fallot (TOF) patients with significant pulmonary regurgitation (PR). We aim to study the relationship between exercise capacity and CMR in these patients.

Methods: The study is a single-centre retrospective analysis of 36 operated TOF patients [median 21.4 (interquartile range 16.4, 26.4) years post-repair; 30 NYHA I, 6 NYHA II; median age 25.2 (interquartile range 19.5-31.7) years, 29 males] with significant PR on CMR who underwent CPET within 15 [median 2.0 (interquartile range 0.8-7.2)] months from CMR. CPET parameters were compared with 30 age- and sex-matched healthy controls [median age 27.8 (interquartile range 21.0-32.8) years; 24 males].

Results: Peak systolic blood pressure (177 versus 192 mmHg, $p = 0.007$), Mets (7.3 versus 9.9, $p < 0.001$), peak oxygen consumption (VO_2max) (29.2 versus 34.5 ml/kg/min, $p < 0.001$) and peak oxygen pulse (11.0 versus 13.7 ml/beat, $p = 0.003$) were significantly lower in TOF group versus control. Univariate analyses showed negative correlation between PR fraction and anaerobic threshold. There was a positive correlation between indexed left (LV) and right (RV) ventricular end-diastolic volumes, as well as indexed LV and effective RV stroke volumes, on CMR and VO_2max and Mets achieved on CPET. These remained significant after adjustment for age and sex.

Conclusions: TOF subjects have near normal exercise capacity but significantly lower Mets, VO_2max and peak oygen pulse achieved compared to controls. Increased PR fraction in TOF subjects was associated with lower anaerobic threshold. Higher indexed effective RV stroke volume, a measure of LV preload, was associated with higher VO_2max and Mets achieved, and may potentially be used as a predictor of exercise capacity.

Keywords: Exercise capacity, Cardiac magnetic resonance imaging, Tetralogy of Fallot

* Correspondence: tan.ru.san@nhcs.com.sg
[1]Department of Cardiology, National Heart Centre Singapore, 5 Hospital Drive, Singapore 169609, Singapore
[2]Duke-NUS Graduate Medical School, Singapore, 8 College Rd, Singapore 169857, Singapore

Background

Long-term outcomes of patients with tetralogy of Fallot (TOF) have improved with advances in surgical techniques [1]. However, pulmonary regurgitation (PR) resulting from repair to the right ventricular outflow tract is a common consequence of the primary surgery. This is usually well tolerated initially, but leads to increased right ventricular (RV) dilatation, dysfunction and worsening exercise intolerance over time, and may result in arrhythmia and sudden cardiac death [2-4].

The optimal timing of pulmonary homograft valve replacement (PVR) in operated TOF patients with significant PR is unclear. The decision for PVR is usually a fine balance between avoiding permanent remodeling of the right ventricle [5,6] and reducing the need for repeat procedures throughout one's lifetime in these often young patients. Cardiopulmonary exercise testing (CPET) and cardiac magnetic resonance (CMR) are two important tools often used by clinicians to help guide this difficult management decision [5,6].

Poor exercise capacity identifies patients at higher risk of hospitalization and mortality [7-9] and guidelines have listed decreasing exercise tolerance as a strong indication for PVR [10-12]. The American College of Cardiology/American Heart Association (ACC/AHA) 2008 guidelines recommend PVR as a Class I indication in operated TOF patients with severe PR and decreased exercise tolerance [12]; exercise testing is a useful adjunct. A Class IIa indication for PVR is in patients with severe PR and moderate to severe RV enlargement [12]. The exact definition of moderate to severe RV dysfunction/enlargement is not clear. The European Society of Cardiology (ESC) 2010 guidelines have similar recommendations but suggest using a RVEDVi cut-off of 160 ml/m2, beyond which normalization of RV becomes unlikely [10]. The Canadian Cardiovascular Society (CCS) 2009 guidelines recommend as a Class IIa indication that PVR should be considered in TOF patients with severe PR who have either a deterioriating exercise performance or moderate to severe RV enlargement (RVEDVi >170 ml/m^2) [11]. A RVEDVi cut-off of 150 ml/m2 is sometimes used clinically [13]. A recent study found similar exercise capacity and stroke volumes in patients below and above the threshold, thus raising questions about the utility of RVEDVi as the main basis for deciding on timing for PVR [14].

The relationship between CMR parameters and actual exercise capacity remains unclear. Understanding the relationship between exercise capacity and CMR parameters is important and may better help rationalize the clinical decision for PVR. We aim to study the exercise capacity in TOF patients with significant PR late (>10 years) after repair and its relationship with CMR parameters.

Methods

Study design and patient population

In our institution, operated adult TOF patients with significant (at least moderate) PR on TTE will undergo CMR and CPET as part of their clinical management. The study is a retrospective review of all consecutive patients with surgically corrected TOF and known significant (moderate to severe) PR on TTE, who underwent CMR and CPET at our institution from Apr 2005 to Mar 2013. All patients were older than 15 years of age and had undergone corrective surgery for TOF more than 10 years previously [median 21.4 years (IQR 16.4, 26.4)]. Patients with residual pulmonary stenosis pressure gradient on Doppler echocardiography, associated atrioventricular septum defect, double outlet right ventricle of Fallot type, pulmonary atresia with ventricular septum defect, TOF with absent pulmonary valve, or patients who had undergone pulmonary valve replacement (PVR) were excluded. Clinical data were obtained from review of patients' case-files and electronic medical records.

CMR and CPET data were recorded. CPET data were also obtained from age- and sex-matched healthy controls. The study was approved by the SingHealth Centralised Institutional Review Board (SingHealth, Singapore).

Cardiac MRI

Study subjects underwent CMR on a 1.5 T Avanto scanner (Siemens). In each patient, fast imaging in steady-state precession (trueFISP) cine MR images were acquired in the left ventricular (LV) long axes (2-, 3- and 4-chamber views), RV outflow tract (RVOT) (oblique sagittal and coronal) planes as well as a parallel contiguous stack of 8 mm ventricular short-axis cine slices. Retrospective ECG-triggering was employed, achieving typical frame rates of about 25 per cardiac cycle. Throughplane flow measurements in planes across the aortic root and main pulmonary trunk were performed using velocity-encoded gradient-echo pulse sequences.

Calculation of left and right ventricular end-diastolic (EDV) and end-systolic (ESV) volumes, LV mass and ejection fractions (EF) was performed using CMRTools (London, UK). All volumes and LV mass measurements were then indexed to body surface area. The presence of RVOT aneurysm, defined as akinesia or dyskinesia (outward movement) during systole of part of the RVOT assessed from the basal ventricular short-axis cine images, was recorded. PR fraction (diastolic reverse flow expressed as a percentage of forward flow) was assessed from anterograde and retrograde flow in the main pulmonary artery (ARGUS software, Siemens, Erlangen). Effective right ventricular stroke volume (RVSV) was calculated as the difference between the total RV forward flow and the pulmonary regurgitant flow [15,16]. Restrictive RV physiology was ascertained by presence of end-diastolic forward pulmonary flow, consistent with severely limited RV capacitance during right atrial contraction.

Cardiopulmonary exercise testing

Cardiopulmonary exercise tests were performed on a Hewlett-Packard Cosmos treadmill machine. A maximal ramp protocol with fixed treadmill speed but constantly increasing incline gradient to provide an increasing workload was employed. Exercise speed was determined at the performing physician's discretion. Patients were encouraged to exercise until symptoms were intolerable, i.e. when Rating of Perceived Exertion reached 18/20. Heart rate was monitored continuously, and non-invasive blood pressure was taken every 2 minutes with both manual and automatic blood pressure. Oxygen saturation was monitored by a finger probe pulse oximeter. Oxygen uptake (VO_2), minute ventilation (VE), and carbon dioxide output (VCO_2) were measured breath by breath. The anaerobic threshold (AT) was chosen as the VO_2 at which respiratory exchange ratio reached 1.0 and when there was a sudden and sustained precipitous rise in VCO_2. Peak VO_2 was defined as the value of averaged data during the final 15 seconds of exercise. The VE/VCO_2 slope was determined as the linear regression slope of VE and VCO_2.

Statistical analysis

Data was analysed using STATA version 11.1 (College Station, Texas, USA). All values were presented as median and interquartile range for continuous data and frequency and percentage for categorical data. Comparisons between groups were made with Mann–Whitney U test, or the Fisher's exact test as appropriate. The linear correlation, *r*, between exercise testing and CMR parameters were initially assessed using Pearson correlation coefficient with 95% confidence interval (CI). Significant relationships were subsequently assessed by multiple linear regression technique adjusting for age and gender. Scatter plots with linear fit were produced. For all analyses, a two-tailed *P* value of <0.05 was considered significant.

Results

Baseline clinical characteristics

Of the 119 TOF patients on clinical follow-up at our institution at the beginning of the study, 36 had significant PR on echocardiography. The latter underwent CPET and CMR testing and were included in this study. Thirty controls were also recruited. There was no significant difference in age, sex and indexed body mass between patients and controls. Six TOF patients had NYHA II functional status; the rest of the study TOF population were either asymptomatic or NYHA I (Table 1).

CPET parameters

Compared to controls, TOF patients achieved significantly lower maximum systolic blood pressure (177 versus 192 mmHg, p = 0.007), Mets (7.3 versus 9.9, p < 0.001), peak oxygen consumption (29.2 versus 34.5 ml/kg/min, p < 0.001) and peak oxygen pulse pressure (11.0 versus 13.7 ml/beat, p = 0.003). These differences were significant even after adjusting for age and sex. There were no significant difference in the rest of the CPET parameters (Table 1). 7 TOF patients experienced arrhythmia during CPET, all consisting of occasional isolated premature ventricular complexes. No malignant arryhtmia was noted.

Medication, Surgical and CMR findings in TOF patients

The majority of the TOF patients were not on any cardiac medications: one patient was on beta-blocker and ACE inhibitor; one patient, ACE inhibitor and diuretics; and one patient, beta-blocker alone. The median age at which surgical repair was performed was 3.7 years (IQR 2.3-6.9) and the median time from surgical repair was 21.4 years (IQR 16.4-26.4). Ten patients (27.8%) had undergone transannular patch repair (Table 2). All patients were in sinus rhythm.

The median RVEDVi, RVESVi, RVEF, RVSVi, effective RVSVi and PR fraction were 167.7 ml/m^2 (IQR 142.5-178.5), 87.2 ml/m^2 (IQR 75.8-98.4), 45.6% (IQR 39.2-50.0), 73.5 ml/m^2 (IQR 61.8-82.9), 41.1 ml/m^2 (37.9-44.3) and 45.0% (IQR 35.5-52), respectively. The median LVEDVi, LVESVi, LVEF and LVSVi were 73.1 ml/m^2 (IQR 66.6-82.5), 30.4 ml/m^2 (IQR 26.9-35.3), 58.7% (IQR 52.9-62.3) and 43.1 ml/m^2 (IQR 39.0-48.1), respectively. All patients had LVEF >40%, with five (13.9%) patients having LVEF between 40-50%. Twenty-six (72.2%) had restrictive RV physiology; and 20 (55.6%), RVOT aneurysms (Figure 1).

Relationship between CPET and CMR parameters in TOF patients

The median time between CPET and CMR was 2.0 months (IQR 0.8-7.2); there was no change in clinical status between CPET and CMR for all patients. Larger RVEDVi (*r* = 0.36, 95% CI 0.03-0.62, p = 0.035), RVESVi (*r* = 0.35, 95% CI 0.01-0.61, p = 0.042) and LVEDVi (*r* = 0.39, 95% CI 0.06-0.64, p = 0.021) were associated with significantly higher Mets achieved during exercise testing. Larger RVEDVi (r = 0.35, 95% CI 0.03-0.61, p = 0.037) and LVEDVi (*r* = 0.35, 95% CI 0.03-0.61, p = 0.030) were associated with higher peak oxygen consumption achieved during exercise testing. Larger LVSVi (*r* = 0.37, 95% CI 0.04-0.62, p = 0.030) and effective RVSVi (*r* = 0.53, 95% CI 0.24-0.73, p = 0.001) were associated with significantly higher Mets achieved. Larger LVSVi (*r* = 0.35, 95% CI 0.02-0.61, p = 0.037) and effective RVSVi (*r* = 0.53, 95% CI 0.24-0.73, p < 0.001) were associated with significantly higher peak oxygen consumption. Greater PR fraction was

Table 1 Demographics and CPET parameters of study population (n = 66)

	TOF (n = 36)	Control (n = 30)	*P value*	*Adjusted P value**
Demographics				
Age	25.2 (19.5, 31.7)	27.8 (21.0, 32.8)	0.20	
Male	29 (80.6)	24 (80.0)	1.00	
BMI (kg/m2)	22.8 (21.0, 26.3)	23.2 (19.6, 25.6)	0.39	
Asymptomatic/NYHA I	30 (83.3)	30 (100.0)	0.03	
CPET parameters				
Max HR (beats/min)	172.5 (159, 178)	176.5 (168, 181)	0.257	0.429
Heart rate reserve (beats/min)	26.5 (8, 39)	15.5 (7, 20)	0.117	0.183
Max SBP (mmHg)	177 (150, 184)	192 (168, 210)	**0.007**	**0.010**
Max DBP (mmHg)	86 (78, 93)	82 (76, 97)	0.575	0.964
Max breathing reserve (L/min)	38 (21, 72.1)	47.8 (34.5, 61.3)	0.540	0.602
Mets	8.3 (7.1, 9.4)	9.9 (8.6,11.7)	**<0.001**	**<0.001**
% predicted Mets (%)	85.0 (74.8, 93.9)	102.7 (91.1, 114.5)	**<0.001**	**<0.001**
Peak oxygen consumption (ml/kg/min)	29.2 (25.5, 33.0)	34.5 (30.0, 41.0)	**<0.001**	**<0.001**
% predicted peak oxygen consumption (%)	83.0 (72.0, 93.5)	102.7 (91.1, 114.8)	**<0.001**	**<0.001**
Anaerobic threshold (ml/min)	1395 (1170, 1574)	1501.5 (1255, 1700)	0.231	0.211
Oxygen pulse pressure (ml/beat)	11.0 (8.8, 13.2)	13.7 (11.9, 16.2)	**0.003**	**0.002**
VE/VCO$_2$ slope	26.0 (23.6, 27.3)	25.6 (24.1, 27.2)	1.00	0.576
Arrhythmias**	7 (19.4)	4 (13.3)	0.742	0.492

Median and interquartile ranges are reported for continuous data and frequency and percentage for categorical data.
*Adjusted for age and gender.
**All were occasional ventricular or atrial ectopics.

associated with lower AT ($r = -0.40$, 95% CI −0.65 to 0.07, p = 0.020)(see Table 3). After adjusting for age and sex, all these relationships remained significant (Table 4, Figure 2). Of note, there was no significant correlation between exercise data and either RVEF or RVSV. Comparing TOF patients with and without restrictive RV physiology, no significant difference in CPET parameters was observed. This was the same among those with and without RVOT aneurysms. There was also no significant association between the rest of the CMR parameters and CPET observations.

Table 2 Medication, Surgical and CMR Data of TOF patients (n = 36)

	TOF (n = 36)
Medication data	
Beta-blockers	2 (5.6%)
ACE Inhibitors	2 (5.6%)
Diuretics	1 (2.8%)
Digoxin	0
Surgical data	
Age of surgical repair	3.69 (2.26, 6.93)
Time from surgical repair	21.4 (16.4, 26.4)
Transannular patch*	10 (27.8)
Pulmonary outflow patch*	4 (11.1)
RV to pul artery conduit*	4 (11.1)
Previous palliative shunt	4 (11.1)

Median and interquartile ranges are reported for continuous data and frequency and percentage for categorical data.
*Complete surgical data missing in 6 patients.

Discussion

Our operated TOF patients with significant PR had near normal exercise capacity, albeit lower than that of normal

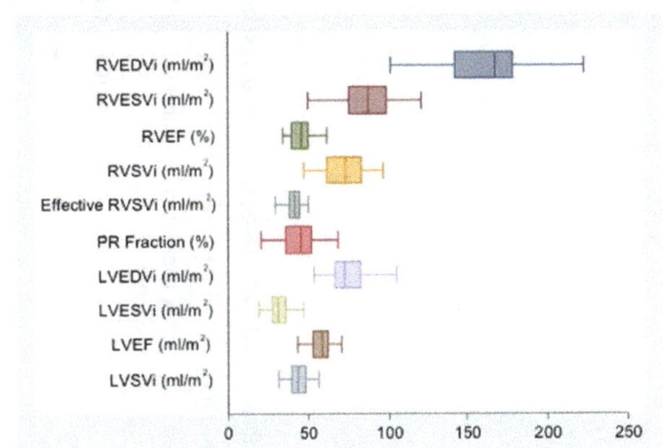

Figure 1 Box plot showing distribution of CMR data.

Table 3 Relationship between exercise testing and RV and LV function/volume in TOF patients (n = 36)

CMR parameters	CPET parameters							
	Max breathing reserve	Mets	% predicted mets	Peak oxygen consumption	% Predicted peak oxygen consumption	Anaerobic threshold	Oxygen pulse pressure	VE/VCO_2 slope
RVEDVi	0.15 (−0.20, 0.46)	**0.36 (0.03, 0.62)***	0.31 (−0.04, 0.59)	**0.35 (0.03, 0.61)***	0.24 (−0.10, 0.52)	−0.03 (−0.36, 0.31)	−0.02 (−0.35, 0.31)	−0.15 (−0.46, 0.20)
RVESVi	0.25 (−0.10, 0.54)	**0.35 (0.01, 0.61)***	0.28 (−0.07, 0.57)	0.31 (−0.02, 0.58)	0.18 (−0.16, 0.48)	0.12 (−0.23, 0.44)	−0.08 (−0.40, 0.26)	−0.16 (−0.47, 0.19)
RVEF	−0.31 (−0.59, 0.03)	−0.16 (−0.47, 0.18)	−0.10 (−0.43, 0.25)	−0.12 (−0.43, 0.22)	−0.01 (−0.34, 0.32)	−0.25 (−0.54, 0.10)	0.15 (−0.19, 0.46)	0.09 (−0.26, 0.42)
RVSVi	−0.13 (−0.45, 0.22)	0.16 (−0.18, 0.47)	0.18 (−0.17, 0.50)	0.18 (−0.15, 0.48)	0.18 (−0.15, 0.48)	−0.26 (−0.55, 0.09)	0.10 (−0.23, 0.42)	−0.05 (−0.38, 0.29)
Effective RVSVi	−0.18 (−0.49, 0.16)	**0.53 (0.24, 0.73)****	**0.45 (0.13, 0.69)****	**0.53 (0.24, 0.73)****	**0.53 (0.24, 0.73)****	0.20 (−0.15, 0.50)	0.28 (−0.06, 0.55)	−0.12 (−0.44, 0.23)
PR Fraction	0.07 (−0.27, 0.40)	−0.33 (−0.60, 0.004)	−0.24 (−0.54, 0.12)	−0.30 (−0.57, 0.03)	−0.33 (−0.59, 0.002)	**−0.40 (−0.65, −0.07)***	−0.18 (−0.48, 0.16)	0.02 (−0.32, 0.36)
LVEDVi	0.19 (−0.16, 0.50)	**0.39 (0.06, 0.64)***	0.05 (−0.30, 0.38)	**0.35 (0.03, 0.61)***	0.11 (−0.23, 0.42)	0.23 (−0.12, 0.53)	−0.02 (−0.35, 0.31)	−0.11 (−0.43, 0.24)
LVESVi	0.18 (−0.17, 0.49)	0.27 (−0.07, 0.55)	−0.06 (−0.40, 0.29)	0.23(−0.11, 0.52)	−0.05 (−0.37, 0.28)	0.20 (−0.15, 0.50)	−0.03 (−0.36, 0.30)	−0.02 (−0.36, 0.32)
LVEF	−0.07 (−0.40, 0.28)	−0.06 (−0.39, 0.28)	0.13 (−0.22, 0.45)	−0.04 (−0.36, 0.29)	0.19 (−0.15, 0.49)	−0.13 (−0.45, 0.22)	0.04 (−0.29, 0.36)	−0.09 (−0.42, 0.26)
LVSVi	0.11(−0.23, 0.43)	**0.37 (0.04, 0.62)***	0.18 (−0.17, 0.50)	**0.35 (0.02, 0.61)***	0.28(−0.05, 0.56)	0.15 (−0.20, 0.47)	0.01 (−0.32, 0.34)	−0.20 (−0.50, 0.15)

Pearson correlation coefficient, *r*, with 95% CI shown.
*p < 0.05.
**p < 0.01.

Table 4 Correlates of CPET parameters on CMR parameters with multiple linear regression analysis adjusting for age and gender

CPET	MRI	Adjusted *r*	95% CI	*P*	R^2,%
Mets	RVEDVi	0.41	(0.07, 0.67)	0.019	40.3
	RVESVi	0.35	(0.0004, 0.62)	0.047	37.2
	Effective RVSVi	0.57	(0.28, 0.77)	0.001	51.9
	LVEDVi	0.36	(0.02, 0.63)	0.036	38.1
	LVSVi	0.39	(0.04, 0.65)	0.026	39.2
% predicted Mets	Effective RVSVi	0.42	(0.08, 0.68)	0.017	23.3
Peak oxygen consumption	RVEDVi	0.40	(0.06, 0.65)	0.019	43.7
	Effective RVSVi	0.58	(0.29, 0.77)	<0.001	55.4
	LVEDVi	0.35	(0.003, 0.62)	0.045	41.1
	LVSVi	0.37	(0.04, 0.64)	0.029	42.4
% predicted peak oxygen consumption	Effective RVSVi	0.52	(0.21, 0.73)	0.002	28.2
Anaerobic threshold	PR Fraction	−0.40	−0.66, −0.05	0.023	41.2

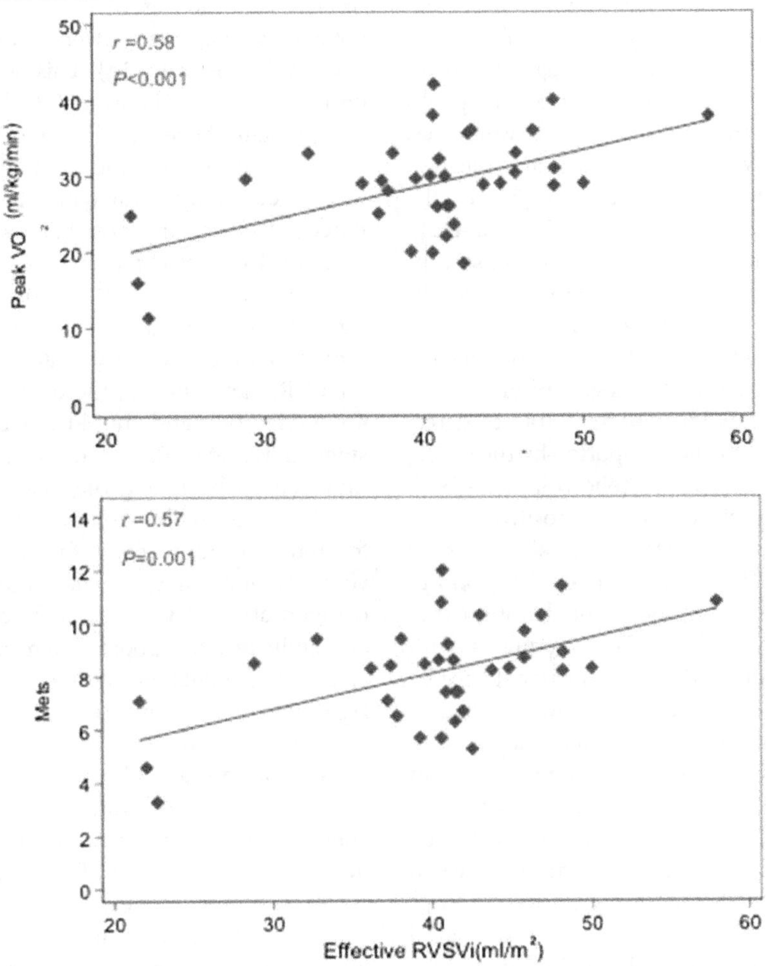

Figure 2 Scatter plots with linear fit showing relationship between CPET and CMR parameters (r and P value were adjusted for age and gender).

healthy controls. Although direct comparison is difficult because of differences in cohort characteristics, the exercise capacity in our operated TOF patients with significant PR is fairly similar to a published series [8] and better compared to others [7,17]. These latter studies included patients with all degrees of PR, unlike our study in which only patients with significant PR on echocardiography were studied with CMR and CPET. In clinical practice, only patients with significant PR routinely undergo surveillance cardiac MR. Our study thus provides clinically-relevant data in the subset of patients with significant PR.

We demonstrated a negative correlation between PR fraction and AT, implying a possible deleterious effect on exercise capacity of worsening PR per se. The AT is decreased in patients with heart disease and is an important functional limit: physiological responses to exercise are different above and below the AT [18]. While low AT in heart failure patients is associated with increased mortality [19], the prognostic value of AT in TOF patients has not been previously studied.

In our study, we found that higher effective RV stroke volume correlated significantly with higher Mets and peak oxygen consumption. In contrast, we found no significant correlation between exercise capacity and either RVEF or RV stroke volume, which is in keeping with reported studies [14,20]. In our TOF cohort, which has similar distribution of RV and LV volume and ejection fraction parameters to that of other studies [14,21], the majority had normal LV function. Conceivably, the main determinant of cardiac output (and thereby exercise capacity) would thus be LV preload. In patients with significant PR, LV preload may best be assessed by effective RVSVi as LV preload is determined by the actual net RV forward flow, taking into account the degree of PR.

That LV preload may play an important role in determining exercise capacity is further supported by the observation that both RV and LV end-diastolic volumes - both indirect estimates of LV preload - showed positive correlation with Mets achieved and peak VO2, albeit not as strong a correlation as effective RVSVi. This appears to be counter-intuitive to the commonly held notion that increasingly dilated ventricular volumes equates with worsening exercise capacity. However, our results are by no means unique. There was a trend towards higher peak VO2 with increasing biventricular diastolic volumes in another study [20]. Similar to our findings, a recent study of 55 operated TOF patients found significant positive correlation between LVEDVi and peak work achieved [14]. They also found that exercise capacity between patients with and without RV dilation was similar. Supporting this notion, another study comparing treated pulmonary stenosis and TOF patients found similar exercise capacities and biventricular function in both groups, despite worse PR and larger RV volumes in TOF patients [22]. Our observations, as well as as those of other investigators, call into question the presumption that RV dilation necessarily means impaired exercise tolerance.

Questions have been raised regarding the use of RV size as a primary parameter in deciding the timing of PVR. Studies have found that exercise capacity and stroke volume are preserved late after tetrology repair, despite severe right ventricular dilation [14]. There are several postulations for this. Firstly, this may represent adaptive LV and RV remodeling in well-compensated TOF subjects. Of note, our TOF subjects had near-normal exercise capacities, indicating a good degree of compensation, despite their significant PR. Furthermore, our study has shown that exercise capacity correlates with stroke volumes, supporting the notion that proper adaptation to volume overload of RV could be helpful for preservation of functional capacity. This phenomenon is well recognized in left ventricular physiology among elite athletes [23,24]. Secondly, PR results in a dilated but not hypertrophied RV. RV dilation exerts lesser impact on oxygen saturation and LV function, so long as RV stroke volume is maintained. Hence, exercise capacity is relatively well preserved [14]. This notion is supported by our observation that effective RV stroke volume is a significant determinant of exercise capacity. The potential of effective RVSVi as an indirect indicator of LV preload, and therefore cardiac output (in patients with largely normal LV function), raises the possibility of this parameter being used for decisions regarding the optimal timing of PVR.

In our study, we have shown that effective RVSVi significantly correlates with exercise capacity and maybe a potentially useful additional parameter in the decision for PVR. Nevertheless, the decision for timing of PVR is a complex one and should not be based primarily on a single parameter. Rather, each case should be considered individually: balancing the need to intervene before the point of irreversible remodeling against the likelihood for repeat procedures in future. The use of ventricular volumes alone may not take into account the degree of compensation of ventricular function. Many factors may also influence the poorer exercise performance in operated TOF patients: not only residual PR, but also residual right ventricular outflow tract obstruction, impaired biventricular function and presence of ventricular or atrial arrhythmias [25].

Abnormal cardiac function and and haemodynamic abnormalities secondary to residual PR and other residual defects may only appear after longer periods of follow-up. As time passes, PR leads eventually to worsening right ventricle enlargement and dysfunction, with consequent biventricular dyssynchrony, progression to heart failure, and poor performance at physical exercise. The challenge is to identify the optimal timing prior to irreversible decompensation for intervention. Presence of arryhythmia is another important consideration in the decision for PVR. Ventricular and atrial arrhythmias occur not uncommonly after correction of TOF and are one of the causes for sudden cardiac death in this group of patients [1,26]. Both the ESC and CCS guidelines recommend PVR in the presence of sustained atrial or ventricular arrhythmias [10,11]. In our cohort of repaired TOF patients, none had any malignant arrhythmias necessitating PVR.

The strength of our study lies in the unique set of data on exercise capacity in operated TOF patients with significant PR, which provides insights into the relationship between exercise capacity and CMR findings in this group of patients. The main limitations of our study is its retrospective and cross-sectional design, with lack of longitudinal CPET and CMR data. The longitudinal relationship between exercise capacity and biventricular volumes and function were not addressed and are best studied in a prospective cohort. The retrospective nature of our study also did not allow us to collect data on exercise habits and behavior which may be significant in this group of young patients and could better help explain our findings. Further, most subjects had near normal exercise capacity, which limits extrapolation of the findings to TOF cases with end-stage symptoms. Finally, our study had been performed in a single centre with relatively few patient number. This could have inadvertently introduced some bias and affect the generalizability of our results.

Conclusion

Although the majority of our TOF subjects had near normal exercise capacity; objective measures of Mets achieved, VO_2max and peak oygen pulse were significant lower than controls. Increased PR fraction in TOF patients was associated with lower AT. Indexed effective RV stroke volume, which we postulate to be a measure of LV preload in the presence of significant PR, was positively associated with VO_2max and Mets achieved. This may potentially be used as a predictor of exercise capacity in repaired TOF with significant PR.

Abbreviations

TOF: Tetralogy of Fallot; RV: Right ventricle; CPET: Cardiopulmonary exercise testing; CMR: Cardiac magnetic resonance imaging; ACC?AHA: American College of Cardiology/American Heart Asscoiation; ESC: European Society of Cardiology; CCS: Canadian Cardiovascular Society; PVR: Pulmonary valve replacement; PR: Pulmonary regurgitation; EDV: End diastolic volume; ESV: End systolic volume; i: indexed; LV: Left ventricle; RVOT: Right ventricular outflow tract; EF: Ejection fraction; SV: Stroke volume; VO2: Oxygen uptake; VE: Minute ventilation; VCO2: Carbon dioxide output; AT: Anaerobic threshold; CI: Confidence interval.

Competing interests

The authors declare that they have no competing interests.

Authors' contributions

JY was involved in the design of the project, acquisition of data, analysis of the results and drafting of the manuscript. JLT, SYT and RST were involved in the design of the project, analysis of the results and drafting of the manuscript. TTL, FG, LZ and RL were involved in the acquisition of data, analysis of results and revision of the manuscript. All authors have read and approved the final manuscript.

Acknowledgements

The authors would like to acknowledge the efforts of the nurses of the cardiopulmonary exercise testing unit for helping to collate the data of the cardiopulmonary exercise testing. The authors have no sources of funding to declare.

References

1. Murphy JG, Gersh BJ, Mair DD, Fuster V, McGoon MD, Ilstrup DM, McGoon DC, Kirklin JW, Danielson GK: **Long-term outcome in patients undergoing surgical repair of tetralogy of fallot.** *N Engl J Med* 1993, **329:**593–599.
2. Zahka KG, Horneffer PJ, Rowe SA, Neill CA, Manolio TA, Kidd L, Gardner TJ: **Long-term valvular function after total repair of tetralogy of Fallot: relation to ventricular arrhythmias.** *Circulation* 1988, **78**(suppl III):14–19.
3. Redington AN, Oldershaw PJ, Shinebourne EA, Rigby ML: **A new technique for the assessment of pulmonary regurgitation and its application to the assessment of right ventricular function before and after repair of tetralogy of Fallot.** *Br Heart J* 1988, **60:**57–65.
4. Gatzoulis MA, Till JA, Somerville J, Redington AN: **Mechanoelectrical interaction in tetralogy of Fallot: QRS prolongation relates to right ventricular size and predicts malignant ventricular arrhythmias and sudden death.** *Circulation* 1995, **92:**231–237.
5. Therrien J, Provost Y, Merchant N, Williams W, Colman J, Webb G: **Optimal timing for pulmonary valve replacement in adults after tetralogy of Fallot repair.** *Am J Cardiol* 2005, **95:**779–782.
6. Oosterhof T, van Straten A, Vliegen HW, Meijboom FJ, van Dijk AP, Spijkerboer AM, Bouma BJ, Zwinderman AH, Hazekamp MG, de Roos A, Mulder BJ: **Preoperative thresholds for pulmonary valve replacement in patients with corrected tetralogy of Fallot using cardiovascular magnetic resonance.** *Circulation* 2007, **116:**545–551.
7. Diller GP, Dimopoulos K, Okonko D, Li W, Babu-Narayan SV, Broberg CS, Johansson B, Bouzas B, Mullen MJ, Poole-Wilson PA, Francis DP, Gatzoulis MA: **Exercise intolerance in adult congenital heart disease: comparative severity, correlates, and prognostic implication.** *Circulation* 2005, **112:**828–835.
8. Buys R, Van De Bruaene A, De Meester P, Budts W, Vanhees L: **Predictors of mid-term event-free survival in adults with corrected tetralogy of Fallot.** *Acta Cardiol* 2012, **67:**415–421.
9. Giardini A, Specchia S, Tacy TA, Coutsoumbas G, Gargiulo G, Donti A, Formigari R, Bonvicini M, Picchio FM: **Usefulness of cardiopulmonary exercise to predict long-term prognosis in adults with repaired tetralogy of Fallot.** *Am J Cardiol* 2007, **99:**1462–1467.
10. Baumgartner H, Bonhoeffer P, De Groot NM, de Haan F, Deanfield JE, Galie N, Gatzoulis MA, Gohlke-Baerwolf C, Kaemmerer H, Kilner P, Meijboom F, Mulder BJ, Oechslin E, Oliver JM, Serraf A, Szatmari A, Thaulow E, Vouhe PR, Walma E, Task Force on the Management of Grown-up Congenital Heart Disease of the European Society of Cardiology (ESC); Association for European Paediatric Cardiology (AEPC); ESC Committee for Practice Guidelines (CPG): **ESC Guidelines for the management of grown-up congenital heart disease (new version 2010).** *Eur Heart J* 2010, **31:**2915–2957.
11. Silversides CK, Kiess M, Beauchesne L, Bradley T, Connelly M, Niwa K, Mulder B, Webb G, Colman J, Therrien J: **Canadian Cardiovascular Society 2009 Consensus Conference on the management of adults with congenital heart disease: outflow tract obstruction, coarctation of the aorta, tetralogy of Fallot, Ebstein anomaly and Marfan's syndrome.** *Can J Cardiol* 2010, **26:**e80–e97.
12. Warnes CA, Williams RG, Bashore TM, Child JS, Connolly HM, Dearani JA, del Nido P, Fasules JW, Graham TP Jr, Hijazi ZM, Hunt SA, King ME, Landzberg MJ, Miner PD, Radford MJ, Walsh EP, Webb GD, Smith SC Jr, Jacobs AK, Adams CD, Anderson JL, Antman EM, Buller CE, Creager MA, Ettinger SM, Halperin JL, Hunt SA, Krumholz HM, Kushner FG, Lytle BW, *et al*: **ACC/AHA 2008 guidelines for the management of adults with congenital heart**

disease: a report of the American College of Cardiology/American Heart Association Task Force on Practice Guidelines (Writing Committee to Develop Guidelines on the Management of Adults With Congenital Heart Disease). Developed in Collaboration With the American Society of Echocardiography, Heart Rhythm Society, International Society for Adult Congenital Heart Disease, Society for Cardiovascular Angiography and Interventions, and Society of Thora/cic Surgeons. *J Am Coll Cardiol* 2008, **52:**e143–e263.

13. Dave HH, Buechel ER, Dodge-Khatami A, Kadner A, Rousson V, Bauersfeld U, Prêtre R: **Early insertion of a pulmonary valve for chronic regurgitation helps restoration of ventricular dimensions.** *Ann Thorac Surg* 2005, **80:**1615–1620. discussion 1620–1.
14. O'Meagher S, Munoz PA, Alison JA, Young IH, Tanous DJ, Celermajer DS, Puranik R: **Exercise capacity and stroke volume are preserved late after tetralogy repair, despite severe right ventricular dilatation.** *Heart* 2012, **98:**1595–1599.
15. Ghez O, Tsang VT, Frigiola A, Coats L, Taylor A, Van Doorn C, Bonhoeffer P, De Leval M: **Right ventricular outflow tract reconstruction for pulmonary regurgitation after repair of tetralogy of Fallot. Preliminary results.** *Eur J Cardiothorac Surg* 2007, **31:**654–658.
16. Coats L, Khambadkone S, Derrick G, Hughes M, Jones R, Mist B, Pellerin D, Marek J, Deanfield JE, Bonhoeffer P, Taylor AM: **Physiological consequences of percutaneous pulmonary valve implantation: the different behaviour of volume- and pressure-overloaded ventricles.** *Eur Heart J* 2007, **28:**1886–1893.
17. Kempny A, Dimopoulos K, Uebing A, Moceri P, Swan L, Gatzoulis MA, Diller GP: **Reference values for exercise limitations among adults with congenital heart disease. Relation to activities of daily life–single centre experience and review of published data.** *Eur Heart J* 2012, **33:**1386–1396.
18. Wasserman K: **The anaerobic threshold: definition, physiological significance and identification.** *Adv Cardiol* 1986, **35:**1–23.
19. Gitt AK, Wasserman K, Kilkowski C, Kleemann T, Kilkowski A, Bangert M, Schneider S, Schwarz A, Senges J: **Exercise anaerobic threshold and ventilatory efficiency identify heart failure patients for high risk of early death.** *Circulation* 2002, **106:**3079–3084.
20. Kempny A, Diller GP, Orwat S, Kaleschke G, Kerckhoff G, Bunck AC, Maintz D, Baumgartner H: **Right ventricular-left ventricular interaction in adults with Tetralogy of Fallot: a combined cardiac magnetic resonance and echocardiographic speckle tracking study.** *Int J Cardiol* 2012, **154:**259–264.
21. Spiewak M, Małek LA, Petryka J, Mazurkiewicz L, Marczak M, Biernacka EK, Kowalski M, Hoffman P, Demkow M, Miśko J, Rużyłło W: **Determinants of left- and right ventricular ejection fractions in patients with repaired tetralogy of Fallot: a cardiac magnetic resonance imaging study.** *Pol Arch Med Wewn* 2013, **123:**539–546.
22. Luijnenburg SE, de Koning WB, Romeih S, van den Berg J, Vliegen HW, Mulder BJ, Helbing WA: **Exercise capacity and ventricular function in patients treated for isolated pulmonary valve stenosis or tetralogy of Fallot.** *Int J Cardiol* 2012, **158:**359–363.
23. Pelliccia A, Culasso F, Di Paolo FM, Maron BJ: **Physiologic left ventricular cavity dilatation in elite athletes.** *Ann Intern Med* 1999, **130:**23–31.
24. Barbier J, Ville N, Kervio G, Walther G, Carré F: **Sports-specific features of athlete's heart and their relation to echocardiographic parameters.** *Herz* 2006, **31:**531–543.
25. Bassareo PP, Saba L, Solla P, Barbanti C, Marras AR, Mercuro G: **Factors influencing adaptation and performance at physical exercise in complex congenital heart diseases after surgical repair.** *Biomed Res Int* 2014, **2014:**862372.
26. Harrison DA, Harris L, Siu SC, MacLoghlin CJ, Connelly MS, Webb GD, Downar E, McLaughlin PR, Williams WG: **Sustained ventricular tachycardia in adult patients late after repair of tetralogy of Fallot.** *J Am Coll Cardiol* 1997, **30:**1368–1373.

15

Diagnostic accuracy of cardiovascular magnetic resonance for patients with suspected cardiac amyloidosis

Lei Zhao, Zhuang Tian and Quan Fang*

Abstract

Background: This study is a systematic review and meta-analysis of the diagnostic value of cardiovascular magnetic resonance (CMR) in cardiac amyloidosis (CA).

Methods: A wide variety of electronic databases were searched for studies of CMR that reported the diagnostic accuracy in patients with suspected CA. Research manuscripts were subjected to further systematic review and meta-analysis. Methodological evaluation was performed under the guidance of the Quality Assessment of Diagnostic Accuracy Studies –2 (QUADAS–2). Heterogeneity was assessed, and a random-effects model was used to assess the diagnostic effects of CMR on pooled sensitivity, pooled specificity, and summary receiver operating characteristics (SROC).

Results: Seven studies that reported the performance of CMR for CA were included in the present systematic review, among which five studies (257 patients) that evaluated the diagnostic accuracy of late gadolinium enhancement (LGE) CMR were analyzed in the present meta-analysis. Heterogeneity was observed only in specificity. A summary sensitivity and specificity of 85 % (95 % CI: 77–91 %) and 92 % (95 % CI: 83–97 %) indicated a high diagnostic accuracy of LGE for CA. The AUC of SROC curve was 0.9530, suggesting that LGE is an effective way of diagnosing patients with possible cardiac involvement in amyloidosis.

Conclusions: LGE–CMR seems to have a relatively high diagnostic accuracy for amyloidosis patients with possible cardiac involvement. Combined CMR techniques may provide important information for the selection of suitable therapy.

Keywords: Cardiac amyloidosis, Cardiac magnetic resonance, LGE, Meta-analysis

Background

The heart, like any organ in the body is susceptible to amyloid deposition. When this occurs in the heart, cardiac amyloidosis (CA) results. Although more than 30 types of protein can cause amyloid, only two types commonly deposit in the ventricular myocardium: amyloid light chain (AL) and amyloid transthyretin (ATTR). The heart is sometimes the only or early manifestation of systemic amyloidosis [1]. Deposition of amyloid precursor proteins which then aggregate into amyloid fibrils in the extracellular space causes separation and distortion of the existing tissues and eventually causes irreversible cardiac dysfunction [2, 3]. This may occur in the myocardium, pericardium, small vessels and conduction system. The result is a restrictive cardiomyopathy with early diastolic dysfunction and later systolic dysfunction, conduction disease including sudden death and, occasionally ischaemia (with arterial involvement) [4].

CA is relatively under-diagnosed, especially wild type ATTR in older people with multisystem diseases. One potential reason is that the symptoms and signs of CA

* Correspondence: quanfangxjn2013@163.com
Department of Cardiology, Peking Union Medical College Hospital, Peking Union Medical College and Chinese Academy of Medical Sciences, No.1 Shuaifuyuan, WangfujingDongcheng District, Beijing 100730, China

such as fatigue, low exercise tolerance and occasionally syncope with progressive diastolic and systolic dysfunction may be nonspecific, particularly in the early phases, resulting in delayed diagnosis and potentially missed therapeutic options. New treatments are available targeting the precursor proteins, including newer chemotherapy regimes and a variety of approaches to reduce transthyretin as a precursor, with further developments in the preclinical phase [5, 6]. For this reason, earlier diagnosis of CA is a major clinical goal [7].

Currently, the main steps in the clinical evaluation of patients with CA involve suspicion, detection, and classification. Suspicion may be raised by multisystem involvement (carpal tunnel, renal impairment etc.). Laboratory investigations may confirm the diagnosis, classify the CA, trace the specific protein precursor and appraise the stage of cardiac involvement including pump function [8]. Currently, the most common examination procedures used to evaluate patients or conditions associated with CA include endomyocardial biopsy (EMB), electrocardiography (ECG), echocardiography and cardiac magnetic resonance (CMR) with some nuclear tests contributing (bone scintigraphy for ATTR, SAP scan for AL - but these are not widely available).

In CA, myocardial tissue histology stands as the gold standard, revealing the accumulation of amyloid proteins and fibers in the extracellular space. Histologically, EMB is initially stained using Congo Red where deposits may look pale red but show apple-green birefringence under cross-polarized light. Immunohistochemistry (IHC) or mass-spectrocopy can definitively subtype the amyloid fibrils [4]. However, the invasive nature of EMB and related high-risk complications are barriers, as is the specialist nature of IHC and mass spectroscopy. Besides, as the lack of standardization on the definition of what constitutes CA, in some cases these is a need to use some ancillary imaging and clinical findings to ensure the pathological diagnosis. In addition, EMB is classified in the class IIa recommendation [9].

ECG Low -voltages is a classical feature of CA [10]. But it provides a low -sensitivity and -specificity diagnosis of CA. This may be due in part to interference from other coexisting conditions, such as obesity, hypothyroidism, and pulmonary diseases, but up to 25 % of ATTR subjects have left ventricular hypertrophy. Under echocardiograph, the CA classical feature (a "brilliant" speckled appearance of myocardium) is a poor discriminator. Biventricular hypertrophy with disproportionate long axis impairment and restriction is more specific, but still has overlap, particularly in early disease [11].

CMR, a noninvasive mean of assessing amyloid burden, makes use of a superconducting magnet with ECG gating to measure the structure and function of the heart analogous to echocardiography. In addition, myocardial tissue characterisation detects tissue pathology [12]. In particular, the late gadolinium enhancement (LGE) has a characteristic pattern in amyloid with subendocardial, later transmural LGE and difficulty nulling. This latter issue appears resolved with the phase-sensitive inversion recovery (PSIR) LGE sequence and it has potential to be a key technique for the diagnosis of patients with potential CA [13]. Several studies have compared the diagnostic accuracy of CMR to that of EMB. However, they focused on different parameters and used different cutoff values in diagnostic tests, which limit their usefulness in the assessment of CA. For this reason, a systematic review was conducted to help evaluate the diagnostic aspects of CMR in patients with suspected CA.

Methods

Data sources

This systematic review was carried out under the guideline of the Cochrane Collaboration's Diagnostic Test Accuracy Group. Search strategies were developed to identify all the relevant studies published in the Pubmed, Embase, the Cochrane Library, Biosis Preview, ISI Web of Science, and China National Knowledge Infrastructure up to April 20, 2015. Medical subject headings and full text were searched for references to CA and magnetic resonance imaging to systematically locate these publications in any language. The details of the search strategies are provided in the additional files. The citations of eligible publications and reviews were also checked. Requirements were limited to human trials.

Study selection and data collection

The first author (LZ) conducted the initial literature search of titles and abstracts. Upon further scrutiny, two reviewers (LZ, ZT) led the retrieval of the full texts of relevant manuscripts independently. A third reviewer (QF) resolved all the disagreements and discrepancies that occurred during these processes through deep discussions. The following inclusion criteria were defined in advance: (1) a diagnostic accuracy test was included; (2) patients with at least suspected CA; (3) the diagnostic accuracy of CMR was evaluated regardless of acquisition protocol used; (4) EMB, clinical criteria, or both served as the reference tests; (5) the absolute numbers of true positive, false positive, true negative, and false negative results could be derived. All the articles that met these criteria were considered eligible. Duplicate and overlapping publications were excluded. Conference abstracts and research manuscripts that could not be obtained in their entirety or from which essential information was missing were also excluded. Diagnostic accuracy details, study methods, results, and additional information on

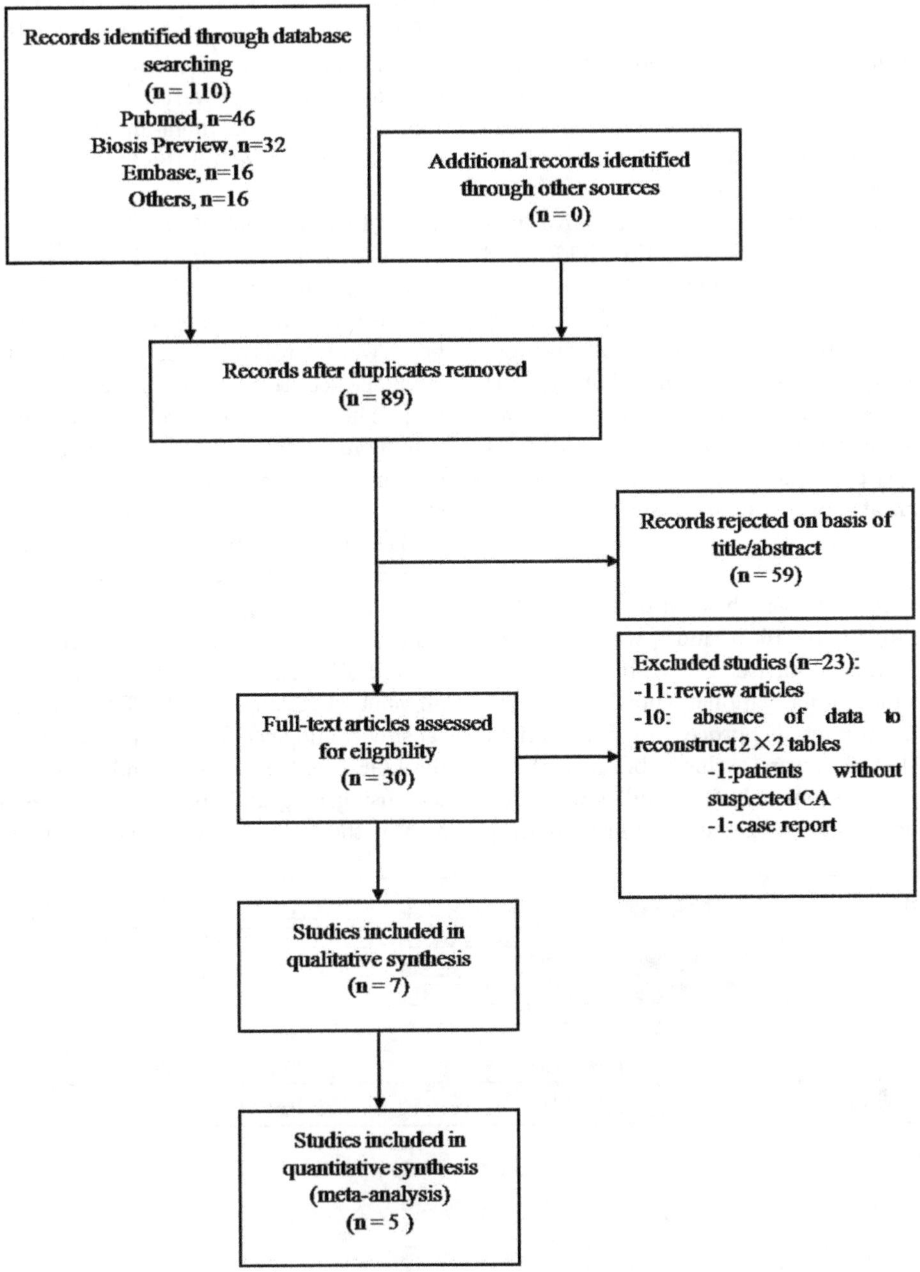

Fig. 1 Flow chart of selection process

patients and procedures were extracted from each primary study independently by two reviewers (LZ, ZT).

Assessment of risk of bias

Two reviewers (LZ, ZT) appraised the methodological quality based on the form suggested by the Quality Assessment of Diagnostic Accuracy Studies–2 (QUADAS–2), which has main parts: patient selection, index test, reference standards, and the flow and timing [14]. Each part involves the assessment of risk of bias (low, high, or unclear) and first 3 parts also need to evaluate the clinical applicability. In cases of disagreement, 2 reviewers would reach a consensus after a thorough discussion with a third person (QF).

Statistical analysis

Statistical analyses were conducted using MetaDisc 1.4 software and Review Manager software version 5.3. First, heterogeneity in included manuscripts was assessed in terms of Cochran Q chi-square tests and I^2 statistics. In cases of significant heterogeneity, the random-effects model was suitable to pool several parameters and sensitivity analysis was used to investigate potential sources targeting risk bias calculated by QUADAS–2. In other cases, the Mantel-Haenszel method was used to establish a fixed-effects model during the evaluation process. In cases of implicit threshold effects, the Spearman rank correlation was taken into consideration. Subgroup analysis determined if there was a correlation between sensitivity and specificity. Second, positive likelihood ratios (PLR), negative likelihood ratios (NLR), and diagnostic odds ratio (DOR), and their 95 % confidence intervals (CI) were estimated based on pooled sensitivity and specificity. In order to estimate the overall diagnostic effect, a summary receiver operating characteristic (SROC) curve was established, with pertinent areas. Whenever a study's data contained zero counts, 0.5 was added as a continuity correction. Any significantly statistical calculating was at a two-sided 0.05 level.

Results

The systematical electronic search identified 110 publications, of which 46, 32, 16, 10, 5, and 1 were found in Pubmed, Biosis Preview, Embase, ISI Web of Science, Cochrane Library and China National Knowledge Infrastructure. Figure 1 outlines the process of manuscripts screening. Here, 21 studies were excluded because of duplicate records. After the removal of 59 studies whose titles or abstracts did not meet the inclusion criteria, only 30 full-text articles were retained for further evaluation. Of the 30 potentially appropriate publications, only 7 were included in the systematic review [15–21]. Most of the excluded studies were reviews or did not provide absolute figures. The meta-analysis was performed on 5 studies that focused on the LGE performance [17–21].

Methodological evaluation

Figure 2 shows the graphs of risk bias and concerns about clinical application evaluated by QUADAS–2. In the patient selection domain, one report did not state that patients were enrolled in a consecutive pattern [20]. Another study lacked relevant information on patient sampling [16]. The Karamitsos and Hosch studies both used a case–control design [15]. In terms of an inappropriate exclusion, both Karamitsos and Hosch's studies were unclear. Regarding interpretation of the CMR results, 2 studies did not clearly state whether they were conducted before knowing the results of EMB, the one by Karamitsos and another one by Austin [19]. LGE–CMR was used in 6 studies, and one study used MR-relaxometry to evaluate T1 and T2 relaxation time (RT), which established a cutoff value of 1273 ms of T1-RT to diagnose CA with a high sensitivity and specificity [15]. The other 6 studies detailed the LGE-CMR procedures and defined amyloid LGE pattern using long and short axes images in the ventricular area without coronary artery distribution [16–21]. No

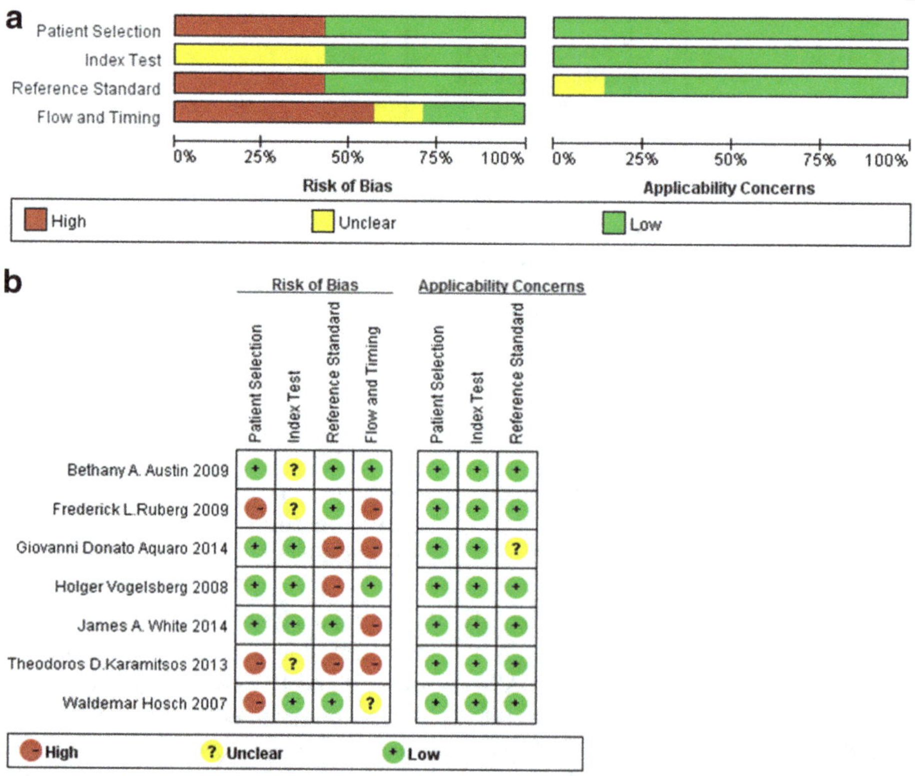

Fig. 2 Assessment of methodological quality according to QUADAS-2

concerns about the included patients going against the inclusion criteria.

There were 2 studies that did not clearly report that the EMB evaluation was blinded to CMR results [19, 21]. Another study stated it was done without blindness [17]. In terms of the reference tests, some patients could not be classified clearly using clinical criteria alone [16, 21]. This kind of study involved high risk bias and uncertainty regarding use in the reference domain.

One study was discarded because of incomplete data for 2 × 2 table [16]. The interval between CMR and the reference test were only clearly stated in 3 studies [17, 19, 21]. But these 3 studies together did not use the same reference test on all the patients. Some patients were evaluated by EMB and others were clinically assessed using ECG, echocardiography, or both. In the study by White, only 25 (28 %) patients with suspected CA were included in the final diagnostic evaluation [18].

Overall, all the included studies involved little concerns regarding applicability and remaining 5 studies were here considered methodologically correct regardless of risk bias [17–21].

Study characteristics

The baseline characteristics of these included studies are shown in Table 1 [15–21]. A total of 485 subjects were recruited in the final systematic analysis. These manuscripts were published during the period from 2007 to 2014 and four of them were prospective studies [15, 18, 20, 21]. Patients involved in individual studies are summarized concisely in Table 1. The sample size ranged from 28 to 106 and the mean age was similarly around 62 years old. Mean time intervals were only available in three studies [17, 19, 21]. Six studies used EMB as a reference test [15, 17–21]. Another one used echocardiography and clinical features as to classify patients [16]. All studies used 1.5-T scanners to perform the CMR, but

Table 1 Characteristics of included studies

Study	Year	Country	Study design	Population	Age, yrs	Male, n	Mean time interval[a]	Blind[b]	Reference test	Index measured using CMR	Field strength
Hosch et al.	2007	Germany	PC	19 with newly diagnosed CA and 9 patients with systemic amyloidosis but without CA and 10 healthy, age-matched control	59 ± 6.1	14	NA	Y	EMB	T1 and T2 RT	1.5 T
Vogelsberg et al.	2008	Germany	NA	33 subjects with suspected CA	64 ± 13	NA	Same day	Y	EMB	Amyloid LGE pattern	1.5 T
Austin et al.	2009	USA	RC	47 subjects with suspected CA	62	33	24–48 h	N	EMB	LGE; DHE	1.5 T
Ruberg et al.	2009	USA	PC	28 patients with systemic AL amyloidosis	62 ± 11	20	NA	Y	EMB or clinical criteria	LGE	1.5 T
Karamitsos et al.	2013	UK/ Canada	NA	53 patients with systemic (primary) AL amyloidosis and 17 patients with aortic stenosis and 36 normal volunteers	63 ± 10[c]	69	NA	Y	Echocardiography and clinical features	Noncontrast T1 mapping; LGE	1.5 T
Aquaro et al.	2014	Italy	PC	59 patients with a previous diagnosis of systemic AL amyloidosis and 20 healthy control subjects	69 ± 10	36	Same day	Y	Echocardiographic criteria and/or ECG criteria or EMB	SID; conventional LGE	1.5 T
White et al.	2014	USA	PC	90 patients with suspected CA and 64 hypertensive patients with LVH	62 ± 13	52	NA	Y	EMB	LGE pattern: Global HE	1.5 T

AL amyloid light-chain, *CA* cardiac amyloidosis, *DHE* delayed hyper-enhancement, *ECG* echocardiography, *HE* hyperenhancement, *EMB* endomyocardial biopsy, *LGE* late gadolinium enhancement, *LVH* left ventricular hypertrophy, *N* no, *NA* not available, *PC* prospective cohort, *RC* retrospective cohort, *RT* relaxation times, *SID* signal intensity decay

[a]Time interval between reference tests and cardiac magnetic resonance

[b]The CMR results were interpreted blind to the results of the reference tests or the reference tests were performed without knowing the results of cardiac magnetic resonance

[c]Amyloid patients with definite cardiac involvement

only five of them evaluated the diagnostic accuracy of LGE by calculating sensitivity and specificity [17–21]. No adverse events were reported in the examinations.

Diagnostic performance of CMR for CA

Five studies contained absolute figures for 2 × 2 tables with respect to LGE and were included in the meta-analysis (Table 2) [17–21]. Individual studies are shown on forest plots focusing on sensitivity and specificity. The χ^2 test for sensitivity and specificity produced a P value of 0.2003 and 0.0581 with I^2 values of 33.2 % and 56.1 %, respectively. In cases with a detectable threshold effect, the Spearman rank correlation between the sensitivity and 1-specifity was performed and the correlation coefficient was 0.8 with a P value 0.104 (Additional files 1 and 2). Because the inconsistency index I^2 was used to quantify the heterogeneity, an I^2 value of 56.1 % was considered moderate (50–74 %). For this reason, the random-effects model was used for the meta-analysis.

As shown in Fig. 3, the pooled sensitivity and specificity of LGE-CMR were 85 % (95 % CI: 77–93 %) and 92 % (95 % CI: 83–97 %). The pooled positive likelihood ratio was 7.481 (95 % CI: 2.835–19.739) and the negative one was 0.183 (95% CI: 0.121–0.277). Figure 4 shows the SROC curve for LEG-CMR, suggesting the LGE is an effective mean of diagnosing patients with amyloidosis and potential cardiac involvement. These results also corresponded to the pooled diagnostic odd ratio (Fig. 5). There was some residual heterogeneity in the diagnostic accuracy. Sensitivity analysis was conducted to determine the source of heterogeneity. After removing the study by Aquaro which involved high risk bias in the methodological evaluation, results showed the specificity have an I^2 value of 9.3 % and P value of 0.3467 [21]. However, this did not change the direction or magnitude of the pooled estimates, which means that the results of relatively good quality. Because only 5 publications were included, no funnel plot was constructed to assess publication bias.

Discussion

Amyloidosis, when it affects the heart, has a poor prognosis. Better diagnostic tests would permit earlier detection and therefore targeted intervention to improve outcomes. Many modalities have been used in clinical settings to detect and evaluate CA [22]. The most common methods are ECG and echocardiography. These tools are convenient and available in most medical facilities in which the EMB is not in common use. However, both methods detect CA with a relatively low accuracy. ECG evaluation is not suitable for patients with pulmonary disorders but many patients with cardiomyopathy, especially elderly patients, are likely to be involved in cardiopulmonary diseases. Echocardiography can detect the advanced cases [23]. However, it cannot easily assess earlier cases or differentiate CA from hypertrophic cardiomyopathy because the characteristics in echocardiography are thick-walled ventricles with speckled myocardia [4, 23]. EMB is considered the gold standard in the diagnosis of CA. However, the unavailability, relatively high risks and clinical complications may hinder its widespread use in clinical settings. CMR provides a third option in the evaluation of the heart's structure and assessment of its diastolic function. It is more precise and more accurate, which are regarded as the hallmarks of good non-invasive methods capable of assessing myocardial scars [13, 24].

The key advantage of using CMR to detect the CA is its unique ability to describe the characteristics of heart, which can be done particularly using LGE [25]. After taking the gadolinium-based contrast, patients with CA presented typical global subendocardial enhancement patterns, which are closely associated with interstitial amyloid burden and often used to qualitatively detect focal fibrosis [26]. This meta-analysis of LGE–CMR

Table 2 Cardiac magnetic resonance evaluation of the included studies in the systematic review

Study	Number of subjects	Index measured using CMR	TF	FP	FN	TN	Sensitivity (%)	Specificity (%)	PPV (%)	NPV (%)	AUC
Hosch et al.	38	T1-RT	16[a]	0[a]	3[a]	10[a]	84[a]	100[a]	NA[a]	NA[a]	0.96[a]
			16[b]	1[b]	3[b]	8[b]	84[b]	89[b]	NA[b]	NA[b]	0.89[b]
Vogelsberg et al.	33	LGE	12	1	3	17	80	94	92	85	NA
Austin et al.	47	LGE	15	2	2	19	88	90	88	90	NA
Ruberg et al.	28	LGE	18	1	3	6	86	86	95	67	NA
Karamitsos et al.	106	Noncontrast T1 mapping	36	6	3	61	92	91	NA	NA	NA
Aquaro et al.	79	SID	51	2	1	26	98	93	96	96	NA
		LGE	42	0	10	27	81	100	100	73	NA
White et al.	154	LGE	15	3	0	7	93	70	NA	NA	NA

AUC area under receiver-operating characteristic curve, *FN* false negative, *FP* false positive, *TN* true negative, *TP* true positive, *PPV* positive predictive value, *NA* not available, *NPV* negative predictive value, *LGE* late gadolinium enhancement, *RT* relaxation time, *SID* signal intensity decay

[a]CA patients compared with the healthy, age-matched control group

[b]CA patients compared with the patient group with systemic amyloidosis but without cardiac involvement

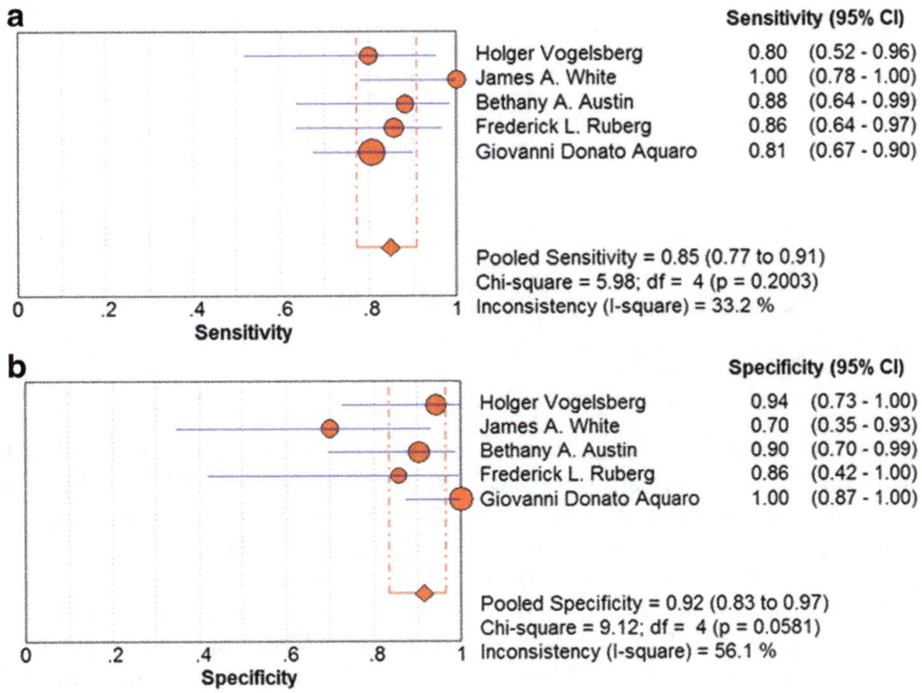

Fig. 3 Forest plot evaluating the sensitivity and specificity of diagnostic performance of late gadolinium enhancement in included studies. CI, confidence interval

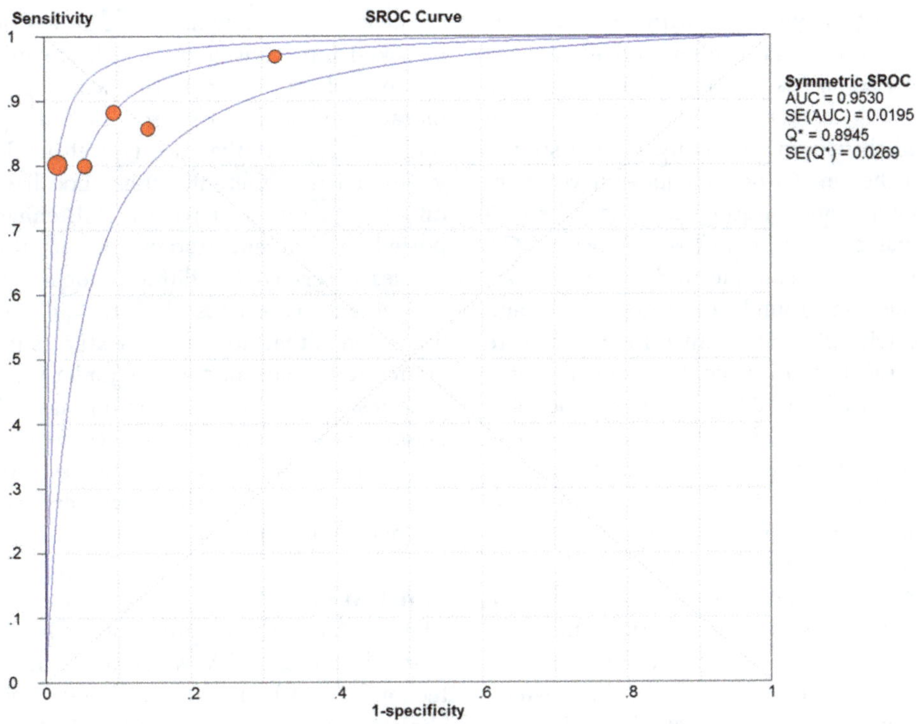

Fig. 4 Summary receiver operator characteristics (SROC) of late gadolinium enhancement on summary estimates of sensitivity and specificity. AUC, area under the curve; SE, standard error

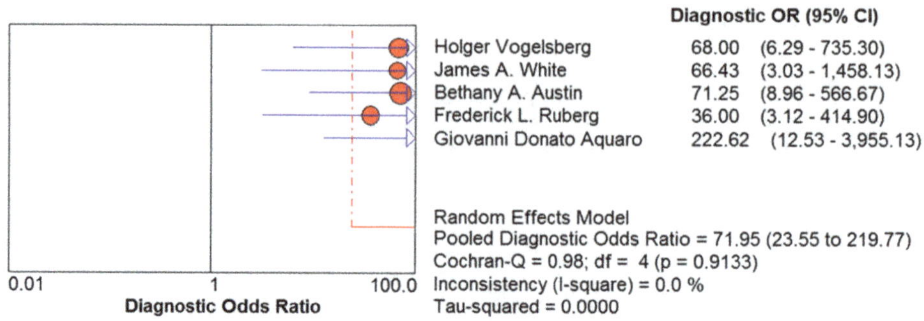

Fig. 5 Forest plot presenting the pooled diagnostic odds ratio of late gadolinium enhancement. CI, confidence interval

showed that the diagnostic accuracy increased with a summary sensitivity of 85 % and a summary specificity of 92 %. In terms of the heart tissue characterization, LGE can distinguish CA patients from healthy controls with a summary positive likelihood ratio of 7.481 (95 % CI: 2.835–19.739). The summary diagnostic odds ratio of 71.945 detected here (95 % CI: 23.552–219.77) indicated that expressed the test was more accurate in the differential diagnosis of CMR than other types of diagnosis. In this way, the values of LR+ and DOR favor of LEG–CMR in patients with suspected CA before EMB. Heterogeneity was observed across studies in terms of specificity, but not sensitivity. This could be partially due to the methodological quality of involved publications on reference tests choosing and flow and timing.

AL and ATTR are two types of amyloidosis typically associated with the heart. ATTR is often underdiagnosed and can be fatal. It also has particular variants in specific ethnic populations, which makes diagnosing and typing both necessary and challenging. Recently, several studies have reported that the new CMR techniques have better diagnostic accuracy in demonstrating the range of structural and functional changes in different types of CA [27]. T1 mapping, a new technique measuring myocardial intrinsic signal, was found to diagnose AL and ATTR very accurately [28, 29]. Native T1 levels were higher in ATTR patients than in controls and the area under the AUC for ATTR and AL patients with possible or definite cardiac involvement was 0.85 (95 % CI: 0.79–0.92) [29]. One study reviewed here evaluated the non-contrast myocardial T1, and the cut-off of 1020 ms yielded 92 % accuracy for identifying CA [16]. T1–RT reported by Hosch also diagnosed CA with a high sensitivity (84 %) and specificity (>89 %) with a cut-off value of ≥1273 ms [15]. The measurement of extracellular volume (ECV) measurement is popular in some centers [30, 31]. ECV is elevated in both AL and ATTR, which helps the evaluation of amyloid burden. It is also elevated in patients where routine examinations, including LGE, indicated no heart involvement. In the present systematic review, one study analyzed the myocardial signal intensity decay (SID) at the subendocardial level after gadolinium injection, showing a greater accuracy (96 %) and sensitivity (98 %) for CA assessment than LGE with a 269 HB threshold [21]. T1 values were higher in AL amyloid than in ATTR, but ECV was higher in ATTR [12]. This suggests that combined T1 and ECV techniques may attach more diagnostic accuracy to patients with cardiac involvement, quantify the amyloid burden to evaluate the pathologic conditions, and distinguish types of CA to help clinicians select the most appropriate treatment for each patient. When LGE combine with these advanced techniques, CMR could be a main technique for the diagnosis of patients with potential CA.

The current review has some limitations, which should be taken into consideration. The main one is the small number of studies included, which restricted deep exploration of potential sources of heterogeneity. The second limitation is that the typical amyloid LGE pattern varies across different series. Localized enhancement, diffuse transmural or patchy LGE enhancement was reported in different studies. In this review, only three studies described the diffuse, global subendocardial enhancement pattern as the amyloid pattern. The third limitation is that not all of the studies used the same reference tests. Not all patients underwent the same reference tests, introducing selection bias in the final results. Despite these limitations, the current work can present the current state of diagnostic tests of CMR for CA, which may help medical workers choose diagnostic methods efficiently and effectively.

Conclusion

The current work indicates that the LGE is more accurate in the diagnosis of CA, which makes it valuable in the detection of amyloid deposit. However, when considering clinical cost-effectiveness and patients with claustrophobia, implanted cardiac devices and renal failure, CMR application value in CA needs further investigation.

Abbreviations

AL, amyloid light chain; ATTR, amyloid transthyretin; AUC, area under the curve; CA, cardiac amyloidosis; CI, confidence intervals; CMR, Cardiovascular magnetic resonance; DOR, Diagnostic odds ratio; ECG, Electrocardiography; ECV, extracellular volume; EMB, Endomyocardial biopsy; LGE, late gadolinium enhancement; NLR, negative likelihood ratios; PLR, positive likelihood ratios; PSIR, phase-sensitive inversion recovery; QUADAS-2, Quality Assessment of Diagnostic Accuracy Studies-2; RT, relaxation time; SID, signal intensity decay; SROC, Summary receiver operating characteristics

Funding

This research received no grant from any funding agency in the public, commercial or not-for-profit sectors.

Author's contributions

LZ participated in the study design and data analysis and drafted the manuscript. ZT helped in the coordination and helped draft the manuscript. QF helped draft the manuscript. All authors read and approved the final manuscript.

Competing interests

The authors declare that they have no competing interests.

References

1. Rapezzi C, Lorenzini M, Longhi S, Milandri A, Gagliardi C, Bartolomei I, Salvi F, Maurer MS. Cardiac amyloidosis: the great pretender. Heart Fail Rev. 2015;20:117–24.
2. Sipe JD, Benson MD, Buxbaum JN, Ikeda S, Merlini G, Saraiva MJ, Westermark P. Amyloid fibril protein nomenclature: 2012 recommendations from the Nomenclature Committee of the International Society of Amyloidosis. Amyloid. 2012;19:167–70.
3. Gertz MA, Dispenzieri A, Sher T. Pathophysiology and treatment of cardiac amyloidosis. Nat Rev Cardiol. 2015;12:91–102.
4. Mohty D, Damy T, Cosnay P, Echahidi N, Casset-Senon D, Virot P, Jaccard A. Cardiac amyloidosis. Updates in diagnosis and management. Arch Cardiovasc Dis. 2013;106:528–40.
5. Yusuf SW, Solhpour A, Banchs J, Lopez-Mattei JC, Durand J, Iliescu C, Hassan SA, Qazilbash MH. Cardiac amyloidosis. Expert Rev Cardiovasc Ther. 2014;12:265–77.
6. Sharma N, Howlett J. Current state of cardiac amyloidosis. Curr Opin Cardiol. 2013;28:242–8.
7. Quarta CC, Solomon SD, Uraizee I, Kruger J, Longhi S, Ferlito M, Gagliardi C, Milandri A, Rapezzi C, Falk RH. Left ventricular structure and function in transthyretin-related versus light-chain cardiac amyloidosis. Circulation. 2014;129:1840–9.
8. Sher T, Gertz MA. Recent advances in the diagnosis and management of cardiac amyloidosis. Futur Cardiol. 2014;10:131–46.
9. Yancy CW, Jessup M, Bozkurt B, Butler J, Casey DE, Drazner MH, Fonarow GC, Geraci SA, Horwich T, Januzzi JL, Johnson MR, Kasper EK, Levy WC, Masoudi FA, McBride PE, McMurray JJ, Mitchell JE, Peterson PN, Riegel B, Sam F, Stevenson LW, Tang WH, Tsai EJ, Wilkoff BL, American College of Cardiology Foundation, American Heart Association Task Force on Practice Guidelines. 2013 ACCF/AHA Guideline for the Management of Heart Failure. J Am Coll Cardiol. 2013;62:e147–239.
10. Murtagh B, Hammill SC, Gertz MA, Kyle RA, Tajik AJ, Grogan M. Electrocardiographic findings in primary systemic amyloidosis and biopsy-proven cardiac involvement. Am J Cardiol. 2005;95:535–7.
11. Cappelli F, Baldasseroni S, Bergesio F, Perlini S, Salinaro F, Padeletti L, Attana P, Paoletti PA, Moggi PA, Grifoni E, Fabbri A, Marchionni N, Gensini GF, Perfetto F. Echocardiographic and biohumoral characteristics in patients with AL and TTR amyloidosis at diagnosis. Clin Cardiol. 2015;38:69–75.
12. Fontana M, Chung R, Hawkins PN, Moon JC. Cardiovascular magnetic resonance for amyloidosis. Heart Fail Rev. 2015;20:133–44.
13. Syed IS, Glockner JF, Feng D, Araoz PA, Martinez MW, Edwards WD, Gertz MA, Dispenzieri A, Oh JK, Bellavia D, Tajik AJ, Grogan M. Role of Cardiac Magnetic Resonance Imaging in the Detection of Cardiac Amyloidosis. J Am Coll Cardiol Img. 2010;3:155–64.
14. Whiting PF, Rutjes AW, Westwood ME, Mallett S, Deeks JJ, Reitsma JB, Leeflang MM, Sterne JA, Bossuyt PM. QUADAS-2: a revised tool for the quality assessment of diagnostic accuracy studies. Ann Intern Med. 2011;155:529–36.
15. Hosch W, Bock M, Libicher M, Ley S, Hegenbart U, Dengler TJ, Katus HA, Kauczor HU, Kauffmann GW, Kristen AV. MR-relaxometry of myocardial tissue: significant elevation of T1 and T2 relaxation times in cardiac amyloidosis. Invest Radiol. 2007;42:636–42.
16. Karamitsos TD, Piechnik SK, Banypersad SM, Fontana M, Ntusi NB, Ferreira VM, Whelan CJ, Myerson SG, Robson MD, Hawkins PN, Neubauer S, Moon JC. Noncontrast T1 Mapping for the Diagnosis of Cardiac Amyloidosis. J Am Coll Cardiol Img. 2013;6:488–97.
17. Vogelsberg H, Mahrholdt H, Deluigi CC, Yilmaz A, Kispert EM, Greulich S, Klingel K, Kandolf R, Sechtem U. Cardiovascular Magnetic Resonance in Clinically Suspected Cardiac Amyloidosis. J Am Coll Cardiol. 2008;51:1022–30.
18. White JA, Kim HW, Shah D, Fine N, Kim K, Wendell DC, Al-Jaroudi W, Parker M, Patel M, Gwadry-Sridhar F, Judd RM, Kim RJ. CMR Imaging With Rapid Visual T1 Assessment Predicts Mortality in Patients Suspected of Cardiac Amyloidosis. J Am Coll Cardiol Img. 2014;7:143–56.
19. Austin BA, Tang WHW, Rodriguez ER, Tan C, Flamm SD, Taylor DO, Starling RC, Desai MY. Delayed Hyper-Enhancement Magnetic Resonance Imaging Provides Incremental Diagnostic and Prognostic Utility in Suspected Cardiac Amyloidosis. J Am Coll Cardiol Img. 2009;2:1369–77.
20. Ruberg FL, Appelbaum E, Davidoff R, Ozonoff A, Kissinger KV, Harrigan C, Starling RC, Desai MY. Diagnostic and Prognostic Utility of Cardiovascular Magnetic Resonance Imaging in Light-Chain Cardiac Amyloidosis. Am J Cardiol. 2009;103:544–9.
21. Aquaro GD, Pugliese NR, Perfetto F, Cappelli F, Barison A, Masci PG, Passino C, Emdin M. Myocardial signal intensity decay after gadolinium injection: a fast and effective method for the diagnosis of cardiac amyloidosis. Int J Cardiovasc Imaging. 2014;30:1105–15.
22. Di Bella G, Pizzino F, Minutoli F, Zito C, Donato R, Dattilo G, Oreto G, Baldari S, Vita G, Khandheria BK, Carerj S. The mosaic of the cardiac amyloidosis diagnosis: role of imaging in subtypes and stages of the disease. Eur Heart J Cardiovasc Imaging. 2014;15:1307–15.
23. Nakahashi T, Arita T, Yamaji K, Inoue K, Yokota T, Hoshii Y, Fukunaga M, Nomura A, Watanabe H, Miura S, Isotani A, Soga Y, Ando K, Iwabuchi M, Yokoi H, Nosaka H, Yamagishi M, Nobuyoshi M. Impact of clinical and echocardiographic characteristics on occurrence of cardiac events in cardiac amyloidosis as proven by endomyocardial biopsy. Int J Cardiol. 2014;176:753–9.
24. Deux JF, Damy T, Rahmouni A, Mayer J, Plante-Bordeneuve V. Noninvasive detection of cardiac involvement in patients with hereditary transthyretin associated amyloidosis using cardiac magnetic resonance imaging: a prospective study. Amyloid. 2014;21:246–55.
25. Maceira AM. Cardiovascular Magnetic Resonance in Cardiac Amyloidosis. Circulation. 2005;111:186–93.
26. Syed IS, Glockner JF, Feng D, Araoz PA, Martinez MW, Edwards WD, Gertz MA, Dispenzieri A, Oh JK, Bellavia D, Tajik AJ, Grogan M. Role of cardiac magnetic resonance imaging in the detection of cardiac amyloidosis. JACC Cardiovasc Imaging. 2010;3:155–64.
27. Dungu JN, Valencia O, Pinney JH, Gibbs SD, Rowczenio D, Gilbertson JA, Lachmann HJ, Wechalekar A, Gillmore JD, Whelan CJ, Hawkins PN, Anderson LJ. CMR-based differentiation of AL and ATTR cardiac amyloidosis. JACC Cardiovasc Imaging. 2014;7:133–42.
28. Banypersad SM, Fontana M, Maestrini V, Sado DM, Captur G, Petrie A, Piechnik SK, Whelan CJ, Herrey AS, Gillmore JD, Lachmann HJ, Wechalekar AD, Hawkins PN, Moon JC. T1 mapping and survival in systemic light-chain amyloidosis. Eur Heart J. 2015;36:244–51.
29. Fontana M, Banypersad SM, Treibel TA, Maestrini V, Sado DM, White SK, Pica S, Castelletti S, Piechnik SK, Robson MD, Gilbertson JA, Rowczenio D, Hutt DF, Lachmann HJ, Wechalekar AD, Whelan CJ, Gillmore JD, Hawkins PN, Moon JC. Native T1 mapping in transthyretin amyloidosis. JACC Cardiovasc Imaging. 2014;7:157–65.
30. Banypersad SM, Sado DM, Flett AS, Gibbs SD, Pinney JH, Maestrini V, Cox AT, Fontana M, Whelan CJ, Wechalekar AD, Hawkins PN, Moon JC. Quantification of myocardial extracellular volume fraction in systemic AL amyloidosis: an equilibrium contrast cardiovascular magnetic resonance study. Circ Cardiovasc Imaging. 2013;6:34–9.
31. Mongeon FP, Jerosch-Herold M, Coelho-Filho OR, Blankstein R, Falk RH, Kwong RY. Quantification of extracellular matrix expansion by CMR in infiltrative heart disease. JACC Cardiovasc Imaging. 2012;5:897–907.

16

Speckle tracking echocardiography in the diagnosis of early left ventricular systolic dysfunction in type II diabetic mice

Rong-juan Li[1,2], Jiao Yang[1,2], Ya Yang[1,2*], Ning Ma[1,2], Bo Jiang[1,2], Qi-wei Sun[1,2] and Yi-jia Li[1,2]

Abstracts

Background: The leptin receptor-deficient db/db mouse is a well-established type II diabetes animal model used to investigate diabetic cardiomyopathy. Previous reports have documented diabetic cardiomyopathy is accompanied by cardiac structural and functional abnormalities. To better elucidate early or subtle changes in cardiac performance in db/db mice, we used speckle tracking echocardiography to assess systolic myocardial strain in vivo with diabetic db/db mice in order to study early changes of left ventricle contractile function in type II diabetes model.

Methods: Male diabetic db/db mice and age-matched control mice from C57BL/6J strain at 8,12 and 16 weeks of age were subjected to echocardiography. At the midpapillary level in the parasternal left ventricular short-axis view, end diastolic and systolic left ventricular diameter, interventricular septal thickness and posterior wall thicknesses, ejection fraction, fractional shortening were determined by M-mode echocardiography. Using speckle-tracking based strain analysis of two-dimensional echocardiographic images acquired from the parasternal short-axis views at the mid-papillary level, systolic global radial and circumferential strain values were analyzed.

Results: There was no significant difference in interventricular septal thickness, posterior wall thicknesses, end diastolic and systolic left ventricular diameter, ejection fraction and fractional shortening between db/db and age-matched control mice at 8,12 or 16 weeks of age ($P > 0.05$). At 8 and 12 weeks of age, there was no significant difference in left ventricular radial strain and circumferential strain between db/db mice and age-matched controls ($P > 0.05$). But at 16 weeks of age, the left ventricular radial strain and circumferential strain in db/db mice were lower than in control mice ($P < 0.01$).

Conclusion: The present study shows that speckle tracking echocardiography can be used to evaluate cardiac functional alterations in mouse models of cardiovascular disease. Radial and circumferential strain are more sensitive and can be used for detection of early left ventricular contractile dysfunction in db/db type II diabetic mice.

Keywords: Diabetic cardiomyopathy, db/db mice, Echocardiography, Strain, Cardiac function

Background

The most prevalent form (90%) of diabetes mellitus is Type II (non-insulin-dependent) diabetes [1]. Epidemiological and clinical evidence shows that type II diabetes mellitus is a prevalent disease that results in a marked increase in cardiovascular complications that are in part due to a specific cardiomyopathy, characterized by ventricular dysfunction in the absence of atherosclerotic coronary heart disease or hypertension [2,3]. Abnormalities in cardiac function and structure in diabetic subjects have been demonstrated in animal [4-7] and human studies [8-11]. However, there is still controversy regarding the severity or time of appearance of cardiac impairment following the appearance of type II diabetes.

Most reports of diabetes-induced cardiac dysfunction have used insulin-deficient (TypeI) models [12-14]. Relatively few studies on cardiac function have been conducted with type II diabetic animal models [15]. The leptin receptor-deficient db/db mouse is a well established model of type II diabetes, with obesity and insulin resistance

* Correspondence: rong4020@126.com
[1]Department of Echocardiography, Beijing Anzhen Hospital, Capital Medical University, Beijing, China
[2]Beijing Institute of Heart, Lung and Blood Vessel Disease, Beijing, China

[16,17]. In vivo evidence for left ventricle structure and dysfunction in diabetic mice is commonly obtained from conventional echocardiography (M-mode, 2D, Doppler) [18,19], which is typically considered late manifestations of disease and insensitive to detect subtle left ventricle dysfunction. The presence of resting abnormalities of sensitive indices of myocardial function measured by speckle tracking echocardiography (STE) has been attributed to a subclinical diabetic cardiomyopathy. Tracking the movement of myocardial tissue, STE is used to determine longitudinal strain, radial and circumferential strain for detecting global and regional myocardial dysfunction [20]. Therefore, the objective of this study was to use STE to assess systolic myocardial strain in vivo with diabetic db/db and control mice in order to study early changes of left ventricle contractile function in type II diabetes model.

Methods

All studies have been approved by Beijing Anzhen Hospital Ethics Committee and performed in accordance with the ethical standards.

Animals

Experiments were performed on 8-, 12- and 16-wk male homozygous diabetic (db/db) ($n = 8$ in each week) and age-matched heterozygote non-diabetic (Control) mice ($n = 8$ in each week), obtained from Beijing University (Beijing, China). The control and diabetic mice (Figure 1) used in this study were the C57BL/6J strain. The mice were housed in groups and allowed ad libitum access to water and standard laboratory mouse chow. All the experimental procedures described below adhered strictly to the guidelines set forth by the National Science and Technology Commission of China and approved by the institutional ethics committee. The experiment conformed to the Animal Research: Reporting In Vivo Experiments (ARRIVE) guidelines.

Conventional echocardiographic measurements

Before examination, all mice were anesthetized in a closed chamber with 3% isoflurane in oxygen for 2 to 5 minutes until immobile. Each mouse was weighed, carefully shaved and taped supine to ECG electrodes on a heated procedure board with isoflurane (at 2%) supplied by a nose cone connected to the anesthesia machine. Warm ultrasound transmission gel was liberally applied to ensure optimal image quality. Echocardiography was performed using a 18 to 38 MHz linear-array transducer with a digital ultrasound system (Vevo2100 Imaging System, VisualSonics, Toronto, Canada). Standard two-dimensional gray-scale image and M-mode image at the mid-papillary level in the parasternal left ventricle short-axis view were obtained during each echocardiographic examination. Conventional echocardiographic image measurements were performed offline. All image acquisitions and offline measurements were conducted by a single investigator who was blinded to animal groups. All M-mode measurements were performed in end-diastole and end-systole according to the leading edge-to-leading edge method of the American Soiety of Echocardiography [21]. Conventional measurements of the left ventricle (LV) included: end-diastolic diameter (LVEDD), end-systolic diameter (LVESD), interventricular septal thickness (IVST) and posterior wall thicknesses (LVPWT), ejection fraction (LVEF), fractional shortening (LVFS).

$LV\ mass = 1.053 \times [(LVEDD + LVPWT + IVST)^3 - LVEDD^3]$. All data are the average of at least two separate scans, each scan representing the average of three selected beats.

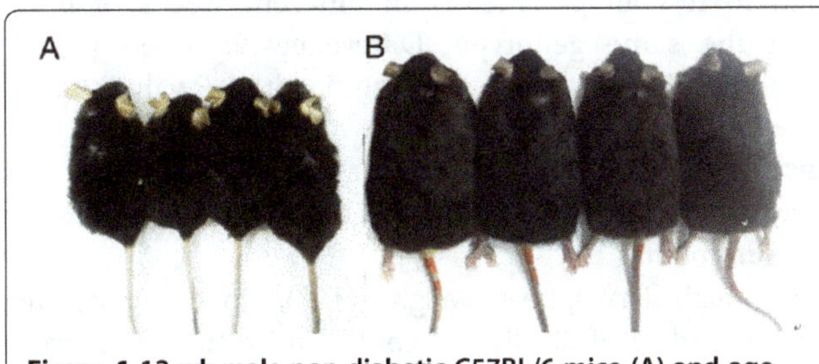

Figure 1 12-wk male non-diabetic C57BL/6 mice (A) and age-matched diabetic db/db mice (B).

Novel speckle tracking echocardiography (STE) based strain measures of myocardial deformation

Using STE based strain analysis of 2D gray scale echocardiographic images acquired from the parasternal short-axis views (at the mid-papillary level), strain analyses were quantified in the radial and circumferential axes. All images were acquired at a frame rate of >200 frames per second and at an average depth of 11 mm. Strain analyses were conducted by the same trained investigator on all animals according to the protocol detailed in the Online Data Supplement and using a speckle-tracking algorithm provided by VisualSonics (VevoStrain, VisualSonics). In brief, suitable B-mode loops were selected from digitally acquired echocardiographic images based on adequate visualization of the endocardial border and absence of image artifacts. Three consecutive cardiac cycles were selected for analysis based on image quality. Semiautomated tracing of the endocardial and epicardial borders were performed and verified over all 3 cardiac cycles and then corrected as needed to achieve good quality tracking throughout each cine loop. Tracked images were then processed in a frame-by-frame manner for strain measurements. Strain measures were averaged over the obtained cardiac cycles, resulting in curvilinear strain data (Figures 2 and 3). Short-axis view of the LV myocardium was divided into 6 standard anatomic segments for regional speckle-tracking based strain analysis throughout the cardiac cycle. Peak radial and circumferential strain measurements were recorded from each of the 6 standard

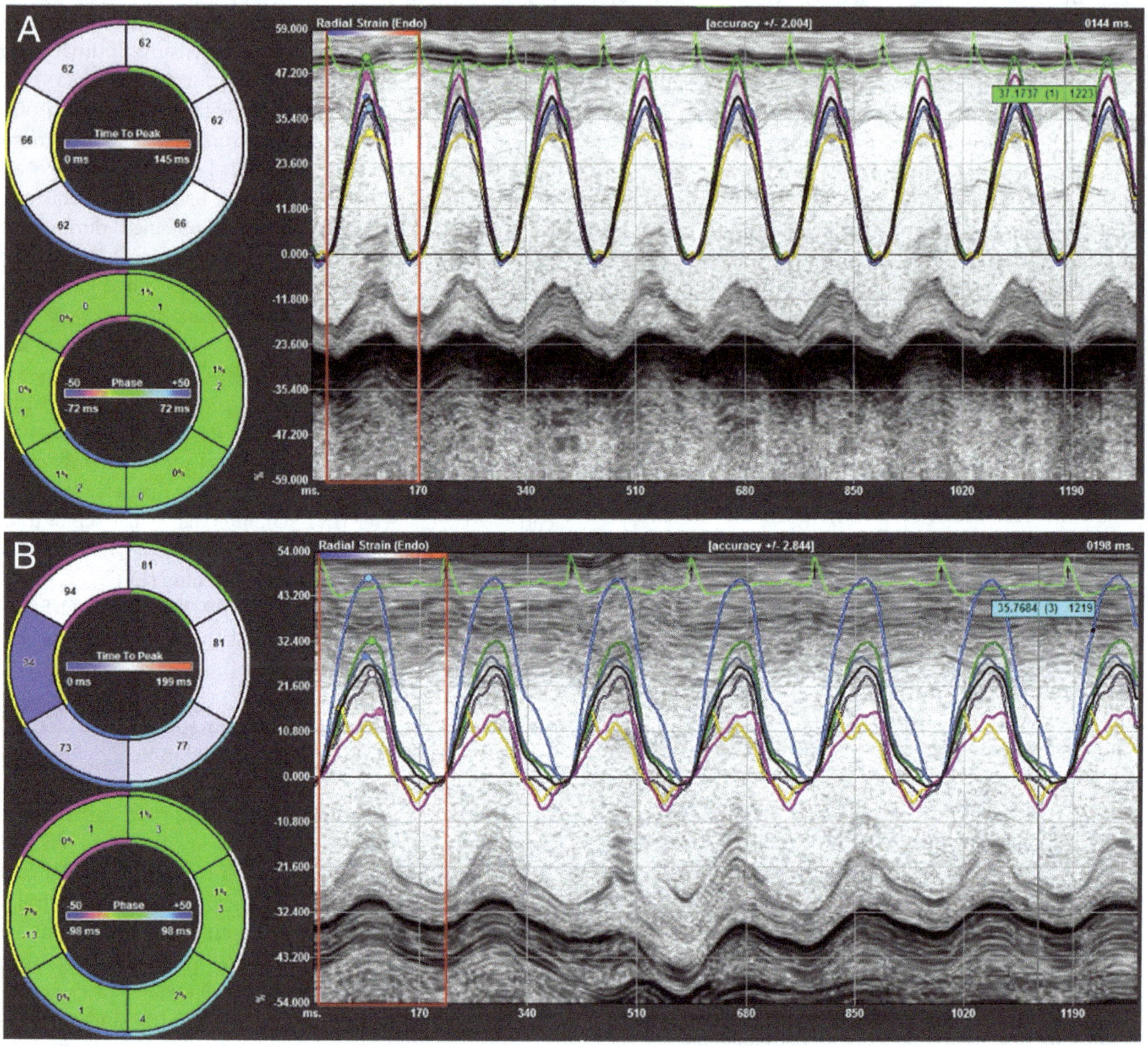

Figure 2 Radial strain curves in 16-wk non-diabetic C57BL/6 mice (A) and age-matched diabetic db/db mice (B).

segments in each view, providing regional strain values. For global radial and circumferential strain values, peak strain measurements were averaged across all 6 segments.

Glucose, heart weight and body weight measurements

Mice were fasted for 8-hrs during the light cycle and blood was drawn from the tail vein. Blood glucose was measured using the glucometer (Johnson & Johnson).

After ultrasound detection, mice were sacrificed. Immediately after death, wet heart weight (HW) and body weight (BW) were measured.

Statistical analysis

All analyses were performed with the use of SPSS 16.0 software. Resulting values are expressed as mean ± SD. Differences in conventional echocardiographic parameters and strain parameters between diabetic (db/db) and control mice of the same age were determined by means of an unpaired t test. Unpaired one-way ANOVA was used to test all parameters in different weeks of mice from the same genotype. Differences between means were regarded as statistically significant at P value <0.05.

Results

Body weight, heart weight, blood glucose and heart rate measurements

Body weight (BW), heart weight (HW), blood glucose and heart rate data of db/db and control mice (n = 8 for each group) were summarized in Table 1. The diabetic mice had larger body weight and fasting blood glucose compared to

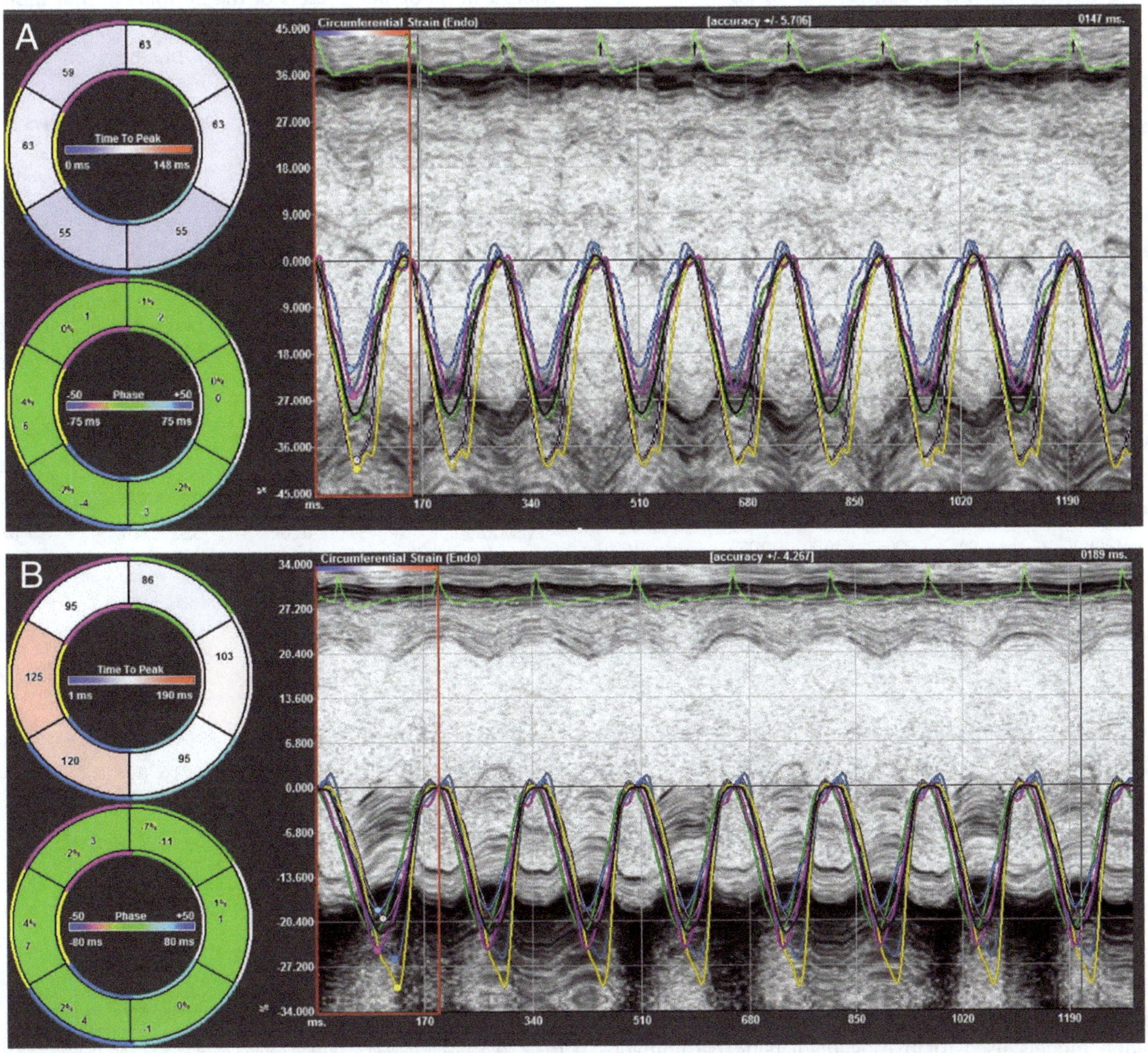

Figure 3 Circumferential strain curves in 16-wk non-diabetic C57BL/6 mice (A) and age-matched diabetic db/db mice (B).

control mice at 8, 12 or 16 weeks of age. There were no difference in heart weight and heart rate between db/db mice and age-matched controls (P > 0.05). HW/BW of db/db mice significantly decreased compared to age-matched controls because of increased BW (P < 0.01).

Conventional echocardiographic measurements of left ventricle structure and systolic function

Conventional echocardiographic parameters of left ventricle structure and systolic function in db/db and control mice were summarized in Table 2. Echocardiography showed that the thickness of interventricular septum and posterior wall were similar at 8, 12 or 16 weeks of age between db/db and control mice (P > 0.05). There was no significant difference in LVEDD, LVESD, LVEF, LVFS and LV mass at the same weeks of age between db/db and control mice (P > 0.05).

LVAWT, LVPWT, LVEDD, LVESD, LVEF and LVFS did not change with age for both dbdb and C57BL/6 mice (P > 0.05).

STE measurements of myocardial deformation

Using speckle tracking echocardiography, systolic global radial and circumferential strain values from the parasternal short-axis views at the mid-papillary level in db/db and control mice were obtained (Table 3 and Figure 4). At 8 and 12 weeks of age, there was no significant difference in left ventricular radial strain and circumferential strain between db/db mice and controls. But at 16 weeks of age, the left ventricular radial

Table 1 Characteristics of control and db/db mice

Variables	Control	Db/db	*P* value
8 weeks			
Body Weight (g)	22.26 ± 1.08	40.19 ± 1.96	*P < 0.0001*
Heart Weight (g)	0.12 ± 0.01	0.12 ± 0.01	*P > 0.05*
HW/BW	0.005 ± 0.0009	0.003 ± 0.0004	*P < 0.0001*
fasting blood glucose(mmol/L)	2.52 ± 0.50	7.62 ± 1.15	*P < 0.0001*
12 weeks			
Body Weight (g)	25.71 ± 1.41	47.82 ± 2.67	*P < 0.0001*
Heart Weight (g)	0.13 ± 0.01	0.13 ± 0.01	*P > 0.05*
HW/BW	0.005 ± 0.0002	0.003 ± 0.0002	*P < 0.0001*
fasting blood glucose(mmol/L)	2.15 ± 0.57	8.12 ± 1.22	*P < 0.0001*
16 weeks			
Body Weight (g)	27.14 ± 1.95	43.42 ± 2.05	*P < 0.0001*
Heart Weight (g)	0.13 ± 0.02	0.12 ± 0.01	*P > 0.05*
HW/BW	0.005 ± 0.0006	0.002 ± 0.0002	*P < 0.0001*
fasting blood glucose(mmol/L)	2.66 ± 0.29	12.71 ± 2.47	*P < 0.0001*

The table shows the diabetic mice have larger body weight and fasting blood glucose compared to control mice at 8, 12 or 16 weeks of age.

Table 2 M-mode parameters of the LV (parasternal short-axis view) in control and db/db mice

Variables	Control	Db/db	*P* value
8 weeks			
Heart Rate(bmp)	397.50 ± 25.46	378.22 ± 37.25	*P > 0.05*
IVST(mm)	0.71 ± 0.05	0.66 ± 0.05	*P > 0.05*
LVPWD(mm)	0.69 ± 0.06	0.68 ± 0.05	*P > 0.05*
LVEDD(mm)	3.79 ± 0.23	3.68 ± 0.28	*P > 0.05*
LVESD(mm)	2.41 ± 0.27	2.26 ± 0.23	*P > 0.05*
LVEF(%)	66.25 ± 7.43	69.15 ± 7.25	*P > 0.05*
LVFS(%)	36.44 ± 5.13	38.39 ± 5.58	*P > 0.05*
LV mass(mg)	90.39 ± 11.15	83.32 ± 10.89	*P > 0.05*
12 weeks			
Heart Rate(bmp)	392.50 ± 44.99	388.77 ± 39.02	*P > 0.05*
IVST(mm)	0.68 ± 0.06	0.71 ± 0.05	*P > 0.05*
LVPWD(mm)	0.70 ± 0.06	0.69 ± 0.06	*P > 0.05*
LVEDD(mm)	3.90 ± 0.26	3.82 ± 0.18	*P > 0.05*
LVESD(mm)	2.49 ± 0.31	2.37 ± 0.20	*P > 0.05*
LVEF(%)	65.91 ± 7.54	68.51 ± 5.25	*P > 0.05*
LVFS(%)	36.01 ± 5.38	37.99 ± 4.53	*P > 0.05*
LV mass(mg)	93.21 ± 9.52	92.24 ± 13.44	*P > 0.05*
16 weeks			
Heart Rate(bmp)	381.25 ± 21.94	391.44 ± 39.81	*P > 0.05*
IVST(mm)	0.72 ± 0.03	0.71 ± 0.03	*P > 0.05*
LVPWD(mm)	0.69 ± 0.04	0.69 ± 0.05	*P > 0.05*
LVEDD(mm)	3.94 ± 0.19	3.77 ± 0.35	*P > 0.05*
LVESD(mm)	2.53 ± 0.21	2.36 ± 0.28	*P > 0.05*
LVEF(%)	66.78 ± 4.17	67.55 ± 7.79	*P > 0.05*
LVFS(%)	36.57 ± 3.30	37.25 ± 6.05	*P > 0.05*
LV mass(mg)	97.81 ± 8.31	90.98 ± 14.37	*P > 0.05*

The diagram shows no significant difference in the measurements of heart rate, left ventricular dimensions, thickness and function parameters by M-mode echocardiography in dbdb and control mice at 8,12 and 16 weeks of age (P > 0.05).

strain and circumferential strain in db/db mice were lower than in control mice (P < 0.01).

Left ventricular radial strain and circumferential strain did not change with age for C57BL/6J mice (P > 0.05). Comparison of 8- and 12-wk db/db mice, left ventricular radial strain and circumferential strain were significantly reduced in 16-wk db/db mice (P < 0.01).

Discussion

Diabetic db/db mice provide one of more commonly used animal models used to investigate diabetic cardiomyopathy, with obesity and insulin resistance [16,17]. In the literature, db/db mice develop severe dabetes by 8 weeks of age [22,23]. Our study showed at 8, 12 and 16 weeks of age, diabetic (db/db) mice weighed significantly more than control mice. As expected, at 8 weeks of age diabetic mice had significantly elevated fasting blood glucose with hyperglycemia.

Diabetic cardiomyopathy is accompanied by functional, structural and pathologic cardiac characteristics. Echocardiography is a noninvasive method that can assess cardiac function in mice [24-26]. We used M-mode measurements of LV dimensions in end systole and end diastole and myocardium thickness to provide information on morphology and systolic function. However, we observed that left ventricular dimensions and myocardium thickness in db/db mice were not significantly increased until 16 weeks of age compared to control mice. The parameters reflecting the left ventricular systolic function such as LVEF and LVFS could not be detected unchanged in db/db mice. These findings were supported by Barouch and colleages as they reported echocardiographically in 24-week-old db/db mice on C57BL/6J background an unchanged LVEF and FS [27]. However, conventional echocardiographic measures lack sensitivity for capturing subtle variations in left ventricular (LV) performance. Changes in LV structure and global function, when detected by conventional echocardiographic parameters, are typically considered late manifestations of disease.

Speckle tracking echocardiography (STE) is a novel, non-Doppler-based technique used to detect myocardial wall motion and myocardial deformation. In clinical studies

Table 3 Radial and circumferential strain values in control and db/db mice by STE measurements

Variables	Control	Db/db	*P* value
8 weeks			
Radial strain(%)	43.43 ± 7.03	42.73 ± 6.77	*P > 0.05*
Circumferential strain(%)	-29.92 ± 2.47	-29.95 ± 4.01	*P > 0.05*
12 weeks			
Radial strain(%)	45.43 ± 8.36	45.14 ± 9.75	*P > 0.05*
Circumferential strain(%)	-30.20 ± 3.83	-28.75 ± 4.82	*P > 0.05*
16 weeks			
Radial strain(%)	42.37 ± 4.40	31.19 ± 3.95	*P < 0.01*
Circumferential strain(%)	-30.71 ± 2.24	-22.54 ± 3.57	*P < 0.01*

The table shows at 8 and 12 weeks of age, there was no significant difference in left ventricular radial strain and circumferential strain between db/db mice and age-matched controls ($P > 0.05$). At 16 weeks of age, radial strain and circumferential strain in db/db mice were lower than in control mice ($P < 0.01$).

STE based on tissue deformation has provided an improved accuracy of myocardial contractility and quantification of global and regional myocardial function. Cardiovascular risk factors result in impaired strain measures before the development of decreased LVEF or ventricular dilatation [28,29]. In experimental studies, the adoption of strain analysis in small animal models has been limited, primarily because of technical differences in imaging mice versus humans, including limited echocardiographic views, translational motion during image acquisition, and the effect of very high heart rates. However, recently developed speckle-tracking based techniques now allow for angle-independent, reproducible, and accurate strain measurements that may be applied to mice. STE can accurately predict pathophysiology during the evolution of MI [30,31] and TAC-induced heart failure in mice [32]. LV contraction is a complex process involving deformation resulting in shortening in 3 normal directions; longitudinal, radial strain (RS) and circumferential strain (CS). RS and CS are more influenced by transmural fiber dysfunction (especially the midmyocardium), and are generally more suited for identifying dysfunction in ventricles with reduced left ventricle systolic function. Therefore our study used STE to assess systolic myocardial radial strain and circumferential strain with diabetic db/db and control mice. With the use of STE, we were able to detect lower myocardial radial and circumferential strain in db/db mice at 16 weeks of age, indicating LV contractile function was indeed abnormal in this type II diabetic mice. Our study showed that subtle abnormalities in strain were associated with the presence of diabetic cardiomyopathy even in the setting of normal cardiac structure and function by conventional measures. In other words, the present study therefore indicate that radial and circumferential strain are more sensitive and can be used for detection of early LV contractile dysfunction in this type II diabetic mice model.

It should be mentioned that the HRs play an important role in the determination of cardiac function in mice by echocardiography. Inhalation anesthesia with isoflurane has currently been considered ideal and useful for experimental studies in the mouse because of its rapid conduction, easy control of the depth of anesthesia, and stable HRs during observations [33,34]. Usually, the range of HRs in anesthetic mice for echocardiography is 300 to 550 beats per minute (bpm), as reported [35]. In our experiment HRs were not significantly different between db/db mice and age-matched controls. Heart rate values of our mice were low but in this range. It may be related to anesthesia time.

Conclusion

The present study shows that speckle tracking echocardiography can be used to evaluate cardiac functional alterations in mouse models of cardiovascular disease. Radial and circumferential strain are more sensitive and can be used for detection of early left ventricular contractile dysfunction in db/db type II diabetic mice.

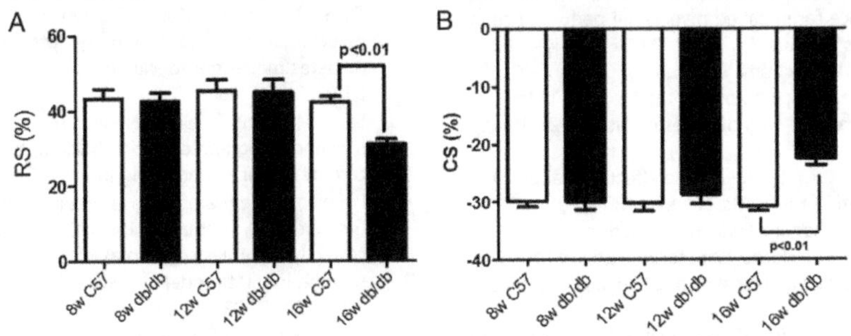

Figure 4 The graphs shows at 8 and 12 weeks of age, there was no significant difference in left ventricular radial strain (A) and circumferential strain (B) between db/db mice and age-matched controls (P > 0.05). At 16 weeks of age, radial strain **(A)** and circumferential strain **(B)** in db/db mice were lower than in control mice ($P < 0.01$). RS indicates radial strain; CS, circumferential strain; C57, non-diabetic C57BL/6 mice; db/db, db/db mice.

Competing interests
The authors declare that they have no competing interests.

Authors' contributions
RJL was involved in the conception, design of the study, doing the experiment, the analysis and interpretation of raw data and writing the article. JY participated in the design of the study, performed data entry, parts of the statistical analysis and helped to draft the manuscript. YY participated in the design of the study, reviewed and edited the manuscript. NM, BJ, QWS, LYJ were substantially participated in doing the experiment and critical revision of the article prior to submission. All authors read and approved the final manuscript.

Acknowledgements
This work was supported by grants from the Natural Science Foundation (No. 81201110, 81171351 and 81201111) and the Basic-Clinical Scientific Research Foundation Program of the Capital Medical University in China (No. 12JL55).We are indebted to the medical and technical staff members of Department of Echocardiography in Beijing An Zhen Hospital, Capital Medical University and Beijing Institute of heart and lung disease.

References
1. Cavaghan MK, Ehrmann DA, Polonsky KS: **Interactions between insulin resistance and insulin secretion in the development of glucose intolerance.** *J Clin Invest* 2000, **106**:329–333.
2. Shehadeh A, Regan TJ: **Cardiac consequences of diabetes mellitus.** *Clin Cardiol* 1995, **18**:301–305.
3. Taffet GE, Hartley CJ, Wen X, Pham T, Michael LH, Entman ML: **Noninvasive indexes of cardiac systolic and diastolic function in hyperthyroid and senescent mouse.** *Am J Physiol Heart Circ Physiol* 1996, **270**:H2204–H2209.
4. Fein FS, Kornstein LB, Strobeck JE, Capasso JM, Sonnenblick EH: **Altered myocardial mechanics in diabetic rats.** *Circ Res* 1980, **47**(6):922–933.
5. Joffe II, Travers KE, Perreault-Micale CL, Hampton T, Katz SE, Morgan JP, Douglas PS: **Abnormal cardiac function in the streptozotocin-induced non-insulin-dependent diabetic rat: noninvasive assessment with doppler echocardiography and contribution of the nitric oxide pathway.** *J Am Coll Cardiol* 1999, **34**(7):2111–2119.
6. Hoit BD, Castro C, Bultron G, Knight S, Matlib MA: **Noninvasive evaluation of cardiac dysfunction by echocardiography in streptozotocin-induced diabetic rats.** *J Card Fail* 1999, **5**(4):324–333.
7. Thompson EW: **Structural manifestations of diabetic cardiomyopathy in the rat and its reversal by insulin treatment.** *Am J Anat* 1988, **182**(3):270–282.
8. Rubler S, Dlugash J, Yuceoglu YZ, Kumral T, Branwood AW, Grishman A: **New type of cardiomyopathy associated with diabetic glomerulosclerosis.** *Am J Cardiol* 1972, **30**(6):595–602.
9. Regan TJ, Lyons MM, Ahmed SS, Levinson GE, Oldewurtel HA, Ahmad MR, Haider B: **Evidence for cardiomyopathy in familial diabetes mellitus.** *J Clin Invest* 1977, **60**(4):884–899.
10. Friedman NE, Levitsky LL, Edidin DV, Vitullo DA, Lacina SJ, Chiemmongkoltip P: **Echocardiographic evidence for impaired myocardial performance in children with type I diabetes mellitus.** *Am J Med* 1982, **73**(6):846–850.
11. Nunoda S, Genda A, Sugihara N, Nakayama A, Mizuno S, Takeda R: **Quantitative approach to the histopathology of the biopsied right ventricular myocardium in patients with diabetes mellitus.** *Heart Vessels* 1985, **1**(1):43–47.
12. Penpargkul S, Schaible T, Yipintsoi T, Scheuer J: **The effect of diabetes on performance and metabolism of rat hearts.** *Circ Res* 1980, **47**:911–921.
13. Tomlinson KC, Gardiner SM, Hebden RA, Bennett T: **Functional consequences of streptozotocin-induced diabetes mel-litus, with particular reference to the cardiovascular system.** *Pharmacol Rev* 1992, **44**:103–179.
14. Yu Z, Tibbits GL, McNeill JH: **Cellular functions of diabetic cardiomyocytes: contractility, rapid-cooling contracture, and ryanodine binding.** *Am J Physiol Heart Circ Physiol* 1994, **266**:H2082–H2089.
15. Pierce GN, Maddaford TG, Russell JC: **Cardiovascular dysfunction in insulin-dependent and non-insulin-dependent an-imal models of diabetes mellitus.** *Can J Physiol Pharmacol* 1997, **75**:343–350.
16. Aasum E, Hafstad AD, Severson DL, Larsen TS: **Age-dependent changes in metabolism, contractile function, and ischemic sensitivity in hearts from db/db mice.** *Diabetes* 2003, **52**:434–441.
17. Carley AN, Semeniuk LM, Shimoni Y, Aasum E, Larsen TS, Berger JP, Severson DL: **Treatment of type 2 diabetic db/db mice with a novel PPAR agonist improves cardiac metabolism but not contractile function.** *Am J Physiol Endocrinol Metab* 2004, **286**:E449–E455.
18. Le Quang K, Bouchareb R, Lachance D, Laplante MA, Husseini DE, Boulanger MC, Fournier D, Fang XP, Avramoglu RK, Pibarot P, Deshaies Y, Sweeney G, Mathieu P, Marette A: **Early development of calcific aortic valve disease and left ventricular hypertrophy in a mouse model of combined dyslipidemia and type 2 diabetes mellitus.** *Arterioscler Thromb Vasc Biol* 2014, **34**(10):2283–2291.
19. Semeniuk LM, Kryski AJ, Severson DL: **Echocardiographic assessment of cardiac function in diabeticdb/db and transgenic db/db-hGLUT4 mice.** *Am J Physiol Heart Circ Physiol* 2002, **283**:H976–H982.
20. Cognet T, Vervueren PL, Dercle L, Bastié D, Richaud R, Berry M, Marchal P, Gautier M, Fouilloux A, Galinier M, Carrié D, Massabuau P, Berry I, Lairez O: **New concept of myocardial longitudinal strain reserve assessed by a dipyridamole infusion using 2D-strain echocardiography: the impact of diabetes and age, and the prognostic value.** *Cardiovasc Diabetol* 2013, **12**:84.
21. Sahn DJ, De Maria A, Kisslo J, Weyman A: **Recommendations regarding quantitation in M-mode echocardiography: results of a survey of echocardiographic measurements.** *Circulation* 1978, **58**:1072–1083.
22. Belke DD, Larsen TS, Gibbs EM, Severson DL: **Altered metabolism causes cardiac dysfunction in perfused hearts from diabetic (db/db) mice.** *Am J Physiol* 2000, **279**:E1104–E1113.
23. Aasum E, Belke DD, Severson DL, Riemersma R, Cooper M, Andreassen M, Larsen TS: **Cardiac function and metabolism in type 2 diabetic mice after treatment with BM 17.0744, a novel PPAR-α activator.** *Am J Physiol* 2002, **283**:H949–H957.
24. Hoit BD: **Echocardiographic characterization of the cardiovascular phenotype in rodent models.** *Toxicol Pathol* 2006, **34**:105–110.
25. Lairez O, Lonjaret L, Ruiz S, Marchal P, Franchitto N, Calise D, Fourcade O, Mialet-Perez J, Parini A, Minville V: **Anesthetic regimen for cardiac function evaluation by echocardiography in mice: comparison between ketamine, etomidate and isoflurane versus conscious state.** *Lab Anim* 2013, **47**(4):284–290.
26. van Bilsen M, Daniels A, Brouwers O, Janssen BJ, Derks WJ, Brouns AE, Munts C, Schalkwijk CG, van der Vusse GJ, van Nieuwenhoven FA: **Hypertension is a conditional factor for the development of cardiac hypertrophy in type 2 diabetic mice.** *PLoS One* 2014, **9**(1):e85078.
27. Barouch LA, Berkowitz DE, Harrison RW, O'Donnell CP, Hare JM: **Disruption of leptin signaling contributes to cardiac hypertrophy independently of body weight in mice.** *Circulation* 2003, **108**(6):754–759.
28. Ng AC, Delgado V, Bertini M, van der Meer RW, Rijzewijk LJ, Hooi Ewe S, Siebelink HM, Smit JW, Diamant M, Romijn JA, de Roos A, Leung DY, Lamb HJ, Bax JJ: **Myocardial steatosis and biventricular strain and strain rate imaging in patients with type 2 diabetes mellitus.** *Circulation* 2010, **122**(24):2538–2544.
29. Ernande L, Rietzschel ER, Bergerot C, De Buyzere ML, Schnell F, Groisne L, Ovize M, Croisille P, Moulin P, Gillebert TC, Derumeaux G: **Impaired myocardial radial function in asymptomatic patients with type 2 diabetes mellitus: a speckle-trackingimaging study.** *J Am Soc Echocardiogr* 2010, **23**(12):1266–1272.
30. Bauer M, Cheng S, Jain M, Ngoy S, Theodoropoulos C, Trujillo A, Lin FC, Liao R: **Echocardiographic speckle-tracking-based strain imaging for rapid cardiovascular phenotyping in mice.** *Circ Res* 2011, **108**:908–916.
31. Popovic ZB, Benejam C, Bian J, Mal N, Drinko J, Lee K, Forudi F, Reeg R, Greenberg NL, Thomas JD, Penn MS: **Speckle-tracking echocardiography correctly identifies segmental left ventricular dysfunction induced by scarring in a rat model of myocardial infarction.** *Am J Physiol Heart Circ Physiol* 2007, **292**:H2809–H2816.
32. Peng Y, Popovic ZB, Sopko N, Drinko J, Zhang Z, Thomas JD, Penn MS: **Speckle tracking echocardiography in the assessment of mouse models of cardiac dysfunction.** *Am J Physiol Heart Circ Physiol* 2009, **297**:H811–H820.
33. Butterfield NN, Graf P, Ries CR, MacLeod BA: **The effect of repeated isoflurane anesthesia on spatial and psychomotor performance in young and aged mice.** *Anesth Analg* 2004, **98**:1305–1311.

17

Two-dimensional speckle-tracking echocardiography for evaluation of dilative ascending aorta biomechanics

Monika Bieseviciene[1*], Jolanta Justina Vaskelyte[1], Vaida Mizariene[1], Rasa Karaliute[1], Vaiva Lesauskaite[2] and Raimonda Verseckaite[1]

Abstract

Background: Two-dimensional (2D) echocardiography is one of the most feasible, noninvasive methods for assessing the aortic diameter and biomechanical changes. We studied possible interfaces between noninvasive biomechanical and speckle-tracking (ST) echocardiographic data from dilated aortas.

Methods: Altogether, 44 patients with dilative pathology of ascending aorta (DPAA) were compared with subjects without ascending aortic dilation (diameter <40 mm). DPAA patients formed two groups based on diameter size: group 1, ≤45 mm diameter; group 2, >45 mm. Conventional and 2D-ST echocardiography were performed to evaluate peak longitudinal strain (LS), longitudinal (LD) and transverse (TD) displacement, and longitudinal velocity (VL). Aortic strain, distensibility, elastic modulus, stiffness index β of Valsalva sinuses and ascending aorta were also evaluated. SPSS version 20 was used for all analyses.

Results: All linear diameters of the ascending aorta were increased in group 2 (>45 mm diameter) ($p < 0.05$). LD of the anterior aortic wall ($p < 0.05$) and TD of both aortic walls ($p < 0.001$) were least in group 2. VL of the posterior and anterior walls diminished in group 2 ($p = 0.01$). Aortic strain and distensibility were least ($p = 0.028$ and $p = 0.001$, respectively) and elastic modulus and stiffness index β values were greatest in group 2, although without statistical significance.

Conclusions: Ascending aortas of both DPAA groups had reduced elasticity and increased stiffness. The greatest changes in biomechanical parameters occurred in ascending aortas >45 mm. Longitudinal ascending aortic wall motion was mostly impaired in patients with aortas >45 mm (i.e., anterior aortic wall LD, VL of the posterior and anterior walls. TD of the posterior and anterior aortic walls was significantly lower in >45 mm aortic diameter patients. TD of 5.2 mm could predict aortic dilation >45 mm (area under the curve 0.76, $p < 0.001$, confidence interval 0.65–0.87; sensitivity 87%; specificity 63%). Greater aortic dilation is associated with reduced aortic stiffness parameters and increased elastic modulus and stiffness index β. Lower LD and LS were associated with less aortic strain and distensibility. There were no significant differences in 2D-ST echocardiographic or stiffness parameters between patients with tricuspid or bicuspid aortic valves.

Keywords: Ascending aorta, Biomechanics of aorta, Speckle-tracking echocardiography, Stiffness

* Correspondence: monika.bieseviciene@gmail.com
[1]Department of Cardiology, Medical Academy, Lithuanian University of Health Sciences, Eivenių Str. 2, Kaunas 50009, Lithuania
Full list of author information is available at the end of the article

Background

Aortic dilation is the most frequent pathology of the ascending aorta and a well-known risk factor for dissection. An aneurysm has been defined as localized dilation of an artery, with at least a 50% increase in the diameter compared with the expected normal diameter. Because of the increased risk of aortic dissection, surgical repair is recommended for patients with an ascending aorta aneurysm [1].

According to the 2014 European Society of Cardiology guidelines on the diagnosis and treatment of aortic disease, surgery is indicated for an aortic root aneurysm in the following patients: those with Marfan syndrome (IC class) with a maximum aortic diameter of 50 mm; those with Marfan syndrome with a 45 mm aortic diameter and risk factors; those with a 50 mm aortic diameter, a bicuspid valve, and risk factors; those with a 55 mm aortic diameter and no elastopathy [2].

The possibility of defining biomechanical properties of an aortic wall more precisely has increased in recent years, which could help improve our understanding of aortic wall properties and the potential risk for rupture [3]. Two-dimensional (2D) echocardiography is one of the most feasible and the oldest method for diagnosing this pathology. More precisely, it can be used not only for diameter assessment but also for noninvasive measurement of biomechanical changes in the aorta.

Arterial stiffness parameters (e.g., distensibility, stiffness β, an elastic modulus, aortic strain) can also be evaluated by 2D echocardiography. Arterial stiffness is one of the earliest detectable manifestations of adverse structural and functional changes in the vessel wall [4]. Arterial stiffness, which increases with age [5], is an important predictor of cardiovascular morbidity and mortality [6]. Changes in arterial stiffness may have global consequences (i.e., affecting the whole arterial system, such as age-related stiffening). Changes could also be more localized, however, as in the case of arterial pathology (e.g., an aortic aneurysm) [7].

A novel method—2D speckle-tracking echocardiography (2D-ST)—is a bedside approach to assessing human aortic wall strain and motion. Up to now there have been few data available regarding the use of 2D-ST echocardiography for evaluating the ascending aorta.

2D-ST echocardiography is able to identify specific acoustic markers (i.e., speckles) in grey-scale images and track them frame-by-frame throughout the cardiac cycle. The results enable independent calculations of motion and deformation variables, such as velocity, displacement, strain (e), and strain rate [8, 9].

We therefore investigated the elastic and mechanical properties of the ascending aorta using the novel 2D-ST method. The aim was to find interfaces between noninvasively measured biomechanical data from a dilated aorta using different echocardiographic techniques.

Methods

Study population

The current study included 44 patients with dilative pathology of the ascending aorta (DPAA; 78.3% men; mean age 55.41 ± 14.69 years) and 53 controls (51.9% men; mean age 58.64 ± 7.50 years). The control group consisted of subjects without ascending aorta dilation (diameter >40 mm). The DPAA group was subdivided into two groups according to the diameter of the ascending aorta: group 1, ≤45 mm diameter; group 2, >45 mm.

All DPAA patients were treated in the Cardiology Department at the Hospital of Lithuanian University of Health Sciences during 2012–2014. Inclusion criteria were an ascending aorta or sinus dilation ≥40 mm with or without aortic valve pathology, good-quality echocardiographic images, sinus rhythm, and the absence of hemodynamically significant coronary artery disease shown by coronary angiography (stenosis <50%). We excluded patients with acute aortic syndrome, aortic coarctation, an implanted pacemaker, atrial fibrillation/flutter, and/or a history of coronary artery bypass surgery.

Clinical evaluation and 2D and 2D-ST echocardiography were performed prior to cardiac surgery. All participants gave their informed written consent, and the Kaunas Regional Biomedical Research Ethics Committee approved the study (ref. number BE-2-12).

2D and 2D-ST echocardiography

Both conventional (2D) and 2D-ST echocardiography were performed using a Vivid 7 (GE-Vingmed Ultrasound AS, Horten, Norway) ultrasonography machine with a M3S probe. M-mode, 2D, Doppler, and 2D-ST echocardiography examinations were performed to obtain standard parasternal and apical views. To minimize the variability of measurements, all echo/Doppler evaluations were performed and analyzed by a single physician. The linear data were measured and averaged over three heartbeats. The diameters of the heart chambers and aortic diameters were measured according to the last published guidelines for cardiac chamber quantification in adults. The left ventricular (LV) volumes and ejection fractions were calculated from apical two- and four-chamber views using the biplane Simpson's disc summation method. Aortic diameters were measured as absolute values and as values indexed to the body surface area. The aortic diameters ratio was determined as ratio of the observed diameter to expected diameter [10].

For the aortic 2D-ST analysis, tissue harmonic images were used. The mean frame rate was adjusted to 50–90 frames per second, and the cine-loop of three consecutive heartbeats was stored and transferred to a workstation for off-line ST analysis (EchoPac PC; GE Vingmed). Before analysis, the timing of an aortic valve and a mitral valve opening and closing was assessed using pulsed-wave Doppler recordings of aortic and transmitral flow, respectively.

The echocardiographic images of the ascending aorta were obtained from the long-axis parasternal view. The shortest distance from the aortic annulus with good visibility was 3 cm. Manual tracing of the inner contour of the aortic root and the proximal ascending aorta was performed during systole. Dedicated software tracked the contour on all other frames automatically. Because the tracking software was created for use in the left ventricle, we used the two-chamber analysis option and then changed the six segments to four, thus dividing the aortic wall into four segments: anterior sinus, anterior ascending aorta, posterior sinus, posterior ascending aorta. For the aortic evaluation, we excluded the "LV apical segment" analysis. After manual correction of the region of interest, correct tracking was verified.

We then evaluated the peak longitudinal strain (LS), which is considered the change in segment length/resting segment length—i.e., deformation of an object relative to its original length (a dimensionless ratio expressed as a percent); longitudinal (LD) and transverse (TD) displacements, defined as a change in the position of an object; and longitudinal velocity (VL), displacement of an object per time unit—of the Valsalva sinuses and the ascending part of the aorta (Fig. 1).

For all of the subjects, arterial blood pressure was measured using a sphygmomanometer at the brachial artery. Aortic stiffness describes the elastic resistance that the aorta sets against distension [7]. The parameters of the ascending aorta stiffness and elasticity were calculated using previously described formulas [11, 12].

Aortic diameter change (mm): SD – DD
Aortic strain: (SD – DD)/DD
Aortic distensibility: 2 × (change in aortic diameter)/(diastolic aortic diameter) × (change in aortic pressure)
Elastic modulus: (SBP – DBP)/strain
Stiffness index β: ln (SBP/DBP)/strain

where DD is the diastolic aortic diameter, SD is the systolic aortic diameter, DBP is the diastolic blood pressure, SBP is the systolic blood pressure, and ln is a natural logarithm.

Statistical analysis

SPSS version 20 (SPSS, Chicago, IL, USA) was used for all data analyses. The continuous variables are expressed as the mean ± standard deviation (SD). Normal distribution of the continuous values was assessed by the Kolmogorov–Smirnov test. The categorical variables are expressed as absolute numbers and percentages. The statistical test used

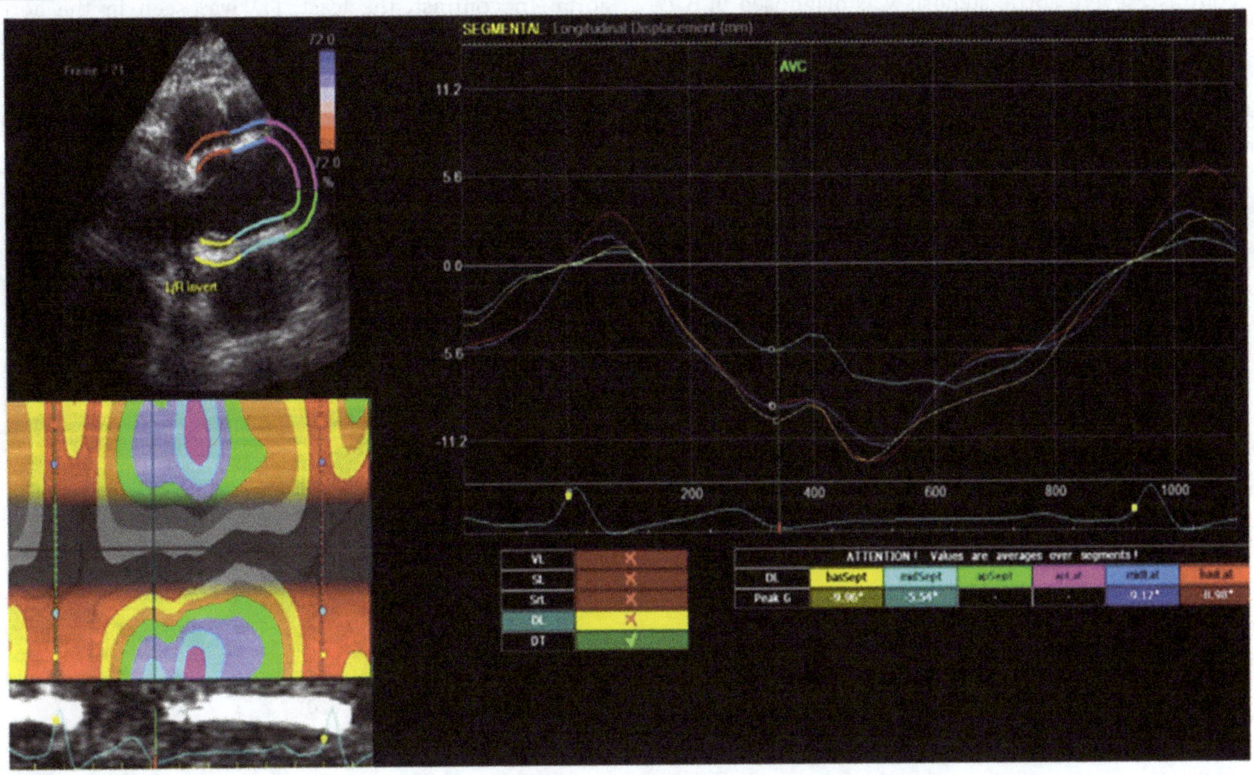

Fig. 1 Example parasternal long axis view of a two-dimensional speckle-tracking echocardiographic image of longitudinal displacement of the ascending aorta

in these cases was the χ^2 test. The means were compared using the two-tailed unpaired Student test or Mann–Whitney test. The relation between the variables was estimated using Pearson's correlation (r). A receiver operating characteristic (ROC) curve was used to determine the sensitivity and specificity of strains for predicting a dilated aorta. A value of $p < 0.05$ was regarded as indicating statistical significance.

Results

The demographic, clinical, and conventional echocardiographic data of the study groups are shown in Tables 1 and 2. More men were enrolled in the study, but there were no differences between the sex distribution, age, or body surface area in the groups. More hypertensive patients (89.3%) were included in group 2 than in group 1 or the controls. Systolic blood pressure was highest in group 2, and diastolic blood pressure was highest in the controls.

The LV diameters did not differ between the DPAA groups but were significantly smaller in the controls. Statistically significantly larger LV ejection fractions were observed in group 1 and the controls. The linear absolute and indexed values of diameters of the ascending aorta were largest in group 2.

There were no aortic valves with hemodynamically significant stenosis or insufficiency in the control group. In contrast, severe aortic stenosis was diagnosed in 6.2% of patients in group 1 and in 15.4% in group 2. Overall, 50% of group 1 and 53.8% of group 2 patients had severe aortic insufficiency. There was no difference in the frequency of aortic regurgitation between the two DPAA groups. All of the control patients had an anatomically tricuspid aortic valve, whereas 62.5% of group 1 patients and 30.4% of group 2 patients had a bicuspid aortic valve (BAV) ($p < 0.04$). The2D-ST echocardiographic parameters of the ascending aorta of the study groups are shown in Table 2. 2D-ST echocardiographic parameters of the ascending aorta of the study groups are shown in Table 2. The 2D-ST echocardiographic parameters of the ascending aorta of the study groups are shown in Table 3.

The LD of an anterior aortic wall (both the sinus and ascending part) was greatest in group 1. Group 2 had significantly less LD of the anterior aortic wall than the controls or group 1. There was no statistically significant difference between the LD values of a posterior wall among the groups, but there was a tendency toward lower values in group 2 than in the controls or group 1.

Both the anterior and posterior walls of the ascending aorta during systole had statistically significantly greater TD in group 1 and the control group than in group 2. The largest TD of the posterior wall was recorded in group 1.

There was a tendency toward greater LD and TD values for the anterior aortic wall than the posterior wall in both DPAA groups. The largest LD values were observed in an anterior sinus segment and the smallest in the posterior aorta. In contrast, the least TD was seen in the aortic posterior sinus and the most in the anterior sinus.

Table 1 Demographic and clinical data for the study population

Parameter	Controls	Diameter of ascending aorta		p		
		Group 1 (≤45 mm)	Group 2 (>45 mm)	Controls vs. group 1	Controls vs. group 2	Group 1 vs. group 2
Age (years)	58.2 ± 7.1	52.9 ± 13.8	60.1 ± 12.2	NS	NS	NS
Sex (F/M) (%)	43.3/56.7	18.8/81.2	25.0/75.0	NS	NS	NS
Body surface area (m^2)	1.91 ± 0.2	2.01 ± 0.2	2.0 ± 0.2	NS	NS	NS
Arterial hypertension (%)	65.2	60.0	89.3	NS	0.02	0.02
Blood pressure (mmHg)						
Systolic	134.6 ± 13.7	138.8 ± 17.7	145.8 ± 23.5	NS	0.01	NS
Diastolic	84.1 ± 9.6	73.4 ± 13.0	78.8 ± 11.8	0.003	0.03	NS
Antihypertensive Rx (%)						
β-Blockers	25.5	85.7	77.8	<0.05	0.001	NS
ACE-I	22.0	64.3	55.6	<0.05	0.002	NS
ARB	17.6	7.7	18.5	NS	NS	NS
Smokers (%)	28.8	0	7.4	<0.05	0.02	NS
Aortic valve pathology (%)						
Aortic valve insufficiency	0	50.0	53.8	<0.001	<0.001	NS
Stenosis	0	6.2	15.4	NS	0.002	NS
Bicuspid	0	62.5	30.4	0.001	0.001	0.04

ACE-I angiotensin-converting enzyme inhibitors, *ARB* angiotensin receptor blockers, *NS* not significant, *Rx* treatment, Values are mean (SD) unless otherwise indicated

Table 2 Conventional echocardiographic data for the study population

Parameter	Controls	Diameter of ascending aorta		p		
		Group 1 (≤45 mm)	Group 2 (>45 mm)	Controls vs. group 1	Controls vs. group 2	Group 1 vs. group 2
LV diastolic diameter (mm)	46.9 ± 4.6	55.9 ± 7.3	55.3 ± 8.9	<0.001	<0.001	NS
LVEDDi (mm/m²)	24.1 ± 2.2	28.0 ± 3.9	27.5 ± 4.2	<0.001	<0.001	NS
Interventricular septum (mm)	10.7 ± 1.5	12.5 ± 1.6	13.5 ± 2.3	<0.001	<0.001	NS
LV posterior wall (mm)	10.1 ± 1.4	11.1 ± 1.5	11.9 ± 2.0	0.02	<0.001	NS
LV ejection fraction (%)	57.2 ± 2.1	54.6 ± 3.4	50.2 ± 8.9	NS	<0.05	0.029
Ascending aorta diameter (mm)						
Aortic annulus	22.5 ± 3.2	27.8 ± 3.2	26.5 ± 2.8	<0.001	<0.001	NS
Sinus at Valsalva level	35.0 ± 3.6	44.8 ± 7.6	47.2 ± 8.2	<0.001	<0.001	NS
Sinotubular junction	30.2 ± 3.1	37.6 ± 5.3	43.1 ± 8.8	<0.001	<0.001	NS
Ascending aorta in end-diastole	33.9 ± 3.3	42.8 ± 2.8	53.2 ± 6.0	<0.001	<0.001	<0.001
Cross sectional area in systole	8.6 ± 1.6	14.5 ± 1.7	21.7 ± 6.7	<0.001	<0.001	<0.001
Cross sectional area in diastole	7.7 ± 1.5	12.8 ± 1.6	19.9 ± 6.3	<0.001	<0.001	<0.001
Aortic diameter/BSA (mm/m²)						
Aortic annulus	11.6 ± 1.7	13.8 ± 1.5	13.4 ± 1.4	<0.001	<0.001	NS
Sinus at Valsalva	18.2 ± 1.9	22.2 ± 2.9	23.5 ± 3.6	<0.001	<0.001	NS
Sinotubular junction	15.6 ± 1.5	18.6 ± 1.5	21.7 ± 4.0	<0.001	<0.001	0.01
Ascending aorta in end-diastole	17.3 ± 1.7	21.5 ± 2.8	27.0 ± 5.5	<0.001	<0.001	<0.001
Aortic diameter index (ratio): observed/expected values						
Aortic annulus	0.89 ± 0.1	1.0 ± 0.1	1.02 ± 0.1	<0.001	<0.001	NS
Sinus at Valsalva level	1.0 ± 0.1	1.29 ± 0.2	1.35 ± 0.2	<0.001	<0.001	NS
Sinotubular junction	1.0 ± 0.1	1.24 ± 0.1	1.44 ± 0.2	<0.001	<0.001	0.01
Ascending aorta in end-diastole	1.1 ± 0.1	1.4 ± 0.2	1.76 ± 0.3	<0.001	<0.001	<0.001

BSA body surface area, *LV* left ventricular, *LVEDDi* left ventricular end-diastolic diameter index, Values are mean (SD) unless otherwise indicated

There was a tendency toward lower LS in group 2, although the differences were not statistically significant. Interestingly, the LS in group 1was highest in the aortic posterior sinus and anterior ascending aorta segments compared with those of the controls but without statistical significance.

VL values for the anterior aortic wall were statistically significantly lower in group 2 than in group 1 and were lower than the control values without a significant difference. In contrast, the posterior aortic wall had lower VL values than the controls. VL values in the anterior sinus were greatest in group 1.

After excluding patients with severe aortic stenosis and severe aortic insufficiency from the analysis, we obtained similar results. There were no differences in the 2D-ST mechanical parameters between the controls and group 1. Less LD and TD of the anterior aortic wall and lower VL of the posterior sinus was found in group 2 than in the controls ($p < 0.05$). Lower LD values were found in the anterior aortic wall of the group 2 than in group 1 ($p < 0.05$).

We analyzed 2D-ST echocardiographic and stiffness parameters (aortic strain, elastic modulus, stiffness index β, distensibility) between patients with tricuspid or BAVs in both DPAA groups. No significant differences were found. Only LS of the aortic posterior sinus was higher in the BAV population (8.9 ± 10.4 vs. 18.8 ± 14.4, $p = 0.02$) (Table 4). The biomechanical aortic parameters (strain, distensibility) were reduced in group 2 compared with those in the controls and group 1. The elastic modulus and stiffness index β values were higher in group 2 than in the controls but without a statistically significant difference (Table 5).

Correlations between the 2D-ST echocardiographic results and the arterial biomechanical parameters of the ascending aorta were calculated for the whole patient population. The LD of both the anterior and posterior aortic walls had a negative correlation with the aortic strain ($r = -0.267$ and $r = -0.211$). LD values were mathematically negative, and the lower LD was associated with less aortic strain.

Less aortic distensibility was associated with reduced LD and LS of the anterior aortic wall. The lower the LD of the anterior aortic wall, the worse was the estimated aortic distensibility.

Table 3 Speckle-tracking echocardiographic parameters of the ascending aorta

Parameter	Controls	Diameter of ascending aorta		*p*		
		Group 1 (≤45 mm)	Group 2 (>45 mm)	Controls vs. group 1	Controls vs. group 2	Group 1 vs. group 2
Longitudinal displacement (mm)						
Aortic posterior sinus	−5.3 ± 4.0	−6.2 ± 4.4	−4.3 ± 3.7	NS	NS	NS
Posterior ascending aorta	−3.3 ± 3.1	−2.6 ± 4.4	−3.3 ± 3.0	NS	NS	NS
Anterior ascending aorta	−9.8 ± 4.3	−11.5 ± 5.3	−6.8 ± 5.3	NS	0.01	0.018
Aortic anterior sinus	−11.7 ± 6.1	−13.9 ± 6.5	−9.6 ± 5.2	NS	NS	0.04
Aortic PW	−4.3 ± 3.4	−4.4 ± 4.1	−3.7 ± 2.8	NS	NS	NS
Aortic AW	−10.7 ± 4.9	−12.7 ± 5.7	−8.2 ± 4.8	NS	0.042	0.02
Transverse displacement (mm)						
Aortic posterior sinus	5.7 ± 2.0	3.8 ± 3.0	3.6 ± 2.0	0.009	<0.001	NS
Posterior ascending aorta	5.4 ± 1.9	6.5 ± 3.0	4.0 ± 1.8	NS	0.002	0.003
Anterior ascending aorta	−5.6 ± 1.9	−5.7 ± 2.0	−3.9 ± 3.1	NS	0.01	NS
Aortic anterior sinus	−8.8 ± 2.2	−9.5 ± 2.6	−6.3 ± 4.1	NS	0.01	0.02
Aortic PW	5.6 ± 1.7	6.2 ± 2.1	3.8 ± 1.8	NS	<0.001	0.002
Aortic AW	−7.2 ± 2.0	−6.8 ± 2.5	−5.4 ± 2.9	NS	0.003	NS
Longitudinal strain (%)						
Aortic posterior sinus	18.9 ± 19.1	19.8 ± 10.3	13.8 ± 16.4	NS	NS	NS
Posterior ascending aorta	17.8 ± 13.8	17.6 ± 14.6	13.54 ± 9.9	NS	NS	NS
Anterior ascending aorta	23.0 ± 17.6	29.0 ± 17.1	19.5 ± 10.9	NS	NS	NS
Aortic anterior sinus	12.5 ± 16.5	10.0 ± 13.4	11.8 ± 18.9	NS	NS	NS
Aortic PW	18.4 ± 15.1	18.4 ± 9.6	13.9 ± 12.1	NS	NS	NS
Aortic AW	17.6 ± 15.6	19.3 ± 11.7	14.8 ± 14.2	NS	NS	NS
Longitudinal velocity (cm/s)						
Aortic posterior sinus	−7.6 ± 2.0	−6.3 ± 2.9	−5.9 ± 2.5	NS	0.002	NS
Posterior ascending aorta	−5.9 ± 2.0	−6.1 ± 2.9	−5.4 ± 2.1	NS	NS	NS
Anterior ascending aorta	−5.6 ± 1.8	−6.4 ± 1.8	−4.8 ± 1.4	NS	NS	0.009
Anterior sinus	−5.0 ± 2.0	−5.8 ± 1.9	−4.3 ± 2.3	NS	NS	NS
Aortic PW	−6.8 ± 1.7	−6.2 ± 2.0	−5.6 ± 1.7	NS	0.01	NS
Aortic AW	−5.3 ± 1.6	−6.1 ± 1.7	−4.5 ± 1.5	NS	NS	0.01

AW anterior wall, *PW* posterior wall, *TD* transverse displacement, Values are mean (SD) unless otherwise indicated

The LS of the anterior aortic wall directly correlated positively with aortic strain and distensibility: the lower the LS, the lower were the aortic strain and distensibility (respectively, $r = 0.22$ and $r = 0.283$). No correlations between the VL and the stiffness parameters of the ascending aorta were observed (Table 6).

Because the 2D-ST-derived aortic wall motion parameters were higher in group 1 patients, the correlation between these parameters and the aortic diameters (including patients from both DPAA groups) were analyzed. The results are shown in Table 7. Negative correlations were found between the aortic dimensions and wall motion. That is, the higher/greater aortic dimensions were associated with reduced absolute values of the LD and TD of the posterior aortic wall and reduced LS of both the anterior and posterior aortic walls.

ROC analysis showed that a value of 5.2 mm for TD of the posterior aortic wall [area under the curve (AUC) 0.76, $p < 0.001$, confidence interval (CI) 0.65–0.87; sensitivity 87%; specificity 63%] predicted aortic dilation >45 mm (Fig. 2).

Discussion

For a long time, the most important determinant of ascending aorta rupture was the size of the aneurysm [13, 14]. More recent data, however, indicate that the absolute size may not be the only factor. Less aortic dilation may lead to dissection, whereas a larger aneurysm

Table 4 Comparison of echocardiographic and stiffness parameters between patients with tricuspid or bicuspid aortic valves in the two DPAA groups

Parameter	Tricuspid aortic valve	Bicuspid aortic valve	*p*
Aortic annulus (mm)	26.3 ± 2.8	28.4 ± 3.8	NS
Sinus at Valsalva level (mm)	48.9 ± 9.6	43.8 ± 6.5	NS
Sinotubular junction (mm)	43.8 ± 8.5	38.5 ± 4.9	0.02
Ascending aorta in end-diastole (mm)	50.8 ± 7.4	46.0 ± 5.0	0.02
Aortic annulus (mm/m^2)	13.6 ± 1.4	14.2 ± 1.3	NS
Sinus at Valsalva level (mm/m^2)	25.2 ± 5.0	22.0 ± 2.9	0.02
Sinotubular junction (mm/m^2)	22.6 ± 4.3	19.3 ± 2.4	0.004
Ascending aorta in end-diastole (mm/m^2)	26.6 ± 6.7	23.2 ± 3.1	NS
2D-ST echocardiographic parameters			
Longitudinal displacement (mm)			
Aortic posterior sinus	−4.6 ± 4.4	−4.7 ± 3.5	NS
Posterior ascending aorta	−3.5 ± 3.8	−2.5 ± 3.1	NS
Anterior ascending aorta	−6.7 ± 5.4	−9.5 ± 5.0	NS
Aortic anterior sinus	−10.0 ± 5.1	−11.7 ± 5.6	NS
Aortic PW	−4.0 ± 3.6	−3.9 ± 2.9	NS
Aortic AW	−8.3 ± 4.8	−10.5 ± 5.1	NS
Transverse displacement (mm)			
Aortic posterior sinus	3.1 ± 2.4	4.0 ± 2.6	NS
Posterior ascending aorta	4.0 ± 3.2	5.4 ± 1.6	NS
Anterior ascending aorta	−3.4 ± 2.9	−4.8 ± 2.9	NS
Aortic anterior sinus	−6.4 ± 4.2	−7.7 ± 3.5	NS
Aortic PW	4.2 ± 2.7	4.8 ± 2.0	NS
Aortic AW	−4.8 ± 2.5	−6.3 ± 3.1	NS
Longitudinal strain (%)			
Aortic posterior sinus	8.9 ± 10.4	18.8 ± 14.4	0.02
Posterior ascending aorta	13.7 ± 11.4	15.1 ± 11.5	NS
Anterior ascending aorta	21.2 ± 11.3	24.8 ± 16.3	NS
Aortic anterior sinus	11.5 ± 20.9	10.9 ± 12.7	NS
Aortic PW	11.4 ± 9.3	16.9 ± 11.3	NS
Aortic AW	15.1 ± 14.0	17.8 ± 12.1	NS
Longitudinal velocity (cm/s)			
Aortic posterior sinus	−5.9 ± 2.6	−5.8 ± 2.6	NS
Posterior ascending aorta	−5.6 ± 2.1	−6.1 ± 3.0	NS
Anterior ascending aorta	−5.2 ± 1.8	5.5 ± 1.3	NS
Anterior sinus	−4.7 ± 2.2	−4.8 ± 2.1	NS
Aortic PW	−5.8 ± 1.7	−6.0 ± 2.0	NS
Aortic AW	−4.9 ± 1.8	−5.2 ± 1.5	NS
Arterial stiffness parameters			
Aortic diameter change (mm)	2.5 ± 1.2	2.4 ± 1.4	NS
Aortic strain (%)	5.3 ± 2.8	5.6 ± 3.2	NS
Elastic modulus (mmHg)	19.8 ± 13.8	23.4 ± 29.6	NS
Stiffness index β	0.2 ± 0.1	0.2 ± 0.3	NS
Aortic distensibility (mmHg)$^{-1}$	0.2 ± 0.1	0.2 ± 0.1	NS

2D-ST two-dimensional speckle tracking, *AW* anterior wall, *PW* posterior wall, Values are mean (SD) unless otherwise indicated

Table 5 Arterial stiffness parameters of the ascending aorta estimated by echocardiography

Parameter	Patient groups			p		
	Controls	Group 1 (≤45 mm)	Group 2 (>45 mm)	Controls vs. group 1	Controls vs. group 2	Group 1 vs. group 2
Aortic diameter change (mm)	1.9 ± 1.3	2.6 ± 1.3	2.2 ± 1.2	NS	NS	NS
Aortic strain (%)	6.3 ± 4.8	6.6 ± 3.4	4.4 ± 2.4	NS	0.028	0.03
Elastic modulus (mmHg)	13.1 ± 11.9	14.2 ± 10.6	23.9 ± 24.2	NS	NS	NS
Stiffness index β	0.1 ± 0.1	0.1 ± 0.1	0.2 ± 0.3	NS	NS	NS
Aortic distensibility ($mmHg^{-1}$)	0.3 ± 0.3	0.2 ± 0.1	0.1 ± 0.1	NS	0.001	NS

Values are mean (SD) unless otherwise indicated

may remain stable. Thus, risk parameters for rupture, other than size, should be considered. Locally confined changes in aortic wall motion or an increase in local strain may be additional indicators [7].

Since 2008, 2D-ST studies have successfully assessed local aortic vascular wall properties [15]. We presented here a bedside approach to assessing human aortic wall biomechanics. We used the 2D strain imaging technique for evaluating LV myocardial strain and adapted it to imaging the ascending aorta. So far, we do not have sufficient data regarding the 2D-ST method for evaluating the ascending aorta to make definitive conclusions.

The main finding of our study was that the 2D-ST parameters of the ascending aorta were most impaired in patients with larger aortas (group 2, >45 mm aortic diameter). During systole, the ascending aorta stretches lengthwise, and all segments of the anterior aortic wall move forward from the aortic annulus. Longitudinal wall motion—i.e., LD of all of the anterior aortic wall and VL of both (anterior and posterior) walls—was diminished in group 2. There was a tendency toward lower LS values for both aortic walls in group 2. The TD of both aortic walls was also decreased in the larger-aorta group. Accordingly, LD of both aortic walls was greatest in group 1 (≤45 mm diameter).

Yurdakul et al. [16] demonstrated that the peak LS, the strain rate, and total LD values were significantly impaired in patients with BAVs, compared with the controls. In our study, only LS of the aortic posterior sinus was greater in the BAV population, with no significant difference between the other 2D-ST parameters. These results could have been influenced by the larger ascending aortic dimensions of tricuspid valve patients compared with those of the BAV patients. It seems that 2D-ST parameters are more dependent on the linear diameters of the aorta than on the type of aortic valve.

Strain imaging of the normal ascending and abdominal aortas, as well as their aneurysms, has demonstrated heterogeneous systolic strain distributions in all aortic segments [7]. Our study showed that four regions of the proximal aorta move differently. The largest LD values were observed in the anterior sinus segment, and the smallest were in the posterior ascending aorta. The TD was least in the aortic posterior sinus and most in the

Table 6 Correlation between speckle-tracking echocardiographic and arterial stiffness parameters of the ascending aorta for the total study population

Parameter	Aortic strain	Aortic distensibility
Longitudinal displacement (mm)		
Aortic AW	−0.267**	−0.290**
Aortic PW	−0.211*	−0.185
Transverse displacement (mm)		
Aortic AW	−0.132	−0.169
Aortic PW	−0.059	−0.016
Longitudinal strain (%)		
Aortic AW	0.220*	0.283*
Aortic PW	0.076	0.105
Longitudinal velocity (cm/s)		
Aortic AW	−0.003	−0.047
Aortic PW	0.077	0.007

AW anterior wall, *PW* posterior wall
**Correlation is significant at the $p < 0.01$ level. *Correlation is significant at the $p < 0.05$ level

Table 7 Correlation between the speckle-tracking echocardiographic parameters and aortic diameters

Parameter	Aortic sinus diameter	Ascending aorta diameter	Aortic cross sectional area
Longitudinal displacement (mm)			
Aortic AW	0.23*	NS	NS
Aortic PW	0.22*	NS	NS
Transverse displacement (mm)			
Aortic AW	0.33**	0.28**	0.33**
Aortic PW	−0.22*	−0.37**	−0.41**
Longitudinal strain (%)			
Aortic AW	−0.23*	NS	NS
Aortic PW	−0.27*	NS	NS
Longitudinal velocity (cm/s)			
Aortic AW	NS	NS	NS
Aortic PW	NS	0.22*	NS

AW anterior wall, *PW* posterior wall
**Correlation is significant at the $p < 0.01$ level. *Correlation is significant at the $p < 0.05$ level

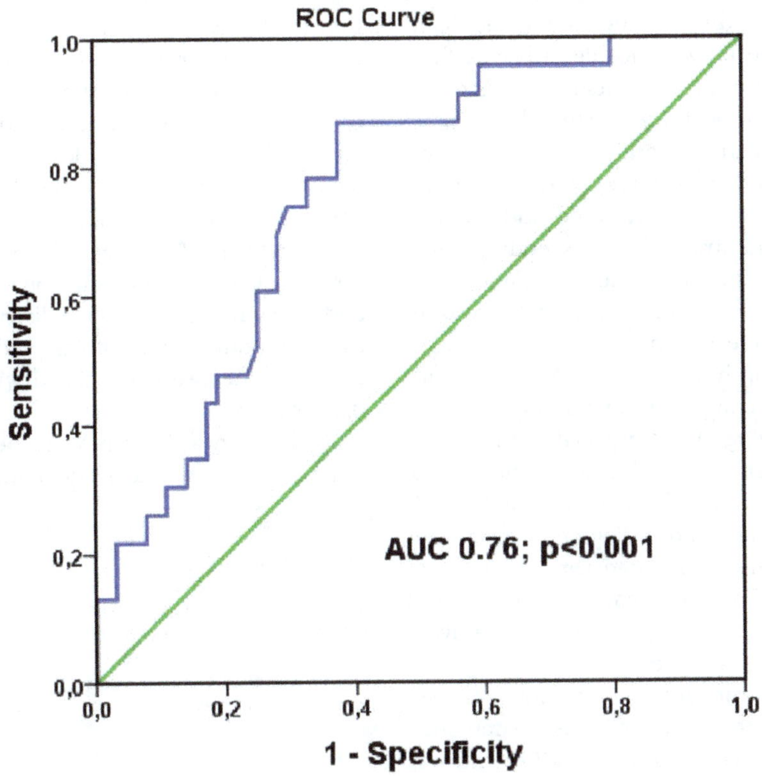

Fig. 2 Receiver operating characteristic curve of transverse displacement of the aortic posterior wall, which predicts aortic dilation

anterior sinus. We determined that a TD value of 5.2 mm is able to predict aortic dilation >45 mm.

The human aorta is often modeled mechanically as a hollow cylinder loaded with pulse pressure, resulting in a completely homogeneous strain distribution in the aortic wall [17]. During systole, the substantial proximal aortic axial displacement produces LS. Analyzing the LS parameters showed that there was a tendency toward lower LS rates in group 2, although we did not determine if there was a statistically significant difference.

We observed intermediate values among the 2D-ST data for the control group compared with those of groups 1 and 2 (i.e., values were lower than in group 1). We assumed that the ascending aorta at the beginning of the dilation process (to 45 mm) compensates for stretching during systole, and the biomechanical 2D-ST findings are thus higher than those for the controls.

In the present study, we measured aortic biomechanics by recording LS curves of the ascending aorta using 2D-ST imaging in addition to the 2D ultrasonographic images for arterial stiffness assessment. It is known that the elasticity of the aorta incorporate both - the property of dilating and the property of recoiling to its initial shape during systole and diastole. Also aortic stiffness describes the elastic resistance that the aorta sets against distension [18]. According to our data, significantly less aortic strain (aortic diameter change) and distensibility parameters of the ascending aorta were observed in the patients with aortas >45 mm. The elastic modulus and stiffness index β values were higher in group 2 than in the controls.

Oishi et al. adapted the same 2D-ST method for evaluating the abdominal aorta. Their study showed that the circumferential aortic strain and the strain rate were significantly lower, and the abdominal aortic stiffness parameter β was significantly greater, in older subjects than in the young/middle-aged group [15]. In our study, there were no age differences between the groups, and the stiffness index β and elastic modulus were greatest in group 2.

In the Yurdacul et al. study, aortic strain and distensibility were significantly impaired in patients with BAVs, compared with that of the control group, and aortic stiffness was markedly increased in the patients with BAVs [16]. We did not observe statistically significant differences between the tricuspid and BAV patients in regard to stiffness parameters of the ascending aorta. This lack of a great difference could be due to smaller aortic dimensions in the BAV group and a higher rate of aortic insufficiency in this group. We established higher LS values for the aortic posterior sinus only in BAV patients.

The same findings were presented in the Ozdemir study of hypertensive non-dipper patients, but the diameters of the ascending aorta were not described [19]. In our study, more of the group 2 patients had a history of systemic hypertension, although the diastolic blood pressure was lower than that in the controls. Approximately half of the patients in both DPAA groups had aortic regurgitation. This group showed increased stiffness and reduced distensibility and strain of the ascending aorta. These changes could result from aortic dilation and arterial hypertension. Both factors seem to be responsible for changes in aortic elastic properties.

Recently, more attention has been paid to complex imaging modalities, such as computed tomography (CT) and magnetic resonance imaging (MRI), especially in regard to imaging the aortic arch and descending aorta, because of the methodological limitations of echocardiography. It is important to note that the echocardiographic data concerning aortic biomechanics correlated with the CT and MRI results. Although CT and MRI have the advantage of being noninvasive, they remain expensive, and the availability of scanning facilities is limited.

We obtained weak to moderate correlation between the 2D-ST indices and the aortic stiffness parameters and aortic dimensions. A wider aorta was stiffer and was associated with lower absolute values for wall motion in longitudinal and transverse directions. This finding confirms that the dilated aorta cannot produce normal movement during several cardiac cycles, which could be a predictor of possible mechanical complications.

Study limitations

Our study had some limitations. About 20% of all of the investigated persons were not included in the study because of a poor acoustic window. In the cases of inadequate quality of echocardiographic images, the software could not perform SP analysis properly, which reduced the ability to perform analysis in all the patients. The offline software for the ST images was created for analyzing the left ventricle, so this effort is simply a pilot study of 2D-ST imaging of the aorta.

We analyzed only the feasibility of 2D-ST echocardiography as a tool for assessing aortic biomechanics. We did not expand our work to determine if it could provide a prognosis for patients with aortic dilation or dissection.

In the present study we investigated a small group of patients, but we presume that a larger size of sample would show more precise results.

Conclusions

Both DPAA groups (ascending aortic diameters >40 mm) had reduced elasticity and increased stiffness of the ascending aorta. The most marked changes of the biomechanical parameters were seen in patients whose ascending aortic diameter was >45 mm. The longitudinal wall motion of the ascending aorta was mostly impaired in patients whose aorta was >45 mm (i.e., LD of the anterior aortic wall and LV of the posterior and anterior walls). TD of the posterior and anterior aortic walls also occurred statistically significantly less in patients whose aortic diameter was >45 mm. A TD value of 5.2 mm predicts aortic dilation >45 mm (AUC 0.76, $p < 0.001$, CI 0.65–0.87; sensitivity 87%; specificity 63%).

More extensive aortic dilation is associated with reduced aortic parameters (strain, distensibility) and increased elastic modulus and stiffness index β values. Lower LD and LS values were associated with less aortic strain and distensibility.

2D-ST echocardiography can be applied in daily clinical practice for evaluating aortic biomechanics.

Abbreviations

2D-ST: Two-dimensional speckle-tracking echocardiography; BAV: Bicuspid aortic valve; DBP: Diastolic blood pressure; DD: Diastolic aortic diameter; DPAA: Dilative pathology of the ascending aorta; EF: Ejection fraction; LD: Longitudinal displacement; LS: Longitudinal strain; LV: Left ventricle; SBP: Systolic blood pressure; SD: Systolic aortic diameter; STJ: Sinotubular junction; TD: Transversal displacement; VL: Longitudinal velocity

Acknowledgements

The authors are grateful to Miss Kristina Vasiljevaite and Miss Gabriele Legotaite for the acquisition of anamnestical data, to Miss Simona Plienaityte for reviewing the English manuscript.

Funding

Not applicable.

Authors' contributions

MB wrote the draft manuscript, made a literature review; has been involved in echocardiographic data acquisition and analysis, speckle-tracking measurements; VM has been involved in echocardiographic data analysis, participated in the design of the study and performed the statistical analysis, revised the manuscript; JJV, VL has been involved in critical revision of the manuscript; RK, RV has been involved echocardiographic data analysis, in speckle-tracking measurements. All authors read and approved the final manuscript.

Competing interests

The authors declare that they have no competing interests.

Author details

[1]Department of Cardiology, Medical Academy, Lithuanian University of Health Sciences, Eivenių Str. 2, Kaunas 50009, Lithuania. [2]Institute of Cardiology at Lithuanian University of Health Sciences, Kaunas, Lithuania.

References

1. Hiratzka LF, Bakris GL, Beckman JA, Bersin RM, Carr VF, Casey DE, Eagle KA, Hermann LK, Isselbacher EM, Kazerooni EA, Kouchoukos NT, Lytle BW, Milewicz DM, Reich DL, Sen S, Shinn JA, Svensson LG, Williams DM. 2010

ACCF/AHA/AATS/ACR/ASA/SCA/SCAI/SIR/STS/SVM guidelines for the diagnosis and management of patients with thoracic aortic disease: executive summary. J Am Coll Cardiol. 2010;55:1509–44.
2. Erbel R, Aboyans V, Boileau C, Bossone E, Bartolomeo RD, Eggebrecht H, Evangelista A, Falk V, Frank H, Gaemperli O, Grabenwoger M, Haverich A, Iung B, Manolis AJ, Meijboom F, Nienaber CA, Roffi M, Rousseau H, Sechtem U, Sirnes PA, Allmen RS V, Vrints CJM, Zamorano JL, Achenbach S, Baumgartner H, Bax JJ, Bueno H, Dean V, Deaton C, Erol C, et al. 2014 ESC Guidelines on the diagnosis and treatment of aortic diseases. Eur Heart J. 2014;35:2873–926.
3. Avanzini A, Battini D, Bagozzi L, Bisleri G. Biomechanical evaluation of ascending aortic aneurysms. Biomed Res Int. 2014;2014:820385.
4. Izzo JL. Arterial stiffness and the systolic hypertension syndrome. Curr Opin Cardiol. 2004;19:341–52.
5. O'Rourke M, Staessen J, Viachopoulos C, Duprez D, Plante G. Clinical application of arterial stiffness; definition and reference values. Am J Hypertens. 2002;15(5):426–44.
6. Mattace-Raso FUS, Van Der Cammen TJM, Hofman A, Van Popele NM, Bos ML, DH SMA, Asmar R, Reneman RS, Hoeks APG, Breteler MMB, Witteman JCM. Arterial stiffness and risk of coronary heart disease and stroke: the Rotterdam study. Circulation. 2006;113:657–63.
7. Karatolios K, Wittek A, Nwe TH, Bihari P, Shelke A, Josef D, Schmitz-Rixen T, Geks J, Maisch B, Blase C, Moosdorf R, Vogt S. Method for aortic wall strain measurement with three-dimensional ultrasound speckle tracking and fitted finite element analysis. Ann Thorac Surg. 2013;96:1664–71.
8. Teixeira R, Monteiro R, Baptista R, Barbosa A, Leite L, Ribeiro M, Martins R, Cardim N, Gonçalves L. Circumferential vascular strain rate to estimate vascular load in aortic stenosis: a speckle tracking echocardiography study. Int J Card Imaging. 2015;31(4):681–9.
9. Geyer H, Caracciolo G, Abe H, Wilansky S, Carerj S, Gentile F, Nesser HJ, Khandheria B, Narula J, Sengupta PP. Assessment of myocardial mechanics using speckle tracking echocardiography: fundamentals and clinical applications. J Am Soc Echocardiogr. 2010:23(4):351–69.
10. Lang RM, Badano LP, Mor-Avi V, Afilalo J, Armstrong A, Ernande L, Flachskampf FA, Foster E, Goldstein SA, Kuznetsova T, Lancellotti P, Muraru D, Picard MH, Rietzschel ER, Rudski L, Spencer KT, Tsang W, Voigt JU. Recommendations for cardiac chamber quantification by echocardiography in adults: an update from the American society of echocardiography and the European association of cardiovascular imaging. Eur Heart J Cardiovasc Imaging. 2015;16:233–71.
11. Stefanadis C, Stratos C, Boudoulas H, Kourouklis C, Toutouzas P. Distensibility of the ascending aorta: comparison of invasive and non-invasive techniques in healthy men and in men with coronary artery disease. Eur Heart J. 1990;11:990–6.
12. Nemes A, Geleijnse ML, Sluiter W, Vydt TCG, Soliman OII, van Dalen BM, Vletter WB, ten Cate FJ, Smeets HJM, de Coo RFM. Aortic distensibility alterations in adults with m.3243A > G MELAS gene mutation. Swiss Med Wkly. 2009;139:117–20.
13. Clouse WD, Hallett JW, Schaff HV, Gayari MM, Ilstrup DM, Melton LJ. Improved prognosis of thoracic aortic aneurysms: a population-based study. JAMA. 1998;280:1926–9.
14. Juvonen T, Ergin MA, Galla JD, Lansman SL, Nguyen KH, McCullough JN, Levy D, de Asla RA, Bodian CA, Griepp RB. Prospective study of the natural history of thoracic aortic aneurysms. Ann Thorac Surg. 1997;63:1533–45.
15. Oishi Y, Mizuguchi Y, Miyoshi H, Iuchi A, Nagase N, Oki T. A novel approach to assess aortic stiffness related to changes in aging using a two-dimensional strain imaging. Echocardiography. 2008;25(1540–8175 (Electronic)):941–5.
16. Yurdakul S, Cengiz B, Sahin T, Bozkurt SA A. Impairment in aortic elastic properties and mechanics of ascending aorta in patients with bicuspid aortic valve. 2013.
17. Kassab GS. Biomechanics of the cardiovascular system: the aorta as an illustratory example. J R Soc Interface. 2006;3:719–40.
18. Nemes A, Geleijnse ML, Forster T, Soliman OII, Ten Cate FJ, Csanády M. Echocardiographic evaluation and clinical implications of aortic stiffness and coronary flow reserve and their relation. Clin Cardiol. 2008;31:304–9.
19. Ozdemir E, Yildirimturk O, Cengiz B, Yurdakul S, Aytekin S. Evaluation of carotid intima-media thickness and aortic elasticity in patients with nondipper hypertension. Echocardiography. 2014;31:663–8.

18

Novel functional advanced echocardiography for the assessment of myocardial mechanics in children with neurocardiogenic syncope – a blinded prospective speckle tracking head-up tilt-table challenge study

Kai O. Hensel[1,2*], Markus Roskopf[1], Francisca Abellan Schneyder[1] and Andreas Heusch[1]

Abstract

Background: Data on left ventricular (LV) function in patients with neurocardiogenic syncope (NS) is conflicting in adults and lacking in children. The aim of this study was to analyze LV myocardial performance in children with NS at rest and during head-up tilt-table (HUTT) testing.

Methods: This is the first study to combine HUTT and speckle-tracking echocardiography (STE) in children with NS. 43 consecutive normotensive pediatric patients with NS (mean age 13.9 ± 2.6 years, 51% female) and 41 sex- and age-matched healthy controls were included in the study. The study groups consisted of 21 patients with a positive HUTT reaction (HUTT+) and 22 with a negative HUTT reaction (HUTT-). STE was used to analyze peak systolic LV myocardial strain and strain rate.

Results: Conventional echocardiographic parameters were similar in all analyzed groups. When compared to healthy controls, children with NS had depressed levels of circumferential strain rate ($p = 0.032$) and significantly depressed longitudinal strain rate ($p < 0.001$) at rest. Interestingly, during HUTT testing LV global strain and strain rate were similar in both groups. LV strain rate was lowest in HUTT+ followed by HUTT- and control subjects both at rest and during HUTT.

Conclusions: Resting LV longitudinal strain rate is attenuated in children with NS, especially in those with a positive HUTT response. This is further evidence that NS patients feature altered cardiac mechanics rendering them prone to vasovagal perturbations that can ultimately result in collapse.

Keywords: Vasovagal syncope, Collapse, Pediatric echocardiography, Functional autonomic response test, Strain rate, LV function

* Correspondence: kai.hensel@uni-wh.de
[1]HELIOS University Medical Center Wuppertal, Children's Hospital, Center for Clinical & Translational Research (CCTR), Faculty of Health, Center for Biomedical Education & Research (ZBAF), Witten/Herdecke University, Faculty of Health, Heusnerstr. 40, D-42283 Wuppertal, Germany
[2]University of Cambridge, Addenbrooke's Hospital, Department of Paediatrics, Cambridge, UK

Background

Syncope is a sudden, brief loss of postural tone and consciousness followed by spontaneous recovery [1]. Up to 15% of children experience an episode of syncope to the end of adolescence [2, 3]. While a few underlying etiologies include potentially life-threatening cardiogenic conditions such as cardiac arrhythmia and structural heart disease, most cases of syncope are of benign origin. Vasovagal syncope - also known as situational, reflex or neurocardiogenic syncope (NS) - is the most common cause of pediatric syncope accounting for more than 50% of cases [4–6]. The development of effective therapies for NS is hindered by the vague and yet conflicting knowledge of the underlying pathophysiologic processes. Sympathetic failure/withdrawal is thought to play a role leading to decreased cardiac contractility and peripheral vascular tone [7]. The "ventricular hypothesis" on the other hand is based on an increase in left ventricular (LV) contractility – i.e. due to ventricular underfilling, sympathetic overactivity or hypovolemia. This may result in LV mechanoreceptor activation, the Bezold-Jarisch reflex, which in turn causes systemic hypotension, peripheral vasodilation and severe bradycardia [8]. However, the origin of the precipitating hemodynamic changes and the specific underlying pathomechanisms resulting in vasovagal syncope in children yet remain a subject of considerable speculation.

Advanced echocardiography techniques – including tissue-Doppler echocardiography (TDI) and speckle-tracking echocardiography (STE) – are promising modalities for the real-time quantitative evaluation of myocardial performance without the disadvantages of adverse effects or high costs. Based on TDI studies, cardiac mechanics such as left atrial and LV filling and contractility are postulated to be altered in neurocardiogenic syncope in adults [9, 10]. STE is reproducible tool for the detection of myocardial strain and strain rate [11, 12]. It has been successfully used to detect subclinical myocardial dysfunction in a variety of clinical settings such as arterial hypertension [13], systemic inflammatory disease [14], diabetes mellitus [15] and short-term alterations of glucose metabolism [16]. In 2013, the "ventricular theory" was fundamentally questioned by Goel et al. as they reported a paradoxical decrease of LV strain in adults with neurally mediated syncope and a positive head-up tilt-table (HUTT) exam utilizing STE [17]. However, echocardiographic assessment of cardiac strain was not performed at the same time as tilt-testing and LV strain rate – which, other than strain, is less dependent of cardiac loading conditions and therefore a better parameter to reflect LV contractility [18] - was not measured. This is the first study utilizing speckle-tracking imaging to shine a light on real-time cardiac mechanics in HUTT testing in children with vasovagal syncope.

Methods

Study population

In this prospective study, we altogether enrolled 84 children – 43 consecutive normotensive pediatric patients aged 13.9 ± 2.6 years (51% female) with a history of vasovagal syncope and 41 healthy sex- and age-matched controls (13.3 ± 3. 1 years, 53% female) without medical problems and with a normal transthoracic echocardiogram. A priori, the study group was further sub-categorized according to their HUTT exam reaction. Inclusion criteria for the study group were a typical history of NS, age < 18 years and a written informed consent signed by the patient and their legal guardian. Moreover, the presence of any acute or chronic condition that might affect the cardiovascular system (e.g. infections, metabolic conditions such as diabetes mellitus, inflammatory disease, renal disease), ECG abnormalities, chronic medication use and the lack of cooperation to participate in this voluntary HUTT study were strict exclusion criteria. 60 patients were excluded from the study due to various reasons: 53 were incompliant regarding the HUTT challenge, 2 patients were obese (BMI > 30), 2 had insufficient image quality at baseline and in 3 patients the continuous ECG signal was corrupted due to technical difficulties which made consecutive speckle tracking post-processing impossible. The study was carried out in accordance with the declaration of Helsinki's ethical principles for medical research involving human subjects and approved by the Witten/Herdecke University ethics committee (*clinical study number: 73/2014*).

Conventional echocardiography

The study took place in a calm room with dimmed lights and at normal room temperature. We performed a comprehensive spectral and color flow Doppler echocardiographic study in all included children according to the current guidelines of the American Heart Association [19]. We used an S5–1 Sector Array transducer (Sector 1–5 MHz) and the commercially available ultrasound device iE33 by Phillips Ultrasound Inc., USA. Echocardiographic images were acquired using a standardized protocol. First, the images and cine loops were digitally recorded in the apical 4-, 3- and 2-chamber views, the parasternal long axis view and in two short axis views at the mitral level and at the level of the papillary muscles. Subsequently, the raw data was transferred to a separate offline workstation for later analysis. XCelera Version 3. 1.1.422 by Phillips Ultrasound Inc., USA was used for conventional echocardiographic parameter analyses. M-mode images were recorded and analyzed according to the standardized American Society Echocardiography (ASE) protocol [20]. For the assessment of LV diastolic function pw-Doppler and pw-TDI were utilized and E/A-ratio, E/E'-ratio and mitral deceleration time were measured as previously described [21]. Z-scores were used to evaluate all conventional echocardiographic parameters [22].

Speckle tracking echocardiography

STE was performed using standard cross-sectional 2D grayscale LV B-mode images to measure strain and strain rate as described previously by our group [23]. Briefly, circumferential strain and strain rate were measured in the standard parasternal short-axis at the papillary muscle plane and longitudinal strain and strain rate were measured in standard apical 4-chamber view. Frame rate was adjusted to 60–90 frames/second and three to five consecutive cardiac cycles synchronized to a continuous ECG were recorded. Caution was paid to minimize artifacts during echocardiographic image acquisition. QLAB Version 10 was used on an off-line workstation to postprocess the anonymized digitally stored DICOM data. Importantly, all involved echocardiographic examiners and interpreters were blinded to the study group status of each participant. Throughout, we verified tissue tracking quality frame-by-frame, in real-time and full thickness coverage of the entire myocardial wall from the endocardial to the epicardial contours was readjusted by hand, where necessary.

Head-up tilt-table challenge

To unmask potential abnormalities in myocardial performance that might remain undiscovered at rest and to study cardiac mechanics during HUTT gravitational challenge, after the resting conventional and STE exam we additionally exposed the study population to a HUTT test and performed STE simultaneously. The HUTT exam was carried out according to the standard Newcastle protocol as previously described [24]. Specifically, patients were fasted for 2–3 h prior to the study and were first reclined in a flat lying position for at least 10 min. Subsequently, the table was tilted to a 70-degree angle in less than 10 s. Patients were kept in that position for a maximum of 30 min. A positive HUTT test (HUTT+) was defined as the development of presyncope with a significant drop in blood pressure (< 70 mmHg systolic) and the production of clinical symptoms such as dizziness, severe nausea or the sudden loss of consciousness. Strict termination criteria were the patient's wish to end the exam or the occurrence of a syncope or presyncope. Echocardiographic images were repeatedly acquired in the 70-degrees "hanging" position according to the same standardized scheme of consecutive viewing planes used for the above-mentioned baseline STE assessment. To achieve comparable hemodynamic circumstances for all patients, we analyzed the last recorded echocardiographic images prior to the termination of the study. Peripheral blood pressure measurements were obtained at 2-min intervals and a 12-channel ECG was continuously monitored. The reported hemodynamic parameters (i.e. heart rate, blood pressure) reflect the time at which the echocardiographic images were recorded. After the HUTT test, patients were kept in a lying position for at least 10 min or until the completely recovered (e.g. post-syncopal).

Biostatistical analyses

Demographic data, baseline clinical parameters, hemodynamics and echocardiographic aspects are presented as mean and standard deviation. Analysis of variance (ANOVA) testing was used to compare clinical, hemodynamic and echocardiographic data of the analyzed groups. Strain and strain rate are displayed as box-whisker-plots. Bonferroni correction was applied to exclude multiple testing bias. Hence, p-values < 0.0025 constituted statistical significance. Microsoft Excel Version 16.0 for PC and GraphPad Prism Version 6 (GraphPad Software, Inc., La Jolla, CA, USA) were utilized for all statistical tests.

Results

Patient characteristics

Baseline clinical characteristics are outlined in Table 1. Children with NS and a positive HUTT exam (HUTT+) were aged 13.4 ± 2.8 years, HUTT- group mean age was 14.4 ± 2.3 years and healthy controls were 13.3 ± 3.1 years old ($p = 0.318$). Height ($p = 0.375$), body weight ($p = 0.101$), body mass index (p = 0.1) and body surface area ($p = 0.165$) were not statistically different between the three groups. All these values were within normal limits as evaluated by Z-scores. HUTT response was positive in 21 of the 43 patients with NS and 2 of the 41 healthy controls ($p < 0.001$). Hemodynamic parameters, e.g. heart rate and arterial blood pressure did not differ between the three groups neither at rest nor at the moment of STE assessment during HUTT testing ($0.2 < p < 0.964$).

Conventional echocardiographic parameters

Standard 2D derived conventional echocardiographic parameters were similar in all groups (Table 2). In detail, M-mode measurements yielded comparable LA/Ao ratio ($p = 0.480$), fractional shortening ($p = 0.760$), LV dimensions ($p \geq 0.15$) and LV mass ($p = 0.578$). LV stroke volume was lowest in the HUTT+ group (46.7 ± 17.3 vs. 53.5 ± 21.3 vs. 53.8 ± 17.6 ml) when compared to HUTT- and healthy control subjects. However, this difference was not statistically different ($p = 0.796$). Moreover, LV ejection fraction (EF) was 54.3 ± 2.9% in syncope HUTT + patients, 54.7 ± 6.6% in HUTT- and 56.7 ± 4.4% in healthy controls ($p = 0.263$). Furthermore, diastolic function as reflected by E/A ratio and E/E' did not differ significantly between the analyzed groups ($p \geq 0.352$). Mitral deceleration time was longer in the HUTT- group

Table 1 Baseline clinical characteristics and hemodynamics of the study population

		Syncope (HUTT+) (*n* = 21)	Syncope (HUTT-) (*n* = 22)	Control (*n* = 41)	*p*-value (ANOVA)
	Age (years)	13.43 ± 2.84	14.43 ± 2.31	13.30 ± 3.06	0.318
	Height (cm)	160.14 ± 20.49	164.24 ± 17.06	157.65 ± 15.67	0.375
	Weight (kg)	56.29 ± 21.49	60.10 ± 19.28	49.95 ± 15.34	0.101
	Female gender (%)	66.7%	40.9%	53.66%	0.184
	Body surface (m^2)	1.57 ± 0.39	1.65 ± 0.34	1.48 ± 0.29	0.165
	Body mass index (kg/m^2)	21.07 ± 4.66	21.65 ± 3.62	19.62 ± 3.2	0.1
	Positive tilt-table test (n)	21	0	2	0.001
Baseline	Heart rate (bpm)	81.18 ± 18.39	82.27 ± 23.38	80.42 ± 13.33	0.964
	BP systolic (mmHg)	113.12 ± 26.42	122.02 ± 52.76	111.29 ± 19.02	0.436
	BP diastolic (mmHg)	76.02 ± 24.96	77.64 ± 35.85	64.02 ± 18.36	0.2
HUTT	Heart rate (bpm)	93.24 ± 26.7	101.41 ± 27.19	96.82 ± 16.03	0.605
	BP systolic (mmHg)	133.16 ± 45.09	133.71 ± 41.63	128.70 ± 13.56	0.866
	BP diastolic (mmHg)	85.94 ± 34.98	87.06 ± 32.33	77.97 ± 18.09	0.580

(0.20 ± 0.07 s, $p = 0.028$) but similar in HUTT+ patients with NS and healthy controls (0.17 ± 0.07 vs. 0.16 ± 0.06 s). However, these values were still within normal limits as evaluated by population-based age-specific reference values [25].

Speckle tracking echocardiography

At rest, median peak systolic LV circumferential strain rate (– 1.46 ± 0.47 vs. -1.59 ± 0.69 vs. -1.75 ± 0.47 s^{-1}, $p = 0.032$) and median peak systolic longitudinal strain rate (– 1.08 ± 0.45 vs. -1.16 ± 0.18 vs. -1.39 ± 0.49 s^{-1}, $p < 0.001$) were lowest in children with NS and a positive HUTT exam (HUTT+) as compared to the HUTT- group and healthy controls (Table 3, Fig. 1). In contrast, there was no statistically significant difference between patients with NS and healthy controls regarding peak LV global circumferential strain or global longitudinal strain at baseline.

During HUTT testing, longitudinal strain rate was lower in children with NS (HUTT+ < HUTT-) than in the control group, but the difference was not statistically different ($p = 0.144$, Fig. 2). Peak LV global circumferential strain and global longitudinal strain were similar in all groups during HUTT testing (Fig. 2). The combination of STE and HUTT was feasible in 15 (72%) HUTT + patients, 14 (63%) HUTT- patients and 16 (39%) healthy controls. A representative echocardiographic image sample of STE assessment in a child with NS is given in Fig. 3.

While the overall comparison to healthy controls revealed LV myocardial strain rate at rest to be significantly lower in patients with neurocardiogenic syncope, we also observed a heterogeneous distribution of LV

Table 2 Conventional echocardiographic parameters derived from two-dimensional and Doppler imaging

	Syncope (HUTT+) (*n* = 21)	Syncope (HUTT-) (*n* = 22)	Control (*n* = 41)	*p*-value (ANOVA)
LA/AoR	1.08 ± 0.13	1.15 ± 0.17	1.07 ± 0.15	0.480
Fractional shortening (%)	34.48 ± 9.65	33.65 ± 9.18	34.02 ± 3.14	0.760
Interventricular septal end-diastolic diameter (cm)	0.97 ± 0.36	0.86 ± 0.29	0.83 ± 0.14	0.150
LV end-diastolic diameter (cm)	4.35 ± 1.26	4.24 ± 1.31	4.41 ± 0.76	0.764
LV posterior wall diameter. Diastolic (cm)	1.01 ± 0.32	0.98 ± 0.31	0.9 ± 0.24	0.244
LV mass (g)	149.65 ± 74.99	130.55 ± 63.00	128.41 ± 60.62	0.578
LV end-diastolic volume (ml)	91.08 ± 29.21	93.59 ± 36.73	94.92 ± 30.29	0.937
Ejection fraction (%)	54.25 ± 2.94	54.69 ± 6.59	56.66 ± 4.43	0.263
Stroke volume (ml)	46.76 ± 17.34	53.49 ± 21.29	53.79 ± 17.61	0.796
E-Wave / A-Wave	2.12 ± 0.68	2.16 ± 0.85	1.95 ± 0.65	0.352
Mitral deceleration time (s)	0.17 ± 0.07	0.20 ± 0.07	0.16 ± 0.06	0.028
E/E' (cm/s)	7.46 ± 1.11	7.56 ± 2.35	7.25 ± 1.84	0.833

Table 3 Speckle tracking derived peak systolic LV strain rate at rest and during head-up tilt table testing

		Syncope (HUTT+) (*n* = 21)	Syncope (HUTT-) (*n* = 22)	Control (*n* = 41)	*p*-value (ANOVA)
Baseline	Circumferential strain rate (s^{-1})	−1.46 ± 0.47	−1.59 ± 0.69	−1.75 ± 0.47	0.032
	Longitudinal strain rate (s^{-1})	−1.08 ± 0.45	− 1.16 ± 0.18	− 1.39 ± 0.49	< 0.001
	Circumferential strain (%)	−21.9 ± 7.24	−22.99 ± 7.82	−24.00 ± 5.89	0.186
	Longitudinal strain (%)	−21.31 ± 8.9	−20.94 ± 1.94	−20.48 ± 5.21	0.468
		(*n* = 15)	(*n* = 14)	(*n* = 16)	
HUTT	Circumferential strain rate (s^{-1})	−1.46 ± 0.69	−1.51 ± 0.54	− 1.49 ± 0.25	0.860
	Longitudinal strain rate (s^{-1})	−1.03 ± 0.52	− 1.07 ± 0.28	−1.14 ± 0.59	0.144
	Circumferential strain (%)	−22.24 ± 10.69	−21.98 ± 7.71	− 22.46 ± 3.67	0.915
	Longitudinal strain (%)	−20.48 ± 10.47	−20.86 ± 5.54	− 20.93 ± 10.98	0.926

deformation in those patients. Interestingly, a subset of patients with NS had high LV circumferential (*n* = 4) or longitudinal strain rate values (*n* = 2; both had also increased circumferential strain rate) at rest (≥ top quartile of healthy controls). Interestingly, all of these patients were in the HUTT- group. One of the four patients was female and one had a history of more than one syncopal episode. The average blood pressure of this subgroup was 121 ± 9 mmHg systolic and 68 ± 2 mmHg diastolic and the average heart rate was 74 ± 10 bpm at. None of the patients with NS and a positive tilt-table response had resting LV longitudinal or circumferential strain rate values ≥ the top quartile of the healthy control group.

Discussion

This is the first study to simultaneously perform speckle-tracking echocardiography (STE) and head-up tilt-table (HUTT) testing in children with NS. Interestingly, we found LV resting longitudinal strain rate to be significantly lower in NS patients than in healthy

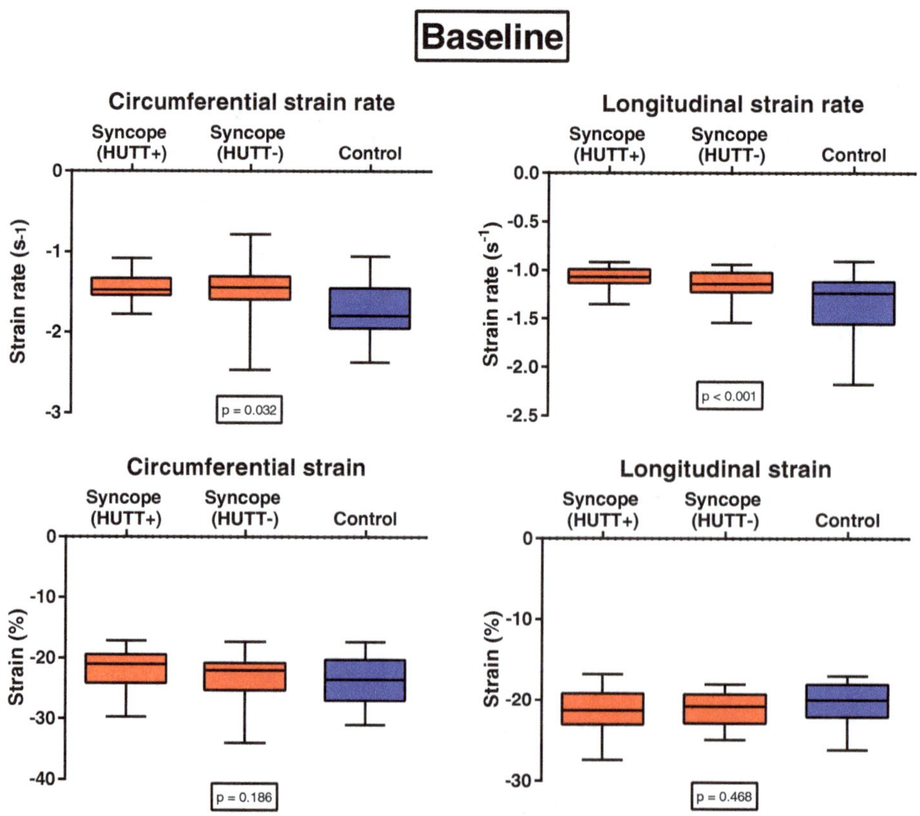

Fig. 1 Left ventricular circumferential and longitudinal strain and strain rate at baseline. *p*-values were calculated using the Mann-Whitney-U test

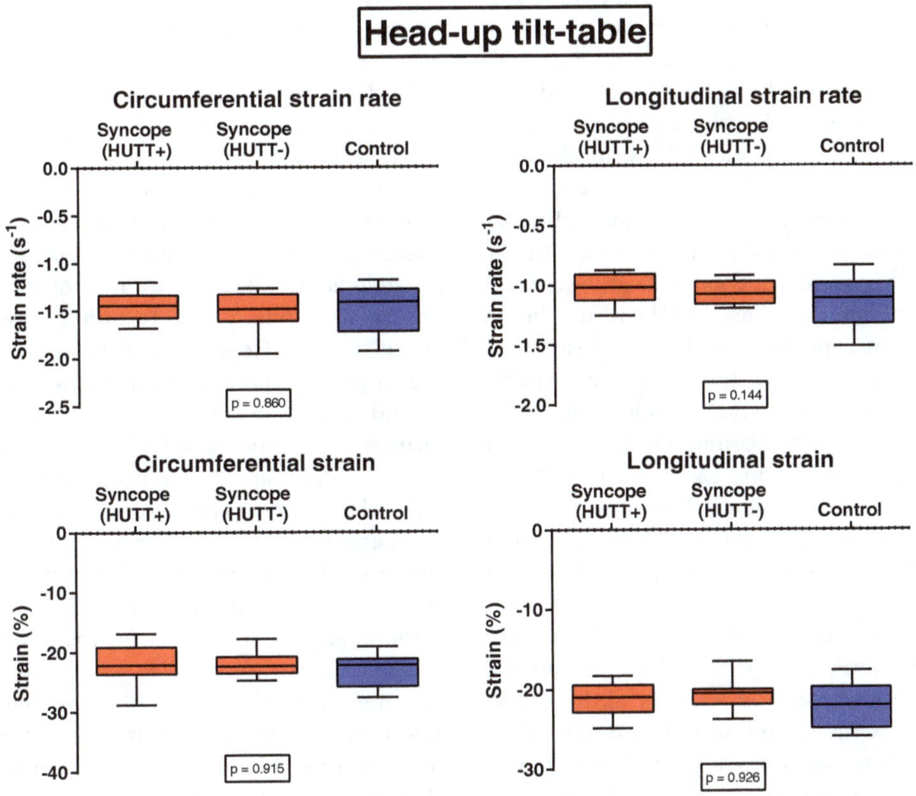

Fig. 2 Left ventricular circumferential and longitudinal strain and strain rate during head-up tilt testing. *p*-values were calculated using the Mann-Whitney-U test

controls with a more pronounced decrease in the HUTT + group. During HUTT challenge we found a similar but not statistically significant tendency of lower longitudinal strain rate in patients with NS. This is in line with findings from Kojo et al., who utilized a Doppler flow meter during HUTT testing and found reduced carotid artery blood flow in pediatric patients with NS [26]. Our findings are furthermore in agreement with results from Sucu and colleagues, who detected atrial conduction delay in adolescents and young adults with NS [27]. Moreover, our data is in accordance with a HUTT echocardiography study in adults reporting that vigorous

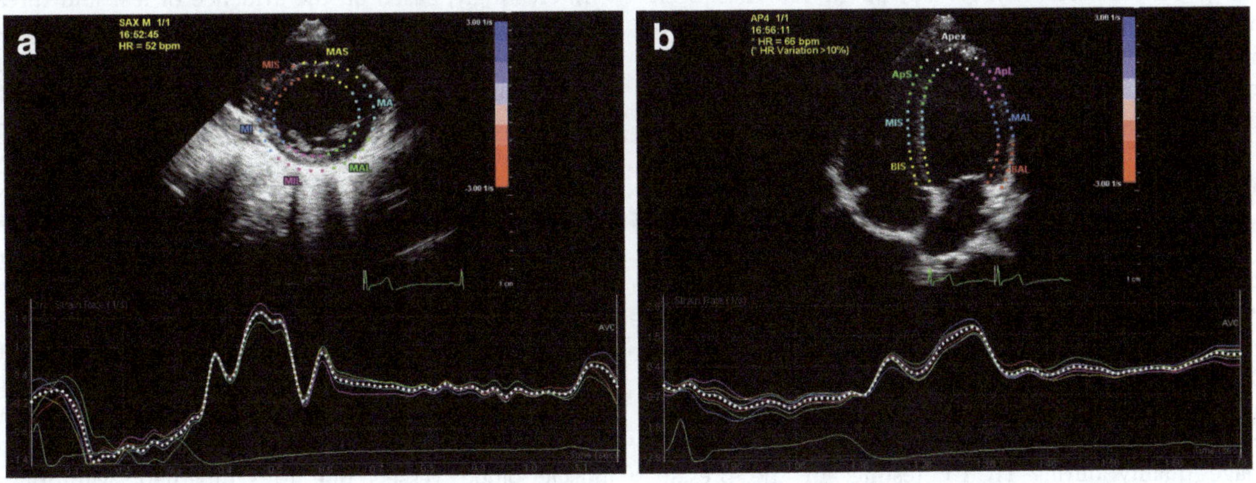

Fig. 3 Echocardiographic image examples of speckle tracking derived left ventricular circumferential (**a**) and longitudinal (**b**) strain rate analyses in a patient with neurocardiogenic syncope

contraction is probably less responsible for vasovagal syncope release than left ventricle volume reduction [28]. Similarly, HUTT+ NS patients had reduced end-systolic stress, LV volume, and chamber function during HUTT testing in another study, which provides further evidence that if paradoxic activation of LV mechanoreceptors has a role in mediating NS, it is not triggered by increased systolic wall stress or LV hypercontractility [8].

On the other hand, our findings are counterintuitive in the light of the "ventricular theory" in that we did not measure an increase but a decrease in LV contractility in patients with NS and a positive HUTT response. This, however, apart from the fact that the ventricular hypothesis is far from being established conclusively, is in agreement with a similarly performed study by Goel et al., who report attenuated resting LV strain in HUTT+ patients and conclude that – other than previously believed – increased resting LV contractility is not a prerequisite for the development of NS [17]. Notably, even though the authors have measured a similar phenomenon as we did in this study, their study bares significant technical limitations which gives incremental value to our observations. Firstly, Goel et al. have performed STE measurements on a different day then HUTT challenge. Moreover, they utilized LV strain as a measure for LV contractility; strain rate was not assessed. Importantly, STE-derived strain rate has been shown to be more robust to dynamic ventricular unloading than strain in several well-performed animal experimental studies [29–31]. In humans, LV strain has been shown to be affected by changes in cardiac loading conditions such as hemodialysis [32] or gravitational gradients [33]. Furthermore, other than strain, strain rate has been demonstrated to be unaffected by preload and correlate well with end systolic elastance as verified by invasive catheterization [18]. In addition, utilizing a stress testing echocardiography set up, strain rate has been shown to reflect myocardial contractility demonstrating a positive force-frequency relationship in both children and young piglets [34]. In conclusion, our study closes that gap as we performed STE and HUTT on the same occasion and detected LV strain rate in addition to LV strain.

The cardiac autonomic response pattern of patients with NS during HUTT challenge has been distinguished between HUTT+ and HUTT- patients in previous studies [35]. In line with this, we measured more attenuated longitudinal strain rate in HUTT+ patients. The lack of statistical significance for circumferential strain rate and longitudinal strain rate during HUTT is most probably a result of the limited sample size as well as suboptimal image quality during HUTT testing. In the present study, we further found HUTT+ patients to have a lower LV stroke volume when compared to HUTT- and healthy control subjects. This is in accordance with the findings from Moon et al., who described decreased left atrial volumes in HUTT+ patients and concluded a limited intracardiac volume reserve to play an important role in the mechanism of NS [36]. A subset of patients with NS had increased strain rate values – corresponding to a "hyperdynamic" type of NS. Interestingly, none of those patients had a positive response during HUTT challenge. While one could speculate about the pathophysiologic significance of this observation, the small sample size underlying this finding should be taken into consideration. Hence, no definite conclusion can be drawn from this observation at this point. Future studies should further investigate the different types of LV deformation in patients with NS with a specific focus on hemodynamics and cardiomechanics.

Another unresolved issue regarding the enigmatic pathogenesis of NS is the factor age. Even though younger and older patients react differently on the HUTT, especially in the early phase [37], the role of the autonomic nervous system for the etiology of NS seems to be similarly important in adults and children [38]. In extreme cases, the cardioinhibitory effect of the adult autonomous nervous system can reach an extent that can cause death, i.e. cardiac arrest due to extensive inhibitory vagal reflex following a laryngoscopic procedure [39]. Neither has a definite origin in the pathogenesis of neurally mediated syncope been identified, nor do previous studies point toward a definite answer for the "chicken or egg" question. While the "ventricular theory" is centered on the heart as the primarily malfunctioning source, arterial distensibility was also shown to be decreased in patients with recurrent episodes of NS [40]. Similarly, Sucu and colleagues have reported increased aortic stiffness as expressed by altered aortic strain in mid-aged adults with NS and a positive HUTT response [41].

Interestingly, based on the evidence of fear and threat bradycardia in animals and the beneficial vasovagal reflex during hemorrhagic shock in humans and animals, some researchers suggest NS not to be a recently evolved human-only disease but rather the remnant of an ancient defense mechanism that has once reduced myocardial oxygen consumption and supported hemostasis before the development of larger blood losses [42–44]. Under this assumption, it is well imaginable, that this trait is now differentially passed on to subsequent generations and therefore despite being common it is variously pronounced which could explain the different response patterns during HUTT challenge. The principle mechanism during the actual faint is an impaired ability to maintain vasomotor tone in the skeletal muscle blood vessels due to sympathetic withdrawal [45]. While – due to the technical design of this study – we did not perform STE during the event of fainting

(HUTT+ group), we assessed LV performance at rest and during HUTT testing before termination of the challenge. The detected lower strain rate may reflect a lower sympathetic tone and thus decreased LV performance which may be a relevant factor in the etiology of NS.

Limitations

Despite the incremental value of these findings, this study design bares important limitations. Firstly, while STE has been implemented in specific clinical practice of pediatric cardiology, i.e. to monitor cardiotoxicity in chemotherapy patients [46], it is still mostly used in experimental settings. Solid cut-off points for pathologic values, especially for strain rate, are still missing and the technique is subject to relevant inter-vendor inconsistency [47, 48]. Interpretation of STE derived myocardial performance parameter is complex and limited by a variety of factors [49]. Secondly, the combination of STE and HUTT is challenging both for the patient and the involved examiner. When performed according to a standardized protocol, HUTT testing has been shown to be highly reproducible [50]. However, reliable STE measurements require optimal image quality, the absence of artifacts and thorough noise-reduction. We proceeded as previously suggested by limiting deformation analysis to subjects with adequate imaging quality to achieve favorable accuracy [51]. Consequently, as substandard echocardiographic image quality is unavoidable during HUTT testing when the patient is placed in a 70-degree hanging position, not to mention the important factor of patient compliance – especially in children – the results of STE during HUTT challenge must be interpreted with caution. Nevertheless, the most important observation of this study was detected at baseline under normal imaging conditions.

Conclusion

This study provides further evidence that decreased LV resting performance may be a relevant factor in the etiology of neurocardiogenic syncope in children. Further experimental animal and human studies should be designed to investigate LV contractility in children and adults with NS under different cardiac loading conditions at baseline and in the context of HUTT challenge.

Abbreviations

ECG: electrocardiogram; EF: ejection fraction; HUTT: head-up tilt-table; HUTT-: pediatric patients with a history of neurocardiogenic syncope and a negative head-up tilt-table response; HUTT+: pediatric patients with a history of neurocardiogenic syncope and a positive head-up tilt-table response; LV: left ventricle; NS: neurocardiogenic syncope; TDI: tissue-Doppler echocardiography

Acknowledgements

The authors thank all enrolled volunteers for participating in the study and Johanna Buttenberg for her assistance regarding the echocardiographic image acquisition.

Funding

This study was supported with a research grant awarded to Dr. Kai O. Hensel by Witten/Herdecke University. The funding body provided financial support only (no participation in the design of the study, collection, analysis, or interpretation of data, nor in writing the manuscript).

Authors' contributions

KOH designed and supervised the study, prepared the tables and figures, interpreted the data and wrote the manuscript. MR and FAS performed the echocardiographic studies and post-processing analyses. MR performed biostatistical analyses and helped preparing the tables and figs. AH helped performing echocardiographic examinations and critically reviewed the manuscript. All authors have read and approved the final version of the manuscript.

Competing interests

The authors declare that they have no competing interests.

References

1. Kapoor WN. Syncope. N Engl J Med. 2000;343(25):1856–62. https://doi.org/10.1056/NEJM200012213432507.
2. Friedman KG, Alexander ME. Chest pain and syncope in children: a practical approach to the diagnosis of cardiac disease. J Pediatr. 2013;163(3):896–901 e1–3. https://doi.org/10.1016/j.jpeds.2013.05.001.
3. Lewis DA, Dhala A. Syncope in the pediatric patient. The cardiologist's perspective. Pediatr Clin N Am. 1999;46(2):205–19.
4. Massin MM, Bourguignont A, Coremans C, Comte L, Lepage P, Gerard P. Syncope in pediatric patients presenting to an emergency department. J Pediatr. 2004;145(2):223–8. https://doi.org/10.1016/j.jpeds.2004.01.048.
5. Pratt JL, Fleisher GR. Syncope in children and adolescents. Pediatr Emerg Care. 1989;5(2):80–2.
6. Romme JJ, van Dijk N, Boer KR, Dekker LR, Stam J, Reitsma JB, et al. Influence of age and gender on the occurrence and presentation of reflex syncope. Clinical autonomic research : official journal of the Clinical Autonomic Research Society. 2008;18(3):127–33. https://doi.org/10.1007/s10286-008-0465-0.
7. Moak JP, Bailey JJ, Makhlouf FT. Simultaneous heart rate and blood pressure variability analysis. Insight into mechanisms underlying neurally mediated cardiac syncope in children. J Am Coll Cardiol. 2002;40(8):1466–74.
8. Liu JE, Hahn RT, Stein KM, Markowitz SM, Okin PM, Devereux RB, et al. Left ventricular geometry and function preceding Neurally mediated Syncope. Circulation. 2000;101(7):777–83. https://doi.org/10.1161/01.cir.101.7.777.
9. Folino AF, Russo G, Buja G, Iliceto S. Contribution of decreased atrial function in the pathogenesis of neurally mediated syncope. Am J Cardiol. 2006;97(7):1017–24. https://doi.org/10.1016/j.amjcard.2005.10.041.
10. Folino AF, Russo G, Porta A, Buja G, Cerutti S, Iliceto S. Autonomic modulation and cardiac contractility in vasovagal syncope. Int J Cardiol. 2010;139(3):248–53. https://doi.org/10.1016/j.ijcard.2008.10.030.
11. Leischik R, Dworrak B, Hensel K. Intraobserver and interobserver reproducibility for radial, circumferential and longitudinal strain echocardiography. Open Cardiovasc Med J. 2014;8:102–9. https://doi.org/10.2174/1874192401408010102.
12. Marcucci C, Lauer R, Mahajan A. New echocardiographic techniques for evaluating left ventricular myocardial function. Semin Cardiothorac Vasc Anesth. 2008;12(4):228–47. https://doi.org/10.1177/1089253208328581.

13. Hensel KO, Jenke A, Leischik R. Speckle-tracking and tissue-Doppler stress echocardiography in arterial hypertension: a sensitive tool for detection of subclinical LV impairment. Biomed Res Int. 2014;2014:472562. https://doi.org/10.1155/2014/472562.
14. Hensel KO, Abellan Schneyder FE, Wilke L, Heusch A, Wirth S, Jenke AC. Speckle tracking stress echocardiography uncovers early subclinical cardiac involvement in pediatric patients with inflammatory bowel diseases. Sci Rep. 2017;7(1):2966. https://doi.org/10.1038/s41598-017-03255-1.
15. Hensel KO, Grimmer F, Roskopf M, Jenke AC, Wirth S, Heusch A. Subclinical alterations of cardiac mechanics present early in the course of pediatric type 1 diabetes mellitus: a prospective blinded speckle tracking stress echocardiography study. J Diabetes Res. 2016;2016:2583747. https://doi.org/10.1155/2016/2583747.
16. Hensel KO, Grimmer F, Jenke AC, Wirth S, Heusch A. The influence of real-time blood glucose levels on left ventricular myocardial strain and strain rate in pediatric patients with type 1 diabetes mellitus - a speckle tracking echocardiography study. BMC Cardiovasc Disord. 2015;15(1):175. https://doi.org/10.1186/s12872-015-0171-5.
17. Goel R, Caracciolo G, Wilansky S, Scott LR, Narula J, Sengupta PP. Effect of head-up tilt-table testing on left ventricular longitudinal strain in patients with neurocardiogenic syncope. Am J Cardiol. 2013;112(8):1252–7. https://doi.org/10.1016/j.amjcard.2013.06.020.
18. Schlangen J, Petko C, Hansen JH, Michel M, Hart C, Uebing A, et al. Two-dimensional global longitudinal strain rate is a preload independent index of systemic right ventricular contractility in hypoplastic left heart syndrome patients after Fontan operation. Circ Cardiovasc Imaging. 2014;7(6):880–6. https://doi.org/10.1161/circimaging.114.002110.
19. Lopez L, Colan SD, Frommelt PC, Ensing GJ, Kendall K, Younoszai AK, et al. Recommendations for quantification methods during the performance of a pediatric echocardiogram: a report from the pediatric measurements writing Group of the American Society of echocardiography pediatric and congenital heart disease council. J Am Soc Echocardiogr. 2010;23(5):465–95; quiz 576-7. https://doi.org/10.1016/j.echo.2010.03.019.
20. Lang RM, Badano LP, Mor-Avi V, Afilalo J, Armstrong A, Ernande L, et al. Recommendations for cardiac chamber quantification by echocardiography in adults: an update from the American Society of Echocardiography and the European Association of Cardiovascular Imaging. J Am Soc Echocardiogr. 2015; 28(1):1–39 e14. https://doi.org/10.1016/j.echo.2014.10.003.
21. Nagueh SF, Appleton CP, Gillebert TC, Marino PN, Oh JK, Smiseth OA, et al. Recommendations for the evaluation of left ventricular diastolic function by echocardiography. Eur J Echocardiogr. 2009;10(2):165–93. https://doi.org/10.1093/ejechocard/jep007.
22. Chubb H, Simpson JM. The use of Z-scores in paediatric cardiology. Ann Pediatr Cardiol. 2012;5(2):179–84. https://doi.org/10.4103/0974-2069.99622.
23. Hensel KO, Wilke L, Heusch A. Transthoracic Speckle Tracking Echocardiography for the Quantitative Assessment of Left Ventricular Myocardial Deformation. Journal of Visualized Experiments. 2016:e54736 (in press). https://doi.org/10.3791/54736.
24. Kenny RA, O'Shea D, Parry SW. The Newcastle protocols for head-up tilt table testing in the diagnosis of vasovagal syncope, carotid sinus hypersensitivity, and related disorders. Heart. 2000;83(5):564–9.
25. Shojaeifard M, Esmaeilzadeh M, Maleki M, Bakhshandeh H, Parvaresh F, Naderi N. Normal reference values of tissue Doppler imaging parameters for right ventricular function in young adults: a population based study. Research in cardiovascular medicine. 2013;2(4):160–6. https://doi.org/10.5812/cardiovascmed.9843.
26. Kojo M, Wada M, Akiyoshi K, Inutsuka M, Izumi T. Reduction of carotid artery blood flow in pediatric patients with syncope: evaluation with head-up tilt test. Neuropediatrics. 2001;32(4):169–75. https://doi.org/10.1055/s-2001-17369.
27. Sucu M, Ercan S, Uku O, Davutoglu V, Altunbas G. Atrial electromechanical conduction delay in patients with neurocardiogenic syncope. Pacing Clin Electrophysiol. 2014;37(5):597–602. https://doi.org/10.1111/pace.12300.
28. Kozlowski D, Byrdziak P, Krupa W, Gawrysiak M, Piwko G, Kubica J, et al. Left ventricle systolic volume in vasovagal syncope patients. Folia Morphol (Warsz). 2003;62(3):175–8.
29. Urheim S, Edvardsen T, Torp H, Angelsen B, Smiseth OA. Myocardial strain by Doppler echocardiography. Validation of a new method to quantify regional myocardial function. Circulation. 2000;102(10):1158–64.
30. Dahle GO, Stangeland L, Moen CA, Salminen PR, Haaverstad R, Matre K, et al. The influence of acute unloading on left ventricular strain and strain rate by speckle tracking echocardiography in a porcine model. Am J Physiol Heart Circ Physiol. 2016;310(10):H1330–9. https://doi.org/10.1152/ajpheart.00947.2015.
31. Weidemann F, Jamal F, Sutherland GR, Claus P, Kowalski M, Hatle L, et al. Myocardial function defined by strain rate and strain during alterations in inotropic states and heart rate. Am J Physiol Heart Circ Physiol. 2002;283(2): H792–9. https://doi.org/10.1152/ajpheart.00025.2002.
32. Choi JO, Shin DH, Cho SW, Song YB, Kim JH, Kim YG, et al. Effect of preload on left ventricular longitudinal strain by 2D speckle tracking. Echocardiography. 2008;25(8):873–9. https://doi.org/10.1111/j.1540-8175.2008.00707.x.
33. Negishi K, Borowski AG, Popovic ZB, Greenberg NL, Martin DS, Bungo MW, et al. Effect of gravitational gradients on cardiac filling and performance. J Am Soc Echocardiogr. 2017;30(20):1180–8. https://doi.org/10.1016/j.echo.2017.08.005.
34. Alvarez SV, Fortin-Pellerin E, Alhabdan M, Lomelin JS, Kantoch M, Atallah J, et al. Strain rate in children and young piglets mirrors changes in contractility and demonstrates a force-frequency relationship. J Am Soc Echocardiogr. 2017;30(8):797–806. https://doi.org/10.1016/j.echo.2017.04.001.
35. Vallejo M, Hermosillo AG, Infante O, Cardenas M, Lerma C. Cardiac autonomic response to active standing in adults with vasovagal Syncope. J Clin Neurophysiol. 2015;32(5):434–9. https://doi.org/10.1097/wnp.0000000000000204.
36. Moon J, Shim J, Park JH, Hwang HJ, Joung B, Ha JW, et al. Small left atrial volume is an independent predictor for fainting during head-up tilt test: the impact of intracardiac volume reserve in vasovagal syncope. Int J Cardiol. 2013;166(1):44–9. https://doi.org/10.1016/j.ijcard.2011.09.076.
37. Ruiz GA, Madoery C, Arnaldo F, Menendez C, Tentori MC. Frequency-domain analysis of heart rate variability during positive and negative head-up tilt test: importance of age. Pacing Clin Electrophysiol. 2000;23(3):325–32.
38. Kochiadakis GE, Papadimitriou EA, Marketou ME, Chrysostomakis SI, Simantirakis EN, Vardas PE. Autonomic nervous system changes in vasovagal syncope: is there any difference between young and older patients? Pacing Clin Electrophysiol. 2004;27(10):1371–7. https://doi.org/10.1111/j.1540-8159.2004.00641.x.
39. Suarez-Penaranda JM, Cordeiro C, Rodriguez-Calvo M, Vieira DN, Munoz-Barus JI. Cardiac inhibitory reflex as a cause/mechanism of death. J Forensic Sci. 2013;58(6):1644–7. https://doi.org/10.1111/1556-4029.12212.
40. Alan B, Teke M, Hattapoglu S, Alan S. Importance of arterial distensibility in patients with vasovagal syncope. Eur Rev Med Pharmacol Sci. 2015;19(21): 4111–8.
41. Sucu MM, Davutoglu V, Akcay M, Yigiter R, Al B. Aortic elastic properties of patients with neurocardiogenic syncope. Pacing Clin Electrophysiol. 2009; 32(11):1417–21. https://doi.org/10.1111/j.1540-8159.2009.02485.x.
42. Alboni P, Alboni M, Bertorelle G. The origin of vasovagal syncope: to protect the heart or to escape predation? Clin Auton Res. 2008;18(4):170–8. https://doi.org/10.1007/s10286-008-0479-7.
43. Diehl RR. Vasovagal syncope and Darwinian fitness. Clin Auton Res. 2005; 15(2):126–9. https://doi.org/10.1007/s10286-005-0244-0.
44. Levi M. Vasovagal fainting as an evolutionary remnant of the fight against hemorrhage. Clin Auton Res. 2005;15(2):69–70. https://doi.org/10.1007/s10286-005-0252-0.
45. Wieling W, Smit AA, de Jong-de Vos van Steenwijk CC, van Lieshout JJ, Karemaker JM. Pathophysiological mechanisms underlying vasovagal syncope in young subjects. Pacing Clin Electrophysiol. 1997;20(8 Pt 2):2034–8.
46. Tran JC, Ruble K, Loeb DM, Chen AR, Thompson WR. Automated functional imaging by 2D speckle tracking echocardiography reveals high incidence of abnormal longitudinal strain in a cohort of pediatric oncology patients. Pediatr Blood Cancer. 2016;63(6):1075–80. https://doi.org/10.1002/pbc.25938.
47. Shiino K, Yamada A, Ischenko M, Khandheria BK, Hudaverdi M, Speranza V, et al. Intervendor consistency and reproducibility of left ventricular 2D global and regional strain with two different high-end ultrasound systems. Eur Heart J Cardiovasc Imaging. 2017;18(6):707–16. https://doi.org/10.1093/ehjci/jew120.
48. Badano LP, Cucchini U, Muraru D, Al Nono O, Sarais C, Iliceto S. Use of three-dimensional speckle tracking to assess left ventricular myocardial mechanics: inter-vendor consistency and reproducibility of strain measurements. Eur Heart J Cardiovasc Imaging. 2013;14(3):285–93. https://doi.org/10.1093/ehjci/jes184.

49. Gayat E, Ahmad H, Weinert L, Lang RM, Mor-Avi V. Reproducibility and inter-vendor variability of left ventricular deformation measurements by three-dimensional speckle-tracking echocardiography. J Am Soc Echocardiogr. 2011;24(8):878–85. https://doi.org/10.1016/j.echo.2011.04.016.
50. Hohnloser SH, Klingenheben T, van de Loo A, Hablawetz E, Bartsch S, Just H. Intra-individual reproducibility of tilt table studies in diagnosis of vasovagal syncope. Z Kardiol. 1993;82(6):352–7.
51. Nesser HJ, Mor-Avi V, Gorissen W, Weinert L, Steringer-Mascherbauer R, Niel J, et al. Quantification of left ventricular volumes using three-dimensional echocardiographic speckle tracking: comparison with MRI. Eur Heart J. 2009; 30(13):1565–73. https://doi.org/10.1093/eurheartj/ehp187.

19

The unique value of cardiovascular magnetic resonance in patients with suspected acute coronary syndrome and culprit-free coronary angiograms

Roman Panovský[1,2]*, Júlia Borová[3], Martin Pleva[3], Věra Feitová[1,4], Petr Novotný[1,2], Vladimír Kincl[1,2], Tomáš Holeček[1,4], Jaroslav Meluzín[1,2], Ondřej Sochor[1,2] and Radka Štěpánová[5]

Abstract

Background: Patients with chest pain, elevated troponin, and unobstructed coronary disease present a clinical dilemma. The purpose of this study was to investigate the incremental diagnostic value of cardiovascular magnetic resonance (CMR) in a cohort of patients with suspected acute coronary syndrome (ACS) and unobstructed coronary arteries.

Results: Data files of patients meeting the inclusion criteria in two cardiology centres were searched and analysed. The inclusion criteria included: 1) thoracic pain suspected with ACS; 2) a significant increase in the high-sensitive Troponin T value; 3) ECG changes; 4) coronary arteries without any significant stenosis; 5) a CMR examination included in the diagnostic process; 6) an uncertain diagnosis before the CMR exam; and 7) the absence of known CMR and contrast media contraindications. Special attention was paid to the benefits of CMR in determining the final diagnosis.

In total, 136 patients who underwent coronary angiography for chest pain were analysed. The most frequent underlying causes were myocarditis (38%) and perimyocarditis (18%), followed by angiographically unrecognised acute myocardial infarction (18%) and Takotsubo cardiomyopathy (15%). The final diagnosis remained unclear in 6% of the patients. The contribution of CMR in determining the final diagnosis determination was crucial in 57% of the patients. In another 35% of the patients, CMR confirmed the suspicion and, only 8% of the CMR examinations did not help at all and had no influence on diagnosis or treatment.

Conclusion: CMR provided a powerful incremental diagnostic value in the cohort of patients with suspected ACS and unobstructed coronary arteries. CMR is highly recommended to be incorporated as an inalienable part of the diagnostic algorithms in these patients.

Keywords: Cardiac magnetic resonance, Acute coronary syndrome, Normal coronary angiography

* Correspondence: panovsky@fnusa.cz

[1]The Department of Cardiovascular Diseases, International Clinical Research Centre, St. Anne's Faculty Hospital, Brno, Czech Republic

[2]The 1st Department of Internal Medicine/Cardioangiology, International Clinical Research Centre – ICRC, St. Anne's Hospital, Masaryk University, Pekařská 53, 656 91 Brno, Czech Republic

Full list of author information is available at the end of the article

Background

Coronary artery disease (CAD) and especially acute coronary syndrome (ACS) are among the leading causes of mortality and morbidity. Detailed guidelines are available for the management and treatment of both acute myocardial infarction (AMI) with and without ST-segment elevations [1, 2]. In addition to several clinical, laboratory and electrocardiographic (ECG) parameters, coronary angiography is one of the basic examinations performed on these patients and in most cases, it provides invaluable information when deciding on the subsequent therapy. However, in several trials, coronary angiography without any visible stenoses/occlusions was found in 1–12% of all patients with ACS [3–9]. In contrast to precise recommendations for the management of proven AMI, there are no guidelines for these culprit-free patients. This means that while the management and treatment of ACS with a clear culprit lesion are nearly identical in all centres, a very different approach is applied to a significant portion of other patients. The methods for clarifying diagnoses and the use of imaging modalities vary in different hospitals. Cardiovascular magnetic resonance (CMR) is a great example of a very useful tool that is used in the vast percentage of cases. While some centres are aware of the great contribution of CMR and its irreplaceability in many cases, other teams use it only rarely.

CMR is a robust non-invasive diagnostic tool in cardiology. It is a precise and highly reproducible technique used to assess ventricular volumes, masses and function. CMR can define cardiac anatomy and structure, quantify myocardial perfusion and measure blood flow. CMR images are acquired without using ionizing radiation or iodinated or radioactive contract agents. Oedema visualization and the late gadolinium enhancement (LGE) technique provide the unique opportunity to assess myocardial tissue in vivo – it enables tissue characterization in ischemic and non-ischemic cardiomyopathies and other cardiac diseases. All these advantages can help to refine the diagnostics of patients with unclear diagnoses [10].

The purpose of this study was to investigate the diagnostic value of CMR in a cohort of patients with suspected ACS and unobstructed coronary arteries.

Methods

Patient population and study protocol

The data files of patients meeting the inclusion criteria in two cardiology centres between 2012 and 2016 were searched and analysed. All inclusion criteria had to be fulfilled: 1) thoracic pain suspected with ACS; 2) a significant increase in the high-sensitive Troponin T value over the normal upper limit (value14 ng/l) in at least one value of Troponin T; 3) ECG changes, including at least a 1-mm ST-segment elevation or ST-segment depression or a negative T wave in at least two leads from one coronary artery section; 4) coronary arteries without any significant stenoses (without any atherosclerosis or with a coronary artery stenosis less than 50% in luminal diameter) proven by an admission coronary angiography; 5) a CMR examination included in the diagnostic process; 6) an uncertain diagnosis before the CMR exam; 7) the absence of any known CMR contraindications such as an implanted pacemaker/defibrillator, cochlear implant, ferromagnetic metal parts in the patient's body or claustrophobia; 8) the absence of contrast media associated contraindications such as significant renal insufficiency; 9) no history or symptoms of former cardiac disease; and 10) the absence of severe cardiac arrhythmias. Special attention was paid to the benefits of CMR in determining the final diagnosis. It was made by comparing the interim diagnosis before CMR (using ECG, laboratory, and coronary angiography results) and the final diagnosis after CMR.

Cardiac magnetic resonance imaging

CMR studies were indicated after the inclusion criteria were met and were performed according to the standard protocol using 1.5 T scanners (Ingenia and Achieva, Philips Medical Systems, Best, The Netherlands) equipped with 5- and 32-element phased array receiver coils that allow for the use of parallel acquisition techniques in the supine position in breath-hold. Functional imaging was performed using balanced steady state free precession (SSFP, b-TFE) cine sequences with the following parameters: 3.4 ms repetition time (TR), 1.7 ms echo time (TE), 60° flip angle, 1.67 × 1.67 × 8 mm spatial resolution and a 1.5 Sensitivity Encoding – factor. Standard cine imaging including four-chamber, two-chamber, and LVOT (left ventricular outflow track) long axis views, and a short axis (SAX) stack from the cardiac base to the apex in the perpendicular plane to the LV long axis (spatial resolution 1.67 × 1.67 × 1.67 mm, 0 mm gap). Wall motion abnormalities were assessed. LV functional and morphological parameters were calculated from the SA stack using the summation-of-disc method in accordance with the recommendations by the post-processing evaluation of the Society of CMR [11].

Visualization of myocardial oedema was performed using a T2 weighted black-blood image (T2-STIR; TR – 2 R-r intervals, 100 ms TE, 90°flip angle, 1.8 × 1.8x8mm spatial resolution).

LGE images in all long-axis views and the SAX view were acquired 10 min after application of an intravenous bolus of 0.15 mmol/kg of the gadolinium-based contrast agent gadobutrol (Gadovist, Bayer-Schering Pharma, Germany) using a contrast sensitive segmented rephased turbo field sequence with the slice selective inversion recovery technique (inversion-recovery turbo field echo- IR-TFE). Both 2-dimensional and 3-diamensional data acquisitions were performed in mid-systole with the following parameters: inversion time (TI) 200-300 ms, 3D: TR 4.0, TE 1.3, 15°flip angle, 1.6 × 1.75x5mm spatial resolution; 2D: TR 6.1, TE 3.0, 25° flip angle, 1.6 × 1.9x10mm spatial resolution). The inversion time (TI) for this sequence was optimized on an individual patient basis. LGE was defined as the area of visually identified contrast enhancement that was higher than the mean signal intensity of an adjacent area of the reference myocardium.

The CMR studies were assessed by two experienced interpreters. The information from cine sequences was combined with the T2-weighted imaging and LGE to determine the final diagnosis. All CMR diagnoses - AMI, myocarditis, pericarditis, Takotsubo cardiomyopathy (CMP) and other CMPs were determined according to standard CMR criteria [12]. An increased T2 signal or/and transmural or subendocardial LGE pattern with regional hypokinesia or akinesia in a corresponding coronary artery territory were criteria for unrecognized AMI. For the diagnosis of myocarditis, an increased T2 signal, increased early gadolinium enhancement and non-ischemic (epicardial, mid-wall or patchy) LGE were used as a marker of inflammation. The diagnosis of Takotsubo CMP was made by a combination of transient LV dysfunction (in a typical apical or less frequent mid-ventricular localization) and the absence of LGE.

Statistical analysis

The baseline characteristics were analysed descriptively and compared between the groups. Standard measures of summary statistics were used to describe the data: relative and absolute frequencies for categorical variables, arithmetic mean supplied with standard deviation for continuous variables.

Most variables did not present a normal distribution (Shapiro-Wilk's test), therefore non-parametric tests were applied. To compare all groups with continuous parameters, the Kruskal-Wallis test was conducted. To make a detailed mutual comparison of the groups, the Wilcoxon Rank Sum test was performed. The Chi-square test was applied to compare the groups with categorical data.

Results with a p-value <0.05 were considered statistically significant.

Results

The study included a total of 136 patients: 79 (58%) males and 57 (42%) females. The baseline characteristics of the patients are shown in Table 1 - the mean age of the entire population was 48.7 years. One-third of them suffered from arterial hypertension, 8.5% diabetes mellitus, 17% dyslipidaemia, and 28.5% of them were former or current smokers.

All patients were initially admitted to the coronary unit or the cathlab for chest pain with a suspicion of ACS. The final diagnoses were made after the completion of all examinations, including CMR. CMR was successfully performed in all 136 patients with no adverse events (Table 2). Wall motion abnormalities were found in 62 (47.7%) patients, LV EF was 57.6 ± 12.1%, EDV 130 ± 47 ml, signs of myocardial oedema were diagnosed in 75 (59.1%) patients and myocardial LGE in 94 (72.3%) patients. In 21 (15%) patients, LGE was subendocardial or transmural, while in 73 (54%) patients, LGE was subepicardial, mid-wall or patchy. Twenty-nine patients had pericardial effusion and/or late enhancement of the pericardium. The majority of the patients suffered from inflammatory diseases – myocarditis (n = 52, 38%) or perimyocarditis (n = 24, 18%) (Fig. 1). No patents had pericarditis alone without any myocardial involvement. Angiographically unrecognised AMI was seen on CMR in 25 patients (18%) (Fig. 2). Takotsubo CMP was diagnosed in 21 patients (15%) as a typical apical ballooning (n = 13, 10%) or as the less frequent mid-ventricular form (n = 8, 6%). Other CMPs were detected for the first time in 4 patients – 2 (1%) of them had dilated CMP and 2 (1%) had hypertrophic CMP. In 2 patients (1%), the chest pain was concluded to most probably be vertebrogenous, with an unclear reason for Troponin elevation. Despite maximum efforts, the final diagnosis remained unclear in 8 (6%) patients.

For a detailed analysis, 130 patients were included; patients with infrequent diagnoses (dilated CMP, hypertrophic CMP, and vertebrogenous disorders) were excluded from the comprehensive analysis. In line with the expectations, patients with inflammatory diseases were younger than others and had higher values of C-reactive protein. Takotsubo CMP was found more frequently in women. LV EF measured close to admission was lowest in the Takotsubo group, followed by rapid recovery (lower values in earlier vetriculographic and echocardiographic measurements compared to later CMR).

From the whole cohort, 121 (89%) patients had at least one pathology on CMR, while 15 (11%) patients had a completely normal CMR – 8 patients had unclear diagnoses, 2 had vertebral chest pain, 1 had Takotsubo CMP, 1 had histologically proven myocarditis, and 3 had a final diagnosis of more probable small AMI caused by a coronary artery spasm or small distal embolization despite the absence of a visible oedema or a scar on CMR.

All included patients had uncertain diagnoses before the CMR exam, as this was one of the inclusion

Table 1 Baseline characteristics

	All population (n = 130)	AMI (n = 25)	Myocarditis (n = 52)	Perimyocarditis (n = 24)	Takotsubo CMP (n = 21)	Unclear dg (n = 8)	p among groups
Clinical characteristics							
Age (years)	48.7 ± 18,0	55.9 ± 14.9	41.6 ± 15.8	38.0 ± 17.3	66.2 ± 11.5	58.2 ± 8.9	<0.001*
Female (n)	57 (41.9%)	16 (64.0%)	14 (26.9%)	5 (20.8%)	18 (85.7%)	2 (25.0%)	<0.001*
BMI (kg/m^2)	27.0 ± 5.1	27.8 ± 6.8	27.6 ± 5.0	24.6 ± 3.6	26.7 ± 4.1	28.1 ± 3.9	0.062
Hypertension (n)	43 (33.1%)	12 (48.0%)	8 (15.4%)	5 (20.8%)	15 (71.4%)	3 (37.5%)	<0.001*
DM (n)	11 (8.5%)	3 (12.0%)	3 (5.8%)	1 (4.2%)	3 (14.3%)	1 (12.5%)	0.640
Dyslipidemia (n)	22 (16.9%)	8 (32,0%)	5 (9.6%)	3 (12.5%)	4 (19%)	2 (25.0%)	0.170
Smoking (n)	37 (28.5%)	10 (40.0%)	13 (25.0%)	9 (37.5%)	4 (19.0%)	1 (12.5%)	0.296
Laboratory							
CK (μkat/l)	15.1 ± 59.0	8.3 ± 6.7	24.1 ± 92.9	13.7 ± 13.1	3.5 ± 2.1	13.9 ± 16.0	0.007
CK-MB (μkat/l)	0.94 ± 0.89	0.93 ± 0.78	0.95 ± 0.85	1.00 ± 1.07	0.63 ± 0.45	1.43 ± 1.46	0.847
Troponin T (μg/l)	0.95 ± 1.07	1.44 ± 1.49	0.77 ± 1.61	1.37 ± 1.42	0.60 ± 0.73	0.34 ± 0.50	0.001*
NT-pro-BNP (ng/l)	1891 ± 4762	1880 ± 3158	1663 ± 6227	895 ± 1095	3999 ± 5107	212 ± 169	0.190
CRP (mg/l)	42.9 ± 50.0	21.0 ± 28.9	46.2 ± 55.6	82.2 ± 76.2	15.3 ± 30.4	21.9 ± 52.1	<0.001*
Echocardiography							
LV EF (%)	53.4 ± 11.2	53.7 ± 10.2	56.1 ± 10.4	53.6 ± 10.3	42.2 ± 10.3	61.3 ± 7.9	<0.001*
WM abnormalities (n)	62 (49.2%)	18 (72.0%)	16 (31.4%)	11 (45.8%)	16 (88.9%)	1 (12.5%)	<0.001*
Coronary angiography							
Coronary AS (n)	43 (35.8%)	11 (44.0%)	12 (25.5%)	3 (15.8%)	12 (57.1%)	5 (62.5%)	0.011*
LV EF (RLVG) (%)	51.3 ± 13.7	56.0 ± 11.0	55.9 ± 13.0	51.6 ± 11.9	37.6 ± 9.4	60.0 ± 9.4	<0.001*

Values are expressed as the mean ± standard deviation or the number of subjects with the percentage in parentheses
AMI acute myocardial infarction, *CMP* cardiomyopathy, *dg* diagnosis, *BMI* body mass index, *DM* diabetes mellitus, *smoking* current or prior smoking, *CK* creatine kinase, *CK-MB* creatine kinase-MB isoensyme, *T* Troponin; *NT-pro-BNP* N-terminal fragment of pro-brain natriuretic peptide, *CRP* C-reactive protein, *LV* left ventricle, *EF* ejection fraction, *WM* wall motion, *AS* atherosclerosis, *RLVG* retrograde left ventriculography
* $p < 0.05$ between groups

criteria. On the other hand, all patients were suspected of having some type of pre-CMR diagnosis, but usually there was insufficient data for making such a diagnosis, and it was often poorly defined and chaotic. In 48 (35%) patients, CMR confirmed this previous suspicion and contributed to the diagnostic conclusion. The incremental contribution of CMR for determining the final diagnosis was crucial in 74 (57%) of the patients, where the diagnosis would have remained unclear or incorrect without using CMR - the greatest benefit of CMR was found in patients with unrecognized AMI (76% of them were diagnosed mainly by CMR) and inflammatory diseases (64% of the conclusions were reached only through the use of CMR). Only 11 (8%) CMR examinations did not help at all and had no influence on either the diagnosis or treatment (Table 3).

Discussion

Our study, which evaluated the utility of CMR in a cohort of patients with suspected ACS and unobstructed coronary disease, highlights several important findings. First, it demonstrated that CMR has a high incremental diagnostic value - in more than one-half of the patients, the diagnosis would have remained unclear or incorrect without the use of CMR. Secondly, the study confirmed the results from other trials that the vast majority of patients admitted to hospital with a suspicion of ACS suffered from an inflammatory disease, which should have been the main differential diagnosis. Third, our study showed the importance of CMR in cases of AMI in patients in combination with the absence of coronary artery occlusions or stenoses.

Differently than the other trials describing CMR examination in similar cohorts of patients, our work calculated the incremental contribution of CMR for determining the final diagnosis. In more than one-half of the cases (57%), the final diagnosis was either incorrect or uncertain and the benefit of CMR was absolutely essential. In another one-third of the patients, CMR was useful for confirming the diagnoses. These results strengthen the need for using CMR in unclear ACS cases. As in many centres, CMR has not yet been included into the standard approach for these patients and our study aims to encourage making a change in these procedures, because the final diagnosis influences prescriptions for treatment. In literature, CMR diagnosis is reached in 90–93% of all cases [9, 13–15] and CMR

Table 2 CMR findings

	All population (n = 130)	AMI (n = 25)	Myocarditis (n = 52)	Perimyocarditis (n = 24)	Takotsubo CMP (n = 21)	Unclear dg (n = 8)	p among groups
LV EF (%)	57.6 ± 12.1	57.4 ± 13.0	60.1 ± 10.6	55.2 ± 10.8	50.3 ± 12.4	67.9 ± 10.5	<0.001*
EDV (ml)	130 ± 47	112 ± 55	141 ± 41	149 ± 46	103 ± 40	131 ± 34	<0.001*
WM abnormalities (n)	62 (47.7%)	20 (80.0%)	13 (25.0%)	9 (37.5%)	20 (95.2%)	0 (0%)	<0.001*
Myocardial LGE (n)	94 (72.3%)	21 (84.0%)	50 (96.2%)	21 (87.5%)	2 (9.5%)	0 (0%)	<0.001*
Myocardial oedema (n)	75 (59.1%)	15 (65.2%)	37 (71.2%)	19 (79.2%)	4 (19.0%)	0 (0%)	<0.001*
LV hypertrophy (n)	27 (20.8%)	4 (16.0%)	7 (13.5%)	5 (20.8%)	7 (33.3%)	4 (50%)	0.118
Pericardial effusion and/or LGE (n)	29 (22.3%)	3 (12.0%)	3 (5.8%)	23 (95.8%)	0 (0%)	0 (0%)	<0.001*

Values are expressed as the mean ± standard deviation or the number of subjects with the percentage in parentheses
AMI acute myocardial infarction, *CMP* cardiomyopathy, *dg* diagnosis, *LV* left ventricle, *EF* ejection fraction, *EDV* end-diastolic volume, *WM* wall motion, *LGE* late gadolinium enhancement
* $p < 0.05$ between groups

leads to a change in therapy in 32% of the patients [16]. Making the correct diagnosis is essential for providing adequate treatment and the appropriate risk-stratification of patients. Although the study samples in the trials were heterogeneous, some studies and meta-analysis described even worse prognoses for these patients (4.7% had a 12-months mortality) compared to patients with AMI [17].

In our study, the majority (56%) of the patients suffered from inflammatory diseases – myocarditis or perimyocarditis, while unrecognised AMI was found in 18% of the patients and Takotsubo CMP was present in 15% of the patients. The distribution of diagnoses differs among studies, mainly due to different inclusion criteria, for instance ECG changes or laboratory markers. Despite the differences in the percentage of diseases, unrecognized AMI and myocarditis are consistently the most frequent causes. In concordance with our study, very similar frequencies of diagnoses have been found by several groups. For instance, in a study by Leurent et al. [5], myocarditis was found in 59.9%, Takotsubo syndrome in 14% and myocardial infarction in 15.8% of the patients. Similarly, Stensaeth et al. [6] described myocarditis or pericarditis in 56% and stress CMP in 10% of the patients, while Assomull et al. [18] found myocarditis in 50%, AMI in 11.6% and CMP in 3.4% of the patients in their trial. Laraudogoitia Zaldumbide et al. [19] discovered myocarditis in 63%, AMI in 15% and Takotsubo CMP in 11% of the patients, and Avegliano et al. [20] diagnosed myocarditis in 60.9%, AMI in 18.7% and stress CMP in 12.5% of their patients. All these trials had very similar inclusion criteria and fewer patients than our study. Some other studies differed greatly, such as a study by Steen et al. [13] in which only 17% of the patients had myocarditis and 38% had AMI. These differences can be explained by their different inclusion criteria, especially by the absence of coronary angiography before CMR. The fact that Mahmoudi et al. [21] performed a CMR examination 2 months after coronary angiography together with missing T2 weighted sequences in the protocol, could probably explain their very low number of myocarditis patients (16%) – it could be assumed that most myocarditis patients were not diagnosed by this late CMR examination. From this comparison, we can highlight the necessity for early inclusion of CMR into the diagnostic algorithm.

CMR is an unbeatable non-invasive method for diagnosing myocarditis. The diagnostic process in myocarditis is based mainly on CMR and endomyocardial biopsy and would be very difficult without using them. Myocarditis is the third leading cause of sudden death and up to 30% of the cases can progress to dilated CMP, so that

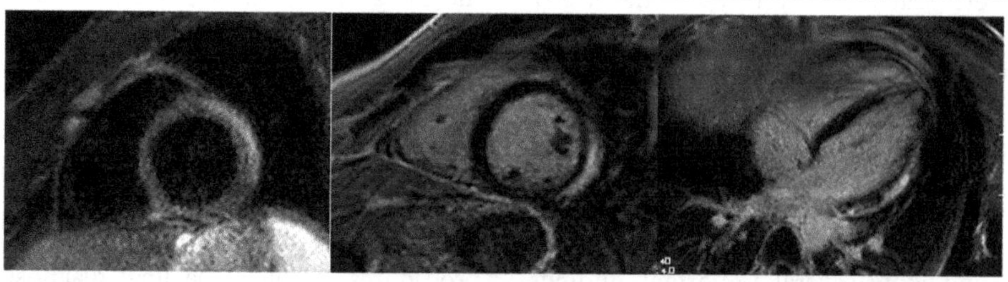

Fig. 1 A patient with myocarditis. Detection of myocardial oedema in the anterolateral wall – **a** a short-axis T2- weighted STIR view; **b** a short-axis delayed enhanced view; **c** a four-chamber delayed enhanced view

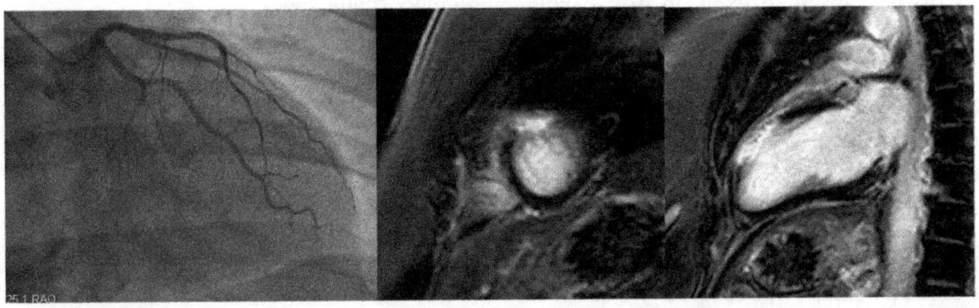

Fig. 2 A patient with culprit-free acute myocardial infarction. **a** Left coronary angiography without any stenoses or occlusions; **b** a short-axis delayed enhanced view with a transmural scar in the anterior wall; **c** a two-chamber delayed enhanced view with a transmural scar in the anterior wall

making the proper diagnosis is crucial for patient management [22, 23]. In our study, 56% of the patients had myocarditis alone or perimyocarditis. Frequently, the first clinical manifestation looks like an AMI, with oppressive chest pain, ECG changes and elevated markers of myocardial damage, so ACS is often the initial diagnosis. CMR provides functional information, but its unique contribution is in the structural information, especially in the detection of regional differences in tissue characteristics. For myocarditis, an increased T2 signal indicating increased water content in an inflamed myocardium, increased early gadolinium enhancement and epicardial, mid-wall, or patchy LGE are typical findings [4, 24]. However, recent data has described a very rapid decrease of CMR oedema markers in just a few weeks with the urgent need for CMR examination at an early stage of the disease [25]. In our study, the mean time interval between the presentation of symptoms and the CMR scan was 7.44 ± 10.03 days, so there is a high probability that all myocarditis patients were captured. The younger age and higher C-reactive protein (CRP) values in myocarditis patients are in concordance with the literature [8].

Culprit-free AMI was the second most common cause in our cohort. The 18% prevalence of these patients is consistent with the published data [8]. Several mechanisms could be proposed to explain these patients, such as coronary spasms, embolisms, atherosclerotic plaque disruptions, or spontaneous recanalization of transitory occlusions. Coronary angiography is a routine examination in patients with ACS. In cases where no visible stenoses/occlusions are found, intravascular ultrasound (IVUS) and/or coronary optical coherence tomography (OCT) can be considered. However, independently of IVUS or OCT results, the diagnosis should be confirmed by other methods. CMR with scar (and/or oedema) visualization is a perfect choice in these situations [26, 27]. A subendocardial or transmural LGE pattern in a corresponding coronary artery section leads to the correct diagnosis with subsequent therapeutic consequences and patient follow-up.

There is no specific CMR pathology for Takotsubo CMP. The diagnosis is usually made by combining transient LV dysfunction and the absence of LGE. Wall motion abnormalities could be apical in typical apical ballooning syndrome, or less frequently as mid-ventricular. Previous studies have shown a prevalence of stress CMP between 11 and 22% [8]; in our cohort, it was 15%.

In a small number of patients (8%), the final diagnosis remained unclear even after using CMR. This number is in keeping with other studies [5]. These patients had lower Troponin T levels compared to other groups and the best LV function among the groups. We could speculate about missing a very small LGE in case of microinfarctions or very mild inflammation due to limited spatial resolution or imaging artefacts. Some cases may be due to an underlying non-cardiac disease. The

Table 3 CMR contribution for the final diagnosis

	All population (n = 130)	AMI (n = 25)	Myocarditis (n = 52)	Perimyocarditis (n = 24)	Takotsubo CMP (n = 21)	Unclear dg (n = 8)	p among groups
Diagnosis made mainly by CMR (n)	74 (56.9%)	19 (76.0%)	31 (59.6%)	18 (75.0%)	6 (28.6%)	0 (0%)	<0.001*
CMR confirmed previous suspicion (n)	45 (34.6%)	4 (16.0%)	20 (38.5%)	6 (25.0%)	15 (74.4%)	0 (0%)	
CMR did not help (n)	11 (8.5%)	2 (8.0%)	1 (1.9%)	0 (0%)	0 (0%)	8 (100%)	

Values are expressed as the number of subjects with the percentage in parentheses
AMI acute myocardial infarction, *CMP* cardiomyopathy, *dg* diagnosis
* $p < 0.05$ between groups

CMR protocol was not designed to exclude non-cardiac reasons for chest pain and biomarker elevation. Further investigation of these patients after excluding a cardiac origin of their troubles was typically not performed in our centre. There is also the possibility of false positive biochemical results.

Study limitations

Even though this is not a prospective study, our unit's policy is to perform CMR in all culprit-free ACS patients. Despite the fact that this is one of the largest cohorts that has been described so far, the relatively small sample size limits the statistical power of our calculations. Another limitation is that the final diagnoses were based on a synopsis of all clinical, ECG, laboratory and imaging findings, including CMR. Individual examinations differed slightly according to each patient's medical history and interim results. Nevertheless, this bias reflects an actual patient workflow.

Especially for patients with AMI, IVUS and/or OCT could help in the understanding of the aetiology, but these procedures were not routinely performed. Furthermore, MR stress first-pass perfusion and cardiac mapping sequences and extracellular volume were not included in the standard CMR protocol. They would certainly provide additional useful information.

Conclusion

Our study demonstrated that CMR had a powerful incremental diagnostic value in a cohort of patients with ACS and unobstructed coronary arteries. CMR is strongly recommended to be included as an inalienable part of diagnostic algorithms in these patients, because making the correct final diagnosis has direct implications on patient management.

Abbreviations

ACS: Acute coronary syndrome; AMI: Acute myocardial infarction; AS: Atherosclerosis; BMI: Body mass index; CAD: Coronary artery disease; CK: Creatine kinase; CK-MB: Creatine kinase-MB isoenzyme; CMP: Cardiomyopathy; CMR: Cardiovascular magnetic resonance; CRP: C-reactive protein; DM: Diabetes mellitus; ECG: Electrocardiography; EDV: End-diastolic volume; EF: Ejection fraction; EGEr: Early gadolinium enhancement ratio; IR-TFE: Inversion-recovery turbo field echo; IVUS: Intravascular ultrasound; LGE: Late gadolinium enhancement; LV: Left ventricle; LVOT: Left ventricular outflow track; NT-pro-BNP: N-terminal fragment of pro-brain natriuretic peptide; OCT: Optical coherence tomography; RLVG: Retrograde left ventriculography; SAX: Short axis; SSFP: Steady state free precession; TE: Echo time; TI: Inversion time; TR: Repetition time; WM: Wall motion

Acknowledgements
Not applicable.

Funding
The work was supported by project no. LQ1605 from the National Program of Sustainability II (MEYS CR). Funding was used for data collection and analysis.

Authors' contributions

RP conceived of the study and was the major contributor in writing the manuscript, RP, MP, PN contributed the study design, JB, VF, VK, TH, JM, and OS cooperated in data collection and processing, RS performed statistical analyses. All authors read and approved the final manuscript.

Authors' information

Not applicable.

Competing interests

The authors declare that they have no competing interests.

Author details
[1]The Department of Cardiovascular Diseases, International Clinical Research Centre, St. Anne's Faculty Hospital, Brno, Czech Republic. [2]The 1st Department of Internal Medicine/Cardioangiology, International Clinical Research Centre – ICRC, St. Anne's Hospital, Masaryk University, Pekařská 53, 656 91 Brno, Czech Republic. [3]The Department of Cardiology, Heart Centre, Hospital Podlesi, Trinec, Czech Republic. [4]The Department of Medical Imaging, St. Anne's Faculty Hospital and Masaryk University, Brno, Czech Republic. [5]International Clinical Research Centre, St. Anne's University Hospital Brno, Brno, Czech Republic.

References

1. Roffi M, Patrono C, Collet JP, Mueller C, Valgimigli M, Andreotti F, et al., on behalf of the ESC Task Force. 2015 ESC guidelines for the management of acute coronary syndromes in patients presenting without persistent ST-segment elevation: Task Force for the management of acute coronary syndromes in patients presenting without persistent ST-segment elevation of the European Society of Cardiology (ESC). Eur Heart J. 2016;37:267–315.
2. Steg PG, James SK, Atar D, Badano LP, Blomstrom Lundqvist C, Borger MA, et al. ESC guidelines for the management of acute myocardial infarction in patients presenting with ST-segment elevation. The Task Force on the management of ST-segment elevation acute myocardial infarction of the European Society of Cardiology (ESC). Eur Heart J. 2012;33:2569–619.
3. Kawecki D, Morawiec B, Monney P, Pellaton C, Wojciechowska C, Jojko J, et al. Diagnostic contribution of cardiac magnetic resonance in patients with acute coronary syndrome and culprit-free angiograms. Med Sci Monit. 2015; 21:171–80.
4. Monney PA, Sekhri N, Burchell T, Knight C, Davies C, Deaner A, et al. Acute myocarditis presenting as acute coronary syndrome: role of early cardiac magnetic resonance in its diagnosis. Heart. 2011;97:1312–8.
5. Leurent G, Langella B, Fougerou C, Lentz PA, Larralde A, Bedossa M, et al. Diagnostic contributions of cardiac magnetic resonance imaging in patients presenting with elevated troponin, acute chest pain syndrome and unobstructed coronary arteries. Arch Cardiovasc Dis. 2011;104:161–70.
6. Stensaeth K, Fossum E, Hoffmann P, Mangschau A, Klow N. Clinical characteristics and the role of early cardiac magnetic resonance imaging in patients with suspected ST-elevation, myocardial infarction, and normal coronary arteries. Int J Cardiovasc Imaging. 2011;27(3):355–65.
7. Chopard R, Jehl J, Dutheil J, Genon VD, Seronde MF, Kastler B, et al. Evolution of acute coronary syndrome with normal coronary arteries and normal cardiac magnetic resonance imaging. Arch Cardiovasc Dis. 2011;104(10):509–17.
8. Tornvall P, Gerbaud E, Behaghel A, Chopard R, Collste O, Laraudogoitia E, et al. Myocarditis or "true" infarction by cardiac magnetic resonance in patients with a clinical diagnosis of myocardial infarction without obstructive coronary disease: a meta-analysis of individual patient data. Atherosclerosis. 2015;241(1):87–91.
9. Collste O, Sorensson P, Frick M, Agewall S, Daniel M, Henareh L, et al. Myocardial infarction with normal coronary arteries is common and associated with normal findings on cardiovascular magnetic resonance - results from the Stockholm myocardial infarction with normal coronaries study. J Intern Med. 2013;273(2):189–96.
10. Panovsky R, Pleva M, Feitova V, Kruzliak P, Meluzin J, Kincl V. The prognostic impact of myocardial late gadolinium enhancement. Cardiol Rev. 2014;22(3):128–39.
11. Schulz-Menger J, Bluemke DA, Bremerich J, Flamm SD, Fogel MA, Friedrich MG, et al. Standardized image interpretation and post processing in

cardiovascular magnetic resonance: Society for Cardiovascular Magnetic Resonance (SCMR). Board of Trustees Task Force on standardized post processing. J Cardiovasc Magn Reson. 2013;15:35.

12. Hundley WG, Bluemke D, Bogaert JG, Friedrich MG, Higgins CB, Lawson MA, et al. Society for Cardiovascular Magnetic Resonance guidelines for reporting cardiovascular magnetic resonance examinations. J Cardiovasc Magn Reson. 2009;11:5.
13. Steen H, Madadi-Schroeder M, Lehrke S, Lossnitzer D, Giannitsis E, Katus HA. Staged cardiovascular magnetic resonance for differential diagnosis of troponin T positive patients with low likelihood for acute coronary syndrome. J Cardiovasc Magn Reson. 2010;12:51.
14. Emrich T, Emrich K, Abegunewardene N, Oberholzer K, Dueber C, Muenzel T, et al. Cardiac MR enables diagnosis in 90% of patients with acute chest pain, elevated biomarkers and unobstructed coronary arteries. Br J Radiol. 2015;88(1049):20150025. doi:10.1259/bjr.20150025.2015.
15. Chu G, Zhang G, Zhu M, Zhang Z, Wu Y, Zhang H. Acute one-stop cardiovascular magnetic resonance imaging for differential diagnosis in patients with acute coronary syndrome and unobstructed coronary arteries. Br J Radiol Med Princ Pract. 2015;24(4):325–31.
16. Gerbaud E, Harcaut E, Coste P, Erickson M, Lederlin M, Labèque JN, et al. Cardiac magnetic resonance imaging for the diagnosis of patients presenting with chest pain, raised troponin, and unobstructed coronary arteries. Int J Cardiovasc Imaging. 2012;28(4):783–94.
17. Pasupathy S, Air T, Dreyer RP, Tavella R, Beltrame JF. Systematic review of patients presenting with suspected myocardial infarction and nonobstructive coronary arteries. Circulation. 2015;131(10):861–70.
18. Assomull RG, Lyne JC, Keenan N, Gulati A, Bunce NH, Davies SW, et al. The role of cardiovascular magnetic resonance in patients presenting with chest pain, raised troponin, and unobstructed coronary arteries. Eur Heart J. 2007;28(10):1242–9.
19. Laraudogoitia Zaldumbide E, Pérez-David E, Larena JA, Velasco del Castillo S, Rumoroso Cuevas JR, Onaindía JJ, et al. The value of cardiac magnetic resonance in patients with acute coronary syndrome and normal coronary arteries. Rev Esp Cardiol. 2009;62:976–83.
20. Avegliano GP, Huguet M, Costabel JP, Kuschnir P, Thierer J, de Lima AA, et al. Cardiac magnetic resonance imaging in patients with chest pain, high troponin levels and absence of coronary artery obstruction. Rev Argent Cardiol. 2011;79(3):227–30.
21. Mahmoudi M, Harden S, Abid N, Peebles C, Nicholas Z, Jones T, et al. Troponin-positive chest pain with unobstructed coronary arteries: definitive differential diagnosis using cardiac MRI. Br J Radiol. 2012;85:e461–6.
22. Maron BJ, Doerer JJ, Haas TS, Tierney DM, Mueller FO. Sudden deaths in young competitive athletes: analysis of 1866 deaths in the United States, 1980–2006. Circulation. 2009;119(8):1085–92.
23. Doolan A, Langlois N, Semsarian C. Causes of sudden cardiac death in young Australians. Med J Aust. 2004;180(3):110–2.
24. Friedrich MG, Sechtem U, Schulz-Menger J, Holmvang G, Alakija P, Cooper LT, et al., International Consensus Group on Cardiovascular Magnetic Resonance in Myocarditis. Cardiovascular magnetic resonance in myocarditis: a JACC white paper. J Am Coll Cardiol. 2009;53(17): 1475–87.
25. Luetkens JA, Homsi R, Dabir D, Kuetting DL, Marx C, Doerner J et al. Comprehensive cardiac magnetic resonance for short-term follow-up in acute myocarditis. J Am Heart Assoc. 2016;5(7); doi: 10.1161/JAHA.116.003603.
26. Panovsky R, Feitova V, Polokova K, Kincl V, Meluzin J, Hlinomaz O, et al. Unusual use of magnetic resonance imaging in diagnosis of myocardial infarction. Cor Vasa. 2011;53:644–8.
27. Dastidar AG, Rodrigues JC, Ahmed N, Baritussio A, Bucciarelli-Ducci C. The role of cardiac MRI in patients with troponin-positive chest pain and unobstructed coronary arteries. Curr Cardiovasc Imaging Rep. 2015;8(8):28.

Interatrial block and atrial remodeling assessed using speckle tracking echocardiography

Juan Lacalzada-Almeida[1*], María Manuela Izquierdo-Gómez[1], Carima Belleyo-Belkasem[1], Patricia Barrio-Martínez[1], Javier García-Niebla[2], Roberto Elosua[3,4], Alejandro Jiménez-Sosa[5], Luis Alberto Escobar-Robledo[6] and Antonio Bayés de Luna[6]

Abstract

Background: To evaluate the possibility of left atrial (LA) remodeling using speckle tracking echocardiography (STE) in patients with interatrial block (IAB).

Methods: We performed a cross-sectional study with three groups of patients: 56 without IAB, 21 with partial IAB (pIAB), and 22 with advanced IAB (aIAB). Transthoracic echocardiographic (TTE) STE was performed and clinical and echocardiographic findings were analyzed.

Results: TTE showed higher LA volume/body surface area in the patients with IAB. With STE, the absolute value of strain rate during atrial booster pump function (SRa) and early reservoir period (SRs) decreased in the pIAB group and even more in the aIAB group, compared to the group without IAB. The independent variables were the echocardiographic measures of LA size and function. After adjusting for confounders, both multiple linear regression and multivariate multinomial regression showed good correlation with dependent variables: longer P-wave duration on electrocardiography and with the type of IAB, respectively. SRa ($p < 0.001$), SRs ($p < 0.001$), and maximal peak LA longitudinal strain in the reservoir period ($p = 0.009$) were independently associated with P-wave duration. SRa was also associated with the presence of pIAB (OR = 11.5; 95% confidence interval (CI): 2.7–49.0; $p = 0.001$) and aIAB, (OR = 98.2; 95% CI: 16–120.4; $p < 0.001$) and SRs was associated with pIAB (OR: 0.03; CI: 0.003–0.29; $p = 0.003$) and with aIAB (OR: 0.008; CI: 0.001–0.12; $p = 0.004$).

Conclusions: IAB correlates directly with structural remodeling and a decrease in the absolute value of LA SRa and SRs determined using STE.

Keywords: Interatrial block, Speckle tracking echocardiography, Strain, Strain rate, Left atrium

Background

Interatrial block (IAB) is an electrical abnormality due to delayed conduction in the Bachmann's bundle region between the two atria. There are two types of IAB, partial (pIAB) and advanced (aIAB) [1]. In the pIAB, the stimulus is delayed but can cross the septum via the Bachmann's bundle [2, 3]. Advanced IAB is produced when electrical stimulus conduction is totally blocked in that region; the activation of the left atrium (LA) is then from the right atrium in the caudo-cranial retrograde direction. The pIAB is characterized by a P-wave duration ≥120 milliseconds (ms) on a 12-lead electrocardiogram (ECG) (Fig. 1a) [2, 3]. The diagnosis of aIAB is made by a P-wave duration ≥120 ms and a biphasic or +/− morphology of the P-wave in leads II, III, and aVF of the ECG (Fig. 1b) [2, 3]. Interatrial block is a marker of electromechanical dysfunction of the LA [4] and a substrate for the development of supraventricular arrhythmias in different scenarios [5, 6], mainly atrial fibrillation (AF), which occurs in a condition referred to as Bayés' Syndrome [7]. Currently, a multicenter registry is tracking these cases to demonstrate this assumption [8].

Several authors have studied alterations in LA wall deformity using speckle tracking echocardiography

* Correspondence: jlacalzada@gmail.com
[1]Department of Cardiology, Hospital Universitario de Canarias, Ofra s/n, La Cuesta, 38320 La Laguna, Tenerife, Spain
Full list of author information is available at the end of the article

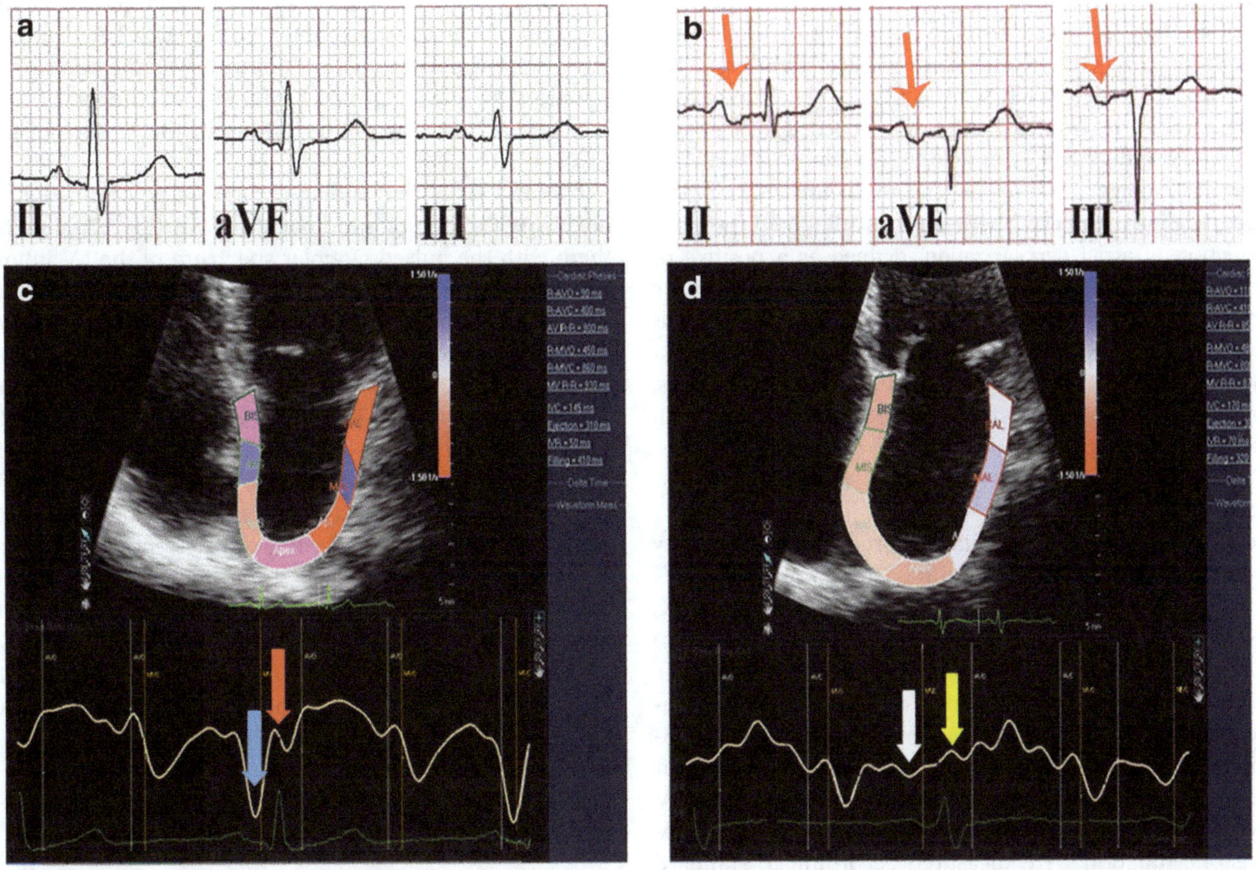

Fig. 1 Comparison of ECG and speckle tracking echocardiography of a normal subject and another with advanced interatrial block. ECG (**a**) and left atrial (LA) strain rate (SR) echocardiography (**c**) in normal subjects, with normal SR of LA contraction (blue arrow) and reservoir (red arrow) phases. ECG with advanced interatrial block (**b**); red arrows show biphasic or +/– P wave morphology and with decreased SR of LA contraction (white arrow) and reservoir (yellow arrow) phases (**d**)

(STE). Patients undergoing STE before ablation of paroxysmal AF (PAF) have shown reduced LA function [9]. Additionally, decreased peak longitudinal strain rate (SR) during the early reservoir period (SRs) of the LA is related to AF recurrence after electrical cardioversion [10]. In addition, decreased peak longitudinal SR during the period of atrial booster pump function (SRa) of the LA is a predictor of new-onset AF [11].

Changes in atrial function and remodeling and their predisposition to present with new-onset AF [12] have been observed using transthoracic echocardiography (TTE) in patients with IAB [2]. However, to date, no studies have described possible alterations in the LA wall using STE. Our hypothesis was that LA remodeling and altered period function could be observed in patients with IAB in sinus rhythm without a history of supraventricular arrhythmias. Our objective was to determine whether there is an association between IAB and atrial remodeling, with possible alterations in the deformation and functionality of the LA wall, determined using STE.

Methods

Study design

We performed a single-cross-sectional study, with prospective and consecutive recruitment of three groups of patients: one group with pIAB, another with aIAB, according to the ECG definition indicated above [2, 3], and a third group without IAB in sinus rhythm (patients with no IAB). Patients with a history of supraventricular arrhythmia verified from their hospital admission, emergency records, or long duration ECG-Holter monitoring were excluded. The study included outpatients aged > 60 years undergoing ECG at our center prospectively between January and May 2016, during the preoperative general surgery assessment. At the same visit, all patients underwent two-dimensional (2D)-Doppler TTE with STE. This study was reviewed and approved by the Clinical Research Ethics Committee of the University Hospital of the Canary Islands (Canary Islands, Tenerife, Spain). Written informed consent was obtained from all patients.

Electrocardiogram

A 12-lead ECG was performed according to established standards [13]. One experienced operator blinded to the TTE and STE data analyzed the ECGs. The P-wave was measured in the frontal plane leads recorded at the same time, with a digitized ECG using GeoGebra 4.2 software. The ECG image was amplified up to 20 times its original size to define the interval between the earliest and the latest detection of atrial depolarization, defined as a positive or negative deflection, respectively, that deviates from the baseline before the QRS complex. The software allowed us to manually draw lines on the ECG and measure the distance between two points, which was then converted to ms. Participants were categorized into three groups of interest, according to the previously given ECG description.

Echocardiographic studies

Echocardiograms were digitally stored and analyzed by two experienced operators blinded to the clinical ECG data, using a commercial system (iE33 xMATRIX, Koninklijke Philips NV, Eindhoven, The Netherlands) with a 2–4 MHz multifrequency transducer. Three consecutive beats were recorded during apnea in a cine-loop format. The analysis was performed using an echocardiographic analysis system (Xcelera R2, Philips). Left atrial and left ventricular (LV) measurements, and LV ejection fraction and Doppler variables to quantify LV diastolic function were measured according to standard echocardiographic methods [14, 15]. The LA area was traced in both the apical four- and two-chamber views in the “frame” prior to the mitral valve opening (MVO), using the bi-plane disk summation algorithm to calculate its volume, similar to that used to measure LV volume, adjusted for body surface area (BSA) [14]. The percentage of atrial systolic contribution to total mitral flow (ASCTMF) was determined as a percentage of the integral wave A velocity-time, with respect to the total area of the diastolic velocity-time curve [16].

For the STE of the LA, standard 2D images from apical 4- and 2-chambers views were acquired, with a narrow sector angle (30°–60°) and a frame-rate of 60–90 frames per second [17]. The LA endocardial border was manually traced in both 4- and 2-chamber views using the point-and-click technique, marking two points at both ends of the mitral annulus and a third at the ceiling of the LA, in end systole. The surface epicardial tracing is automatically generated by the system and can be adjusted manually by the operator in cases of tracking failure. Any segments that subsequently failed to track were excluded. The LA myocardium was divided into 12 segments of interest for analysis [17] and longitudinal strain and SR were measured automatically “offline,” using the QLAB Advanced Tissue Motion Quantification (Philips) Release 8.1, equipped with STE analysis software. Global longitudinal strain and SR were the averages of the 12 values obtained for each LA segment. Since the primary variable of interest was the contractile function of the LA, the beginning of the cycle was arbitrarily chosen as the beginning of the P-wave of the ECG [18, 19].

The periods of the cardiac cycle were determined after obtaining the LA longitudinal strain/SR (Fig. 2), aligning them with the pulsed Doppler spectrum of the LV inflow and outflow tracts, starting at the ECG P-wave. The atrial contraction period (CT) was defined as A-wave duration, the LA reservoir period (R) as the interval between mitral valve closure (MVC) and MVO, and the LA conduit period (CD) as the interval between MVO and the onset of the A-wave. Maximum values of longitudinal strain/SR were measured during the LA CT, R, and CD periods [18–20]. In our study, the following parameters of strain and SR were determined (Fig. 2): (1) peak strain point 1, peak strain point 2, and peak SR point 2′ (SRa), during the CT period, (2) in the LA R period the peak strain point 4 or maximal peak LA longitudinal strain (εs LAmax), and peak SR point 4′ (SRs) on early reservoir period (ER), (3) finally, in the CD period, peak strain point 6 and peak SR point 6′ during LV early filling (EF), and peak strain point 7 during diastasis (D).

Other covariates

Sociodemographic variables and the presence of comorbidities and pharmacological treatments were recorded.

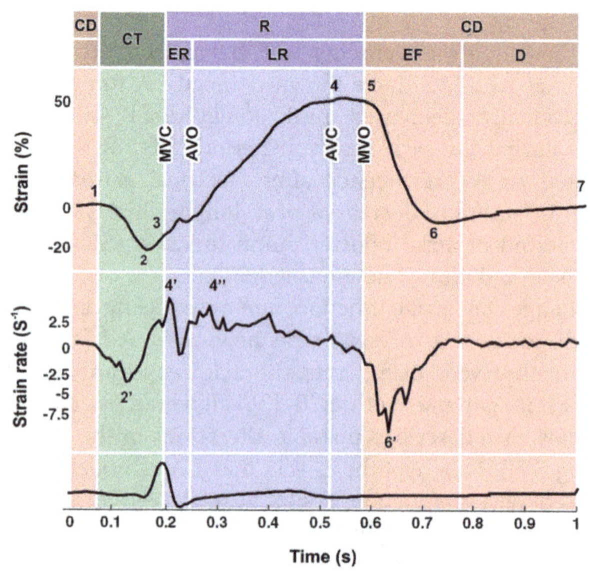

Fig. 2 Normal strain and strain rate echocardiography curves in normal subjects. Atrial periods: CD = conduit period; CT = contraction period; R = reservoir period

Statistical analysis

Continuous variables were reported as means and standard deviations or as medians and interquartile ranges according to the nature of the variables (determined using the Shapiro-Wilk test). Categorical variables were reported as frequencies and percentages. Comparisons of continuous variables between groups were carried out using the one-way ANOVA test. Variables that were not normally distributed were compared using the Kruskal-Wallis test. Comparisons between groups for categorical variables were carried out with the chi-square test. Correlations were obtained using the Spearman rank test. Multivariate linear regression analysis adjusted for potential confounders was performed, the dependent variable being P-wave duration and the independent variables being various measures of LA function. To compare the magnitude of these associations, the standardized regression coefficient (b) was calculated. We also used the multinomial logistic regression model, with the dependent variable taking three values ("pIAB," "aIAB," and "patients with no IAB"). The independent variables were the echocardiographic measures of LA size and function. Both the linear and logistic regression models were adjusted for potential confounders, including those variables that proved significant on univariate analysis: age, gender, arterial hypertension, diabetes mellitus, maximal LA volume indexed to body surface area (LAVImax) (mL/m^2), and ASCTMF. Odds ratio (OR) and 95% confidence intervals (CIs) were calculated as measures of the clinical impact of the predictor variables. Overall differences between models were tested by calculating overall differences in log-likelihood chi-square analysis between models. The ability of the multivariate logistic model to correlate with the presence or absence of IAB was verified using receiver operating characteristic (ROC) curves. The overall accuracy, sensitivity, specificity, and positive and negative predictive values for the optimal cut-off were calculated using the Youden index. Intra- and inter-observer variability was assessed using Bland-Altman analysis. A two-tailed P value of < 0.05 was considered to indicate statistical significance. All statistical analyses were performed using SPSS for Windows, version 23 (SPSS Inc., Chicago, IL, USA).

Results

Of 105 patients initially included, four were excluded due to AF and two because of poor-quality TTE images. The final sample consisted of 99 patients: 21 with pIAB, 22 with aIAB, and 56 were patients with no IAB. ECGs were analyzed by one observer with low intra-observer variability (mean 0.6%; 95% CI 0.3–0.9%). The STE was analyzed in 95% of the acquired segments. Bland-Altman analysis showed good intra- and inter-observer agreement with a non-significant bias. Intra-observer variabilities were mean change 1.20% (95% CI, 1.10–1.31%) for LA global longitudinal strain and 1.36% (95% CI, 1.12–1.51%) for LA global longitudinal SR, and inter-observer variabilities were 1.32% (95% CI, 1.15–1.62%) and 1.6% (95% CI, 1.25–1.92%), respectively. Clinical and TTE characteristics of the patients included in this study are shown in Table 1 and Additional file 1: Table S1. Patients with aIAB were older and had a higher prevalence of diabetes. On TTE, patients with aIAB and pIAB had larger LAVImax compared to the patients with no IAB; Doppler echocardiography showed that the ASCTMF decreased and the E wave to A wave (E/A) ratio increased in the group of patients with pIAB and even more in the group with aIAB, compared to the patients with no IAB group. The values of strain and SR

Table 1 Clinical and Doppler-echocardiographic characteristics

Variable	No [a]IAB (c) ($n = 56$)	[b]pIAB (p) ($n = 21$)	[c]aIAB (a) ($n = 22$)	p ANOVA	p Post Hoc
Age, years	72.2 ± 8.0	69.7 ± 9.9	77.0 ± 7.6	0.014	p vs. $a = 0.013$
Men, n (%)	32 (57)	14 (67)	11 (50)	0.54	
Duration of P wave on ECG (ms)	108 (100–115)	127.5 (123–135.3)	139 (132–149.3)	< 0.001	c vs. $p < 0.001$
					c vs. $a < 0.001$
					p vs. $a < 0.001$
Hypertension, n (%)	37 (66)	17 (81)	19 (86)	0.09	
Diabetes mellitus, n (%)	16 (29)	9 (43)	14 (64)	0.011	
[d]LAVImax	25.6 (21.4–30.3)	33.5 (27.2–45.1)	35.2 (27.1–42.6)	< 0.001	c vs. $p < 0.001$
					c vs. $a < 0.001$
[e]E/A ratio	0.74 (0.66–0.87)	0.96 (0.79–1.3)	1.1 (0.85–1.3)	< 0.001	c vs. $p = 0.011$
					c vs. $a < 0.001$
[f]ASCTMF (%)	47 ± 37	44 ± 10	39 ± 10	0.006	c vs. $a = 0.004$

Clinical and Doppler-echocardiographic characteristics of the sample. Values are presented as mean ± SD or median (interquartile range). [a]*IAB* interatrial block, [b]*pIAB* partial interatrial block, [c]*aIAB* advanced interatrial block, [d]*LAVImax* Maximal left atrial volume indexed to body surface area (mL/m^2), [e]*E/A ratio* E wave to A wave ratio, a measure of the function of the left ventricle, [f]*ASCTMF* atrial systolic contribution to total mitral flow are shown in Table 2, with significant differences between the groups. We observed that the greater the degree of IAB, the lower the absolute values of LA wall deformation during the CT and R period of LA.

Table 3 shows the standardized regression coefficients of the unadjusted simple linear regression model and the adjusted multiple linear regression model for potential confounders' variables. The variables that showed the strongest associations with P-wave duration were LAVImax (direct association) and ASCTMF, εs LAmax, absolute SRa, and SRs (inverse associations). With these variables, we performed a backward stepwise analysis adjusting for age, gender, arterial hypertension, diabetes mellitus, LAVImax, and ASCTMF. The sample size allowed supporting all covariates from the linear model. In the first model, the SRs was associated with P-wave duration (standardized β – 0.345, $p = 0.004$). In the second model, LAVImax (standardized β 0.269, $p = 0.013$) and SRa (standardized β 0.420, $p < 0.001$) remained associated. In the third model, LAVImax (standardized β 0.319, $p = 0.004$) and εs LAmax (standardized β – 0.290, $p = 0.008$) remained associated.

Table 4 shows the variables significantly associated with both types of IAB after univariate multinomial regression analysis. Several multinomial logistic submodels were constructed to avoid saturation and collinearity (Additional file 2: Table S2) of the regression model. The reference model comprised age and diabetes mellitus, which were included in successive models with the following variables introduced one by one: LAVImax, ASCTMF, εs LAmax, SRa, and SRs (Table 5). Comparing the overall differences between five nested models, the models which included LAVImax and SRa proved statistically superior to the others (Fig. 3). The results of the linear and logistic models are similar, suggesting in a robust way the association between P-wave of ECG duration or type of IAB and the mean peak of SRa and SRs. According to the ROC curve analysis (Fig. 4), the best cut-off that identified patients with IAB versus patients with no IAB was absolute SRa ≤ – 1.20 S^{-1} (AUC 0.85, CI 0.77–0.93, $p < 0.001$), with a sensitivity of 70% (CI: 54.6–81.9) and specificity of 78% (CI: 64.8–87.2). On grouping the total sample of SRa by tertiles and observing the distribution, according to the presence or absence of IAB, a linear trend was demonstrated, such that the lower the absolute value of SRa, the greater the number of patients with IAB (Mantel Haenszel Test for tendencies $p < 0.001$) (Additional file 3: Table S3).

Discussion

Our main finding was that a longer duration of the P-wave in the ECG, belonging to the group of patients with pIAB and aIAB, correlated directly with the increase in LAVImax on 2D echocardiogram (2DE) and inversely with the decrease in the absolute value of LA SRa and SRs on STE (Fig. 1d). To our knowledge, our study is the first to describe LA wall deformation alterations determined using STE in patients with IAB. The SRa was especially useful for correlation with the presence or absence of IAB. This indicates the reliable correlation between ECG and STE in patients with IAB.

Several studies using TTE have shown increased LA size and slow and poor contractility in patients with IAB [3, 4, 12]. Similar findings were observed in our patients with IAB, in relation to the LA volume increase, especially in those with aIAB, where ASCTMF was significantly decreased compared to in patients with no IAB. Although IAB and enlarged LA share a similar ECG pattern, a recent study has indicated that they are independent entities [3].

Table 2 Atrial strain and strain rate characteristics

Variable	No [a]IAB (c) (n = 56)	[b]pIAB (p) (n = 21)	[c]aIAB (a) (n = 22)	*p* ANOVA	*p* Post Hoc
[d]ε peak [e]LAc, (%)	– 2.8 (– 3.4 – – 2.1)	–2.9 (– 4.1 – – 1.9)	–1.9 (– 2.5 – – 0.68)	0.003	c vs. *a* < 0.001
					p vs. *a* = 0.011
[f]εs LAmax, (%)	18.0 ± 5.5	15.1 ± 3.0	12.7 ± 4.0	< 0.001	c vs. *p* = 0.020
					c vs. *a* < 0.001
[g]SRa, S^{-1}	–2.12 ± 0.57	– 1.20 ± 0.39	– 0.82 ± 0.26	< 0.001	c vs. *p* < 0.001
					c vs. *a* = 0.027
					p vs. *a* = 0.004
[h]SRs, S^{-1}	1.71 ± 0.27	0.99 ± 0.34	0.62 ± 0.25	< 0.001	c vs. *p* = 0.003
					c vs. *a* < 0.001
[i]SREF, S^{-1}	– 0.99 ± 0.57	– 0.94 ± 0.48	– 0.58 ± 0.22	0.009	c vs. p 0.003
					c vs. *a* < 0.001

Atrial strain and strain rate echocardiographic characteristics of the sample. Values are presented as mean ± SD or median (interquartile range). [a]*IAB* interatrial block, [b]*pIAB* partial interatrial block, [c]*aIAB* advanced interatrial block, [d]*ε* strain, [e]*LAc* left atrial contraction, [f]*εs LAmax* strain in LA reservoir phase, [g]*SRa* strain rate in LA booster pump function phase, [h]*SRs* strain rate in LA reservoir phase, [i]*SREF* strain rate LA in early ventricular filling phase

Table 3 Unadjusted and adjusted standardized linear regression coefficients

	Unadjusted simple regression		Adjusted multiple regression[a]	
Variable	b Coefficient Standardized	P	b Coefficient Standardized	P
Age	0.220	0.029		
Gender	0.003	0.97		
Hypertension	0.181	0.07		
Diabetes mellitus	0.227	0.03		
[b]LAVImax (mL/m^2)	0.353	< 0.001	0.347	< 0.001
[c]ASCTMF	−0.276	0.012	−0.227	0.039
[d]ε onset [e]LAc, (%)	−0.347	< 0.001	− 0.184	0.07
ε peak LAc, (%)	0.152	0.14	0.088	0.40
[f]εs LAmax, %	−0.423	< 0.001	− 0.263	0.009
[g]SRa, S^{-1}	0.520	< 0.001	0.369	< 0.001
[h]SRs, S^{-1}	−0.437	< 0.001	−0.296	< 0.001
[i]SREF, S^{-1}	0.249	0.018	0.161	0.12

Unadjusted and adjusted multiple standardized linear regression coefficients[a]: adjustment for variables age, gender, hypertension, diabetes mellitus, LAVImax, and ASCTMF. [b]*LAVImax* Maximal left atrial volume indexed to body surface area (mL/m^2), [c]*ASCTMF* atrial systolic contribution to total mitral flow, [d]*ε* strain, [e]*LAc* left atrial contraction, [f]*εs LAmax* strain in LA reservoir phase, [g]*SRa* strain rate in LA booster pump function phase, [h]*SRs* strain rate in LA reservoir phase, [i]*SREF* strain rate LA in early ventricular filling phase

The European Association of Cardiovascular Imaging/ European Heart Rhythm Association Expert Consensus for the evaluation of patients with AF indicates that, in this context, measuring LA strain using STE is very promising [21], even in patients with permanent AF [16]. Sun et al. analyzed the effect of aging on the strain of the LA using 2DE STE, noting that, as age increases, the absolute value of SRa increases, regardless of gender. This is due to coupling between LA CT and decreased diastolic function with older age [20]. In our series, patients with aIAB were older than the subjects in the other two groups, despite the fact that their absolute SRa values were pathologically diminished (Tables 1 and 2), probably due to age-related atrial fibrosis [22]. However, not only age must be considered, because the regression analyses adjusted for this and the other confounding variables showed correlations with both types of IAB. In addition, absolute values of SRa showed a linear decrease in the groups of patients with pIAB and aIAB.

Table 4 Multinomial univariate analysis results

	[a]pIAB			[b]aIAB		
Variable[c]	[d]OR	95% [e]CI	P	OR	95% CI	P
Age	0.96	0.91–1.02	0.25	1.1	1.021–1.15	0.026
Gender	0.67	0.23–1.91	0.45	1.3	0.50–3.60	0.57
Hypertension	2.10	0.61–7.04	0.25	4.62	0.97–22.04	0.06
Diabetes mellitus	1.83	0.64–5.18	0.26	4.87	1.66–14.32	0.004
[f]LAVImax(mL/m^2)	1.11	1.05–1.17	< 0.001	1.08	1.03–1.14	0.004
[g]ASCTMF	0.018	0.01–12.7	0.04	0.01	0.001–0.03	0.02
[h]εs LAmax, %	0.90	0.78–0.99	0.04	0.76	0.65–0.88	< 0.001
[i]SRa, S^{-1}	8.03	2.16–29.9	< 0.001	16.5	5.94–46.2	< 0.001
[j]SRs, S^{-1}	0.04	0.04–0.31	< 0.001	0.009	0.001–0.1	< 0.001

[a]*pIAB* partial interatrial block, [b]*aIAB* advanced interatrial block, [c]*Variable* normal ECG group taken as reference category. [d]*OR* odds ratio, [e]*CI* confidence interval, [f]*LAVImax* Maximal left atrial volume indexed to body surface area (mL/m^2), [g]*ASCTMF* atrial systolic contribution to total mitral flow, [h]*εs LAmax* strain in LA reservoir phase, [i]*SRa* strain rate in LA booster pump function phase, [j]*SRs* strain rate in LA reservoir phase

Speckle tracking echocardiography findings of LA deformation similar to ours have been reported in patients with permanent or PAF [16]. Hirose T et al. reported that subjects who develop new-onset non-valvular AF have lower absolute values of SRa and SRs than those who do not [11]. Other authors have evaluated the role of LA deformation imaging as a predictor of a successful second cardiac ablation in PAF, noting that strain and SR during the CT and R periods of the LA were significantly lower in the second cardiac ablation group compared to healthy volunteers and patients undergoing first cardiac ablation without AF recurrence ($p < 0.001$, for all) [23]. It has also been shown that a decrease in the LA global longitudinal strain is an independent predictor of the progression of PAF towards persistent or permanent AF [24].

Atrial fibrosis can be visualized and quantified using cardiac magnetic resonance imaging (CMR) with late gadolinium enhancement (LGE), but it can also manifest as atrial enlargement, decrease in deformation during CT and R periods, determined using LA 2DE STE, even before the occurrence of atrial dilation, as well as higher daily AF load [25]. All these findings have been associated with stroke in patients with AF [26]. One possible application of determining atrial strain could be to predict the risk of AF. This has recently been demonstrated by Mahnkopf et al., who assessed LA fibrosis with LGE-CMR and atrial function using STE before cardiac ablation, creating the Utah classification. They correlated AF recurrence directly with decreased εs LAmax and the highest degree of atrial fibrosis on LGE-CMR [27]. Therefore, the STE 2DE finding of decreased LA deformation in our patients with IAB is identical to that predicting AF in patients with no IAB [2, 22]. Given the direct relationship between decreased deformation and LA fibrosis in PAF, this same relationship could exist between decreased deformation and LA fibrosis in our patients with IAB. The latter, associated with the LA enlargement in the patients with IAB, would indicate that these patients present the two factors that define atrial structural remodeling [28]. The Expert Consensus on Atrial Cardiomyopathy proposed the following as a working definition of this: “any complex of structural, architectural, contractile, or electrophysiological changes affecting the

Table 5 Multinomial multivariate analysis results

	[a]pIAB			[b]aIAB		
Variable[c]	[d]OR	95% [e]CI	*P*	OR	95% CI	*P*
[f]LAVImax (mL/m^2)	1.12	1.05–1.18	< 0.001	1.10	1.04–1.17	0.002
[g]ASCTMF	0.02	0.003–11.1	0.24	0.03	0.004–0.14	0.003
[h]εs LAmax	0.85	0.72–1.01	0.07	0.77	0.64–0.92	0.004
[i]SRa	11.5	2.7–49	0.001	98.2	16–120.4	< 0.001
[j]SRs	0.03	0.003–0.29	0.003	0.008	0.001–0.12	0.004

[a]*pIAB* partial interatrial block, [b]*aIAB* advanced interatrial block, [c]*Variable* normal ECG group taken as reference category. [d]*OR* odds ratio, [e]*CI* confidence interval, [f]*LAVImax* Maximal left atrial volume indexed to body surface area (mL/m^2), [g]*ASCTMF* atrial systolic contribution to total mitral flow, [h]*εs LAmax* strain in LA reservoir phase, [i]*SRa* strain rate in LA booster pump function phase, [j]*SRs* strain rate in LA reservoir phase

atria with the potential to produce clinically-relevant manifestations." It could, therefore, be considered that the contractile alterations of the LA wall and the occurrence of supraventricular arrhythmias in patients with IAB would be a form of atrial cardiomyopathy [28]. The atrial myopathy hypothesis proposes that atrial fibrosis increases the risk of thromboembolism independently of atrial rhythm [29]. Identifying these STE parameters in patients with IAB is important because they indicate alteration of atrial structure and function, even before severe enlargement of the LA occurs, as we have detected in pIAB. It remains to be clarified whether this decrease, as determined using STE in IAB, has a similar ability to predict the development of new-onset AF.

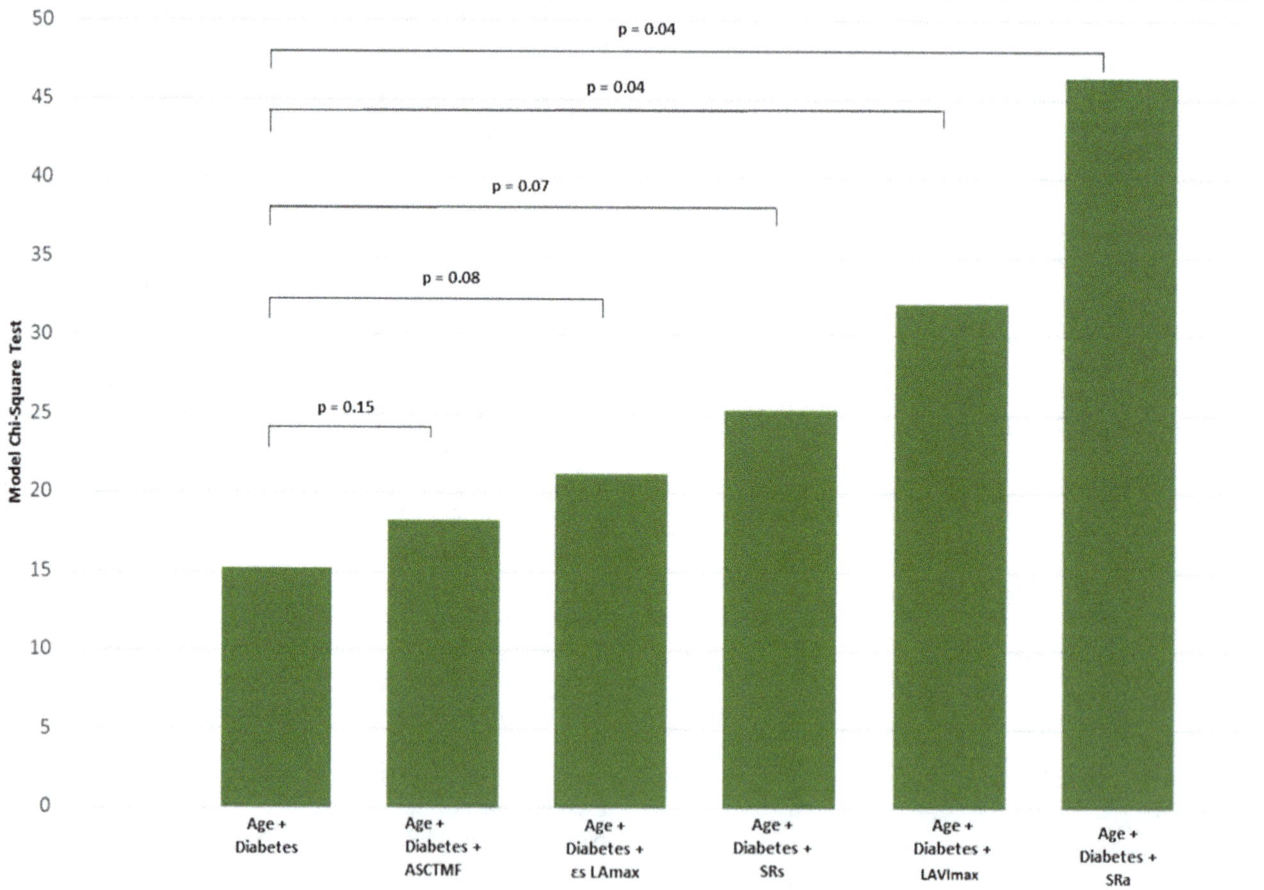

Fig. 3 Comparison of multivariate models. Incremental correlation between interatrial block and echocardiographic variables with respect to age and diabetes mellitus. We used the multinomial logistic regression model, with the dependent variable taking three values ("pIAB," "aIAB," and "patients with no IAB"). pIAB = partial Interatrial Block; aIAB = advanced Interatrial Block; ASCTMF = atrial systolic contribution to total mitral flow; LA = left atrial; εs LAmax = LA strain in reservoir phase; SRs = LA strain rate in reservoir phase; LAVImax = maximal LA volume indexed to body surface area; SRa = LA strain rate in booster pump function phase

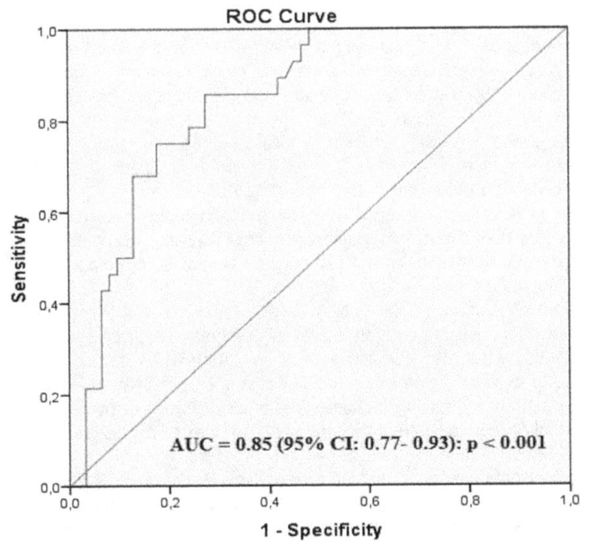

Fig. 4 Receiver operating characteristic curves of the atrial booster pump function phase (SRa) (independent variable) in correlation with presence or not of interatrial block (dependent variable). AUC = area under the curve

Limitations

We have not been able to establish whether IAB is a degenerative process independent of the specific atrial conduction system or associated with atrial fibrosis. We did not measure the LA electromechanical coupling, the LA mechanical dispersion, or the inter- and intra-atrial electromechanical delays. Failure to perform LGE-CMR prevented us from directly correlating the degree of fibrosis with the 2DE STE findings of LA contractile function. The three-dimensional TTE technique could provide useful strain data from multiple sites and a more accurate assessment of atrial volumes. Finally, and because our study was not designed to establish a causal relationship between decreased atrial deformity and AF, a prospective longitudinal design would be needed to determine whether ECG and STE findings in patients with IAB are related to AF and cardioembolic events. Then, establishing the incremental value that STE has on the ECG can provide information regarding prognosis and therapeutic measures in patients with IAB.

Conclusions

To our knowledge, this is the first study to describe LA wall deformation alterations determined using 2D STE in patients with IAB. It demonstrated that SRa and SRs of LA are pathologically diminished in patients with IAB. This finding could indicate the existence of an atrial cardiomyopathy in patients with IAB.

Additional files

Additional file 1: Table S1. Clinical and Doppler-echocardiographic characteristics. Clinical and transthoracic echocardiography characteristics of the patients included in this study. (DOC 47 kb)

Additional file 2: Table S2. Matrix of correlations between P-wave duration on ECG, Doppler- echocardiographic and strain variables. Correlation between continuous variables: P-wave duration on ECG, Doppler- echocardiographic and strain variables. (DOC 41 kb)

Additional file 3: Table S3. Peak left atrial longitudinal strain rate in booster pump function phase in tertiles. Mantel Haenszel Test for tendencies of peak left atrial longitudinal strain rate in booster pump function phase. (DOC 34 kb)

Abbreviations

AF: Atrial fibrillation; ASCTMF: Percentage of atrial systolic contribution to total mitral flow; BSA: Body surface area; CD: LA conduit period;; CIs: 95% confidence intervals; CMR: Cardiac magnetic resonance imaging; CT: LA contraction period; D: Diastasis; EF: LV early filling; ER: Early reservoir period; IAB: Interatrial block; LA: Left atrium; LAVImax: Maximal LA volume indexed to body surface area; LGE: Late gadolinium enhancement; LV: Left ventricular; MVC: Mitral valve closure; MVO: Mitral valve opening; OR: Odds ratio; PAF: Paroxysmal atrial fibrillation; R: LA reservoir period; ROC: Receiver operating characteristic curves; SR: Strain rate; SRa: Peak left atrial longitudinal strain rate in booster pump function phase; SRs: Peak left atrial longitudinal strain rate in early reservoir phase; STE: Speckle tracking echocardiography; TTE: Transthoracic echocardiography; εs LAmax: Maximal peak left atrial longitudinal strain in reservoir phase

Acknowledgements

We thank Michael Mclean for help with the text in English.

Funding

Not applicable

Authors' contributions

JL conceived the study and its design. MI, CB, PB, LE and JL worked on acquisition of data and analysis. JL, JG, RE, AJ and AB worked on interpretation of data and drafting of the manuscript. JL, RE and AB revised the manuscript critically. All authors read and approved the final manuscript.

Competing interests

The authors declare that they have no competing interests.

Author details

[1]Department of Cardiology, Hospital Universitario de Canarias, Ofra s/n, La Cuesta, 38320 La Laguna, Tenerife, Spain. [2]Servicios Sanitarios del Área de Salud de El Hierro, Valle del Golfo Health Center, El Hierro, Spain. [3]Cardiovascular Epidemiology and Genetics Research Group, IMIM (Hospital del Mar Medical Research Institute), Barcelona, Catalonia, Spain. [4]CIBER Cardiovascular Diseases (CIBERCV), Barcelona, Spain. [5]Research Unit, Hospital Universitario de Canarias, La Laguna, Santa Cruz de Tenerife, Spain. [6]Fundación Investigación Cardiovascular, Institut Català Ciències Cardiovasculars, Barcelona, Catalonia, Spain.

References

1. Barbero U, Ho SY. Anatomy of the atria a road map to the left atrial appendage. Herzschrittmacherther Elektrophysiol. 2017;28(4):347–54.
2. Bayés de Luna A, Cladellas M, Oter R, Torner P, Guindo J, Martí V, et al. Interatrial conduction block and retrograde activation of the left atrium and paroxysmal supraventricular tachyarrhythmia. Eur Heart J. 1988;9(10):1112–8.

3. Bayés De Luna A, Platonov P, Cosio FG, Cygankiewicz I, Pastore C, Baranowski R, et al. Interatrial blocks. A separate entity from left atrial enlargement: a consensus report. J Electrocardiol. 2012;45(5):445–51.
4. Goyal SB, Spodick DH. Electromechanical dysfunction of the left atrium associated with interatrial block. Am Heart J. 2001;142(5):823–7.
5. Conde D, Van Oosten EM, Hamilton A, Petsikas D, Payne D, Redfearn DP, et al. Prevalence of interatrial block in patients undergoing coronary bypass graft surgery. Int J Cardiol. 2014;171(3):e98–9.
6. Alexander B, Rodriguez C, de la Isla LP, Islas F, Quevedo PJ, Nombela-Franco L, et al. The impact of advanced interatrial block on new-onset atrial fibrillation following TAVR procedure. Int J Cardiol. 2016;223:672–3.
7. Conde D, Seoane L, Gysel M, Mitrione S, Bayes de Luna A, Baranchuk A. Bayes' syndrome: the association between interatrial block and supraventricular arrhythmias. Expert Rev Cardiovasc Ther. 2015;13(5):541–50.
8. Martinez-Selles M, Baranchuk A, Elosua R, Bayés de Luna A. Rationale and design of the BAYES (interatrial block and yearly events) registry. Clin Cardiol. 2017;40(4):196–9.
9. Sarvari SI, Haugaa KH, Stokke TM, Ansari HZ, Leren IS, Hegbom F, et al. Strain echocardiographic assessment of left atrial function predicts recurrence of atrial fibrillation. Eur Heart J Cardiovasc Imaging. 2016;17(6):660–7.
10. Di Salvo G, Caso P, Lo Piccolo R, Fusco A, Martiniello AR, Russo MG, et al. Atrial myocardial deformation properties predict maintenance of sinus rhythm after external cardioversion of recent-onset lone atrial fibrillation: a color Doppler myocardial imaging and transthoracic and transesophageal echocardiographic study. Circulation. 2005;112(3):387–95.
11. Hirose T, Kawasaki M, Tanaka R, Ono K, Watanabe T, Iwama M, et al. Left atrial function assessed by speckle tracking echocardiography as a predictor of new-onset non-valvular atrial fibrillation: results from a prospective study in 580 adults. Eur Heart J Cardiovasc Imaging. 2012;13(3):243–50.
12. Ariyarajah V, Apiyasawat S, Fernandes J, Kranis M, Spodick DH. Association of Atrial Fibrillation in patients with interatrial block over prospectively followed controls with comparable echocardiographic parameters. Am J Cardiol. 2007;99(3):390–2.
13. Kligfield P, Gettes LS, Bailey JJ, Childers R, Deal BJ, Hancock EW, et al. Recommendations for the standardization and interpretation of the electrocardiogram: part I: the electrocardiogram and its technology: a scientific statement from the American Heart Association electrocardiography and arrhythmias committee, council on clinical cardiology; the American College of Cardiology Foundation; and the Heart Rhythm Society: endorsed by the International Society for Computerized Electrocardiology. Circulation. 2007;115(10):1306–24.
14. Lang RM, Badano LP, Mor-Avi V, Afilalo J, Armstrong A, Ernande L, et al. Recommendations for cardiac chamber quantification by echocardiography in adults: an update from the American Society of Echocardiography and the European Association of Cardiovascular Imaging. J Am Soc Echocardiogr. 2015;28(1):1–39. e14
15. Nagueh SF, Smiseth OA, Appleton CP, Byrd BF, Dokainish H, Edvardsen T, et al. Recommendations for the evaluation of left ventricular diastolic function by echocardiography: an update from the American Society of Echocardiography and the European Association of Cardiovascular Imaging. J Am Soc Echocardiogr. 2016;29(4):277–314.
16. Manning WJ, Leeman DE, Gotch PJ, Come PC. Pulsed Doppler evaluation of atrial mechanical function after electrical cardioversion of atrial fibrillation. J Am Coll Cardiol. 1989;13(3):617–23.
17. Yasuda R, Murata M, Roberts R, Tokuda H, Minakata Y, Suzuki K, et al. Left atrial strain is a powerful predictor of atrial fibrillation recurrence after catheter ablation : study of a heterogeneous population with sinus rhythm or atrial fibrillation. Eur Hear J Cardiovasc Imaging. 2015;16(9):1008–14.
18. Vianna-Pinton R, Moreno CA, Baxter CM, Lee KS, Tsang TSM, Appleton CP. Two-dimensional speckle-tracking echocardiography of the left atrium: feasibility and regional contraction and relaxation differences in normal subjects. J Am Soc Echocardiogr. 2009;22(3):299–305.
19. Todaro MC, Choudhuri I, Belohlavek M, Jahangir A, Carerj S, Oreto L, et al. New echocardiographic techniques for evaluation of left atrial mechanics. Eur Heart J Cardiovasc Imaging. 2012;13(12):973–84.
20. Sun JP, Yang Y, Guo R, Wang D, Lee APW, Wang XY, et al. Left atrial regional phasic strain, strain rate and velocity by speckle-tracking echocardiography: normal values and effects of aging in a large group of normal subjects. Int J Cardiol. 2013;168(4):3473–9.
21. Donal E, Lip GYH, Galderisi M, Goette A, Shah D, Marwan M, et al. EACVI/EHRA expert consensus document on the role of multi-modality imaging for the evaluation of patients with atrial fibrillation. Eur Heart J Cardiovasc Imaging. 2016;17(4):355–83.
22. Martínez-Sellés M, Massó-van Roessel A, Álvarez-García J, García de la Villa B, Cruz-Jentoft AJ, Vidán MT, et al. Interatrial block and atrial arrhythmias in centenarians: prevalence, associations, and clinical implications. Heart Rhythm. 2016;13(3):645–51.
23. Montserrat S, Gabrielli L, Bijnens B, Borràs R, Berruezo A, Poyatos S, et al. Left atrial deformation predicts success of first and second percutaneous atrial fibrillation ablation. Heart Rhythm. 2015;12(1):11–8.
24. Yoon YE, Oh I, Kim S, Park K, Kim SH. Echocardiographic predictors of progression to persistent or permanent atrial fibrillation in patients with paroxysmal atrial fibrillation (E6P study). J Am Soc Echocardiogr. 2015; 28(6):709–17.
25. Rydman R, Shiina Y, Diller G, Niwa K, Li W, Uemura H, et al. Major adverse events and atrial tachycardia in Ebstein ' s anomaly predicted by cardiovascular magnetic resonance. Heart. 2018;104(1):37–44.
26. Longobardo L, Todaro MC, Zito C, Piccione MC, Di Bella G, Oreto L, et al. Role of imaging in assessment of atrial fibrosis in patients with atrial fibrillation: state-of-the-art review. Eur Heart J Cardiovasc Imaging. 2014;15(1):1–5.
27. Mahnkopf C, Badger TJ, Burgon NS, Daccarett M, Haslam TS, Badger CT, et al. Evaluation of the left atrial substrate in patients with lone atrial fibrillation using delayed-enhanced MRI: implications for disease progression and response to catheter ablation. Heart Rhythm. 2010;7(10):1475–81.
28. Goette A, Kalman JM, Aguinaga L, Akar J, Angel J, Ann S, et al. EHRA / HRS / APHRS / SOLAECE expert consensus on atrial cardiomyopathies : definition, characterisation, and clinical implication. J Arrhythmia. 2016;32:247–78.
29. Calenda BW, Fuster V, Halperin JL, Granger CB. Stroke risk assessment in atrial fibrillation: risk factors and markers of atrial myopathy. Nat Rev Cardiol. 2016;13(9):549–59.

21

Systolic characteristics and dynamic changes of the mitral valve in different grades of ischemic mitral regurgitation –insights from 3D transesophageal echocardiography

Caroline Morbach[1,2], Diego Bellavia[1,3], Stefan Störk[2] and Lissa Sugeng[1*]

Abstract

Background: Mitral regurgitation in ischemic heart disease (IMR) is a strong predictor of outcome but until now, pathophysiology is not sufficiently understood and treatment is not satisfying. We aimed to systematically evaluate structural and functional mitral valve leaflet and annular characteristics in patients with IMR to determine the differences in geometric and dynamic changes of the MV between significant and mild IMR.

Methods: Thirty-seven patients with IMR (18 mild (m)MR, 19 significant (moderate+severe) (s)MR) and 33 controls underwent TEE. 3D volumes were analyzed using 3D feature-tracking software.

Results: All IMR patients showed a loss of mitral annular motility and non-planarity, whereas mitral annulus dilation and leaflet enlargement occurred in sMR only. Active-posterior-leaflet-area decreased in early systole in all three groups accompanied by an increase in active-anterior-leaflet-area in early systole in controls and mMR but only in late systole in sMR.

Conclusions: In addition to a significant enlargement and loss in motility of the MV annulus, patients with significant IMR showed a spatio-temporal alteration of the mitral valve coaptation line due to a delayed increase in active-anterior-leaflet-area. This abnormality is likely to contribute to IMR severity and is worth the evaluation of becoming a parameter for clinical decision-making. Further, addressing the leaflets aiming to increase the active leaflet-area is a promising therapeutic approach for significant IMR. Additional studies with a larger sample size and post-operative assessment are warranted to further validate our findings and help understand the dynamics of the mitral valve.

Keywords: Three-dimensional echocardiography, Mitral valve, Functional regurgitation, Dynamic, Leaflet, Coaptation line, Tenting, Ischemic, Therapeutic approach

Background

Mitral regurgitation is a strong predictor of cardiac outcome in patients with ischemic heart disease and is associated with higher mortality [1, 2]. The treatment of mitral regurgitation in ischemic heart disease (IMR) has been debated for several decades: Mitral valve (MV) repair is favored due to lower perioperative morbidity and mortality [3, 4], whereas MV replacement if favored by others due to better long-term outcomes and lower IMR recurrence rates [5–7]. A detailed comprehension of the dynamic mitral valve anatomy and function across the cardiac cycle might help to develop and advance novel and more specific treatment options.

IMR has been subject to detailed investigation using three-dimensional (3D) echocardiography and important changes of the MV apparatus have been found. The mitral annulus has been shown to increase in size, flatten its saddle-like shape and loose its dynamic function with

* Correspondence: lissa.sugeng@yale.edu; Lissa.Sugeng@yale.edu
[1]Yale School of Medicine, Section Cardiovascular Medicine, 330 Cedar Street, P.O Box 208017, New Haven, CT 06511, USA
Full list of author information is available at the end of the article

higher degrees of IMR [8–19]. Nevertheless, little is known about the changes of the dynamic leaflet motion and function in significant IMR and the differences amongst diverse stages of IMR severity. We therefore aimed to systematically evaluate structural and functional mitral valve leaflet and annular characteristics in patients with IMR to determine the differences in geometric and dynamic changes of the MV between significant and mild IMR.

Methods

Study population

We analyzed the stored images of 37 consecutive patients with ischemic heart disease, who had a TEE out of clinical reasons. Inclusion criteria were 1) ischemic heart disease shown by cardiac catheterization, 2) mitral regurgitation of any degree and 3) structurally normal mitral valve in comprehensive echocardiographic evaluation. Exclusion criteria were 1) acute myocardial infarction, 2) contraindications to undergoing TEE, 3) structural mitral valve or subvalvular disease (i.e. degenerative mitral valve disease, prolapse, flail leaflet, cleft, post-endocarditic lesion), 4) significant regurgitation or stenosis of any other cardiac valve, 5) other cardiac disease. IMR severity was determined according to current guidelines [20, 21] and graded into mild (m)MR and significant (s)MR, the latter subsuming moderate and severe IMR. Thirty three subjects without valvular or structural heart disease undergoing TEE for other clinical reasons (i.e. exclusion of endocarditis or search of cardiac source of embolism after ischemic stroke) served as controls.

Echocardiography

TEE was performed according to the American Society of Echocardiography Guidelines [22] using an x-7 T MTEE probe (Philips Medical Systems, Andover, MA) and standard views were acquired. Additionally, 3D volumes of the mitral valve were recorded. A 4-beat wide-angled acquisition using ECG gating created a full-volume scan of about 90°× 90° volume. Left ventricular ejection fraction (LVEF) was determined by the Simpson's biplane method. Wall motion abnormalities (WMA) were determined and patients were scored according to their number of by WMA affected LV regions (septal, lateral, inferior, posterior, anterior, apical).

Offline analysis

Blinded to MR severity, we used custom 3D feature-tracking software (TomTec® Imaging Systems GmbH, Unterschleißheim, Germany) to analyze the datasets. As ECG information is lost when data are exported to the software platform, we identified end-diastole as the first frame when the mitral valve was completely closed and end-systole as the frame preceding mitral valve opening. Initial frame of interest was mid-systole, the mid-frame between end-diastole and end-systole. Mitral annular tracking points were identified in two perpendicular planes in mid-systole. The aortic valve and the apical aortic annulus point were marked and the leaflet coaptation line was defined in a 3-chamber view plane. After defining those landmarks, the program automatically tracked the valve in the initial frame and adjustments of the mitral annulus and the leaflets were performed when necessary (Fig. 1). Subsequently, the program automatically tracked the valve in all frames between end-diastole and end-systole and again, manual adjustments if appropriate. As final step the MV parameters (Figs. 2 and 3) were calculated, saved and exported for further analysis. For quality assurance, a random sample of 10 patients was selected for assessing inter- and intraobserver variability and read in a blinded fashion by an expert in echocardiography once and by another expert twice, more than 4 weeks apart.

Data analysis

Data analysis was performed using Prism6® (GraphPad, LaJolla, CA, USA). Patient characteristics and echocardiography variables are presented as mean ± standard deviation (SD). Inter- and intra-observer variability are expressed as the absolute difference between two measurements as a percentage of their mean values. For categorical variables differences between groups were assessed using Fishers's exact test. The difference in WMA score between mMR and sMR was calculated using Mann-Whitney Test. For continuous variables differences between groups were analyzed by one-way analysis of covariance (ANCOVA), and corrected for multiple testing by the Holm-Sidak method. All variables were assessed for normality using the Shapiro-Wilks test, and non-parametric variables were logarithmically transformed prior to analysis. All tests were two-sided, and p-values < 0.05 were considered statistically significant.

Results

Subject characteristics

Table 1 shows the characteristics of the three groups. Sex, age and height were not significantly different between the three groups. Patients with mMR had a significantly higher weight and body surface area. Left ventricular ejection fraction was significantly lower and left ventricular end-diastolic diameter larger in both patient groups compared to controls, but there was no difference amongst the IMR groups. Owing to the ischemic etiology, wall motion abnormalities were present in both IMR groups with a preponderance in the lateral and inferior wall sections in sMR. In the mMR and sMR group, one and six patients, respectively, had an IMR jet that was oriented in the posterior or posterolateral direction. All other patients had a central IMR jet.

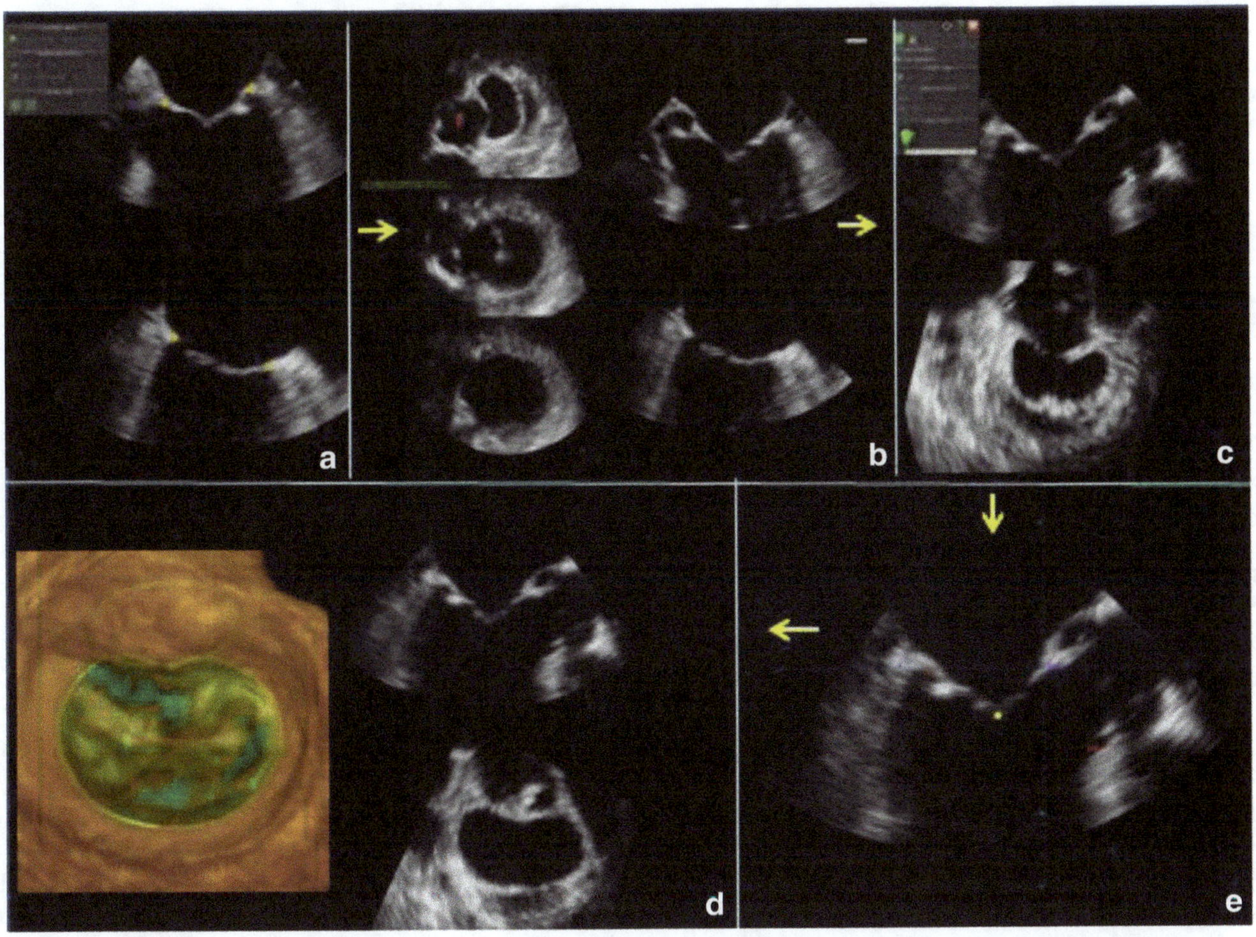

Fig. 1 **a** Opening the 3D study, the system displays a four and a two chamber view where the observer has to manually set a total of four landmarks (orange dots) to indicate the mitral valve annulus in two perpendicular planes; **b** as a second step, the aortic valve has to be identified (red dot); **c** subsequently, a long axis view is displayed where the observer has to indicate the apical aortic annulus point (blue dot); **d** finally, the observer has to mark the mitral leaflets coaptation (yellow dot) in the same long axis view; **e** when all landmarks have been set, the program automatically tracks the mitral valve

Annular displacement (7.5 mm (normal) vs. 5.3 mm (mMR and sMR), $p = 0.042$) and annular displacement velocity (38 mm/s (normal) vs. 25 mm/s (mMR) and 24 mm/s (sMR), $p < 0.0001$), as assessed by 3D analysis, were markedly reduced in both IMR groups with no significant differences between both patients groups. Frame rates were similar amongst all three groups.

Inter- and intraobserver variability

Coefficients of variation were low (≤6%) for all diameters, annulus circumference, non-planar angle and annular displacement and velocity, whereas coefficients of variation were higher for annulus area and anterior and posterior leaflet area (Table 2).

Mitral valve structural characteristics in mid-systole

Initial measurements were performed in mid-systole (Table 3). There were no significant differences in diameters, annulus circumference and area, and anterior and posterior leaflet area between controls and mMR, whereas all parameters were significantly increased in sMR compared to controls and mMR. The proportionate increase between controls and sMR in anterior-posterior (AP) diameter (18%) and anterolateral-posteromedial (AL-PM) diameter (18%) as well as in intercommissural diameter (17%) was of similar magnitude.

The non-planar angle was significantly flattened in both IMR groups compared to controls with no difference between mMR and sMR patients.

The above detailed mid-systolic differences in MV characteristics between IMR groups and controls were present in end-diastole and end-systole, too (Table 3).

Mitral valve dynamics in systole

In controls, we observed an increase in AP diameter, AL-PM diameter, intercommissural diameter, annulus

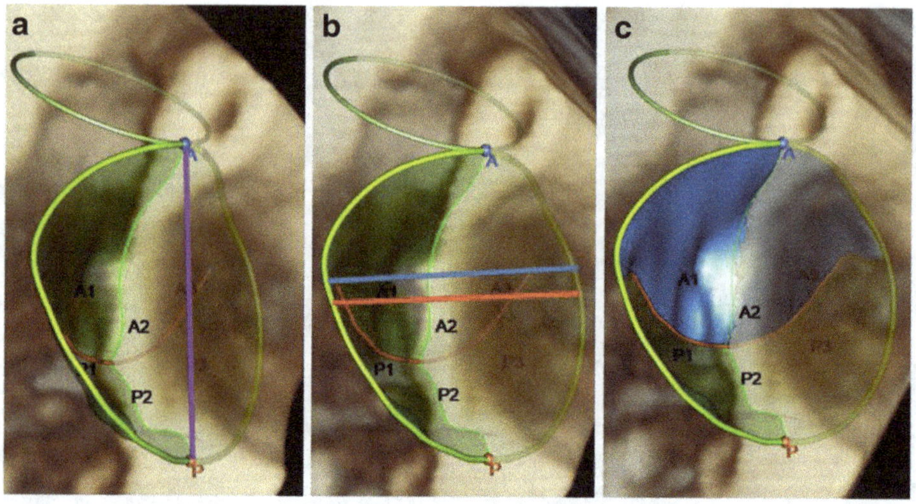

Fig. 2 Parameters of the mitral valve analysis. Anterior view of the mitral valve in mid-systole (3D TEE, surface rendering images). The semi-automated analysis of the mitral valve gives the following results: Panel **a**: scheme of the mitral valve including the mid-anterior point (blue dot), the mid-posterior point (red dot), the anterior-posterior diameter as distance between mid-anterior and mid-posterior point (purple line), and the circumference framing the annulus area (yellow circle line). Panel **b**: the anterolateral-posteromedial diameter gives the maximal distance in the horizontal plane (red line), and the intercommissural diameter gives the horizontal diameter at the commissures' insertion (blue line). Panel **c**: the anterior (blue) and posterior (green) leaflet area is defined as the area between the annulus and the coaptation line (red line) not including the part of the leaflets that form the coaptation zone

circumference and annulus area which primarily occurred in early systole (Table 3, Fig. 4). Furthermore, the anterior leaflet area increased homogenously during systole whereas the posterior leaflet area showed a slight but non-significant decrease in early systole (Table 3, Fig. 4).

The widening of the mitral annulus in early systole occurred in mMR as well, but it occurred later in sMR, which was associated with an increase in anterior leaflet area. A decrease in posterior leaflet area in early systole was seen in all three groups but reached significant values in sMR only.

Leaflet tenting volume and height decreased significantly in early systole in all three groups with a slight but insignificant increase in late systole. This was accompanied by flattening of the non-planar angle, which was most obvious in the sMR group.

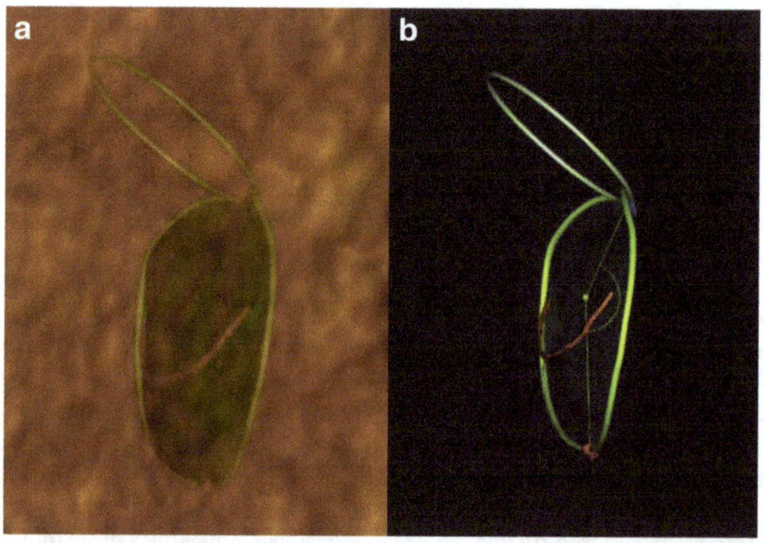

Fig. 3 Non-planar angle. Anterior view of the mitral valve in mid-systole: **a** 3D TEE surface rendering. **b** wire frame images. The non-planar angle is assessed as maximal level of "non-planarity" on the line between mid-anterior (blue) and mid-posterior (red) point

Table 1 Basic characteristics

	Normal	mMR	sMR	P-value		
	$N = 33$	$N = 18$	$N = 19$	Normal vs. mMR	Normal vs. sMR	mMR vs. sMR
Males (%)	42	61	47	ns	ns	ns
Age (years)	58 ± 16	64 ± 11	65 ± 10	ns	ns	ns
Height (cm)	172 ± 12	171 ± 10	166 ± 9	ns	ns	ns
Weight (kg)	82 ± 17	94 ± 20	78 ± 10	0.0394	ns	0.0133
BSA (m^2)	1.95 ± 0.25	2.05 ± 0.24	1.86 ± 0.15	ns	ns	0.0403
Frame rate (Hz)	23 ± 8	22 ± 4	25 ± 7	ns	ns	ns
LVEF (%)	60 ± 7	43 ± 18	38 ± 17	< 0.0001	< 0.0001	ns
LVEDD (mm)	36 ± 4	44 ± 8	46 ± 10	< 0.0001	< 0.0001	ns
WMA septal (%)	–	50	63	–	–	ns
WMA lateral (%)	–	33	74	–	–	0.0217
WMA inferior (%)	–	50	74	–	–	ns
WMA posterior (%)	–	28	58	–	–	ns
WMA anterior (%)	–	33	63	–	–	ns
WMA apical (%)	–	39	63	–	–	ns

mMR mild mitral regurgitation, *sMR* significant mitral regurgitation, vs. versus, *ns* not significant, *LVEF* left ventricular ejection fraction, *LVEDD* left ventricular end-diastolic diameter, *WMA* wall motion abnormalities

Discussion

To our knowledge, this is the first study reporting on the structural and functional dynamic modifications of the mitral valve in different grades of IMR, tracked from end-diastole to end-systole, and assessed by high resolution 3D TEE. The main findings of the present investigation were: 1) as compared to controls or patients with mild valve regurgitation, patients with significant IMR have a bidirectional dilated mitral annulus as well as an increase of the active area of both valve leaflets considered in absolute terms. Furthermore, this group of patients shows 2) loss of the normal mitral non-planar saddle shape, and 3) pronounced reduction of the active-posterior-leaflet-area in early systole as well as 4) delayed dynamic augmentation of the active-anterior-leaflet-area.

Table 2 Intra- and interobserver variability

MV Parameters	Coefficient of variation (%)	
	Interobserver	Intraobserver
AP diameter	4.5	4.5
AL-PM diameter	5.4	4.3
Non planar angle	1.8	3.1
Annulus circumference	4.4	4.2
Annulus area (3D)	9.0	8.3
Annular displacement	3.2	3.2
Annular displacement velocity	3.4	4.7
Anterior leaflet area	8.3	9.1
Posterior leaflet area	14.6	15.4

AP anterior-posterior, *AL-PM* anterolateral-posteromedial, *3D* three dimensional

We observed 37 patients with IMR and subdivided them by IMR severity. We pooled patients with moderate and severe IMR into one group (i.e., sMR) since it is this group for which mitral valve surgery in combination with coronary artery bypass surgery would be considered [23, 24]. By contrast, in subjects with mMR watchful waiting is advised. Both patient groups had a moderately decreased LVEF with similar LV dimensions and alteration of LV function. However, the frequency of wall motion abnormalities was higher in sMR with a preponderance of lateral LV wall hypokinesis and a posteriorly oriented regurgitation jet.

In our study, intra- and interobserver variability for one-dimensional measurements like annular diameters and circumference was excellent and was similar compared to other studies using semi-automated analysis software [9, 10, 25, 26]. The variability was higher for squared values like annulus and valve areas, where minimal measurement differences induce considerable variation.

Mitral valve annulus

Patients with mMR showed no significant differences in anatomical annular parameters (diameters, area and circumference) compared to controls, whereas these parameters were significantly larger in sMR. Applying the Pringle Principle, the significant increase in annular circumference and area in absence of difference in planarity in sMR indicates a real dilation of the mitral annulus, not only a change in shape. We further observed smaller absolute and relative intra-systolic changes in annulus area in both IMR groups as correlate for the mitral annulus' loss of motility, its ability to modify its shape throughout the

Table 3 Dynamic mitral valve characteristics in systole

MV Parameters	End-diastole			Mid-systole			End-systole		
	normal	mMR	sMR	normal	mMR	sMR	normal	mMR	sMR
AP diameter (cm)	2.60s ± 0.48	2.56 ± 0.48	3.18 ± 0.49[a,b]	2.75 ± 0.46[c]	2.75 ± 0.42[c]	3.25 ± 0.49[a,b,c]	2.78 ± 0.47	2.69 ± 0.41	3.33 ± 0.50[a,b,d]
AL-PM diameter (cm)	3.16 ± 0.50	3.21 ± 0.50	3.78 ± 0.62[a,b]	3.23 ± 0.49[c]	3.28 ± 0.46[c]	3.81 ± 0.61[a,b,c]	3.25 ± 0.49[d]	3.29 ± 0.47	3.83 ± 0.60[a,b,d]
Intercommissural diameter (cm)	3.11 ± 0.49	3.18 ± 0.49	3.72 ± 0.66[a,b]	3.18 ± 0.64[c]	3.25 ± 0.45[c]	3.72 ± 0.65[a,b]	3.20 ± 0.48[d]	3.26 ± 0.45	3.77 ± 0.64[a,b,d]
Annulus circumference (cm)	9.85 ± 1.54	9.59 ± 1.47	11.69 ± 1.99[a,b]	10.14 ± 1.47[c]	9.81 ± 1.29[c]	11.75 ± 1.92[a,b]	10.19 ± 1.49	9.85 ± 1.29	11.86 ± 1.94[a,b,d]
Annulus area 3D (cm^2)	7.23 ± 2.29	6.95 ± 2.11	10.40 ± 3.72[a,b]	7.71 ± 2.23[c]	7.27 ± 1.91[c]	10.56 ± 3.67[a,b]	7.82 ± 2.27	7.36 ± 1.91	10.82 ± 3.73[a,b,d]
Anterior leaflet area (cm^2)	4.65 ± 1.29	4.69 ± 1.56	7.23 ± 2.79[a,b]	4.82 ± 1.32[c]	4.75 ± 1.43	7.21 ± 2.78[a,b]	5.00 ± 1.44[d]	4.85 ± 1.42	7.44 ± 2.91[a,b,d]
Posterior leaflet area (cm^2)	3.78 ± 1.65	3.51 ± 1.33	5.36 ± 0.82 [a,b]	3.66 ± 1.51	3.40 ± 1.24	4.88 ± 1.94 [a,b,c]	3.79 ± 1.53	3.46 ± 1.22	5.01 ± 2.15[a,b]
Non planar angle (°)	143 ± 11	155 ± 10[a]	157 ± 10[a]	143 ± 11	154 ± 11[a]	157 ± 10[a]	144 ± 11[d]	155 ± 11[a,d]	160 ± 9[a,d]
Tenting volume (cm^3)	1.62 ± 0.96	1.82 ± 1.03	3.78 ± 2.13[a,b]	1.05 ± 0.89[c]	1.42 ± 0.82[c]	2.98 ± 1.76[a,b,c]	1.33 ± 1.12	1.50 ± 0.82	3.30 ± 2.15[a,b]
Tenting height (mm)	6.86 ± 2.17	6.39 ± 1.75	9.28 ± 2.10[a,b]	5.26 ± 1.80[c]	5.42 ± 1.82[c]	7.74 ± 2.25[a,b,c]	5.68 ± 2.14	5.39 ± 1.41	7.80 ± 2.56[a,b]

AP anterior-posterior, *AL-PM* anterolateral-posteromedial, *mMR* mild mitral regurgitation, *sMR* significant mitral regurgitation, *3D* three dimensional
[a]Significant difference compared to normal in the same phase of cardiac cycle ($p < 0.05$)
[b]Significant difference compared to mild MR in the same phase of cardiac cycle ($p < 0.05$)
[c]Significant difference compared to end-diastolic value in the same patient group ($p < 0.05$)
[d]Significant difference compared to mid-systolic value in the same patient group ($p < 0.05$)

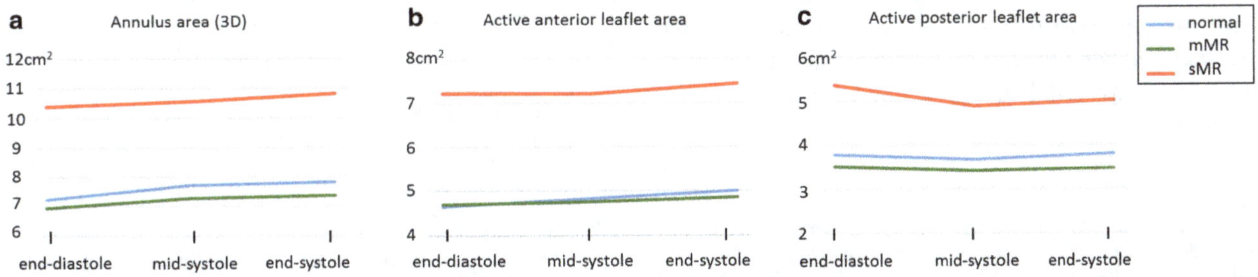

Fig. 4 Intrasystolic changes in **a** mitral valve annulus area as well as in **b** active anterior leaflet area and **c** active posterior leaflet area in patients with ischemic heart disease and functional mild (mMR) and significant (sMR = moderate and severe) mitral regurgitation compared to normal controls

cardiac cycle [9, 11, 13, 27], involving a flattening of the mitral annulus' non-planarity.

The dilation of the mitral annulus confirms reports of previous studies [9, 11, 13, 28] and is the basis of standard surgical treatment of functional MR using reduction annuloplasty with an undersized ring [2, 7]. Nevertheless, this treatment alone is not satisfying with persistently high recurrence rates [2, 5]. This brings forth the question, if, although imaging does not show any of the known abnormalities from degenerative valve disease, the leaflets are altered anyway and therefore significantly contribute to IMR severity and might be a target for successful treatment.

Mitral valve leaflets

Anterior and posterior leaflet areas were significantly larger in sMR compared to controls and mMR. This might be caused by mitral annular enlargement with subsequent augmentation of the leaflets' circumference but leaflet enlargement also occurs as response to hemodynamic stress and chronic tethering [12, 13, 29]. Despite leaflet augmentation, the leaflets' adaptation to the new situation does not seem to be sufficient in patients with sMR, and impaired leaflet adaptation rather than the increase in LV and MV size per se seems to cause IMR [30, 31].

The active-posterior-leaflet-area (measured in the closed MV from the annulus to the coaptation line) showed a decrease in early systole, non-significant in controls and mMR but significant in sMR, most probably due to tethering. In return, controls had a significant and homogenous increase in active-anterior-leaflet-area throughout systole, which occurred only in late systole in sMR. This systolic relocation of the coaptation zone with a posterior movement of the coaptation line in competent MVs implies an "anterior leaflet reserve" to compensate for the posterior movement [32, 33]. The MV is able to maintain competency until there is inadequate anterior leaflet coaptation length [33]. Though IMR is believed to be a primary response to ventricular remodeling, compromised anterior leaflet reserve or failure to increase the anterior leaflet area in sMR - as seen in our study - might be a key aspect in the development of moderate to severe mitral regurgitation in ischemic heart disease.

On the one hand, this finding should trigger the proceeding in the development of novel treatment options like surgical elongation of the anterior mitral leaflet [34] or application of neo-chordae in the presence of "pseudoprolapse" of the anterior leaflet [35] as addendum to conventional annuloplasty [36–39]. On the other hand, this finding seems worth the evaluation as a parameter for clinical decision making regarding the optimal treatment time point and treatment option in larger patient cohorts to achieve the best patient's outcome.

Limitations

Owing to the study design, we had no consistent information on the onset of coronary artery disease, i.e. the duration of the disease and the dynamic development of IMR and IMR severity. Further, not all patients had a recent angiogram, however, we were able to assess wall motion abnormalities as a surrogate of coronary artery disease in the TEE images. Lastly, the intra- and interobserver variability for "squared" parameters, which could be an important limitation for common and easily practical application of the software, was higher when compared to "simple" values but still in the range of previous reports [25].

Conclusions

In addition to a significant enlargement and loss in motility of the MV annulus, patients with significant IMR showed a spatio-temporal alteration of the mitral valve coaptation line due to a delayed increase in active-anterior-leaflet-area. This abnormality is likely to contribute to IMR severity and is worth the evaluation of becoming a parameter for clinical decision-making. Further, addressing the leaflets aiming to increase the active leaflet-area is a promising therapeutic approach for significant IMR. Our observations are based on a small but well characterized patient sample and should therefore be regarded hypothesis-generating; studies with a larger sample size and post-operative assessment are warranted to further validate our findings, explore their pathophysiologic etiology, and help understand the dynamics of the mitral valve.

Abbreviations

3D: Three-dimensional; AL-PM: Anterolateral-posteromedial; AP: Anterior-posterior; IMR: Ischemic mitral regurgitation; LV: Left ventricle; LVEF: Left ventricular ejection fraction; mMR: Mild mitral regurgitation; MV: Mitral valve; SD: Standard deviation; sMR: Significant mitral regurgitation; TEE: Transesophageal echocardiography; WMA: Wall motion abnormalities

Acknowledgements

We acknowledge the contribution of Berthold Klaas, employee of TomTec, who contributed to this project with technical support exceeding the custom support. We further thank Lynn Weinert from the University of Chicago, Chicago, IL, USA, as well as Irena Vaitkeviciute MD, Pramod Bonde MD, Abeel A. Mangi MD, and David Yuh MD from the Yale New Haven Hospital who all contributed to image acquisition and the scientific discussion of the study results.

Funding

The Comprehensive Heart Failure Center, Würzburg, is supported by the German Ministry of Research and Education within the (BMBF 01EO1004 and 01EO1504). This publication was funded by the German Research Foundation (DFG) and the University of Würzburg in the funding programme Open Access Publishing.

Authors' contributions

CM contributed to the conceptualization of the present study, performed the image and parts of the statistical analyses, and drafted the manuscript. DB performed the image double readings for quality control and parts of the statistical analyses, contributed to the scientific discussion and interpretation of the results, and reviewed the manuscript. SS contributed to the scientific discussion and interpretation of the results and reviewed the manuscript. LS contributed to the conceptualization of the present study, to image acquisition, to the scientific discussion and interpretation of the results, and reviewed the manuscript. All authors read and approved the final manuscript.

Competing interests

Analyses have been performed using custom software (ImageArena®, TomTec). Lissa Sugeng and Caroline Morbach are in research cooperation with TomTec. There is no further relationship like grants or personal honoraria. TomTec did not influence the analysis or interpretation of the study results. The other authors have no competing interests regarding this work.

Author details

[1]Yale School of Medicine, Section Cardiovascular Medicine, 330 Cedar Street, P.O Box 208017, New Haven, CT 06511, USA. [2]Comprehensive Heart Failure Center and Department of Internal Medicine I, University of Würzburg, Würzburg, Germany. [3]Istituto Mediterraneo per i Trapianti e Terapie ad Alta Specializzazione (IRCCS-ISMETT), Palermo, Italy.

References

1. Grigioni F, Enriquez-Sarano M, Zehr KJ, Bailey KR, Tajik AJ. Ischemic mitral regurgitation: long-term outcome and prognostic implications with quantitative Doppler assessment. Circulation. 2001;103:1759–64.
2. Timek TA, Miller DC. Another multidisciplinary look at ischemic mitral regurgitation. Semin Thorac Cardiovasc Surg. 2011;23:220–31.
3. Gillinov AM, Wierup PN, Blackstone EH, Bishay ES, Cosgrove DM, White J, et al. Is repair preferable to replacement for ischemic mitral regurgitation? J Thorac Cardiovasc Surg. 2001;122:1125–41.
4. Grossi EA, Goldberg JD, LaPietra A, Ye X, Zakow P, Sussman M, et al. Ischemic mitral valve reconstruction and replacement: comparison of long-term survival and complications. J Thorac Cardiovasc Surg. 2001;122:1107–24.
5. LaPar DJ, Acker MA, Gelijns AC, Kron IL. Repair or replace for severe ischemic mitral regurgitation: prospective randomized multicenter data. Ann Cardiothorac Surg. 2015;4:411–6.
6. Glower DD. Surgical approaches to mitral regurgitation. J Am Coll Cardiol. 2012;60:1315–22.
7. Acker MA, Parides MK, Perrault LP, Moskowitz AJ, Gelijns AC, Voisine P, et al. Mitral-valve repair versus replacement for severe ischemic mitral regurgitation. N Engl J Med. 2014;370:23–32.
8. Saito K, Okura H, Watanabe N, Obase K, Tamada T, Koyama T, et al. Influence of chronic tethering of the mitral valve on mitral leaflet size and coaptation in functional mitral regurgitation. JACC Cardiovasc Imaging. 2012;5:337–45.
9. Daimon M, Saracino G, Fukuda S, Koyama Y, Kwan J, Song JM, et al. Dynamic change of mitral annular geometry and motion in ischemic mitral regurgitation assessed by a computerized 3D echo method. Echocardiography. 2010;27:1069–77.
10. Daimon M, Saracino G, Gillinov AM, Koyama Y, Fukuda S, Kwan J, et al. Local dysfunction and asymmetrical deformation of mitral annular geometry in ischemic mitral regurgitation: a novel computerized 3D echocardiographic analysis. Echocardiography. 2008;25:414–23.
11. Veronesi F, Corsi C, Sugeng L, Caiani EG, Weinert L, Mor-Avi V, et al. Quantification of mitral apparatus dynamics in functional and ischemic mitral regurgitation using real-time 3-dimensional echocardiography. J Am Soc Echocardiogr. 2008;21:347–54.
12. Sprouse C, Mukherjee R, Burlina P. Mitral valve closure prediction with 3-D personalized anatomical models and anisotropic hyperelastic tissue assumptions. IEEE Trans Biomed Eng. 2013;60:3238–47.
13. Little SH, Ben Zekry S, Lawrie GM, Zoghbi WA. Dynamic annular geometry and function in patients with mitral regurgitation: insight from three-dimensional annular tracking. J Am Soc Echocardiogr. 2010;23:872–9.
14. Kwan J, Shiota T, Agler DA, Popovic ZB, Qin JX, Gillinov MA, et al. Geometric differences of the mitral apparatus between ischemic and dilated cardiomyopathy with significant mitral regurgitation: real-time three-dimensional echocardiography study. Circulation. 2003;107:1135–40.
15. Timek TA, Lai DT, Tibayan F, Liang D, Daughters GT, Dagum P, et al. Ischemia in three left ventricular regions: insights into the pathogenesis of acute ischemic mitral regurgitation. J Thorac Cardiovasc Surg. 2003;125:559–69.
16. Gorman JH 3rd, Gorman RC, Jackson BM, Hiramatsu Y, Gikakis N, Kelley ST, et al. Distortions of the mitral valve in acute ischemic mitral regurgitation. Ann Thorac Surg. 1997;64:1026–31.
17. Watanabe N, Ogasawara Y, Yamaura Y, Kawamoto T, Toyota E, Akasaka T, et al. Quantitation of mitral valve tenting in ischemic mitral regurgitation by transthoracic real-time three-dimensional echocardiography. J Am Coll Cardiol. 2005;45:763–9.
18. Watanabe N, Ogasawara Y, Yamaura Y, Yamamoto K, Wada N, Kawamoto T, et al. Geometric differences of the mitral valve tenting between anterior and inferior myocardial infarction with significant ischemic mitral regurgitation: quantitation by novel software system with transthoracic real-time three-dimensional echocardiography. J Am Soc Echocardiogr. 2006;19:71–5.
19. Nguyen TC, Itoh A, Carlhall CJ, Bothe W, Timek TA, Ennis DB, et al. The effect of pure mitral regurgitation on mitral annular geometry and three-dimensional saddle shape. J Thorac Cardiovasc Surg. 2008;136:557–65.
20. Nishimura RA, Otto CM, Bonow RO, Carabello BA, Erwin JP 3rd, Guyton RA, et al. 2014 AHA/ACC guideline for the management of patients with valvular heart disease: executive summary: a report of the American College of Cardiology/American Heart Association task force on practice guidelines. J Am Coll Cardiol. 2014;63(22):2438–88.
21. Mascherbauer J, Rosenhek R, Bittner B, Binder J, Simon P, Maurer G, et al. Doppler echocardiographic assessment of valvular regurgitation severity by measurement of the vena contracta: an in vitro validation study. J Am Soc Echocardiogr. 2005;18:999–1006.
22. Hahn RT, Abraham T, Adams MS, Bruce CJ, Glas KE, Lang RM, et al. Guidelines for performing a comprehensive transesophageal

echocardiographic examination: recommendations from the American Society of Echocardiography and the Society of Cardiovascular Anesthesiologists. J Am Soc Echocardiogr. 2013;26:921–64.
23. Chan KM, Punjabi PP, Flather M, Wage R, Symmonds K, Roussin I, et al. Coronary artery bypass surgery with or without mitral valve annuloplasty in moderate functional ischemic mitral regurgitation: final results of the randomized ischemic mitral evaluation (RIME) trial. Circulation. 2012;126:2502–10.
24. Daimon M, Fukuda S, Adams DH, McCarthy PM, Gillinov AM, Carpentier A, et al. Mitral valve repair with Carpentier-McCarthy-Adams IMR ETlogix annuloplasty ring for ischemic mitral regurgitation: early echocardiographic results from a multi-center study. Circulation. 2006;114:I588–93.
25. Veronesi F, Corsi C, Sugeng L, Mor-Avi V, Caiani EG, Weinert L, et al. A study of functional anatomy of aortic-mitral valve coupling using 3D matrix transesophageal echocardiography. Circ Cardiovasc Imaging. 2009;2:24–31.
26. Mihaila S, Muraru D, Miglioranza MH, Piasentini E, Peluso D, Cucchini U, et al. Normal mitral annulus dynamics and its relationships with left ventricular and left atrial function. Int J Cardiovasc Imaging. 2015;31:279–90.
27. Mihalatos DG, Joseph S, Gopal A, Bercow N, Toole R, Passick M, et al. Mitral annular remodeling with varying degrees and mechanisms of chronic mitral regurgitation. J Am Soc Echocardiogr. 2007;20:397–404.
28. Bartels K, Thiele RH, Phillips-Bute B, Glower DD, Swaminathan M, Kisslo J, et al. Dynamic indices of mitral valve function using perioperative three-dimensional transesophageal echocardiography. J Cardiothorac Vasc Anesth. 2014;28:18–24.
29. Dal-Bianco JP, Aikawa E, Bischoff J, Guerrero JL, Handschumacher MD, Sullivan S, et al. Active adaptation of the tethered mitral valve: insights into a compensatory mechanism for functional mitral regurgitation. Circulation. 2009;120:334–42.
30. Beaudoin J, Handschumacher MD, Zeng X, Hung J, Morris EL, Levine RA, et al. Mitral valve enlargement in chronic aortic regurgitation as a compensatory mechanism to prevent functional mitral regurgitation in the dilated left ventricle. J Am Coll Cardiol. 2013;61:1809–16.
31. Beaudoin J, Thai WE, Wai B, Handschumacher MD, Levine RA, Truong QA. Assessment of mitral valve adaptation with gated cardiac computed tomography: validation with three-dimensional echocardiography and mechanistic insight to functional mitral regurgitation. Circ Cardiovasc Imaging. 2013;6:784–9.
32. Zeng X, Nunes MC, Dent J, Gillam L, Mathew JP, Gammie JS, et al. Asymmetric versus symmetric tethering patterns in ischemic mitral regurgitation: geometric differences from three-dimensional transesophageal echocardiography. J Am Soc Echocardiogr. 2014;27:367–75.
33. Gogoladze G, Dellis SL, Donnino R, Ribakove G, Greenhouse DG, Galloway A, et al. Analysis of the mitral coaptation zone in normal and functional regurgitant valves. Ann Thorac Surg. 2010;89:1158–61.
34. Rabbah JP, Siefert AW, Bolling SF, Yoganathan AP. Mitral valve annuloplasty and anterior leaflet augmentation for functional ischemic mitral regurgitation: quantitative comparison of coaptation and subvalvular tethering. J Thorac Cardiovasc Surg. 2014;148:1688–93.
35. Hashim SW, Youssef SJ, Ayyash B, Rousou AJ, Ragnarsson S, Collazo S, et al. Pseudoprolapse of the anterior leaflet in chronic ischemic mitral regurgitation: identification and repair. J Thorac Cardiovasc Surg. 2012;143:S33–7.
36. Rendon F, Aramendi JI, Rodrigo D, Baraldi C, Martinez P. Patch enlargement of the posterior mitral leaflet in ischemic regurgitation. Asian Cardiovasc Thorac Ann. 2002;10:248–50.
37. Langer F, Rodriguez F, Cheng A, Ortiz S, Nguyen TC, Zasio MK, et al. Posterior mitral leaflet extension: an adjunctive repair option for ischemic mitral regurgitation? J Thorac Cardiovasc Surg. 2006;131:868–77.
38. Dobre M, Koul B, Rojer A. Anatomic and physiologic correction of the restricted posterior mitral leaflet motion in chronic ischemic mitral regurgitation. J Thorac Cardiovasc Surg. 2000;120:409–11.
39. de Varennes B, Chaturvedi R, Sidhu S, Cote AV, Shan WL, Goyer C, et al. Initial results of posterior leaflet extension for severe type IIIb ischemic mitral regurgitation. Circulation. 2009;119:2837–43.

22

Cardiac amyloidosis mimicking severe aortic valve stenosis – a case report demonstrating diagnostic pitfalls and role of dobutamine stress echocardiography

Tim Salinger[1,2], Kai Hu[1,2], Dan Liu[1,2], Sebastian Herrmann[1,2], Kristina Lorenz[3], Georg Ertl[1,2] and Peter Nordbeck[1,2,4*]

Abstract

Background: Aortic valve stenosis is a common finding diagnosed with high sensitivity in transthoracic echocardiography, but the examiner often finds himself confronted with uncertain results in patients with moderate pressure gradients and concomitant systolic heart failure. While patients with true-severe low-gradient aortic valve stenosis with either reduced or preserved left ventricular systolic function are primarily candidates for valve replacement, there is a relevant proportion of patients with pseudo-severe aortic valve stenosis anticipated not to benefit but actually rather deteriorate by interventional therapy or surgery.

Case presentation: In this article we present a case report of a male patient with pseudo-severe aortic valve stenosis due to cardiac amyloidosis highlighting the diagnostic schedule. The patient underwent stress echocardiography because of discrepant findings in transthoracic echocardiography and cardiac catheterization regarding the severity of aortic valve stenosis. After evaluation of the results, it became clear that he had a need for optimum heart failure medication and implantation of a cardiac resynchronization therapy defibrillator.

Conclusion: Due to the pitfalls in conventional as well as invasive diagnostics at rest, Stress echocardiography should be considered part of the standard optimum diagnostic spectrum in all unclear or borderline cases in order to confirm the correct diagnosis and constitute optimal therapy.

Keywords: Aortic valve stenosis (AS), Cardiac amyloidosis, Dobutamine stress echocardiography, Low-gradient AS, Pseudo-severe AS, Case report

Background

Stenosis of the aortic valve (AS) is the most common valvular disease in elderly persons today. Previous studies have reported prevalence for moderate or severe AS of 5–8% in a population older than 74 years [1, 2]. While current guidelines recommend conservative medical treatment in patients with mild and moderate AS [3], severe AS is highly recommended for surgical treatment especially in symptomatic patients, because of the poor prognosis of this disease entity in patients under conservative therapy [3, 4]. In elderly patients ≥80 years with severe AS, 3-year mortality has been described to be approximately 40% [5].

The diagnostic cornerstone in the differentiation between moderate and severe AS is transthoracic echocardiography. By convenient use of this widely available, non-invasive, and cost saving imaging technique, the experienced echocardiographer is able to determine the transvalvular pressure gradients and calculate the valve area with high diagnostic accuracy in most patients [3]. However, diagnostic accuracy can be considerably diminished in certain patients. This particularly refers to patients with a decreased left-ventricular-ejection-fraction (LVEF), occasionally leading to low transvalvular pressure gradients even if the opening area of the valve

* Correspondence: nordbeck_p@ukw.de
[1]Department of Internal Medicine I, University Hospital Würzburg, Würzburg, Germany
[2]Comprehensive Heart Failure Center (CHFC), University of Würzburg, Würzburg, Germany
Full list of author information is available at the end of the article

is indeed severely restricted, as e.g. confirmed by transesophageal echocardiography, usually referred to as low-gradient AS [6]. On the other hand, an echocardiographically confirmed severely diminished aortic valve opening area in this patient group might also be functional due to the profoundly reduced LV stroke volume leading to incomplete opening of the aortic valve, usually referred to as pseudo-severe AS [7]. Some patients may also have low aortic valve pressure gradient and severe AS, but preserved LVEF [8]. This so called paradoxical low-flow, low gradient AS is particularly difficult to diagnose and standard diagnostics often lead to false results and inadequate therapy [9]. While conclusive differentiation of the before mentioned disease entities is highly important for therapy planning in this patient group with high procedural risk during aortic valve replacement (AVR), it often represents a diagnostic dilemma for the cardiologist particularly in case of combined valvular diseases or myocardial comorbidities since even invasive measurements are often inconclusive in such cases.

Case presentation

An 82 year old male patient was referred to our cardiological department for treatment of aortic valve stenosis. The patient was in substantially reduced general condition with dyspnoe on insignificant loads (NYHA III) and edemas of hands and feet. Physical examination revealed a grade 3/6 systolic ejection murmur with radiation to the carotid arteries. There had been multiple hospitalizations in the past 6 month because of recurrent cardiac decompensations. Previously known comorbidities were chronic heart failure for unknown reason, atrial fibrillation, pulmonary hypertension and chronic obstructive pulmonary disease. Cardiovascular risk factors were arterial hypertension, diabetes, and former nicotine abuse. Biochemical tests revealed a moderately decreased glomerular filtration rate (54 ml/min/1.73qm), slightly increased creatinine (1.35 mg/dl) and increased high sensitivity troponin (98.5 pg/ml). NT-proBNP was 5473 pg/ml.

The patient underwent transthoracic echocardiography for staging severity of the aortic valve stenosis, which revealed borderline results (peak aortic jet velocity 2.8 m/s, mean aortic jet velocity 2.1 m/s, peak aortic pressure gradient 31 mmHG, mean aortic pressure gradient 19 mmHG, calculated aortic valve area 0.9 cm^2). Global left ventricular systolic function was highly reduced (LVEF Simpson 4CH = 29%), stroke volume index was 24 ml/qm. Global longitudinal strain was -7.3%. Apical sparing, which could be a sign for cardiac amyloidosis [10] was not present. Transthoracic echocardiography also revealed diastolic dysfunction (e = 1.01 m/s; e' septal = 0.03 m/s; e'lateral = 0.04 m/s; s'septal 0.02 m/s; s'lateral = 0.03 m/s, e/e' = 28.9). The left atrium was moderately, and the right atrium profoundly enlarged (35 cm^2 each, left atrial volume index 67.8 ml/qm). Chest X-ray showed a global enlarged heart, chronic pulmonary congestion, and right-sided pleural effusion (Fig. 1). Coronary angiography showed no significant coronary artery stenosis. Laevocardiography confirmed a highly reduced LVEF and a massively increased left ventricular end-diastolic pressure (33 mmHg), Right heart catheterization showed a normal cardiac output at rest (cardiac index 3.1 l/min*m^2) and post-capillary pulmonary hypertension (pulmonary artery mean pressure 44 mmHG, max 66 mmHg, pulmonary capillary wedge pressure 35 mmHG). Invasively measured aortic valve gradients were 25/16 (max/mean) mmHG and the aortic valve opening area was calculated as 1.9 cm^2. In transesophageal echocardiography, the opening area of the aortic valve was planimetrically determined as 0.8 cm^2, again indicating severe AS (Fig. 2).

Due to discrepant findings in echocardiography and cardiac catheterization regarding the severity of aortic valve stenosis, low-dose dobutamine stress echocardiography was performed (Fig. 3). At rest conditions, there was global hypokinesia with an ejection fraction of 33%. Aortic valve (AV) mean pressure was 16 mmHg referring to a calculated aortic valve opening area of 0,7 cm^2. Under peak dobutamine stress (20 mcg/kg/min), LVEF increased to 47% mean and mean AV pressure gradient to 23 mmHg. Left ventricular outflow tract velocity increased more than aortic valve velocity (LVOT/AV 0.2 at rest vs. 0.25 under stress) referring to an enlarged opening area of the aortic valve under stress conditions from 0.7 cm^2 to 1.1 cm^2. Stroke volume increased by 61.3% to 50 ml. On the basis of these diagnostic findings, AS was classified as pseudo-severe due to systolic dysfunction of the left ventricle with preserved contractile reserve, indicating a non-valvular reason for heart-failure and no indication for valve replacement.

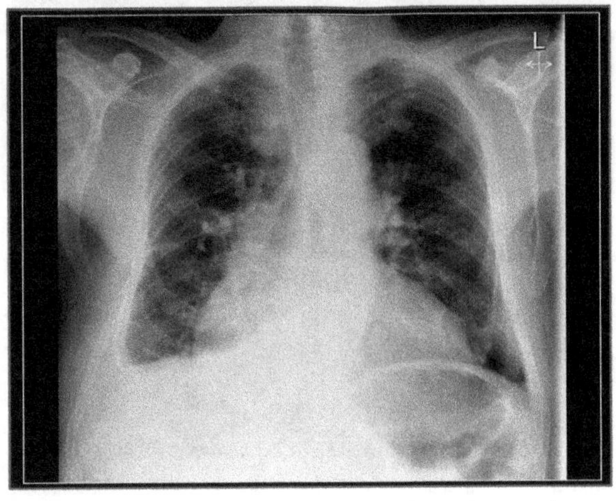

Fig. 1 Chest X-ray depicting a global enlarged heart, chronic pulmonary congestion, and right-sided pleural effusion

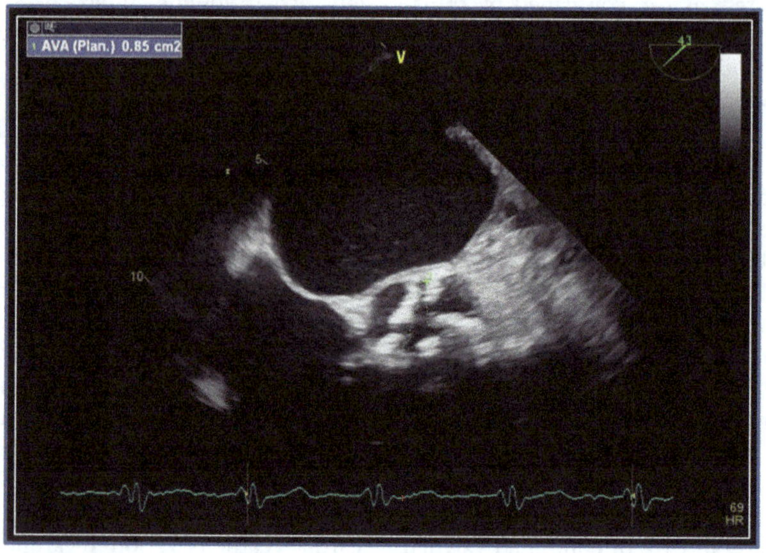

Fig. 2 Morphologic aspect of the aortic valve in transesophageal echocardiography. Aortic valve area is calculated as 0.85 cm^2 by planimetry

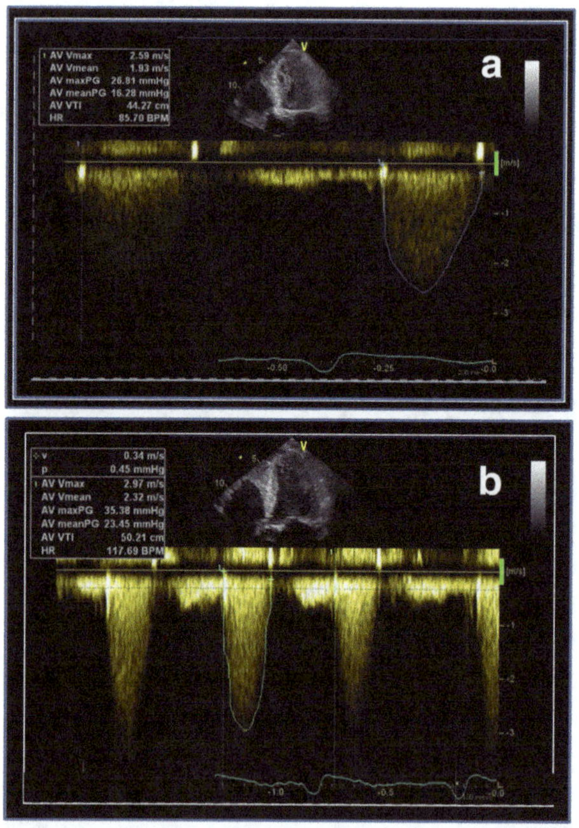

Fig. 3 **a** Stress echocardiography at rest conditions. AV mean pressure is calculated as 16 mmHg. **b** Under stress conditions (20 gamma dobutamine), AV mean pressure did not exceed 23 mmHg

Since the origin of the highly reduced LVEF was still unclear, cardiac MRI was performed, confirming global hypokinesia with a LVEF of 35% and revealing reduced myocardium-to-blood contrast, raising suspicion for presence of a cardiomyopathy (Fig. 4). An endomyocardial biopsy from the intraventricular septum in the right ventricular outflow tract was done, revealing multifocal interstitial transthyretin- related cardiac amyloidosis (ATTR). Because of a newly developed complete left bundle branch block in the ECG (Fig. 5) and the severely reduced LVEF, implantation of a cardiac resynchronization therapy defibrillator (CRT-D), was performed on top of optimum heart failure medication. Regrettably, at short- and medium-term follow-up echocardiography, LVEF did not show relevant improvement, although no signs of cardiac dyssynchrony could be found. However, NYHA improved to NYHA II and in the following 2-year period after device implantation, no more hospitalizations were required. Status of AS in follow-up transthoracic echocardiography 1 year later did not differ from baseline.

Discussion and conclusions

This clinical case highlights the potential value of dobutamine stress echocardiography in anticipated low-grade true-severe AS. After the initial echocardiography showing low LVEF, a mean valvular gradient <40 mmHg and a calculated valve area <1 cm^2, the patient was suspected to have low-flow, low-gradient aortic stenosis [3]. This disease entity would normally lead to valve replacement because of the potential benefits in terms of symptoms and survival gained from this procedure [3, 11], but should also be assessed very carefully when planning valve replacement. The American College of Cardiology recommends AVR for "symptomatic patients with severe

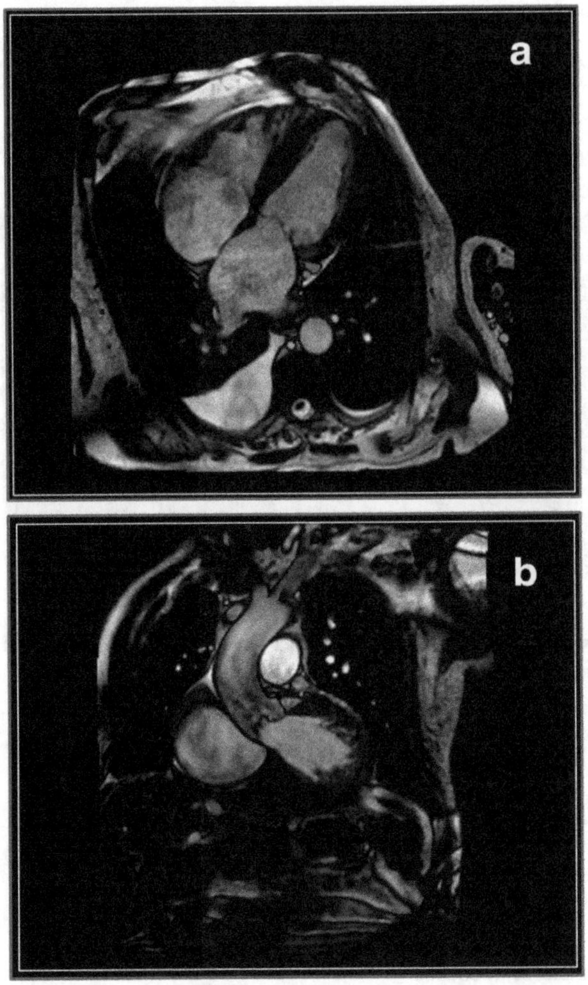

Fig. 4 a Native MRI, 4-chamber view, showing enlarged atria und left ventricular hypertrophy (LA 40 mm^2; RA 41 mm^2, lateral wall thickness 14 mm; septal wall thickness 16 mm) as signs of cardiac amyloidosis. **b** Morphologic aspect of the left ventricular outflow tract and aortic valve in MRI

AS and decreased systolic opening in calcified or congenitally stenotic aortic valves and an aortic velocity of >4.0 m/s or greater, or a mean pressure gradient of 40 mmHg or higher and symptoms of heart failure" [11]. However, in particular patients without contractile reserve have been shown to have exceedingly high operative mortality [12]. Differentiation between patients with low-flow, low-gradient stenosis and those with pseudo-severe stenosis can be very difficult in clinical practice since echocardiographic characteristics might differ only marginally at rest between both groups. Dobutamine stress echocardiography was first used as early as 1995 to distinguish these two subgroups. Based on the results from this study, it was already speculated that a broader use of this method might be clinically useful [13]. In 2001 it was first shown that clinical management of individuals with aortic stenosis and left ventricular dysfunction as well as low or intermediate valve gradients can indeed be improved by dobutamine stress echocardiography, because not only the distinction between patients with severe and non-severe aortic stenosis is improved, but this has indeed relevant implications on clinical outcome [14]. True-severe low-flow, low-gradient stenosis patients primarily benefit from AVR, since the valve itself is the main problem, whereas the primary pathology in pseudo-severe stenosis is located in the myocardium, requiring intensified conservative or specialized treatment based on the underlying disease [15].

In the present case, aortic stenosis of our patient could be clearly classified pseudo-severe by low dose dobutamine stress echocardiography. In the respective guidelines of the European Society of Cardiology, this procedure is not well established, but mentioned as potentially useful for the aforesaid diagnostic indication [3]. It is a widely-used, non-invasive method that can be done not only in-hospital but also in ambulatory patient care. Examination time is actually short and procedural risk has shown to be low [13]. Therefore, the net benefit greatly outweighs potential patient risks, justifying the investment in cases similar to the one described above.

Following stress-echocardiography, we performed cardiac MRI to reveal the origin of high-grade systolic dysfunction in our patient, revealing typical signs of an infiltrative cardiomyopathy such as late gadolinium enhancement [16] and dilated atria as well as a thickened septum and global left ventricular hypertrophy. High sensitive troponin was checked and turned out to be elevated. This serum biomarker has been shown to be a useful but non-specific diagnostic tool in various hereditary or secondary cardiomyopathies such as e.g. Sarcoidosis or Anderson-Fabry disease [17, 18]. In the described case, the final diagnosis ultimately clarifying the etiology of the pathological myocardial findings was made by endomyocardial biopsy from the right ventricle. Histological findings clearly revealed cardiac amyloidosis.

Amyloidosis is a systemic disease which can affect every organ, but especially cardiac involvement is a major determinant in patients prognosis [19]. In general, amyloidosis is considered a rare disease. However, there is a high probability of under-diagnosis particularly in elderly patients, where specific symptoms can be easily misinterpreted as an expression of advanced aging processes. Different studies have also shown that Amyloidosis and AS may occur together in a significant number of patients [20–23]. Today, several diagnostic tools are available to rule out whether a patient is indeed affected by cardiac amyloidosis, including the ECG, serum biomarkers, echocardiography, MRI and nuclear medicine imaging techniques [24, 25]. In cases where additional advanced imaging techniques are not available, standard echocardiographic

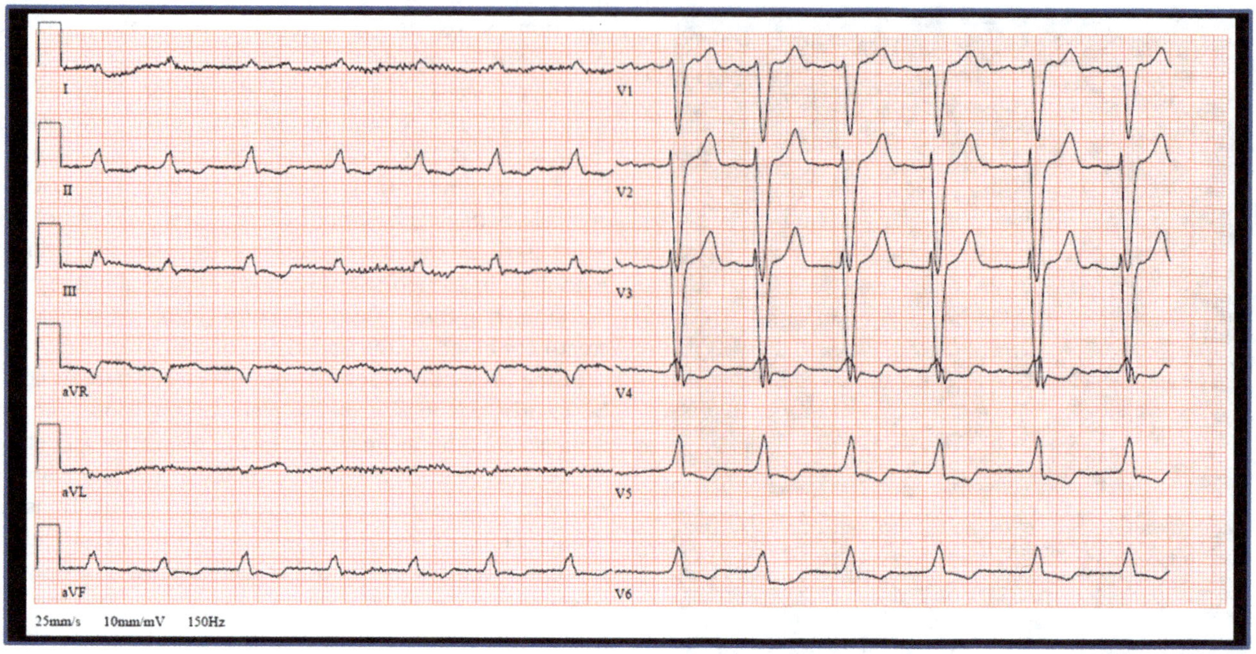

Fig. 5 ECG at admission shows atrial fibrillation at 78 bpm, left bundle branch block and signs of left ventricular hypertrophy

examinations can be expanded by speckle tracking analysis of left ventricular (systolic) function [26]. However, in order to come to a definite diagnosis, current guidelines recommend endomyocardial biopsy [27]. Guidelines for therapy also recommend intensified heart failure therapy in respective patients with mainly systolic dysfunction. However, the impact of device therapy such as CRT-D on top of medical therapy on symptoms and prognosis in cardiac amyloidosis is currently not well investigated.

The presented case highlights some important aspects and pitfalls in diagnosis and treatment of elderly patients with aortic valve stenosis transferred to hospital for aortic valve replacement. While the natural history of low-gradient aortic valve stenosis and concept of optimum therapy including valve replacement is generally better understood today, great care has to be taken not to exaggerate these findings to patients with pseudo-severe aortic valve stenosis. Stress echocardiography should be considered part of the standard optimum diagnostic spectrum in all unclear or borderline cases in order to confirm the correct diagnosis and constitute optimal therapy.

Abbreviations

AS: Aortic stenosis; AV: Aortic valve; AVR: Aortic valve replacement; CRT-D: Cardiac resynchronization therapy defibrillator; LVEF: Left- ventricular- ejection- fraction

Acknowledgements

Not applicable.

Funding

This work was supported by the Federal Ministry for Education and Research of the Federal Republic of Germany (BMBF 01EO1504, MO6 to Peter Nordbeck). There was no role of the funding body in the design of the study and collection, analysis, and interpretation of data and in writing the manuscript.

Authors' contributions

Conception and design: TS, PN; analysis and interpretation of data: TS, KH, DL, SH, KL, GE PN; drafting the article: TS, PN; revising the article: TS, KH, DL, SH, KL, GE, PN. All authors read and approved the final manuscript.

Competing interests

The authors declare that they have no competing interests.

Author details

[1]Department of Internal Medicine I, University Hospital Würzburg, Würzburg, Germany. [2]Comprehensive Heart Failure Center (CHFC), University of Würzburg, Würzburg, Germany. [3]Leibniz-Institut für Analytische Wissenschaften – ISAS, University Duisburg-Essen, Dortmund, Germany. [4]Medizinische Klinik und Poliklinik I – Kardiologie, Universitätsklinikum Würzburg, Oberdürrbacher Str. 6, 97080 Würzburg, Germany.

References

1. Nkomo VT, et al. Burden of valvular heart diseases: a population-based study. Lancet. 2006;368(9540):1005–11.
2. Lindroos M, et al. Prevalence of aortic valve abnormalities in the elderly: an echocardiographic study of a random population sample. J Am Coll Cardiol. 1993;21(5):1220–5.
3. Joint Task Force on the Management of Valvular Heart Disease of the European Society of, C, et al. Guidelines on the management of valvular heart disease (version 2012). Eur Heart J. 2012;33(19):2451–96.
4. Horstkotte D, Loogen F. The natural history of aortic valve stenosis. Eur Heart J. 1988;9(Suppl E):57–64.

5. Rezzoug N, et al. Prevalence and Prognostic Impact of Valve Area-Gradient Patterns in Patients >/=80 Years With Moderate-to-Severe Aortic Stenosis (from the Prospective BELFRAIL Study). Am J Cardiol. 2015;116(6):925–32.
6. Herrmann S, et al. Differences in natural history of low- and high-gradient aortic stenosis from nonsevere to severe stage of the disease. J Am Soc Echocardiogr. 2015;28(11):1270–82. e4.
7. Fougeres E, et al. Outcomes of pseudo-severe aortic stenosis under conservative treatment. Eur Heart J. 2012;33(19):2426–33.
8. Kamperidis V, et al. Low gradient severe aortic stenosis with preserved ejection fraction: reclassification of severity by fusion of Doppler and computed tomographic data. Eur Heart J. 2015;36(31):2087–96.
9. Pibarot P, Dumesnil JG. Aortic stenosis suspected to be severe despite low gradients. Circ Cardiovasc Imaging. 2014;7(3):545–51.
10. Phelan D, et al. Relative apical sparing of longitudinal strain using two-dimensional speckle-tracking echocardiography is both sensitive and specific for the diagnosis of cardiac amyloidosis. Heart. 2012;98(19):1442–8.
11. Nishimura RA, et al. 2014 AHA/ACC guideline for the management of patients with valvular heart disease: a report of the American College of Cardiology/American Heart Association Task Force on Practice Guidelines. J Thorac Cardiovasc Surg. 2014;148(1):e1–e132.
12. Monin J-L, et al. Low-Gradient Aortic Stenosis: Operative Risk Stratification and Predictors for Long-Term Outcome: A Multicenter Study Using Dobutamine Stress Hemodynamics. Circulation. 2003;108(3):319–24.
13. de Filippi CR, et al. Usefulness of dobutamine echocardiography in distinguishing severe from nonsevere valvular aortic stenosis in patients with depressed left ventricular function and low transvalvular gradients. Am J Cardiol. 1995;75(2):191–4.
14. Schwammenthal E, et al. Dobutamine echocardiography in patients with aortic stenosis and left ventricular dysfunction: predicting outcome as a function of management strategy. Chest. 2001;119(6):1766–77.
15. Clavel MA, et al. Validation of Conventional and Simplified Methods to Calculate Projected Valve Area at Normal Flow Rate in Patients with Low Flow, Low Gradient Aortic Stenosis. The Multicenter TOPAS (True Or Pseudo Severe Aortic Stenosis) Study. Cardiology. 2010;115(4):258.
16. Bejar D, et al. Infiltrative Cardiomyopathies. Clin Med Insights Cardiol. 2015;9 Suppl 2:29–38.
17. Baba Y, et al. Usefulness of high-sensitive cardiac troponin T for evaluating the activity of cardiac sarcoidosis. Int Heart J. 2012;53(5):287–92.
18. Seydelmann N, et al. High-Sensitivity Troponin: A Clinical Blood Biomarker for Staging Cardiomyopathy in Fabry Disease. J Am Heart Assoc. 2016;5(6). doi:10.1161/JAHA.115.002839.
19. Patel KS, Hawkins PN. Cardiac amyloidosis: where are we today? J Intern Med. 2015;278(2):126–44.
20. Longhi S, et al. Coexistence of Degenerative Aortic Stenosis and Wild-Type Transthyretin-Related Cardiac Amyloidosis. JACC Cardiovasc Imaging. 2016; 9(3):325–7.
21. Nietlispach F, et al. Pathology of transcatheter valve therapy. JACC Cardiovasc Interv. 2012;5(5):582–90.
22. Galat A, et al. Aortic stenosis and transthyretin cardiac amyloidosis: the chicken or the egg? Eur Heart J. 2016;37(47):3525–3531.
23. Treibel TA, et al. Occult Transthyretin Cardiac Amyloid in Severe Calcific Aortic Stenosis: Prevalence and Prognosis in Patients Undergoing Surgical Aortic Valve Replacement. Circ Cardiovasc Imaging. 2016;9(8). doi:10.1161/CIRCIMAGING.116.005066.
24. Di Bella G, et al. The mosaic of the cardiac amyloidosis diagnosis: role of imaging in subtypes and stages of the disease. Eur Heart J Cardiovasc Imaging. 2014;15(12):1307–15.
25. Hu K, et al. Impact of monitoring longitudinal systolic strain changes during serial echocardiography on outcome in patients with AL amyloidosis. Int J Cardiovasc Imaging. 2015;31(7):1401–12.
26. Ternacle J, et al. Causes and Consequences of Longitudinal LV Dysfunction Assessed by 2D Strain Echocardiography in Cardiac Amyloidosis. JACC Cardiovasc Imaging. 2016;9(2):126–38.
27. Quarta CC, Kruger JL, Falk RH. Cardiac amyloidosis. Circulation. 2012; 126(12):e178–82.

23

Acute myocardial infarction after blunt chest wall trauma with underlying coronary aneurysm

Xu Guo[1], Xiaoou Wang[1], Xinzhong Zhang[1], Ahmed O. Ahmed[1], David H. Hsi[2] and Daqing Zhang[1*]

Abstract

Background: Kawasaki disease is an acute febrile disease with mucocutaneous and cardiovascular involvement affecting infants and young children. Though coronary artery abnormalities are common in Kawasaki disease, no consensus has been reached regarding the treatment of acute coronary artery diseases in this population.

Case presentation: We described a case of myocardial infarction triggered by blunt chest wall trauma in a 20 years old girl. She presented with chest pain and breathlessness with brief syncope, lab results and electrocardiogram findings were consistent with acute myocardial infarction. Chest computer tomography (CT) demonstrated coronary artery calcifications and echocardiography revealed multiple giant left anterior descending aneurysms, suggestive of Kawasaki disease. Subsequent contrast enhanced 3 dimensional coronary computer tomography angiography (CTA) confirmed these findings. We managed this young patient with a conservative strategy. The patient remained symptom free during 2-years follow-ups.

Conclusions: Prompt medical treatment for traumatic myocardial infarction even with underlying giant coronary artery aneurysms can successfully preserve left ventricular function and prevent remodeling with good short term prognosis.

Keywords: Coronary artery aneurysm, Kawasaki disease, Acute coronary syndrome, Echocardiography

Background

Kawasaki disease (KD) is an acute febrile disease with mucocutaneous involvement affecting infants and young children first described in Japan in 1967 [1]. Later, KD was found to target coronary arteries and other cardiovascular structures, making the patients vulnerable to coronary artery aneurysms (CAA) and thrombosis [2]. No consensus has been reached regarding the treatment for acute coronary syndrome (ACS) in this population. Here we describe a case of myocardial infarction (MI) triggered by blunt chest wall trauma in a 20-year old patient with possible underlying KD.

* Correspondence: zhangdaqing@vip.163.com
[1]Department of Cardiology, Shengjing Hospital of China Medical University, #36 Sanhao Street, Heping district, Shenyang City, Liaoning Province 110004, People's Republic of China
Full list of author information is available at the end of the article

Case presentation

A 20-year-old female patient presented to our hospital with a history of severe and dull substernal chest pain and breathlessness after being hit by a baseball to her chest 2 h ago. Immediately after being hit, she had an episode of syncope briefly without convulsion. The symptoms lasted for half-an-hour and resolved spontaneously. Her vital signs showed blood pressure of 95/64 mmHg and pulse of 70 beats/minute. There was no sign of chest wall penetrating injury. Electrocardiogram (ECG) revealed sinus rhythm with QS complexes in leads V2 to V3, ST segment elevation and T-wave inversion in leads V2 to V5 (Fig. 1a). Laboratory tests showed cardiac Troponin I level of 19.03 ng/ml (normal range < 0.01 ng/ml). Chest computer tomography (CT) revealed no traumatic injury but demonstrated coronary artery calcifications (Fig. 2a). Her parents recalled a history of high fever lasting for several days at the age of 5-year-old. The patient was admitted to our hospital diagnosed of acute traumatic MI. Serum Troponin I was peaked to 20.3 ng/ml, creatine phosphokinase(CK) to 1237 U/L and CK-MB to 101 U/L 12 h after

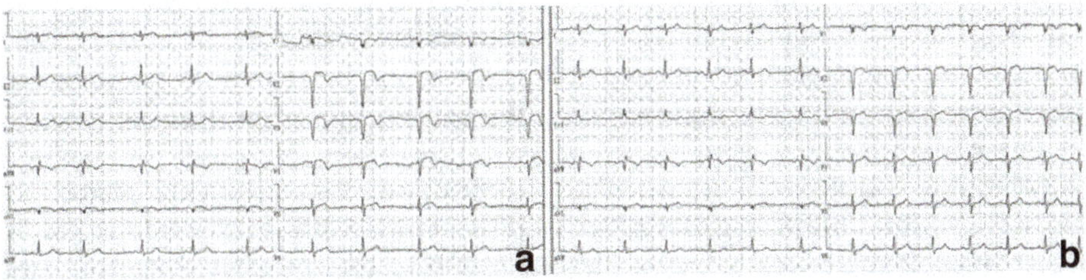

Fig. 1 Dynamic ECG changes after blunt chest wall trauma. **a** ECG on admission: sinus rhythm with QS complexes in leads V2 to V3, ST segment elevations and T-wave inversions in leads V2 to V5. **b** ECG at the 2-month follow-up: leads V2 and V3 with QS complex and resolution of the other acute changes

admission. Serum BNP level was normal at 85.9 pg/ml on admission. During hospitalization, serial ECG changes were consistent with an evolving MI. She had frequent ventricular premature beats on the Holter monitor. Trans-thoracic echocardiography revealed normal left ventricular size and mild anterior hypokinesis. Notably, multiple giant left anterior descending (LAD) aneurysms with diameters from 7.5 to 8.5 mm (Fig. 2b) and slow flow velocity were detected. To further assess CAA, we performed contrast enhanced coronary artery computer tomography angiography (CTA)with three-dimensional (3-D)reconstruction of coronary arteries. A ringed calcification in the proximal portion of LAD artery with multiple aneurysms, thrombi and occlusions were visualized (Fig. 2c). CTA also demonstrated multiple aneurysms with beads-on-string appearance in the LAD artery (Fig. 2d). Antinuclear antibody (ANA) was minimally positive (1:10) with unknown significance. Serum levels of C3 (0.864 g/L), C4 (0.912 g/L), CRP (< 1.0 mg/L), ASO (< 25 IU/ml), ESR (15 mm/h), Rheumatoid Factor (< 25 IU/ml) and ANCA were within normal ranges. Those results did not seem to support active vasculitis, rheumatic or immunologic diseases. Based on the typical images and her childhood fever history, we recognized that the patient's underlying coronary structural abnormality was most likely originated from KD. Considering stable hemodynamic parameters and multiple giant aneurismal dilatations of LAD artery, we managed this young patient with a conservative strategy including dual anti-platelet treatment with aspirin and

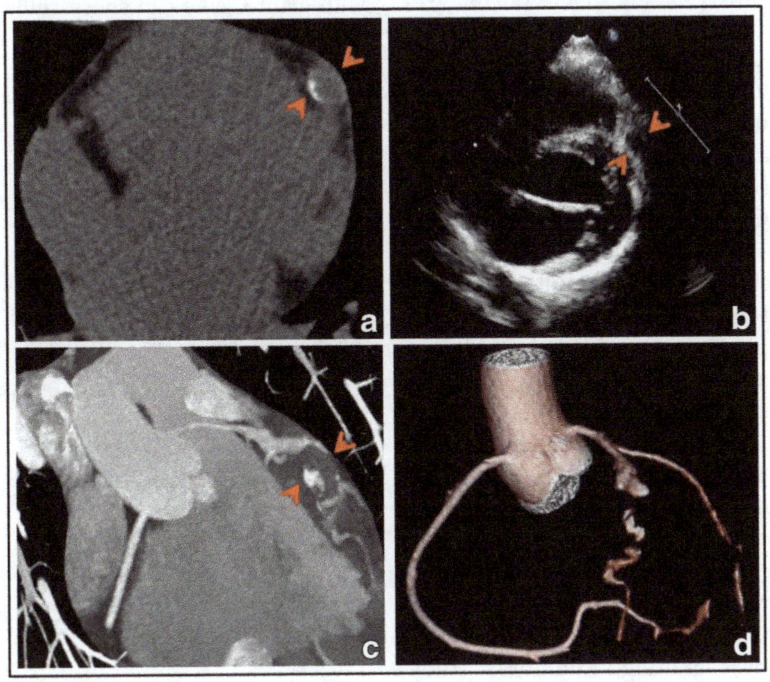

Fig. 2 Coronary artery aneurysm of the left anterior descending artery. **a** Chest computer tomography (CT): ringed calcification with 9.8 mm diameter in the left anterior descending (LAD) artery. **b** Trans-thoracic echocardiography: the proximal aneurismal dilation of the LAD artery. **c** Coronary CT angiography(CTA) image in orthogonal plane: LAD artery aneurysm. **d** Coronary CTA with three-dimensional volume rendering: multiple giant aneurysms with lumen occlusion and distal re-canalization in the LAD artery (arrows)

clopidogrel for at least 1 year, and titrations of captopril and metoprolol to prevent ventricular remodeling. At the 2-month follow-up, the patient remained asymptomatic. ECG showed QS complex only in V2 and V3 leads and other abnormalities were resolved (Fig. 1b). Echocardiography revealed left ventricular diastolic dimension of 48 mm, normal LAD artery velocity, and no ventricular dilatation or akinesis. She remained asymptomatic two year later.

Discussion and conclusions

According to the third universal definition of myocardial infarction [3], the patient's present history, dynamic ECG changes, increased serum myocardial biomarkers, and typical coronary artery images were consistent with an acute traumatic MI. Her syncope might have been due to ventricular arrhythmia when the baseball hit her left chest at the vulnerable period of cardiac cycle mimicking commotio cordis. MI after blunt trauma to the chest is a rare clinical condition. The potential mechanisms include coronary artery intimal tearing and hemorrhage, thrombosis and coronary atherosclerotic plaque rupture. The LAD artery has been reported as the most commonly involved coronary artery during blunt trauma. Considering the patient's stable condition, we performed coronary CTA with 3-D reconstruction. The 3-D coronary CTA images showed this young patient with underlying coronary structural abnormality, which had made her vulnerable for the traumatic MI. Importantly, the large aneurysm calcification in the proximal portion of LAD artery is a typical manifestation of KD [4]. Although coronary angiography, thrombus aspiration and stent placement have been reported to successfully treat patients in critical conditions, serious postoperative complications have also been reported [5, 6]. Giant CAA >8 mm and large thrombus usually cause underestimation of the diameter or the morphological characteristics, resulting in new aneurysm formation, stent malposition and recurrent thrombosis after stent implantation [7, 8]. In addition, the most commonly used stent in the presence of CAAs is polytetrafluoroethylene(PTFE) membrane covered stent, which has high incidence of restenosis, delayed graft reendothelization, neointimal hyperplasia and side branch occlusion [9]. Thus, the long-term outcome of percutaneous intervention in this population is unpredictable. In young patients, it may be prudent to avoid emergent interventional approach except in life-threatening situations requiring rescue operation. As for coronary artery bypass grafting, Kitamura's study demonstrated that cardiac event-free rate at 20 and 25 years were only 67 and 60%, respectively [10]. Considering this patient was young and stable, we recommended a conservative strategy with close follow-up. Interestingly, the ECG changes were eventually improved. Echocardiography also showed normal LAD velocity during the 2-month follow-up. We postulated that the patient might have had spontaneous coronary recanalization after the onset of acute MI. Spontaneous recanalization(SR) in AMI might influence the ECG presentation with smaller infarct size and a better prognosis [11, 12]. At this point, the patient is doing well without any post-MI complications.

If the KD in childhood was not treated early with high-dose intravenous immunoglobulin, 1 in 5 children with KD might develop CAA [13]. Although vascular aneurysms associated with KD in childhood may remain clinically silent until adulthood, stenosis and occlusion could progress over years. Angiographic results show that 90% of patients with CAA mostly involved the LAD artery. Risk of MI from KD is peaked in the first 2 years after the initial presentation [14]. However, our patient suffered an acute anterior-septal MI with LAD artery thrombosis at her 20 years of age. We do want to point out the limitation in this patient's history of febrile illness which could have been due to many other etiologies than KD, in spite of the typical coronary artery aneurysms on the CTA.

It is important to increase the awareness of early identification and appropriate treatment of KD in childhood, which can reduce their future risks of CAAs and MI. Additionally, prompt medical treatment for traumatic MI even with giant CAAs can successfully preserve left ventricular function and prevent remodeling with good prognosis.

Abbreviations

ACS: Acute coronary syndrome; ANA: Antinuclear antibody; CAA: Coronary artery aneurysms; CK: Creatine phosphokinase; CT: Computer tomography; ECG: Electrocardiogram; KD: Kawasaki disease; LAD: Left anterior descending; MI: Myocardial infarction

Authors' contributions

DQZ designed the research protocol. DQZ, XG and AOA analyzed and interpreted the data, drafted the manuscript and made critical revision of the manuscript for important intellectual content. DQZ, XG,XOW and XZZ collected the patient data. DHH provided consultation, participated in the design and coordination of the manuscript. All authors read and approved the final manuscript.

Competing interests

The authors declare that they have no competing interests.

Author details

[1]Department of Cardiology, Shengjing Hospital of China Medical University, #36 Sanhao Street, Heping district, Shenyang City, Liaoning Province 110004, People's Republic of China. [2]Heart& Vascular Institute, Stamford Hospital, Stamford, CT 06904, USA.

References

1. Kawasaki T. Acute febrile mucocutaneous syndrome with lymphoid involvement with specific desquamation of the fingers and toes in children. Arerugi = [Allergy]. 1967;16(3):178–222.

2. Kawasaki T, Kosaki F, Okawa S, Shigematsu I, Yanagawa H. A new infantile acute febrile mucocutaneous lymph node syndrome (MLNS) prevailing in Japan. Pediatrics. 1974;54(3):271–6.
3. Thygesen K, Alpert JS, Jaffe AS, Simoons ML, Chaitman BR, White HD, Katus HA, Lindahl B, Morrow DA, Clemmensen PM, et al. Third universal definition of myocardial infarction. Circulation. 2012;126(16):2020–35.
4. McCrindle BW, Rowley AH, Newburger JW, Burns JC, Bolger AF, Gewitz M, Baker AL, Jackson MA, Takahashi M, Shah PB, et al. Diagnosis, treatment, and long-term Management of Kawasaki Disease: a scientific statement for health professionals from the American Heart Association. Circulation. 2017; 135(17):e927-e999.
5. Sawai T, Tanigawa T, Masuda J, Yamada N, Miyahara M, Nakamura M, Ito M. New coronary aneurysm formation and malapposition after zotarolimus-eluting stent implantation in Kawasaki disease. J Cardiol Cases. 2013;8(3):118–20.
6. Gordon JB, Daniels LB, Kahn AM, Jimenez-Fernandez S, Vejar M, Numano F, Burns JC. The Spectrum of cardiovascular lesions requiring intervention in adults after Kawasaki disease. Jacc Cardiovasc Interv. 2016;9(7):687–96.
7. Lolay GA, Abdel-Latif AK. Trauma induced myocardial infarction. Int J Cardiol. 2016;203:19–21.
8. Tsuda E. Intervention in adults after Kawasaki disease. JACC Cardiovasc Interv. 2016;9(7):697–9.
9. Bitigen A, Cevik C, Turan B, Otahbachi M. Use of PTFE-covered stent in acute myocardial infarction of aneurysmatic coronary artery. Int J Cardiol. 2009;132(2):e72–3.
10. Kitamura S, Tsuda E, Kobayashi J, Nakajima H, Yoshikawa Y, Yagihara T, Kada A. Twenty-five-year outcome of pediatric coronary artery bypass surgery for Kawasaki disease. Circulation. 2009;120(1):60–8.
11. Lee CW, Hong MK, Lee JH, Yang HS, Kim JJ, Park SW, Park SJ. Determinants and prognostic significance of spontaneous coronary recanalization in acute myocardial infarction. Am J Cardiol. 2001;87(8):951–4. a953
12. Abo Y, Yokoi H, Furuta T, Kondo T, Inami O, Kakizawa S, Fujiwara W, Tamura K, Nomura M, Watanabe Y. Electrocardiographic diagnosis of the coronary artery culprit site in ischemic heart disease. Circ J. 2003;67(9):775–80.
13. Newburger JW, Takahashi M, Burns JC. Kawasaki Disease. J Am Coll Cardiol. 2016;67(14):1738–49.
14. Suda K, Iemura M, Nishiono H, Teramachi Y, Koteda Y, Kishimoto S, Kudo Y, Itoh S, Ishii H, Ueno T, et al. Long-term prognosis of patients with Kawasaki disease complicated by giant coronary aneurysms: a single-institution experience. Circulation. 2011;123(17):1836–42.

Prevalence and characteristics of primary left-sided valve disease in a cohort of 15,000 patients undergoing echocardiography studies in a tertiary hospital in Uganda

Joselyn Rwebembera[1*], William Manyilirah[1], Zhang Wan Zhu[1], Juliet Nabbaale[1], Judith Namuyonga[1,2], Isaac Ssinabulya[1,2], Sulaiman Lubega[1], Peter Lwabi[1,2], John Omagino[1] and Emmy Okello[1,2]

Abstract

Background: Although rheumatic heart disease remains the leading cause of valve heart disease (VHD) in developing countries, other forms of valve disease have been over shadowed and not regarded as a public health problem. However, several facts suggest that the role of non-rheumatic VHD as a significant cardiovascular disease should be reconsidered. We aimed to assess the prevalence and characteristics of different forms of primary left sided valve diseases from a series of 15,009 echocardiographic studies.

Methods: This was a retrospective review of echocardiographic reports for studies performed between January 2012 and December 2013 (24 months) at Uganda Heart Institute. All patients with primary left-sided valve disease were classified into one of five major diagnostic categories and in each diagnostic category; patients were sub-classified into stages A-D of primary valve disease as defined by the American College of Cardiology.

Results: Three thousand five hundred eighty-two echocardiography reports qualified for final data analysis. The "sclerotic valve changes with normal valve function", a Stage A sub-class of "degenerative valve disease" overwhelmingly overshadowed all the other diagnostic categories in this stage. "Rheumatic Heart Disease", "Degenerative Valve Disease", "Bicuspid Aortic Valve", "Mitral Valve Prolapse" and "Endomyocardial Fibrosis" diagnostic categories accounted for 53.0%, 41.8%, 2.2%, 1.4% and 1.7% respectively in stages B-D of primary VHD. Rheumatic heart disease disproportionately affected the young, productive age groups. It was the major risk factor for infective endocarditis; and was the indication for valve surgery in 44 of 50 patients who had undergone valve replacement procedures.

Conclusions: We acknowledge that rheumatic heart disease remains a leading cause of progressive and severe primary left-sided valve disease among young adults in Uganda. But we bring to light the contemporary footprints of other forms of primary valve disease that require coordinated multidisciplinary approach to research, education and clinical management to ensure improved patient outcomes.

Keywords: Primary, Left-sided, Valve disease, Rheumatic, Non-rheumatic, Uganda

* Correspondence: joselynr36@gmail.com
[1]Uganda Heart Institute, Kampala, Uganda
Full list of author information is available at the end of the article

Background

Valvular heart disease is classically predominated by rheumatic heart disease (RHD) in the young in low-resource settings and by calcific aortic valvluar disease in the elderly in high-resource settings [1–3]. In the last decade, studies from across the African continent have begun to provide a better understanding of RHD across the continent, with important advances in epidemiology, diagnosis, and outcomes [4–11].

However, the last two decades have witnessed a substantial increase in life expectancy in sub-Saharan Africa [12], and more of the population is living past the 7th decade of life. It stands to reason that the etiology of valvular heart disease may also be shifting, as has been documented in middle-income countries [13–15].

The Uganda Heart Institute (UHI) provides cardiology tertiary referral for the country of Uganda, with diagnostic echocardiography and both pediatric and adult cardiologists with expertise in echocardiographic performance and interpretation. The objective of this study was to classify the burden of primary left-sided valvular heart disease across the lifespan in Uganda, through retrospective study of a large cohort of patients evaluated at UHI over a two-year period.

Methods

Study design

This was a retrospective review of echocardiographic reports for studies performed between January 2012 and December 2013 (24 months) at UHI.

Study site

UHI is a specialized tertiary centre for cardiovascular care in Uganda, located within Mulago Hospital Complex, the country's national referral hospital and teaching hospital for Makerere University Medical School. The adult (≥ 13 years) echocardiography laboratory serves approximately 10,000 patients per year with three fully functional echocardiography machines (2 x GE medical Systems Vivid 7 Dimension - GE Vingmed Ultrasound AS N-3190 Horten, Norway and 1 x Phillips IE33 – Phillips Ultrasound Bothell WA, 98041 USA).

Study population

The study population consisted of adults who had an echocardiogram performed at UHI during the study period. Only the first echocardiographic report from each patient during the study period was utilized for data collection. Retrospective echo report review was performed for all patients ≥13 years. Patients with an incomplete echocardiography report, those found to have no structural heart disease, those with unclear etiology of valvular disease, those with secondary/functional left-sided valvular regurgitation and those with non-valvular cardiac structural abnormalities were excluded from further data analysis (Fig. 1).

Echocardiography procedures

Echocardiograms were performed by adult cardiologists or cardiology fellows in accordance with the American Society of Echocardiography guidelines [16, 17]. Although these echocardiographic studies were performed in 2012 and 2013, we reviewed the valve parameters provided in the echocardiography reports and graded the severities of valve dysfunction (regurgitation and/or stenosis) according to the 2014 and 2017 guidelines for the management of patients with valvular heart disease [18–21] (Table 1). The etiology of the valve dysfunction remained the same as that which was reported in the original reports. Care was always taken during the echocardiography studies to exclude secondary mitral regurgitation due to dilated cardiomyopathy and ischemic heart disease before making a diagnosis of "primary mitral regurgitation" [18, 21].

Diagnostic classification

Patients with primary left-sided valvluar heart disease were categorized into one of 5 major categories:

1. Rheumatic Heart Disease (RHD), which was diagnosed according to the 2012 World Heart Federation criteria [22].
2. Degenerative valve disease (DVD), which represented: a) Sclerotic valve changes but with normal valve function: This required presence of mitral and/or aortic leaflet sclerosis - seen as calcium deposits on the leaflets without involvement of the commissures and without valve incompetence or stenosis [16, 20, 23, 24]; or b) Degenerative valve changes with impaired valve function, which required sclerosis/calcification of the mitral and/or aortic valvular apparatus with resultant mild to severe valve incompetence or stenosis and in the absence of rheumatic features [16–21, 23, 24].
3. Bicuspid Aortic Valve (BAV), which was defined by the finding of fusion of any 2 of the aortic valve cusps with or without a raphe [25, 26]. All aortic valves that met this anatomical definition were included in this diagnostic category regardless of the functional status.
4. Primary mitral valve prolapse (MVP), for which the standard echocardiographic definitions of classic and non-classic MVP were utilized [17, 21, 27, 28].
5. Endomyocardial Fibrosis (EMF), whose diagnosis was based on the typical echocardiographic features that have been described [29, 30].

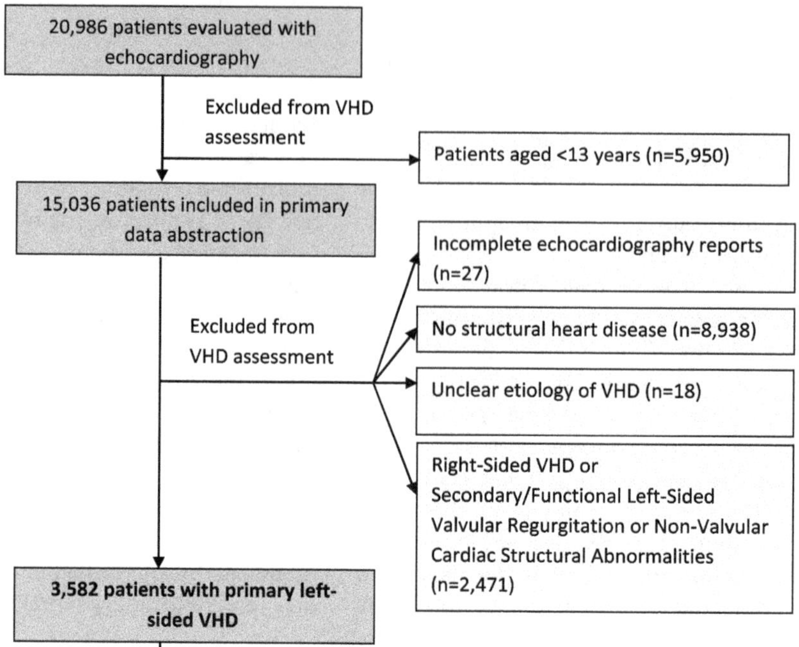

Diagnosis	N (%)
Stage A (At Risk of Progressive VHD)	
Probable Rheumatic Heart Disease (RHD)	28 (1.2%)
Sclerotic Valve Changes with Normal Valve Function (SVC)	2,262 (98.3%)
Bicuspid Aortic Valve (BAV)	01 (0.04%)
Mitral Valve Prolapse (MVP)	05 (0.2%)
Endomyocaial Fibrosis (EMF)	04 (0.17%)
Stage B (Asymptomatic Progressive VHD), Stage C (Asymptomatic Severe VHD), & Stage D (Symptomatic Severe VHD)	
Rheumatic Heart Disease (RHD)	681 (53%)
Degenerative Valve Disease – With Impaired Valve Function (DVD)	537 (41.8%)
Bicuspid Aortic Valve (BAV)	28 (2.2%)
Mitral Valve Prolapse (MVP)	18 (1.4%)
Endomyocardial Fibrosis (EMF)	22 (1.7%)

Fig. 1 Flow chart of the echocardiography study selection process. Legend: Echocardiography report selection was based on age of the patients at the time of the echocardiography study and completeness of the echocardiography reports

In each of these diagnostic categories, patients were further classified according to the 2014 ACC/AHA staging of primary VHD [18].

1. Stage A represents patients with risk factors for development of progressive VHD, and in this series included probable RHD (stage A of RHD), sclerotic valve changes but with normal valve function (stage A of DVD), bicuspid aortic valve with normal valve function, mitral valve prolapse without mitral valve incompetence and endomyocardial fibrosis without mitral/aortic valve dysfunction [18].
2. Stages B, C and D represent mild to moderate asymptomatic VHD, severe asymptomatic VHD, and severe symptomatic VHD respectively [18]. In this series, these stages included mild, moderate and severe valve incompetence and/or stenosis in each of the 5 diagnostic categories. Patients who had undergone surgical procedures for the correction of valve abnormalities were categorized in group D.

Table 1 Grading of mitral and aortic valve regurgitant and stenotic lesions

Valve lesion	Grading method	Mild	Moderate	Severe
Mitral stenosis	Valve area	≥2.0 cm^2	1.6–1.9 cm^2	≤1.5 cm^2
Primary mitral regurgitation	Vena contracta width	< 0.3 cm	0.3–0.69 cm	≥0.7 cm
	Regurgitant fraction	< 30%	30–49%	≥50%
	Regurgitant volume	< 30 mls	30-59 mls	≥60 mls
	Effective regurgitant orifice area	< 0.2 cm^2	0.2–0.39 cm^2	≥0.4 cm^2
Aortic sclerosis	Peak velocity	< 2.5 m/s		
Aortic stenosis	Peak velocity	2.6–2.9 m/s	3.0–4.0 m/s	≥4.0 m/s
	Mean gradient	< 20 mmHg	20-39 mmHg	≥40 mmHg
	Valve area by continuity equation	> 1.5cm^2 or indexed AVA > 0.85 cm^2/m^2	1.0–1.5cm^2 or indexed AVA 0.6–0.85 cm^2/m^2	≤ 1.0cm^2 or indexed AVA ≤ 0.6 cm^2/m^2
Aortic regurgitation	Vena contracta width	< 0.3 cm	0.3–0.6 cm	≥0.6 cm
	Central jet width/LVOT width	< 25%	25–64%	≥65%
	Regurgitant fraction	< 30%	30–49%	≥50%
	Regurgitant volume	<30 mls	30–59 mls	≥60 mls
	Effective regurgitant orifice area	< 0.1 cm^2	0.1–0.29 cm^2	≥0.3 cm^2

Other echocardiographic assessments

Examination of native or prosthetic valves for echocardiographic features of past or current infective endocarditis was performed according to standard guidelines [31, 32]. Prosthetic valves were evaluated according to the 2009 American Society of Echocardiography's Guidelines for the echocardiographic evaluation of prosthetic valves [31].

Data management

Data was initially captured in Epi info 3.0 and later exported to Stata 12.0. Continuous variables are presented as means ± standard deviation. Categorical variables are presented as proportions.

Results

Of 20,986 echocardiographic studies performed during the study period, 3582 were included in the data analysis (Fig. 1). Over 60% of the 3582 patients were females (Table 2). The diagnostic category of "sclerotic valve changes with normal valve function" accounted for 98% of the primary valve diseases in Stage A while rheumatic heart disease accounted for over half of the primary valve diseases in Stages B to D (Fig. 2).

"Stage a" primary left-sided valve diseases

"Sclerotic valve changes with normal valve function" overshadowed all the other valve diseases in this stage (Fig. 2). All of the patients with sclerotic valve changes with normal valve function were aged ≥40 years and 56% were males. There were much smaller numbers of patients "at risk" of progressive RHD, BAV, MVP and EMF-related valve dysfunction.

"Stages b, c and d" primary left-sided valve diseases

RHD was the leading cause of valve disease in these categories and was closely followed by DVD. The other diagnostic categories occurred in much smaller numbers.

a) Rheumatic Heart Disease
Stages B-D of RHD included mild, moderate and severe RHD valve lesions. We also included patients with RHD who had undergone valve replacement procedures for RHD valve dysfunction and those who had undergone mitral valve repair or open mitral commissurotomy for rheumatic mitral valve disease (Fig. 3). Patients who had undergone valve

Table 2 Participant demographics of the 3582 patients

Characteristics of the 3582 patients	Number of participants (%)
Age groups (years)	
13–19	251 (7.0%)
20–29	162 (4.5%)
30–39	128 (3.6%)
40–49	404 (11.3%)
50–59	503 (14.0%)
60–69	612 (17.1%)
70–79	733 (20.5%)
80–89	714 (20.0%)
90–99	70 (2.0%)
≥100	05 (0.1%)
Sex	
Male	1329 (37.1%)
Female	2253 (62.9%)

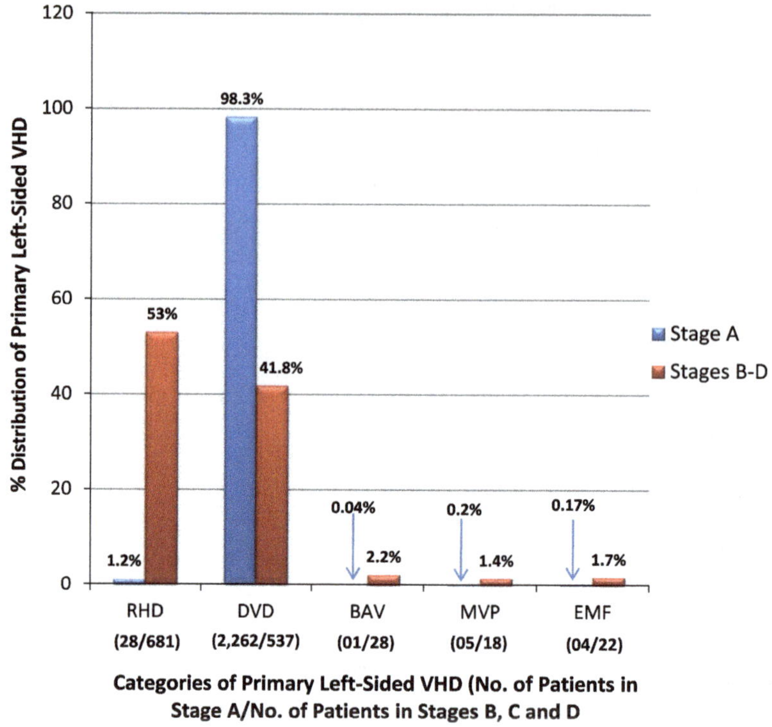

Fig. 2 The 5 major echocardiographic diagnostic categories. Legend: Stage A: Patients with risk factors for development of progressive VHD; Stage B: Progressive VHD (asymptomatic mild to moderate VHD); Stage C: Asymptomatic severe VHD; D: Symptomatic severe VHD

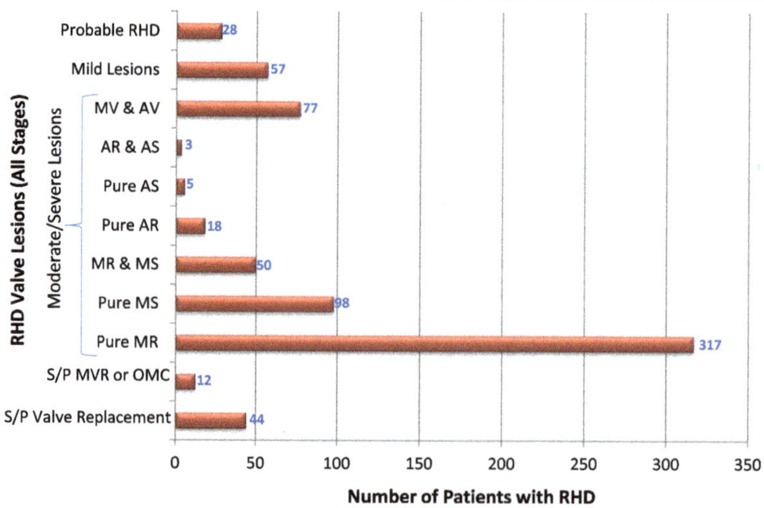

Fig. 3 Number of patients with RHD valve lesions (all stages). Legend: Mild lesions" represented definite RHD with mild mitral and/or aortic valve incompetence and/or stenosis. In the categories of "Pure AS" and "Pure AR", patients always had echocardiographic features of rheumatic involvement of the mitral valve (with trivial to mild mitral valve dysfunction) which supported the diagnosis of RHD. "Pure MR": Isolated moderate to severe mitral regurgitation; "Pure MS": Isolated moderate to severe mitral stenosis; "MR & MS": mixed mitral valve disease – coexistent moderate to severe mitral regurgitation and mitral stenosis; "AR & AS": mixed aortic valve disease – moderate to severe aortic regurgitation and stenosis; "MV & AV": mixed mitral and aortic valve disease - coexistent moderate to severe mitral and aortic valve disease

replacement, mitral valve repair or open mitral commissurotomy were classified as such regardless of the functional status of left sided native or prosthetic valves at the time of echocardiography. Isolated mitral regurgitation was the most common rheumatic valve lesion. RHD disproportionately affected the young under-40 years age group, with the 'number of cases per age group' falling below that of DVD in the 5th decade of life (Fig. 4).

b) Degenerative Valve Disease
Calcific degenerative mild to severe valve disease was the second common diagnostic category, following closely after RHD (Fig. 2). The 'number of cases per age group' increased with age, peaking in the 70–79 year age group (Fig. 4). Mitral regurgitation was the most predominant degenerative valve lesion (Fig. 5).

c) Bicuspid Aortic Valve
Twenty-nine patients were reported to have bicuspid aortic valves. Sixteen (55%) were males, and there was a fair distribution among all the age groups (Fig. 6). Majority of the affected patients had severe aortic valve dysfunction while 1 patient had undergone aortic valve replacement (Fig. 7). Two patients had co-existing coarctation of the aorta, 2 patients had ascending aortic aneurysms – a manifestation of bicuspid aortopathy while 1 patient had echocardiographic evidence of aortic valve endocarditis. There were no reports of other congenital structural valve abnormalities like cleft mitral valve, parachute mitral valve or sub-mitral aneurysms over the 24 months.

d) Primary Mitral Valve Prolapse
Twenty three patients had definite primary classic or non-classic mitral valve prolapse. Majority of these were teenagers (Fig. 8). All the cases were reported to be myxomatous in origin. Three patients were reported to have co-existent aortic leaflet prolapse but with preserved aortic valve function in all the cases. Of the 23 individuals with MVP, 3 had severe, 8 had moderate, 7 had mild while 5 had no mitral valve regurgitation.

e) Endomyocardial Fibrosis
Twenty-two patients had moderate to severe mitral valve regurgitation due to involvement of the mitral valve in left ventricular or biventricular endomyocardial fibrosis. EMF was exclusively diagnosed in the 13–39 years age groups, and 72% of the patients were females.

Other findings

a) Infective Endocarditis
Infective endocarditis is not presented as a separate diagnostic category because there were no reports of "primary" endocarditis. All the cases of left-sided infective endocarditis that were reported were super-imposed on another form of primary valve disease. Echocardiographic evidence of past or active mitral and/or aortic valve infective endocarditis was reported in 39 patients. RHD was the predominant predisposing factor and the mitral valve was most commonly affected (Fig. 9). One patient had an aortic root abscess while the rest of the patients had mitral and/or aortic valve vegetations. A description of further work up to confirm active infection and the causative organisms is beyond the scope of this paper.

b) Prosthetic Valves
Fifty patients had undergone mitral and/or aortic valve replacement procedures. RHD was overwhelmingly the leading indication for valve

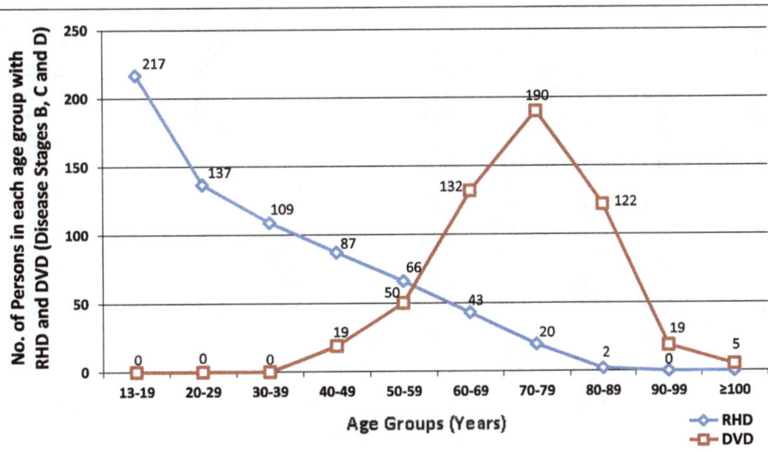

Fig. 4 Number of persons in different age groups with RHD and number of persons in different age groups with DVD. Legend: RHD: Rheumatic Heart Disease, DVD: Degenerative Valvular Disease

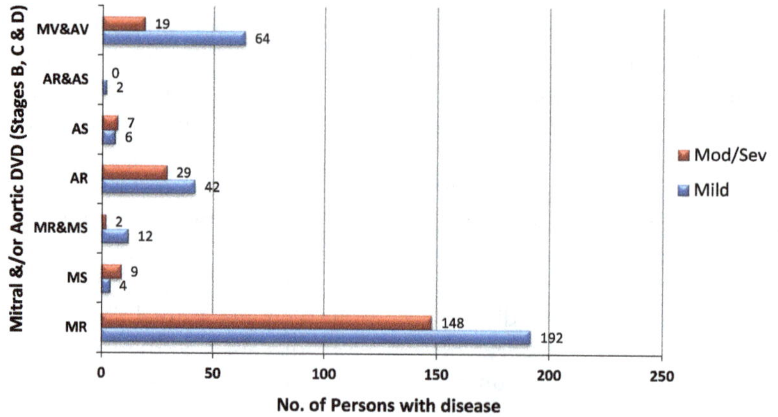

Fig. 5 Frequency of degenerative valve lesions (Stages B-D). Legend: MR: Mitral regurgitation alone; MS: Mitral stenosis alone; MR & MS: Mixed mitral valve regurgitation and stenosis; AR: Aortic regurgitation alone; AS: Aortic stenosis alone; AR & AS: Mixed valve regurgitation and stenosis; MV & AV: Mixed mitral and aortic degenerative valve disease

replacement and mechanical prosthetic valves were mostly utilized (Table 3). The majority of valve replacements were performed when patients were under 30 years of age (Fig. 10). All the prosthetic valves were functioning normally. One patient had evidence of vegetations on a mechanical mitral prosthesis but the valve function was normal.

Discussion

In this study, we describe the burden of a variety of forms of primary left-sided valve disease from a large series of echocardiographic studies in a tertiary cardiac care centre in Uganda.

We demonstrated a large number of patients in this series with "sclerotic valve changes with normal valve function". This early stage of leaflet changes is recognized as "Stage A" or the "initiation stage" of progressive DVD, and indicates a population that is at risk of developing progressive valve stenosis or regurgitation [18–21, 24]. Progressive valve disease develops in approximately 10–15% of patients with valve sclerotic changes, and this category of patients has been shown to have an increased risk of cardiovascular events over 5 years [24]. Although previous randomized clinical trials of lipid-lowering therapy in adults with mild-to-moderate aortic stenosis showed no significant effect on disease progression or aortic-valve events [33], this early "initiation" stage remains a potential opportunity for medical intervention to prevent or delay disease progression.

Rheumatic heart disease was the leading cause of primary left-sided valve disease with valve dysfunction. There is already a bulk of descriptive data on patterns, presentations, and complications of RHD in Africa and – in particular, from the current study site by the same working group [4–11].

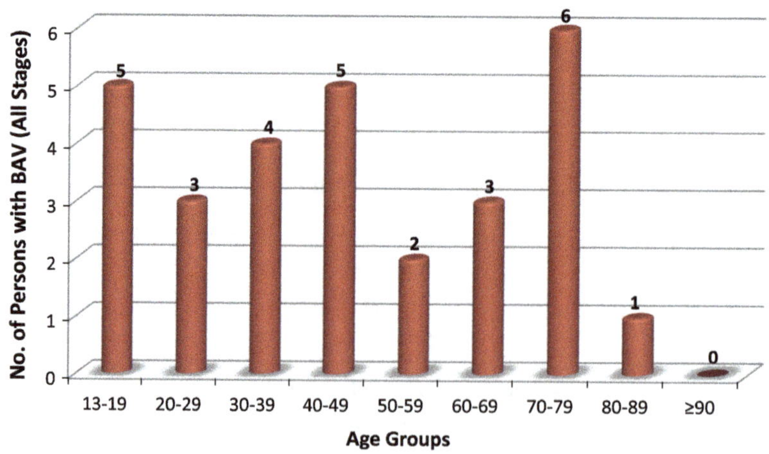

Fig. 6 Age-group distribution of bicuspid aortic valve (all stages). Legend: Number of persons in different age groups with bicuspid aortic valve, with or without valve dysfunction

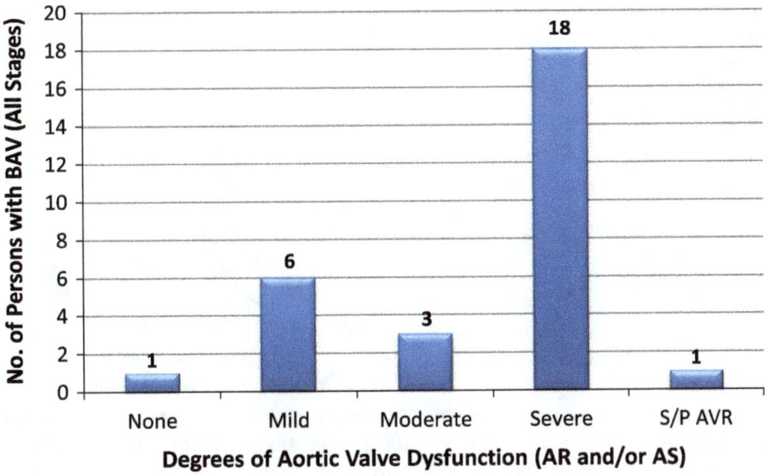

Fig. 7 Functional status of the aortic valve among patients with bicuspid aortic valve (all stages). Legend: AS: Aortic Stenosis; AR: Aortic Regurgitation; S/P AVR: Status Post Aortic Valve Replacement

In high income countries, VHD is typically degenerative and is regarded as an emerging public health problem [2]. Degenerative valve disease closely tallied behind RHD among the diagnostic categories with valve dysfunction in this echocardiographic series. In what appears to be quite a similar black South-African study population, Sliwa et al. [14] reported a prevalence of 21% of DVD among structural valve abnormalities. Differences in reporting methods and slight variations in the study populations do not permit direct comparison, but it is evident that the problem of DVD is not as minor in developing countries as it is assumed to be. With improvement in socioeconomic living conditions and increasing life expectancy in Africa [12]; more cases of DVD should be expected as we experience our share of the epidemiological transition of VHD.

Bicuspid aortic valve (BAV) is the commonest congenital cardiac abnormality in the general population with an estimated prevalence of 1–2% [34]. Although the findings in this study are far from being representative of the general population of Uganda, we bring into the limelight the existence of a pathology in a setting where there is barely any prior literature recording. In Uganda, only a singleton remote documentation by Somers and Rankin in 1962 [35] of a case of aortic coarctation co-existing with BAV can be found. The medical fraternity needs to master its natural progression, as evidenced by the proportions of patients with mild to severe degrees of valve dysfunction, and other clinical components of this pathology such as indications and timing of surgical intervention, infective endocarditis, and bicuspid aortopathy, as demonstrated in this echocardiographic series.

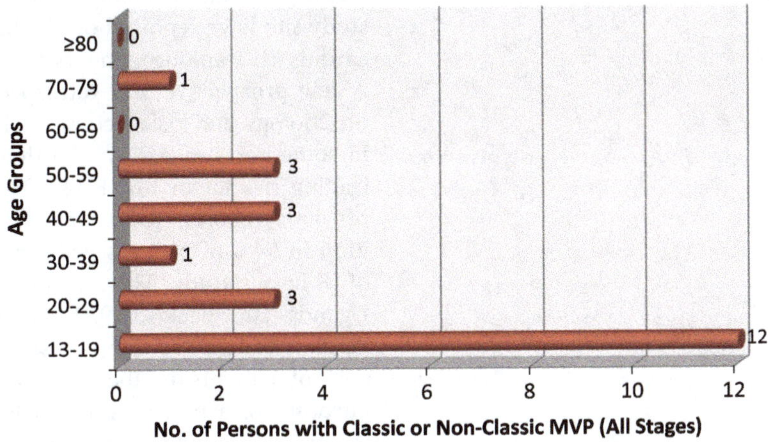

Fig. 8 Age-group distribution of mitral valve prolapse (all stages). Legend: Persons with classic or non-classic mitral valve prolapse, with or without mitral valve regurgitation in different age groups

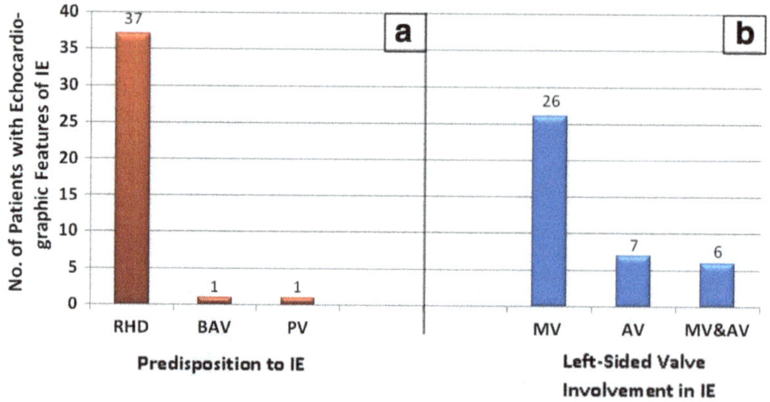

Fig. 9 Risk factors for and patterns of valve involvement in infective endocarditis. Legend: **a**: Cardiac structural abnormalities that likely predisposed patients to infective endocarditis. RHD: Rheumatic Heart Disease, BAV: Bicuspid Aortic Valve, PV: Prosthetic Valves; **b**: Left sided valve involvement in infective endocarditis. MV: Only mitral valve involvement; AV: Only aortic valve involvement; MV & AV: Both mitral and aortic valves involved in infective endocarditis

Primary MVP contributed 1.4% to the pool of primary valve diseases in stages B-D. Despite the study population and reporting differences, our findings rhyme closely with those of Sliwa et al. [14] who reported a prevalence of MVP of 1% among 481 black patients with structural heart disease. Majority of the patients with MVP were young and had mild to moderate mitral regurgitation, similar to what several population-based studies have demonstrated. Severe mitral regurgitation was less common [27, 36].

Table 3 Indications for valve replacement, valve(s) replaced, and types of valves used for replacement

Indications for valve replacement	
Indication	No. of patients
Rheumatic heart disease	44
Aortic root disease with aortic regurgitation	2
Dilated cardiomyopathy with functional mitral regurgitation	1
Bicuspid aortic valve	1
Calcific aortic stenosis	2
Valve(s) replaced	
Valve(s)	No. of patients
Mitral valve only	26
Aortic valve only	10
Mitral & Aortic valves	13
Mitral, aortic and tricuspid valves	1
Types of prosthetic valves	
Type of prosthetic valve	No. of patients
Mechanical valves	44
Bioprosthetic valves	5
Autograft (ross procedure)	1

Recognized as the country where EMF was first described [37, 38], Uganda has remained an endemic region for the disease. EMF is one of the neglected cardiovascular diseases whose etiology and pathogenesis remain elusive, the natural history is incompletely understood and therefore, no effective therapy is currently available [29, 39]. It remains an important cause of heart failure in endemic areas, comparable to rheumatic heart disease. The mechanisms by which heart failure develops are multifactorial with valvular involvement and dysfunction inclusive. Concerted efforts from local scientists, communities, governments and international collaborations are needed for renewed interest in this neglected tropical disease.

Infective endocarditis is an important component of VHD, with the predisposing factors in developing countries strikingly different from those in developed countries. Despite its clinical impact and poor outcomes in our setting, data on this subject are missing or sparse in many low- and middle-income regions [40]. Previous studies in sub-Saharan Africa including the current study site have reported on the burden of infective endocarditis (IE) among patients with RHD [11, 14, 41, 42]. A few prospective and retrospective descriptive studies on etiology and risk factors for IE have been performed in some parts of Africa, and they report RHD to be the leading risk factor for IE [43, 44]. In keeping with these previous reports, RHD was the identifiable predisposition in 94% of patients with echocardiographic features of IE in our study. The only detailed description of IE in Uganda dates back to 1972 [45], at which time a preponderance of RHD as the predisposing factor was found in 65% of patients in the clinically diagnosed series. For purposes of achieving up-to-date local clarity, our team is currently conducting a prospective study of the risk factors and etiology of infective endocarditis in Mulago National Referral Hospital.

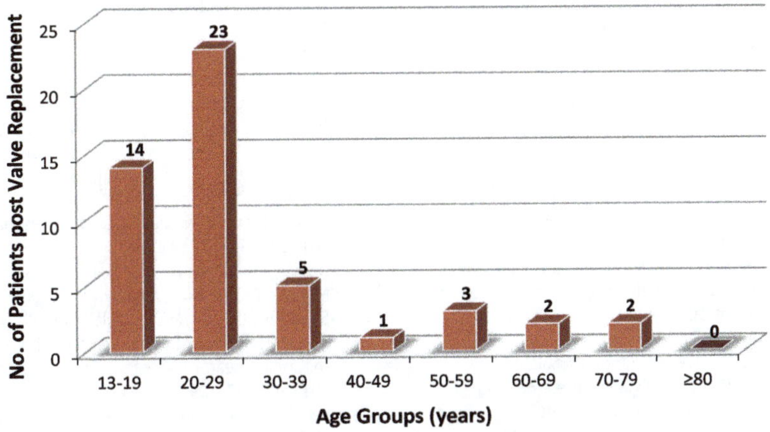

Fig. 10 Number of persons with prosthetic valves in different age groups. Legend: Persons with prosthetic valves (mechanical or bioprosthetic)

RHD was the leading indication for valve surgery in this series as opposed to developed countries where degenerative valve disease takes the lead. Valve surgery is becoming more accessible in Uganda and therefore the number of patients with prosthetic valves is consistently on the rise. By definition, valve disease is still present after interventional therapy and prosthetic valves are a recognized independent entity of valve heart disease. The clinical issues surrounding the timing of valve surgery, prosthetic valve selection, prosthetic valves and pregnancy, anticoagulation and infective endocarditis pose a new frontier in a developing country that all practicing clinicians must get conversant with.

Strengths and limitations

This descriptive study provides vital information that should act as a basis for more focused and analytical studies in the field of valve heart disease in Uganda and developing countries at large. The main limitation of this study is its retrospective nature and thus the inherent shortcoming of incomplete data among others. Also, these findings do not reflect the burden of valve heart disease in the general population of Uganda.

Conclusions

Over the past years, a picture has been painted which gives a reflection that "valve heart disease in Africa is synonymous with rheumatic heart disease in Africa". Our bringing to the limelight by way of publication of the contemporary footprints of other forms of VHD in significant proportions suggests that this assumption is not true. National and continental programs already exist for rheumatic heart disease. A similar coordinated multidisciplinary approach to research, education and clinical management is now needed to ensure improved outcomes for patients with other forms of VHD.

Abbreviations

AR: Aortic regurgitation; AS: Aortic stenosis; BAV: Bicuspid aortic valve; DVD: Degenerative valve disease; EMF: Endomyocardial fibrosis; IE: Infective endocarditis; MR: Mitral regurgitation; MS: Mitral stenosis; MVP: Mitral valve prolapse; RHD: Rheumatic heart disease; UHI: Uganda Heart Institute; VHD: Valve heart disease

Acknowledgements

Special thanks go to the medical records department at the Uganda Heart Institute for searching through all the available systems to avail us a near-complete set of records. We also extend our sincere appreciation to Dr. Andrea Beaton who helped with the medical scientific writing and English revision of this manuscript.

Authors' contributions

JR conceived and designed the project, and drafted the first version of the manuscript. IS, ZWZ, JN1 and JN2 in two pairs read the qualifying echocardiography reports, agreed on protocol-adhering echocardiographic diagnoses and built data sets that were analyzed. SL, PL and JO made substantial contributions to conception and design. EO and WM made substantial contributions to analysis and interpretation of data, and critically revised the manuscript for important intellectual content. All authors read and approved the final manuscript.

Competing interests

The authors declare that they have no competing interests.

Author details

[1]Uganda Heart Institute, Kampala, Uganda. [2]School of Medicine Makerere University, Kampala, Uganda.

References

1. Iung B, Baron G, Butchart EG, et al. A prospective survey of patients with valvular heart disease in Europe: the euro heart survey on Valvular heart disease. Eur Heart J. 2003;24:1231–43.
2. Nkomo V, Gardin JM, Skelton TN, Scott CG, Enriqez-Serano M. Burden of valvular heart disease: a population based study. Lancet. 2006;368:1005–11.
3. Ray S. Changing epidemiology and natural history of valvular heart disease. Clinical Medicine. 2010;2(10):168–71.
4. Okello E, Kakande B, Sebatta E, Kayima J, Kuteesa M, Mutatina B, et al. Socioeconomic and environmental risk factors among rheumatic heart disease patients in Uganda. PLoS One. 2012;7(8):e43917.
5. Okello E, Beaton A, Mondo CK, Kruszka P, Kiwanuka N, Odoi-Adome R, Freers J. Rheumatic heart disease in Uganda: the association between MHC class II HLA DR alleles and disease: a case control study. BMC Cardiovasc Disord. 2014;14:28.
6. Longenecker CT, Okello E, Lwabi P, Costa MA, Simon DI, Salata RA. Management of Rheumatic Heart Disease in Uganda: the emerging epidemic of non-AIDS co-morbidity in resource-limited settings. J Acquir Immune Defic Syndr. 2014;65(2):e79–80.
7. Zhang W, Okello E, Nyakoojo W, Lwabi P, Mondo CK. Proportion of patients in the Uganda rheumatic heart disease registry with advanced disease requiring urgent surgical interventions. Afr Health Sci. 2015;15(4):1182–8.
8. Aliku T, Sable C, Scheel A, Tompsett A, Lwabi P, Okello E, et al. Targeted echocardiographic screening for latent rheumatic heart disease in northern Uganda: evaluating familial risk following identification of an index case. PLoS Negl Trop Dis. 2016;10(6):e0004727.
9. Okello E, Longenecker CT, Beaton A, Kamya MR, Lwabi P. Rheumatic heart disease in Uganda: predictors of morbidity and mortality one year after presentation. BMC Cardiovasc Disord. 2017;17:20.
10. Zhang W, Mondo C, Okello E, Musoke C, Kakande B, Nyakoojo W, Kayima J, Freers J. Presenting features of newly diagnosed rheumatic heart disease patients in Mulago hospital: a pilot study. Cardiovasc J Afr. 2013 Mar;24(2):28–33.
11. Okello E, Zhang W, Musoke C, Kakande B, Mondo C, Freers J, Twalib A, Lwabi P, Wilson NB, Odoi-Odome R. Cardiovascular complications in newly diagnosed rheumatic heart disease patients at Mulago hospital, Uganda. Cardiovasc J Afr. 2013;24(3):82–7.
12. United Nations, Department of Economic and Social Affairs, Population division, population estimates and projections section 2012.
13. Liu F-Z, et al. Five-year epidemiological survey of valvular heart disease: changes in morbidity, etiological spectrum and management in a cardiovascular center of southern China. J Thorac Dis. 2014;6(12):1724–30.
14. Sliwa K, Carrington M, Mayosi BM, Zigiriadis E, Mvungi R, Stewart S. Incidence and characteristics of newly diagnosed rheumatic heart disease in urban African adults: insights from the heart of Soweto study. Eur Heart J. 2010;31:719–27.
15. Essop MR, Nkomo VT. Rheumatic and non-rheumatic valvular heart disease: epidemiology, management and prevention in Africa. Circulation. 2005;112: 3584–91.
16. Baumgartner H, Hung J, Bermejo J, Chambers JB, Evangelista A, et al. Echocardiographic assessment of valve stenosis: EAE/ASE recommendations for clinical practice. J Am Soc Echocardiogr. 2009;1:1–23.
17. Zoghbi WA, Enriquez-Sarano M, Foster E, Grayburn PA, Kraft CD. Recommendations for evaluation of the severity of native valvular regurgitation with two-dimensional and Doppler echocardiography. J Am Soc Echocardiogr. 2003;16(7):777–802.
18. Nishimura RA, Otto CM, Bonow RO, Carabello BA, Erwin JP III, Guyton RA, O'Gara PT, Ruiz CE, Skubas NJ, Sorajja P, Sundt TM III, Thomas JD. 2014 AHA/ACC guideline for the management of patients with valvular heart disease: executive summary: a report of the American College of Cardiology/American Heart Association task force on practice guidelines. Circulation. 2014;129:1–96.
19. Nishimura RA, Otto CM, Bonow RO, Carabello BA, Erwin JP 3rd, Fleisher LA, Jneid H, Mack MJ, McLeod CJ, O'Gara PT, Rigolin VH, Sundt TM 3rd, Thompson A. 2017 AHA/ACC focused update of the 2014 AHA/ACC guideline for the management of patients with valvular heart disease: a report of the American College of Cardiology/American Heart Association task force on clinical practice guidelines. J Am Coll Cardiol. 2017;70:252–89.
20. Baumgartner H, Hung J, Bermejo J, Chambers JB, Edvardsen T, Goldstein S, Lancellotti P, LeFevre M, Miller F Jr, Otto CM. Recommendations on the echocardiographic assessment of aortic valve stenosis: a focused update from the European Association of Cardiovascular Imaging and the American Society of Echocardiography. J Am Soc Echocardiogr. 2017;30: 372–92.
21. Zoghbi WA, Adams D, Bonow RO, Enriquez-Sarano M, Foster E, Grayburn PA, Hahn RT, Han Y, Judy Hung MD, Lang RM, Little SH, Shah DJ, Shernan S, Thavendiranathan P, Thomas JD, Weissman NJ. Recommendations for noninvasive evaluation of native Valvular regurgitation. A report from the American Society of Echocardiography developed in collaboration with the Society for Cardiovascular Magnetic Resonance. J Am Soc Echocardiogr. 2017;30:303–71.
22. Reményi B, Wilson N, Steer A, Ferreira B, Kado J, Kumar K, Lawrenson J, Maguire G, Marijon E, Mirabel M, Mocumbi AO, Mota C, Paar J, Saxena A, Scheel J, Stirling J, Viali S, Balekundri VI, Wheaton G, Zühlke L, Carapetis J. World heart federation criteria for echocardiographic diagnosis of rheumatic heart disease–an evidence-based guideline. Nat Rev Cardiol. 2012;9(5):297–309.
23. Valvular stenosis and valvular regurgitation. In: Otto CM, editor. Textbook of clinical echocardiography. Philadelphia: Elsevier Saunders; 2004. p. 281–328.
24. Otto CM, Prendergast B. Aortic valve stenosis — from patients at risk to severe valve obstruction. N Engl J Med. 2014;371:744–56.
25. Schaefer BM, Lewin MB, Stout KK, Gill E, Prueitt A, Byers PH, Otto CM. The bicuspid aortic valve: an integrated phenotypic classification of leaflet morphology and aortic root shape. Heart. 2008;94(12):1634–8.
26. Bicuspid aortic valve. A comprehensive review. Cardiol Res Pract. 2012;2012: 196037.
27. Freed LA, Levy D, Levine RA, et al. Prevalence and clinical outcome of mitral-valve prolapse. N Engl J Med. 1999;341(1):1–7.
28. Perloff JK, Child JS. Mitral valve prolapse. Evolution and refinement of diagnostic techniques. Circulation. 1989;80(3):710–1.
29. Mocumbi AO. Endomyocardial fibrosis: a form of endemic restrictive cardiomyopathy. Global cardiology Science and Practice. 2012;11. http://dx.doi.org/10.5339/gcsp.2012.11.
30. Mocumbi AO, Carrilho C, Sarathchandra P, Ferreira MB, Yacoub M, Burke M. Echocardiography accurately assesses the pathological abnormalities of chronic endomyocardial fibrosis. Int J Cardiovasc Imaging. 2011;27(7):955–64.
31. Zoghbi WA, Chambers JB, Dumesnil JG, Foster E, Gottdiener JS, Grayburn PA, et al. American Society of Echocardiography's guidelines and standards committee; task force on prosthetic valves. J Am Soc Echocardiogr. 2009;22: 975–1014.
32. Habib G, Hoen B, Tornos P, et al. Guidelines on the prevention, diagnosis, and treatment of infective endocarditis. Eur Heart J. 2009;30:2369–413.
33. Teo KK, Corsi DJ, Tam JW, Dumesnil JG, Chan KL. Lipid lowering on progression of mild to moderate aortic stenosis: meta-analysis of the randomized placebo controlled clinical trials on 2344 patients. Can J Cardiol. 2011;27:800–8.
34. Ward C. Clinical significance of the bicuspid aortic valve. Heart. 2000;83:81–5.
35. Somers K, Rankin AM. Three cases of coarctation of the aorta from an east African hospital. The Central African Journal of Medicine. 1962;8:375–9.
36. Freed LA, Benjamin EJ, Levy D, et al. Mitral valve prolapse in the general population: the benign nature of echocardiographic features in the Framingham heart study. J Am Coll Cardiol. 2002;40:1298.
37. Connor DH, Somers K, MSR H, Manion WC, D'Arbela PG. Endomyocardial fibrosis in Uganda (Davies' disease). An epidemiologic, clinical, and pathological study. Am Heart J. 1967;74:687–709.
38. Shaper AG, MSR H, Coles RM. Necropsy study of endomyocardial fibrosis and rheumatic heart disease in Uganda, 1950-1965. Br Heart J. 1968;30:391–401.
39. Mocumbi AO, Ferreira MB, Sidi D, Yacoub MH. A population study of endomyocardial fibrosis in a rural area of Mozambique. N Engl J Med. 2008; 359:43–9.
40. Bin Abdulhak AA, Baddour LM, Erwin PJ, Hoen B, Chu VH, Mensah GA, Tleyjeh IM. Global and regional burden of infective endocarditis, 1990-2010: a systematic review of the literature. Glob Heart. 2014;9(1):131–43.
41. Sani MU, Karaye KM, Borodo MM. Prevalence and pattern of rheumatic heart disease in the Nigerian savannah: an echocardiographic study. Cardiovasc J Afr. 2007;18:295–9.
42. Nkomo VT. Epidemiology and prevention of valvular heart diseases and infective endocarditis in Africa. Heart. 2007;93:1510–9.

43. Koelenberg CFN, Doubell AF, Orth H, Reuter H. Infective endocarditis in the western Cape Province of South Africa: a three-year prospective study. Q J Med. 2003;96:217–25.
44. Moges T, Gedlu E, Isaakidis P, et al. Infective endocarditis in Ethiopian children: a hospital based review of cases in Addis Ababa. Pan African Medical Journal. 2015;20:75.
45. Somers SK, Patel AK, Steiner I, D'Arbela PG, Hutt MSR. Infective endocarditis: an African experience. Br Heart J. l972;34:1107–12.

25

The evaluation of the aortic annulus displacement during cardiac cycle using magnetic resonance imaging

Tomasz Plonek[1,2*], Mikolaj Berezowski[1], Jacek Kurcz[3], Przemyslaw Podgorski[3], Marek Sąsiadek[3], Bartosz Rylski[4], Andrzej Mysiak[5] and Marek Jasinski[1]

Abstract

Background: The stress in the ascending aorta results from many biomechanical factors including the geometry of the vessel and its maximum dimensions, arterial blood pressure and longitudinal systolic stretching due to heart motion. The stretching of the ascending aorta resulting from the longitudinal displacement of the aortic annulus during the heart cycle has not been examined in the general population so far. The aim of the study is to evaluate this parameter using cardiovascular magnetic resonance (CMR) imaging in the general population in all age groups.

Methods: The cardiac magnetic resonance images of 73 patients were evaluated. The maximum distance to which the ventriculo-aortic junction was pulled by the contracting heart (LDAA – longitudinal displacement of the aortic annulus) was measured in the cine coronal sequences. Moreover, the maximum dimensions of the aortic root and the ascending aorta were assessed.

Results: The LDAA value was on average 11.6 ± 2.9 mm (range: 3-19 mm; 95% CI: 10.9–12.3 mm) and did not differ between males and females (11.8 ± 2.9 mm vs. 11.2 ± 2.9 mm, $p = .408$). The diameter of the ascending aorta was 32 ± 6.3 mm (range: 20-57 mm). The maximal dimension of the aortic root was 35 ± 5.1 mm (range: 18-42 mm). There was a statistically significant negative correlation between the LDAA and the age of patients ($r = -.38$, $p = .001$). There was no significant correlation between the LDAA and aortic root dimension ($r = .1$, $p = .409$) and between the LDAA and diameter of the ascending aorta ($r = .16$, $p = .170$).

Conclusions: Human aortic root and ascending aorta are significantly stretched during systole and the distance to which the aorta is stretched decreases with age. The measurement of the longitudinal displacement of the aortic annulus using the CMR is feasible and reproducible.

Keywords: Aorta, Dissection, Aneurysm, Cardiovascular magnetic resonance

Background

There are several biomechanical factors that influence stress in the wall of the ascending aorta and the risk of aortic dissection. To date, the most common radiographic parameter used to predict this risk is maximum aortic diameter [1–3]. However, recent studies suggest that the aorta usually dissects when its diameter is much lower than the threshold regarded as an indication for surgery [4, 5]. Therefore, new objective parameters to assess the risk of dissection are necessary. Some of them, including the presence of arterial hypertension and genetic predispositions are already taken into account when assessing this risk [2, 3]. Some, new anatomic and radiographic parameters like aortic elongation are being under investigation [6, 7].

The aorta is subjected to circumferential stress since the vessel increases its diameter due to the rise in blood pressure [8, 9]. Moreover, the aortic root and ascending aorta are in close proximity to the heart which pulls and stretches the vessel during systole. This phenomenon results in longitudinal stress [10–12].

* Correspondence: tomaszplonek@gmail.com
[1]Department of Cardiac Surgery, Wroclaw Medical University, Borowska 213, 50-556, Wroclaw, Poland
[2]Department of Cardio-Thoracic Surgery, Onze Lieve Vrouwe Gasthuis, Amsterdam, the Netherlands
Full list of author information is available at the end of the article

The longitudinal displacement of the aortic annulus (LDAA) has not been well examined so far and there are no studies assessing the LDAA with the use of the cardiovascular magnetic resonance (CMR) in the general population [10, 13]. There is only one study that assessed the dynamics of the aorta including the longitudinal strain but included only the elderly population (70 years or older) [14].

This is the first study that uses CMR to evaluate the longitudinal displacement of the aortic annulus in the patients from all age groups. The aim of the study is to estimate the LDAA using magnetic resonance imaging in the general population and assess how it changes with the patients' age, height and weight.

Methods

Patients

This was a retrospective study of all patients who had been referred for cardiovascular magnetic resonance (CMR) between 2015 and 2016 to the Department of General and Interventional Radiology and Neuroradiology at Wroclaw Medical University in Poland. In total, the cardiovascular magnetic resonance images of 89 patients were included for initial assessment. The exclusion criteria were poor quality of the images in the cine coronal view, which resulted mainly from the respiratory movement of the patient (6 patients) or arrhythmia (5 patients). Finally, 73 patients were included in the analysis.

Cardiovascular magnetic resonance imaging

The CMR examinations were carried out on 1.5 T Signa HDxt (General Electric Healthcare, WI, USA) with an eight phased-array coil. All measurements were performed in the ECG-gated coronal cine Fast Imaging Employing Steady-state Acquisition (FIESTA) sequences. The serial images with a nominal resolution of 1.2 × 1.2 mm and 6 mm section thickness were obtained. The images covered a 256 × 256 mm field of view.

Measurements

The CMR images were analyzed in the coronal cine-MRI view. The maximum distance to which the ventriculo-aortic junction (VAJ) was pulled by the contracting heart was measured (LDAA – longitudinal displacement of the aortic annulus). First, the position of the VAJ was established in the maximum systole and diastole, then the distance between the mid-points of the VAJ in systole and diastole was measured. Moreover, the maximum dimensions of the aortic root and the ascending aorta were assessed. The methodology of the measurements is presented in Fig. 1.

Inter- and intraobserver variability

All examinations were evaluated by two observers. For inter-observer variability, the same examinations were analyzed by a second observer blinded to all the measurements performed by the first observer. For intraobserver variability of longitudinal systolic stretching of the aorta, all measurements were retaken by each observer 1 week after the initial assessment.

Statistical analysis

The normality of distribution was assessed using the Shapiro-Wilk test. Based on the distribution, data are

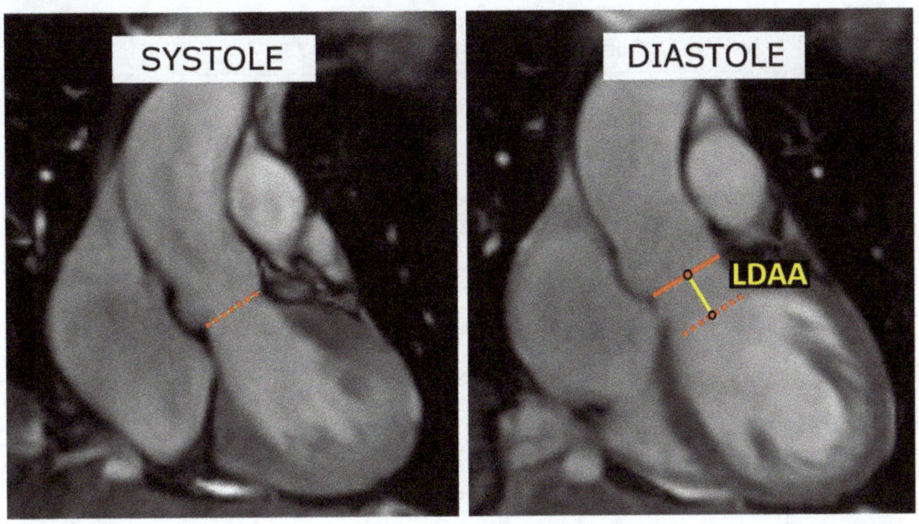

Fig. 1 The measurements taken from the coronal cine-MRI sequences. Left (systole): red dotted line - the position of the ventriculo-aortic junction (VAJ) in systole. Right (diastole): red dotted line - the position of the ventriculo-aortic junction (VAJ) in systole, red line - position of the ventriculo-aortic junction (VAJ) in diastole; yellow line – the longitudinal displacement of the aortic annulus (LDAA)- the line links the mid-points of the VAJ in systole and diastole

presented as mean ± standard deviation or median and range for continuous data. The categorical data are presented as frequencies. The correlations were assessed using the Pearson correlation coefficient. The means were compared using either the student's t-test or the Mann-Whitney U test depending on the normality of the distribution. The inter- and intraobserver variabilities were assessed using the interclass correlation coefficient. The analyses were carried out using Dell Statistica 13 software (Dell, USA).

Results

Longitudinal stretching of the aorta

The mean age of the patients was 45.2 ± 17.3 years and 68% (50 patients) were males. The mean height of the patients was 171.3 ± 14.4 cm and mean weight was 77.2 ± 10.8 kg. The mean BMI was 26.1 ± 3.8. There were 11 patients diagnosed with arterial hypertension and one patient had diabetes mellitus. There were no patients with poor ejection fraction of the left ventricle (< 30%). The diameter of the ascending aorta was 32.0 ± 6.3 mm (range: 20-57 mm) and was comparable between the genders (males: 32.6 ± 6.9 mm vs. females: 30.7 ± 4.8 mm, $p = .256$). The maximum dimension of the aortic root was 35.0 ± 5.1 mm (range: 18-42 mm) and was bigger in males than females (36.4 ± 5.2 mm vs. 31.2 ± 3.4 mm, $p < .001$).

The longitudinal displacement of the aortic annulus (LDAA) was on average 11.6 ± 2.9 mm (range: 3-19 mm; 95% CI: 10.9–12.3 mm) and did not differ between males and females (11.8 ± 2.9 mm vs. 11.2 ± 2.9 mm, $p = .408$). The aortic arch (junction between the innominate artery and the left carotid artery) was displaced on average by 2.9 ± 0.4 mm (range: 0-6 mm; 95% CI: 2.1–3.7 mm). There was a tendency towards lower LDAA values in older patients and a statistically significant negative correlation between the LDAA and the age of patients ($r = -.38$, $p = .001$) was observed (Fig. 2). The values of the LDAA in the age groups were as follows (0-20 yrs.: 14.6 ± 2.7 mm; 21-40 yrs.: 12.1 ± 2.5 mm; 41-60 yrs.: 11.5 ± 2.6 mm; 61-80 yrs.: 9.6 ± 2.8 mm; $p = .002$) and are shown on Fig. 3. There was no statistically significant correlation between the LDAA and the patient's height ($r = .112$, $p = .092$), weight ($r = .096$, $p = .771$) and BMI ($r = .084$, $p = .501$).

The longitudinal displacement of the aortic annulus was not affected by the maximum dimension of the aorta. No significant correlations between the LDAA and aortic root dimension ($r = .1$, $p = .409$) and between the LDAA and diameter of the ascending aorta ($r = .16$, $p = .170$) were found in the examined patients (Fig. 4).

Intra- and inter-observer and variability

The interobserver variability for the longitudinal stretching of the ascending aorta was 0.95 (95% CI: 0.92–0.97) and the intraobserver variability was 0.96 (95% CI: 0.94–0.98).

Discussion

This is the first study to evaluate the longitudinal displacement of the aortic annulus and aortic root using magnetic resonance imaging in patients from all age groups. The longitudinal displacement of the aortic annulus is regarded as an important factor that has an impact on the wall stress in the ascending aorta [10, 12, 13]. The LDAA may be responsible for a transverse intimal entry tear in the ascending aorta that is a common finding in patients with type A aortic dissection [13].

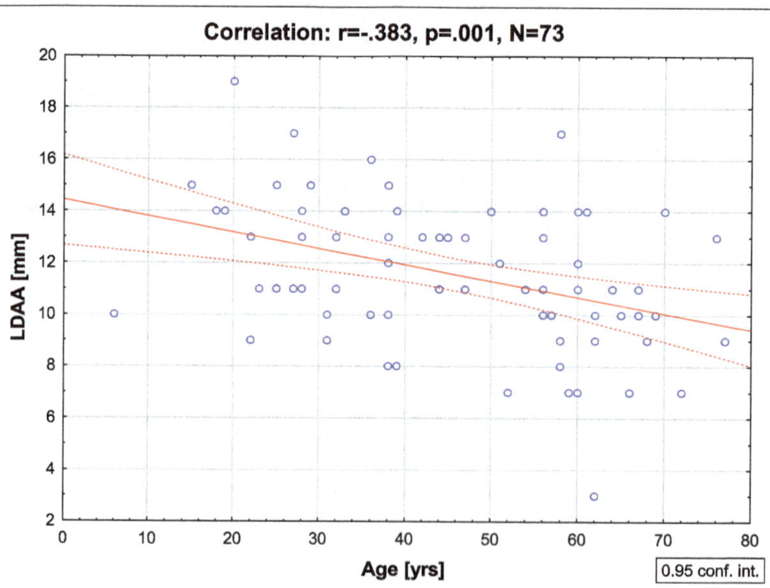

Fig. 2 The correlation between the longitudinal displacement of the aortic annulus (LDAA) and the age of the patients

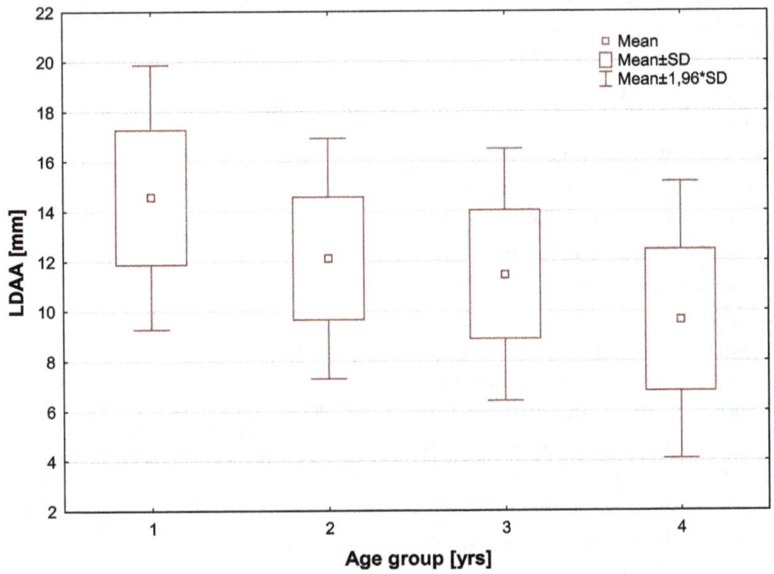

Fig. 3 The longitudinal displacement of the aortic annulus (LDAA) in various age groups

The results of this study can be summarized as follows:

(i) the measurement of the LDAA using the magnetic resonance imaging is feasible,
(ii) human aortic root and ascending aorta are significantly stretched during systole,
(iii) the distance to which the aorta is stretched decreases with age,
(iv) the LDAA does not correlate with the dimensions of aortic root and ascending aorta.

The most common parameter used to evaluate the risk of aortic dissection is the maximum diameter of the vessel [1–3, 15, 16]. There is a correlation between the diameter of the aorta and the risk of dissection, however, most dissections occur in patients with only slightly enlarged aortas [1, 4, 5]. This phenomenon can be explained by the fact that there are potentially many more patients with moderately dilated aortas compared to those with large aneurysms. The risk is lower when the vessel is not very dilated but the overall number of dissections is still much higher in patients with moderately dilated aortas [4, 5]. Thus, new parameters to assess the risk of dissection are needed to better evaluate this risk in patients with moderately dilated aortas.

Human ascending aorta is subjected to many biomechanical factors. Some of them, including the

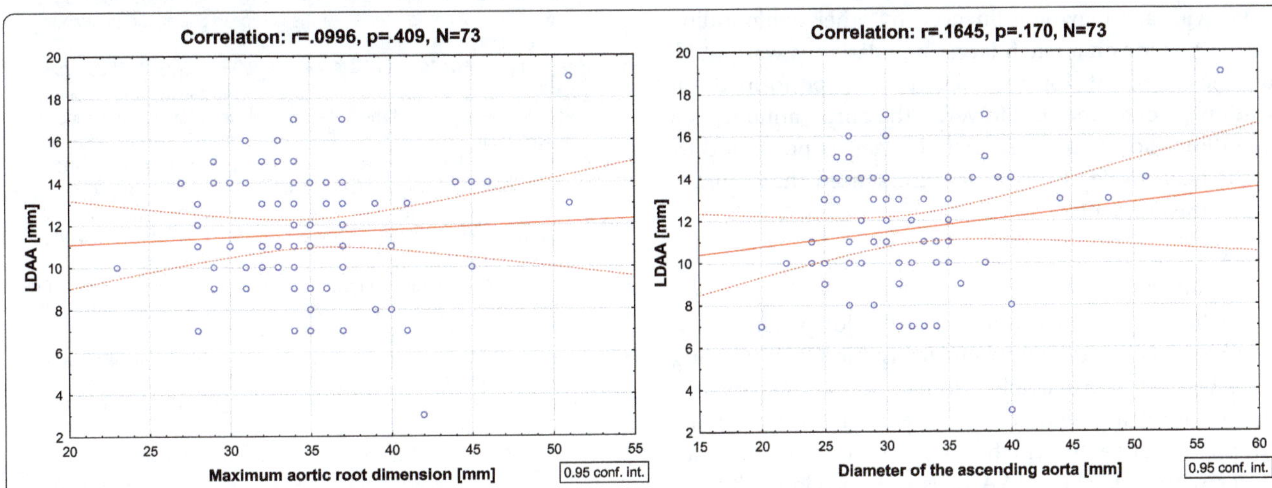

Fig. 4 The correlation between the longitudinal displacement of the aortic annulus (LDAA) and the maximum aortic root dimension (left) and the maximum diameter of the ascending aorta (right)

geometry of the vessel, arterial blood pressure and longitudinal systolic stretching due to heart motion play the key role in the biomechanics of this vessel [13, 17–20].

The longitudinal displacement of the aortic annulus has only been evaluated using the aortography, which is an invasive procedure that requires heart catheterization and contrast injection [10, 11]. In our study, we proposed a method to assess this parameter using the CMR imaging in the coronal cine sequences. The measurements were easy to perform and are reproducible with satisfactory inter- and intraobserver variability.

The LDAA was on average 11.6 mm and did not differ significantly between males and females. The maximum dimension of the vessel did not affect the longitudinal displacement of the aortic annulus. In our study, the LDAA negatively correlated with age. It may be explained by the fact that aortic wall elasticity decreases with age [21]. The LDAA could be used as a parameter to predict the potential loss of elasticity of the ascending aorta, i.e. in young patients. An unusually low value of the LDAA may then indicate that the aorta has lost its normal elasticity and that such a patient should be examined more thoroughly in search for connective tissue disorders. The LDAA could be a reasonable substitute for standard arterial stiffness to examine the elasticity/stiffness of the aorta and not the stiffness of the whole arterial tree. Nevertheless, additional studies are necessary to confirm the correlation between aortic wall elasticity and LDAA.

Study limitations

This is a small cohort study that include normal controls. An additional study assessing the LDAA in patients' with cardiovascular diseases is necessary to evaluate the clinical relevance of the LDAA. Due to a small sample size, one cannot rule out that the significant correlation of the LDAA with age may be influenced by other confounding factors. A study on a much larger population is warranted. The measurements of the LDAA were performed on two-dimensional images. However, the aortic annulus is a three-dimensional structure that changes its position during the heart cycle. It might have influenced the accuracy of the measurements.

Conclusions

In conclusion, the measurement of the longitudinal displacement of the aortic annulus using the CMR imaging is feasible and reproducible. Human aortic root and ascending aorta are significantly stretched during systole and the distance to which the aorta is stretched decreases with age. The LDAA does not correlate with the dimensions of aortic root and ascending aorta. In our opinion, the LDAA is a biomechanical factor that should be taken into account when analyzing the biomechanics of the thoracic aorta.

Abbreviations

CMR: Cardiovascular magnetic resonance; ECG: Electrocardiogram; FIESTA: Fast Imaging Employing Steady-state Acquisition; FOV: Field of view; LDAA: Longitudinal displacement of the aortic annulus; STJ: Sino-tubular junction; VAJ: Ventriculo-aortic junction

Funding

This study was supported by a statutory grant from Wroclaw Medical University (STMC050.16.008).

Authors' contributions

TP: study design, data collection, data analysis, manuscript preparation; MB: data collection, data analysis; JK: data collection, manuscript preparation; PP: data collection, manuscript preparation; MS: data collection, critical review; BR: data collection; critical review; AM: data collection, critical review; MJ: data analysis, critical review. All authors read and approved the final manuscipt.

Competing interests

The authors declare that they have no competing interests.

Author details

[1]Department of Cardiac Surgery, Wroclaw Medical University, Borowska 213, 50-556, Wroclaw, Poland. [2]Department of Cardio-Thoracic Surgery, Onze Lieve Vrouwe Gasthuis, Amsterdam, the Netherlands. [3]Department of General and Interventional Radiology and Neuroradiology, Wroclaw Medical University, Wroclaw, Poland. [4]Department of Cardio-vascular Surgery, Heart Centre Freiburg University, Faculty of Medicine, University of Freiburg, Freiburg, Germany. [5]Department of Cardiology, Wroclaw Medical University, Wroclaw, Poland.

References

1. Elefteriades JA. Beating a sudden killer. Sci Am. 2005;293(2):64–71.
2. Erbel R, et al. ESC guidelines on the diagnosis and treatment of aortic diseases: document covering acute and chronic aortic diseases of the thoracic and abdominal aorta of the adult. The task force for the diagnosis and treatment of aortic diseases of the European Society of Cardiology (ESC). Eur Heart J, 2014. 2014;35(41):2873–926.
3. Hiratzka LF, et al. 2010 ACCF/AHA/AATS/ACR/ASA/SCA/SCAI/SIR/STS/SVM guidelines for the diagnosis and management of patients with Thoracic Aortic Disease: a report of the American College of Cardiology Foundation/American Heart Association Task Force on Practice Guidelines, American Association for Thoracic Surgery, American College of Radiology, American Stroke Association, Society of Cardiovascular Anesthesiologists, Society for Cardiovascular Angiography and Interventions, Society of Interventional Radiology, Society of Thoracic Surgeons, and Society for Vascular Medicine. Circulation. 2010;121(13):e266–369.
4. Pape LA, et al. Aortic diameter >or = 5.5 cm is not a good predictor of type a aortic dissection: observations from the international registry of acute aortic dissection (IRAD). Circulation. 2007;116(10):1120–7.
5. Rylski B, et al. How does the ascending aorta geometry change when it dissects? J Am Coll Cardiol. 2014;63(13):1311–9.
6. Kruger T, et al. Ascending aortic elongation and the risk of dissection. Eur J Cardiothorac Surg. 2016;50(2):241–7.
7. Kruger T, et al. Aortic elongation and the risk for dissection: the Tubingen aortic Pathoanatomy (TAIPAN) projectdagger. Eur J Cardiothorac Surg. 2017; 51(6):1119–26.
8. Kim J, Baek S. Circumferential variations of mechanical behavior of the porcine thoracic aorta during the inflation test. J Biomech. 2011;44(10):1941–7.

9. Okamoto RJ, et al. The influence of mechanical properties on wall stress and distensibility of the dilated ascending aorta. J Thorac Cardiovasc Surg. 2003;126(3):842–50.
10. Beller CJ, et al. Role of aortic root motion in the pathogenesis of aortic dissection. Circulation. 2004;109(6):763–9.
11. Beller CJ, et al. Increased aortic wall stress in aortic insufficiency: clinical data and computer model. Eur J Cardiothorac Surg. 2005;27(2):270–5.
12. Plonek T, et al. The combined impact of mechanical factors on the wall stress of the human ascending aorta - a finite elements study. BMC Cardiovasc Disord. 2017;17(1):297.
13. Martufi G, et al. Is there a role for biomechanical engineering in helping to elucidate the risk profile of the thoracic aorta? Ann Thorac Surg. 2016; 101(1):390–8.
14. Bell V, et al. Longitudinal and circumferential strain of the proximal aorta. J Am Heart Assoc. 2014;3(6):e001536.
15. Elefteriades JA, Farkas EA. Thoracic aortic aneurysm clinically pertinent controversies and uncertainties. J Am Coll Cardiol. 2010;55(9):841–57.
16. Kim EK, et al. Aortic diameter predicts acute type a aortic dissection in patients with Marfan syndrome but not in patients without Marfan syndrome. J Thorac Cardiovasc Surg. 2014;147(5):1505–10.
17. Doyle BJ, et al. Identification of rupture locations in patient-specific abdominal aortic aneurysms using experimental and computational techniques. J Biomech. 2010;43(7):1408–16.
18. Krishnan K, et al. Ascending thoracic aortic aneurysm wall stress analysis using patient-specific finite element modeling of in vivo magnetic resonance imaging. Interact Cardiovasc Thorac Surg. 2015;21(4):471–80.
19. Martin C, Sun W, Elefteriades J. Patient-specific finite element analysis of ascending aorta aneurysms. Am J Physiol Heart Circ Physiol. 2015;308(10): H1306–16.
20. Nathan DP, et al. Increased ascending aortic wall stress in patients with bicuspid aortic valves. Ann Thorac Surg. 2011;92(4):1384–9.
21. Mitchell GF, et al. Changes in arterial stiffness and wave reflection with advancing age in healthy men and women: the Framingham heart study. Hypertension. 2004;43(6):1239–45.

26

Silent myocarditis in systemic sclerosis detected by cardiovascular magnetic resonance using Lake Louise criteria

Sophie Mavrogeni[1*], Loukia Koutsogeorgopoulou[2], Georgia Karabela[3], Efthymios Stavropoulos[3], Gikas Katsifis[3], John Raftakis[4], Sotiris Plastiras[2], Michel Noutsias[5], George Markousis-Mavrogenis[1] and Genovefa Kolovou[1]

Abstract

Background: Systemic sclerosis (SSc) is an autoimmune disease characterized by microvascular abnormalities, inflammation and fibrosis. We hypothesized that myocarditis may be diagnosed in asymptomatic SSc, undergoing routine cardio-vascular magnetic resonance (CMR) for fibrosis assessment, using the Lake Louise criteria: T2 ratio, early (EGE) and late gadolinium enhanced (LGE) images.

Methods: Eighty-two asymptomatic SSc, diagnosed according to American College of Rheumatology criteria, aged 43 ± 5 yrs., 62 with diffuse (dSSc) and 20 with localized (lSSc) systemic sclerosis were evaluated by CMR, performed at 1.5 T scanner, according to Lake Louise criteria.

Results: CMR documented normal biventricular function in all SSc. However, 7/62 (11.2%) with dSSc and 2/20 (10%) with lSSc, had CMR signs of myocarditis according to Lake Louise criteria, without any clinical cardiac symptom. In these 9 patients, T2 ratio, EGE ratio and LGE (positive in all 9 SSc) were 2.8 ± 0.5%, 8 ± 3% and 5 ± 3% of LV mass, respectively. No correlation between CMR and blood inflammatory indices (C-reactive protein and erythrocyte sedimentation rate), cardiac troponin T, disease characteristics or type of SSc was identified. A repeat CMR at 6 months, after treatment with prednisone and azathioprine, showed normalisation of the acute inflammation CMR indices.

Conclusions: Silent myocarditis may be diagnosed using the Lake Louise paper criteria in SSc patients without cardiac symptoms, has no correlation with blood inflammatory indices, cardiac troponin or disease characteristics. CMR is a promising tool to diagnose silent myocarditis in SSc and monitor the response to immunosuppressive treatment.

Keywords: Cardiovascular magnetic resonance, Systemic sclerosis, Myocarditis, Myocardial fibrosis

Background

Systemic sclerosis (SSc) is an autoimmune disease characterized by microvascular abnormalities, inflammation and increased fibrosis of all organs, including the heart [1]. Asymptomatic cardiac disease can be presented in up to 80% of SSc patients [2–6] and is included between the three major causes of death in SSc [4]. However, clinically overt heart disease in SSc is less frequent, and was documented only in 20–25% of them [3].

Myocarditis, fibrosis, pulmonary hypertension and blood vessel abnormalities are considered as the main etiologic factors of cardiac involvement in SSc. Myocarditis is a contributor of recent-onset cardiac disease in SSc, and if timely treated, the progression to further cardiac damage can be avoided by immunosuppression [7]. However, the true incidence of myocarditis in asymptomatic SSc has never been assessed.

Cardiovascular Magnetic Resonance (CMR), a non-invasive, non-radiating, operator independent technique, has been successfully used for the evaluation of myocardial fibrosis in SSc [8, 9]. The ability to perform tissue characterisation makes CMR an excellent diagnostic tool to detect myocarditis either due to infective [10] or connective tissue diseases, including SSc [11–15]. The International Consensus Group on CMR Diagnosis of Myocarditis achieved consensus among CMR experts

* Correspondence: soma13@otenet.gr
[1]Onassis Cardiac Surgery Center, 50 Esperou Street, 175-61 P.Faliro, Athens, Greece
Full list of author information is available at the end of the article

and published the Lake Louise criteria about recommendations on the current state-of-the-art use of CMR for myocarditis. The recommendations include indications for CMR in patients with suspected myocarditis, CMR protocol standards, terminology for reporting CMR findings, and diagnostic criteria for myocarditis [10]. According to Lake Louise criteria, oedema evaluation was based on the ratio of myocardial against skeletal muscle signal intensity in STIRT2 images. Early (EGE) was based on ECG-triggered T1-W multislice spin-echo images obtained in axial orientation with identical parameters before and after an intravenous bolus of 0.1 mmol/kg Gd-DTPA within 1 min of injection in the same area as in STIRT2 images. Finally, late gadolinium-enhanced images (LGE) were assessed from images taken 15 min later after another injection of 0.1 mmol/kg Gd-DTPA using an inversion recovery sequence. The examination was considered as positive for myocarditis if 2/3 examined indices are positive [10]. Given that the expected tissue pathology in active myocarditis includes intracellular and interstitial oedema, capillary leakage, hyperaemia and – in more severe cases - myocytolysis and replacement fibrosis, the Lake Louise criteria provide a reliable diagnostic approach to diagnose myocarditis.

We hypothesized that the Lake Louise criteria for myocarditis [10] may be also positive in asymptomatic SSc patients. The aim of our study was to diagnose the potential presence of CMR indices positive for myocarditis according to Lake Louise criteria in asymptomatic SSc.

Methods

Patients

Eighty-two consecutive SSc without cardiac symptoms, diagnosed according to 2013 American College of Rheumatology criteria [16] (ACR score 13 ± 2), aged 43 ± 5 yrs., 62 with diffuse (dSSc) and 20 with localized (lSSc) systemic sclerosis were evaluated. Disease characteristic were presented in Table 1. Exclusion criteria included contraindications to CMR, heart/renal/liver impairment, severe dyspnoea due to lung involvement, pulmonary hypertension, pregnancy and hypersensitivity to gadolinium. All patients gave a written informed consent and the protocol was approved by the Onassis Cardiac Surgery Center ethics committee.

Methods

The presence of myocarditis and the left ventricular systolic function were evaluated by CMR. Myocarditis was documented using STIR T2-weighted (T2-W), T1-weighted before and early after contrast media injection (EGE) and late enhanced images (LGE). The study was considered as positive for myocarditis, according to Lake Louise criteria [10].

A. CMR evaluation of inflammation

Cardiovascular magnetic resonance examination was performed in a 1.5 T Philips Intera system using STIR T2-weighted (T2-W), T1-weighted (T1-W) before and early after contrast media injection (EGE) and late enhanced images (LGE). ECG-triggered, STIR T2-W multislice spin-echo sequence was performed in axial orientation and the signal ratio was calculated from the left ventricular myocardium and the skeletal muscle in the same slice. ECG-triggered T1-W multislice spin-echo images were also obtained in axial orientation with identical parameters before and after an intravenous bolus of 0.1 mmol/kg Gd-DTPA. Measurements were performed after 1 min of injection of Gd-DTPA for early gadolinium enhancement (EGE) in the same area as in T2-W. Immediately after this, 0.1 mmol/kg Gd-DTPA was given again and late gadolinium-enhanced images (LGE) were taken 15 min later, using an a 3D–T1-TFE sequence, preconditioned with a 180 degrees inversion pulse (flip angle =15°, TE = 1.4 msec, TR = 5.5 ms, TI 225 to 275 ms as individually optimized to null myocardial signal, matrix 256X192 and slice thickness = 5 mm). Images were analyzed according to previously described protocols [10].

B. CMR functional study

For each subject, localizing scans were obtained to define the long (2-chamber) axis of the left ventricle. A mid ventricular short axis view was prescribed, and used to plan a 4-chamber view. The short axis orientation was then defined accurately, perpendicular to both the 2- and 4-chamber views. To cover the entire left ventricle, 10 contiguous (gap = 0 mm) short axis slices were acquired in each study. The imaging sequence was a 2D, multi-phase (16 cardiac phases were acquired per cardiac cycle resulting to a temporal resolution of 47 ms for a heart rate of 80 beats/min), steady-state free-precession (SSFP) sequence (TE = 1.5 ms, TR = 3.1 ms, flip angle = 70°, slice thickness = 8 mm, acquired in-plane spatial resolution = 1.8 mm × 2.0 mm) characterized by the application of balanced gradients in all directions [10].

C. Image analysis

In T2-W the signal ratio was measured from the region of interest covering the left ventricular myocardium as well as within a skeletal muscle in the same slice.

xIn T1-W early enhancement (EGE), which reflects hyperaemia and capillary leak as a marker of inflammation, the early myocardial enhancement was measured from the region of interest covering the left ventricular myocardium as well as within a skeletal muscle in the same slice [10].

Table 1 Disease characteristics of SSc population at the time of CMR evaluation

Disease characteristics	dSSc (*n* = 62)	lSSc (*n* = 20)
Female/Male	55/7	17/3
Age (years)	43 ± 2	38 ± 4
Disease duration (months)	5 ± 3	6 ± 1
Current smokers	5	1
Hypertension	8	1
Diabetes	3	0
Hyperlipidemia	6	0
Lung involvement	50	0
Raynaud phenomenon	58	1
Digital ulcers	45	0
Pulmonary hypertension	0	0
GI involvement	28	0
Arthritis	5	0
ESR, mm/h (normal 3–18)	10 ± 2	13 ± 5
CRP, mg/L (normal 2–8)	4 ± 2	2 ± 3
Cardiac troponin T (cTnT), ng/mL (normal 0.01 ± 0.03)	0.006 ± 0.007	0.008 ± 0.007
mRSS	20 ± 6	-
Anti-centromere antibodies, n (%)	0	12
Anti-topoisomerase 1 antibodies, n (%)	53	0
Calcium channel blockers	57	8
Methotrexate	15	0
Prednizolone	0	0
Azathioprine	3	0
Cloroquine	2	1
NSAID	18	3

ESR Erythrocyte sedimentation rate
CRP C-reactive protein
Mrss Modified Rodnan skin score
NSAID Non-steroidal anti-inflammatory drug

To assess the contrast-enhanced images (LGE), all short-axis slices from base to apex were evaluated for areas of normal (completely nulled) myocardium [9, 10]. Mean signal intensity and standard deviation (SD) was derived and a threshold of >6 SD exceeding the mean was used to define areas of LGE. Summing the planimetered areas of LGE in all short- axis slices yielded the total volume, which was expressed as a proportion of total LV myocardium (% LGE). The LGE analysis was performed by one experienced reader and reviewed and by a second expert reader, with both of the readers blinded to patient's identity and clinical history. Any discrepancies between the 2 readers was then adjudicated by a senior reader with >10 yrs. of CMR experience, also blinded to patient's identity and clinical history [9].

Cine images were used for the evaluation of left and right ventricular ejection fraction (LVEF/RVEF), using the MRI-MASS (Medis, Leiden, the Netherlands) software was used and the readers were blinded to the clinical data [11].

Statistical analysis

All measurements were expressed as mean ± SD. Statistical significance of the differences was investigated using unpaired Student's T-test. Correlation between variables was sought with Pearson's correlation coefficient. For non-parametric data, the Mann-Whitney test and Spearman's correlation coefficient were used respectively. Statistical significance was considered for $p < 0.05$.

Results

In our study, CMR documented normal biventricular function in all SSc evaluated. However, 7/62 with dSSc and 2/20 with lSSc, although they had no cardiac symptoms/signs, were positive for myocarditis, according to Lake Louise criteria [10]. In all 9 SSc patients, 3/3 indices were positive for myocarditis. T2 ratio (Fig. 1), EGE and LGE (Fig. 2) were 2.8 ± 0.5, 8 ± 3 and 5 ± 3% of LV mass, respectively. No patient with 2/3 positive indices was identified. In SSc patients without evidence of myocarditis T2 ratio was 1.6 ± 0.2 and 1.5 ± 0.3, EGE 1.16 ± 0.9 and 0.6 ± 0.4, LGE 1.6 ± 2.8 and 0.7 ± 1.4 for dSSc and lSSc, respectively.

There was no correlation between the CMR findings and the blood inflammatory indices (C-reactive protein/CRP and erythrocyte sedimentation rate/ESR), the cardiac troponin T (cTnT) measured at the time of CMR evaluation, the disease characteristics or type of SSc was identified. CMR findings of SSc were presented in Table 2.

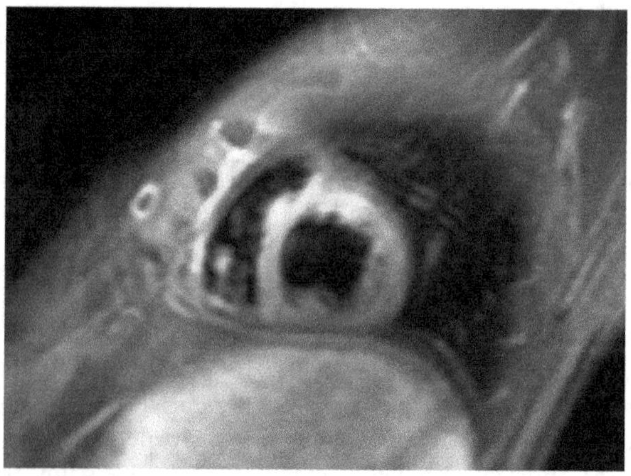

Fig. 1 Short axis STIR T2 showing evidence of oedema in an SSc patient without clinical cardiac symptoms

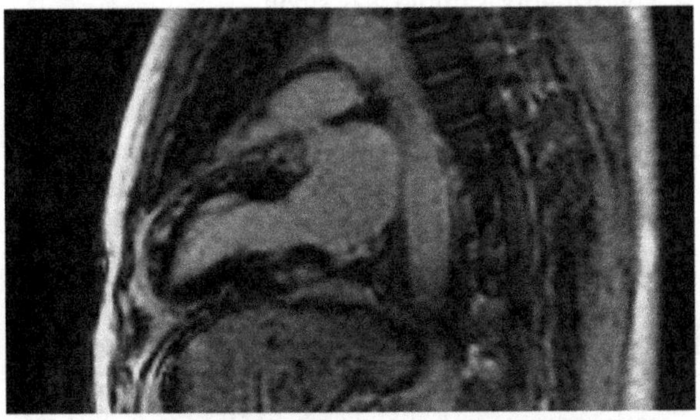

Fig. 2 Two-chamber inversion recovery image showing fibrotic lesions in the anterior and inferior wall of LV, in a patient with SSc, compatible with asymptomatic myocarditis

Treatment with prednisone 20 mg poqd and azathioprine 100 mg poqd started after the positive CMR result for myocarditis was available. A follow up CMR was performed in all SSc patients after 6 months of immunosuppression. These follow up CMR investigations showed complete normalisation of CMR indices indicative of acute myocarditis (T2 ratio = 1.2 ± 2, EGE = 2.5 ± 0.8 and LGE = 3 ± 2% of LV mass).

Discussion

In our study, using the Lake Louise criteria, we documented that 10% of patients with either dSSc or lSSc presented CMR evidence of myocarditis, although they had no cardiac symptoms/signs and positive inflammatory or cardiac biomarkers. No correlation between type of SSc, disease duration, inflammatory indices or cTnT levels and CMR findings was identified. After 6 months of immunosuppression a complete normalization of CMR indices indicative of acute inflammation was identified.

Table 2 CMR findings of the SSc patients studied

Characteristics	dSSc (*n* = 62)	lSSc (*n* = 20)
LVEDV (ml)	117.9 ± 27.9	119.9 ± 19.2
LVESV (ml)	42.6 ± 19.8	40.9 ± 9.5
LVEF (%)	64.7 ± 9.4	63.5 ± 5.7
RVEDV (ml)	110.8 ± 30.9	108.5 ± 21.7
RVESV (ml)	54.4 ± 25.9	46.1 ± 11.8
RVEF (%)	55 ± 11	57 ± 8.5
LGE (%LV)	2 ± 2.9	1 ± 1.77
T2 ratio	1.8 ± 0.4	1.6 ± 0.4
EGE	1.9 ± 2.2	1.4 ± 2.6

LVEDV Left ventricular enddiastolic volume
LVESV Left ventricular endsystolic volume
LVEF Left ventricular ejection fraction
RVEDV Right ventricular enddiastolic volume
RVESV Right ventricular endsystolic volume
RVEF Right ventricular ejection fraction
EGE Early Gd enhancement
LGE Late Gd enhancement

Although myocardial involvement in SSc was usually attributable to non-inflammatory causes, there are early reports presenting SSc patients with evidence of myocarditis and good response to the combination of either corticosteroids and azathioprine [11] or corticosteroids and cyclophosphamide [12]. Our results are in agreement with the majority of previous studies detecting myocarditis in SSc [7–9, 13–15, 17, 18]. However, we identified a significant lower incidence of myocarditis in comparison with other studies [15]. This discrepancy is probably due to the lack of T1, T2 mapping and Extracellular Volume (ECV) assessment. Indeed, native T1 mapping is superior to T2-weighted imaging in detecting myocardial oedema [19]. T1 mapping and ECV can also detect diffuse fibrosis and were well correlated with histology [20]. However, in SSc, it is difficult to distinguish if an increase in T1 mapping is due to myocarditis or to diffuse myocardial fibrosis, which is the "trademark" of the disease, as both can increase native T1 mapping values and ECV. The application of T1 mapping as an oedema index in SSc can potentially lead to overestimation of myocarditis' incidence and "overmedicalisation" of these patients, since it is known that myocarditis in SSc demands prompt treatment with corticosteroids and immunosuppressive drugs [7]. In this context, the application of T2 mapping seems more rational for the detection of recent myocardial inflammation in SSc. This concept is further supported by studies documenting that only T2 mapping seems to be superior, when compared with standard CMR parameters, global myocardial T1, and ECV for assessment of active myocarditis in patients with recent-onset heart failure and reduced LVEF [21]. The application of new CMR indices, mainly of T2 mapping that is the best indicator of myocardial oedema, may further increase the incidence of asymptomatic myocarditis and serve as a prognostic indicator in asymptomatic SSc patients [22].

Although parametric imaging was not available in these SSc patients, recent unpublished data from our group after assessment of 24 SSc patients evaluated by both Lake Louise criteria and parametric imaging in our department showed an increase of T2 mapping in 15/24 SSc with values ranging between 62 and 75 msec, STIR T2 ratio > 2 in 17/24 and native T1 values ranging between 1110 and 1235 mesc in all 22/24 SSc patients. These very preliminary data seem rather support of the use of T2 instead of T1 mapping as an index of recent inflammation in SSc.

Another important issue is the lack of correlation between the blood inflammatory indices and cTnT and CMR indices. However, this is not unusual because lack of such correlation was also identified in both infective [23] and autoimmune myocarditis [8, 13, 24]. This lack of correlation further emphasizes the role of CMR as a powerful diagnostic tool that can provide direct tissue characterization beyond clinical and laboratory findings and potentially modify both rheumatic and cardiac treatment.

Endomyocardial biopsy (EMB), although it carries serious limitations due to its invasive nature, interobserver variability and sampling error, is considered as the diagnostic "gold standard" in clinical scenarios suggestive of myocarditis [25, 26]. Autoimmune myocarditis is likely to be present in our SSc patients, but an overlapping of potential presence of viral myocarditis can not be excluded in the absence of EMB. However, in the clinical setting of our SSc patients, the EMB indication did not fulfil class I or II evidence level [27]. Therefore, we lack a comparative analysis between CMR and EMB in our cases. However, the improvement of CMR indices after immuno-suppressive treatment was strongly supportive of autoimmune myocarditis.

The published literature in the field supports the crucial role of CMR in the diagnosis of myocarditis, as a contributor of heart disease in SSc [7–9, 13–18]. However, there is one study supporting that although CMR is considered as the gold standard in the diagnosis of myocarditis, its role was controversial or falsely negative in half of patients with biopsy-proven myocarditis [28]. Keeping in mind that fibrosis is the hallmark of myocardial disease in SSc, and its pathogenesis is multifactorial, due to microvascular ischemia, spasm and inflammation, this controversy seems rather expectable. Indeed, in SSc, fibrosis may not be used as an independent criterion of myocarditis, since it represents the result of both myocarditis and fibrotic disease independent of inflammatory processes, typical of SSc. On the other hand, the diagnosis of asymptomatic myocarditis in SSc is extremely significant, because it demands prompt rheumatic treatment to avoid future irreversible cardiac lesions [7]; furthermore, although it is easy to diagnose the presence of clinically overt myocarditis, which usually presents with concurrent myositis in SSc [7], it remains rather difficult to achieve this target in asymptomatic cases [8, 13, 18]. The presence of 3 positive CMR indices in all our patients emphasizes the clinical role of Lake Louise criteria in the early detection of asymptomatic myocarditis in SSc. However, due to the pathophysiology of fibrosis in SSc, these criteria may need modifications with regard to myocarditis' diagnosis in SSc. In these patients, maybe all 3 indices should be used for a positive diagnosis and not only the 2/3, as it is the current recommendation of the Lake Louise criteria.

Limitations of the study

The following limitations may be discussed for this study:

1. The patients' sample was small
2. T1 and T2 mapping was not performed, because these sequences were not available at the time of the CMR examination at our center. However, we should mention that although these indices represent an important part of current CMR research, they are not widely available and standardization of the relevant protocols and normal values are still under evaluation [29].
3. Endomyocardial biopsy (EMB) for comparison with CMR findings was not performed, because our patients were not eligible for EMB, due to lack of symptoms and normal biventricular function [30]. Furthermore, the sensitivity of EMB is hampered by e.g. a substantial sampling error due among others to the patchy distribution of this disease (sampling error) [31], and the shortcomings of the currently applied methodology of some laboratories [32].

Conclusions

Silent myocarditis may be diagnosed using the Lake Louise criteria in a considerable percentage of SSc patients presenting without clinical cardiac symptoms, and has no correlation with blood inflammatory indices (CRP, ESR) or further clinical disease characteristics. CMR signs of myocarditis frequently normalize 6 months under after immunosuppressive treatment with corticosteroids and immunosuppressive treatment.

Abbreviations

CMR: Cardiovascular Magnetic Resonance; CRP: C reactive protein; EMB: Endomyocardial biopsy; ESR: Erythrocyte sedimendation rate; JACC: Journal of American Society of Cardiology; LVEF: Left ventricular ejection fraction; SSc: Systemic sclerosis; SSFP: Steady-state free-precession sequence; T1-W: T1- weighted; T2-W: T2- weighted; TE: Echo time; TR: Repetition time

Acknowledgements

Not applicable.

Disclosure of potential conflicts of interest

Author Sophie Mavrogeni declares she is co-editor in BMC CVD. Author Loukia Koutsogeorgopoulou declares that he/she has no conflict of interest. Author Georgia Karabela declares that he/she has no conflict of interest. Author Efthymios Stavropoulos declares that he/she has no conflict of interest. Author Gikas Katsifis declares that he/she has no conflict of interest. Author John Raftakis declares that he/she has no conflict of interest. Author Sotiris Plastiras declares that he/she has no conflict of interest. Author Michel Noutsias declares the following potential conflicts of interest: MN has received grants related to myocarditis (Deutsche Forschungsgemeinschaft through the Sonderforschungsbereich Transregio 19 "Inflammatory Cardiomyopathy" (SFB TR19; TP B2, C6 and Z1); and by the University Hospital Giessen and Marburg Foundation Grant "T cell functionality" (UKGM 10/2009 to MN). MN has been consultant to the IKDT (Institute for Cardiac Diagnosis and Therapy GmbH, Berlin) 2004–2008, and has received honoraria for presentations and/or participated in advisory boards from AstraZeneca, Bayer, Fresenius, Miltenyi Biotech, Novartis, Pfizer and Zoll. Author George Markousis-Mavrogenis declares that he/she has no conflict of interest. Author Genovefa Kolovou declares that he/she has no conflict of interest.

Funding

Not applicable.

Authors' contributions

S M, Patients scanning analysis and paper writing. LK, rheumatic data evaluation and writing. GK, cardiac data evaluation and writing. E S, rheumatic data evaluation and writing. G K, rheumatic data evaluation and writing. J R, rheumatic data evaluation and writing. S P, cardiac data evaluation and writing. M N, paper writing. GMM, study design, scanning analysis and paper writing. GK, paper writing, team coordination. All authors read and approved the final manuscript.

Competing interests

Competing interests for Prof Noutsias (BMC editor).
Dr. S. Mavrogeni (BMC co-editor).

Author details

[1]Onassis Cardiac Surgery Center, 50 Esperou Street, 175-61 P.Faliro, Athens, Greece. [2]Pathophysiology Department, Laikon Hospital, Athens, Greece. [3]Athens Naval Hospital, Athens, Greece. [4]Asklipion Voulas Hospital, Athens, Greece. [5]Department of Internal Medicine III, Division of Cardiology, Angiology and Intensive Medical Care, University Hospital Halle, Martin-Luther-University Halle, Ernst-Grube-Straße 40, D-06120 Halle (Saale), Germany.

References

1. Ferri C, Valentini G, Cozzi F, et al. Systemic sclerosis: demographic, clinical, and serologic features and survival in 1,012 Italian patients. Medicine Baltimore. 2002;81:139–53.
2. Janosik DL, Osborn TG, Moore TL, Shah DG, Kenney RG, Zuckner J. Heart disease in systemic sclerosis. Semin Arthritis Rheum. 1989;19:191–200.
3. Deswal A, Follansbee WP. Cardiac involvement in scleroderma. Rheum Dis Clin N Am. 1996;22:841–60.
4. Lee P, Langevitz P, Alderdice CA, Aubrey M, Baer PA, Baron M, et al. Mortality in systemic sclerosis (scleroderma). Q J Med. 1992;298:139–48.
5. Follansbee WP, Curtiss EI, Medsger TA Jr, Steen VD, Uretsky BF, Owens GR, et al. Physiologic abnormalities of cardiac function in progressive systemic sclerosis with diffuse scleroderma. N Engl J Med. 1984;310:142–8.
6. Candell-Riera J, Armadans-Gil L, Simeon CP, Castell-Conesa J, Fonollosa-Pla V, Garcia-del-Castillo H, et al. Comprehensive noninvasive assessment of cardiac involvement in limited systemic sclerosis. Arthritis Rheum. 1996;39:1138–45.
7. Pieroni M, De Santis M, Zizzo G, Bosello S, Smaldone C, Campioni M, De Luca G, Laria A, Meduri A, Bellocci F, Bonomo L, Crea F, Ferraccioli G. Recognizing and treating myocarditis in recent-onset systemic sclerosis heart disease: potential utility of immunosuppressive therapy in cardiac damage progression. Semin Arthritis Rheum. 2014;43(4):526–35.
8. Mavrogeni SI, Bratis K, Karabela G, Spiliotis G, Kv W, Hautemann D, Reiber JH, Koutsogeorgopoulou L, Markousis-Mavrogenis G, Kolovou G, Stavropoulos E. Cardiovascular magnetic resonance imaging clarifies cardiac pathophysiology in early, asymptomatic diffuse systemic sclerosis. Inflamm Allergy Drug Targets. 2015;14(1):29–36.
9. Mavrogeni S, Karabela G, Koutsogeorgopoulou L, Stavropoulos E, Katsifis G, Plastiras SC, Kitas GD, Panopoulos S, Pentazos G, Tzatzaki E, Markousis-Mavrogenis G, Kolovou G, Sfikakis PP. Pseudo-infarction pattern in diffuse systemic sclerosis. Evaluation using cardiovascular magnetic resonance. Int J Cardiol. 2016;214:465–8.
10. Friedrich MG, Sechtem U, Schulz-Menger J, Holmvang G, Alakija P, Cooper LT, White JA, Abdel-Aty H, Gutberlet M, Prasad S, Aletras A, Laissy JP, Paterson I, Filipchuk NG, Kumar A, Pauschinger M, Liu P. International consensus group on cardiovascular magnetic resonance in Myocarditis. Cardiovascular magnetic resonance in myocarditis: a JACC white paper. J Am Coll Cardiol. 2009;53:1475–87.
11. Kerr LD, Spiera H. Myocarditis as a complication in scleroderma patients with myositis. Clin Cardiol. 1993;16(12):895–9.
12. Stack J, McLaughlin P, Sinnot C, Henry M, MacEneaney P, Eltahir A, Harney S. Successful control of scleroderma myocarditis using a combination of cyclophosphamide and methylprednisolone. Scand J Rheumatol. 2010;39(4):349–50.
13. Mavrogeni S, Sfikakis PP, Gialafos E, Bratis K, Karabela G, Stavropoulos E, Spiliotis G, Sfendouraki E, Panopoulos S, Bournia V, Kolovou G, Kitas GD. Cardiac tissue characterization and the diagnostic value of cardiovascular magnetic resonance in systemic connective tissue diseases. Arthritis Care Res (Hoboken). 2014;66(1):104–12.
14. Ntusi NA, Piechnik SK, Francis JM, Ferreira VM, Matthews PM, Robson MD, Wordsworth PB, Neubauer S, Karamitsos TD. Diffuse myocardial fibrosis and inflammation in rheumatoid arthritis: insights from CMR T1 mapping. JACC Cardiovasc Imaging. 2015;8(5):526–36.
15. Ntusi NA, Piechnik SK, Francis JM, Ferreira VM, Rai AB, Matthews PM, Robson MD, Moon J, Wordsworth PB, Neubauer S, Karamitsos TD. Subclinical myocardial inflammation and diffuse fibrosis are common in systemic sclerosis–a clinical study using myocardial T1-mapping and extracellular volume quantification. J Cardiovasc Magn Reson. 2014;16:21.
16. van den Hoogen F, Khanna D, Fransen J, et al. 2013 classification criteria for systemic sclerosis: an American College of Rheumatology/European league against rheumatism collaborative initiative. Ann Rheum Dis. 2013;72:1747–55.
17. Kobayashi Y, Kobayashi H. T Giles J, Yokoe I, Hirano M, Nakajima Y, Takei M. Detection of left ventricular regional dysfunction and myocardial abnormalities using complementary cardiac magnetic resonance imaging in patients with systemic sclerosis without cardiac symptoms: a pilot study. Intern Med. 2016;55(3):237–43.
18. Mavrogeni S, Sfikakis PP, Karabela G, Stavropoulos E, Spiliotis G, Gialafos E, Panopoulos S, Bournia V, Manolopoulou D, Kolovou G, Kitas G. Cardiovascular magnetic resonance imaging in asymptomatic patients with connective tissue disease and recent onset left bundle branch block. Int J Cardiol. 2014;171(1):82–7.
19. Ferreira VM, Piechnik SK, Dall'Armellina E, Karamitsos TD, Francis JM, Choudhury RP, Friedrich MG, Robson MD, Neubauer S. Non-contrast T1-mapping detects acute myocardial edema with high diagnostic accuracy: a comparison to T2-weighted cardiovascular magnetic resonance. J Cardiovasc Magn Reson. 2012;14:42.
20. Bull S, White SK, Piechnik SK, Flett AS, Ferreira VM, Loudon M, Francis JM, Karamitsos TD, Prendegrast BD, Robson MD, Neubauer S, Moon JC, Myerson SG. Human non-contrast T1 values and correlation with histology in diffuse fibrosis. Heart. 2013;99:932–7.
21. Bohnen S, Radunski UK, Lund GK, Kandolf R, Stehning C, Schnackenburg B, Adam G, Blankenberg S, Muellerleile K. Performance of t1 and t2 mapping cardiovascular magnetic resonance to detect active myocarditis in patients with recent-onset heart failure. Circ Cardiovasc Imaging. 2015;8(6). doi:10.1161/CIRCIMAGING.114.003073. PubMed PMID: 26015267.
22. Spieker M, Haberkorn S, Gastl M, Behm P, Katsianos S, Horn P, Jacoby C, Schnackenburg B, Reinecke P, Kelm M, Westenfeld R, Bönner F. Abnormal T2 mapping cardiovascular magnetic resonance correlates with adverse clinical outcome in patients with suspected acute myocarditis. J Cardiovasc Magn Reson. 2017;19(1):38.
23. Mavrogeni S, Markousis-Mavrogenis G, Kolovou G. How to approach the great mimic? Improving techniques for the diagnosis of myocarditis. Expert Rev Cardiovasc Ther. 2016;14(1):105–15.
24. Mavrogeni S, Markousis-Mavrogenis G, Koutsogeorgopoulou L, Dimitroulas T, Bratis K, Kitas GD, Sfikakis P, Tektonidou M, Karabela G, Stavropoulos E, Katsifis G, Boki KA, Kitsiou A, Filaditaki V, Gialafos E, Plastiras S, Vartela V, Kolovou G. Cardiovascular magnetic resonance imaging pattern at the time of diagnosis of treatment naïve patients with connective tissue diseases. Int J Cardiol. 2017;236:151–6.
25. Noutsias M, Seeberg B, Schultheiss HP, Kühl U. Expression of cell adhesion molecules in dilated cardiomyopathy: evidence for endothelial activation in inflammatory cardiomyopathy. Circulation. 1999;99(16):2124–31.
26. Caforio AL, Pankuweit S, Arbustini E, Basso C, Gimeno-Blanes J, Felix SB, Fu M, Helio T, Heymans S, Jahns R, Klingel K, Linhart A, Maisch B, McKenna W, Mogensen J, Pinto YM, Ristic A, Schultheiss HP, Seggewiss H, Tavazzi L, Thiene G, Yilmaz A, Charron P, Elliott PM, European Society of Cardiology Working Group on M, Pericardial D. Current state of knowledge on aetiology, diagnosis, management, and therapy of myocarditis: a position statement of the European Society of Cardiology Working Group on myocardial and pericardial diseases. Eur Heart J. 2013;34(33):2636–48. 2648a-2648d
27. Cooper LT, Baughman KL, Feldman AM, Frustaci A, Jessup M, Kühl U, Levine GN, Narula J, Starling RC, Towbin J, Virmani R. The role of endomyocardial biopsy in the management of cardiovascular disease: a scientific statement from the American Heart Association, the American College of Cardiology, and the European Society of Cardiology Endorsed by the Heart Failure Society of America and the heart failure Association of the European Society of cardiology. Eur Heart J. 2007;28(24):3076–93.

28. Zizzo G, De Santis M, Bosello S, Peluso G, Alivernini S, Pinnelli M, et al. Myocarditis in systemic sclerosis diagnosed through endomyocardial biopsy. Arthritis Rheum. 2009;60(Suppl 10):1201.
29. von Knobelsdorff-Brenkenhoff F, Prothmann M, Dieringer MA, Wassmuth R, Greiser A, Schwenke C, Niendorf T, Schulz-Menger J. Myocardial T1 and T2 mapping at 3 T: reference values, influencing factors and implications. J Cardiovasc Magn Reson. 2013;15:53.
30. Leone O, Veinot JP, Angelini A, Baandrup UT, Basso C, Berry G, Bruneval P, Burke M, Butany J, Calabrese F, d'Amati G, Edwards WD, Fallon JT, Fishbein MC, Gallagher PJ, Halushka MK, McManus B, Pucci A, Rodriguez ER, Saffitz JE, Sheppard MN, Steenbergen C, Stone JR, Tan C, Thiene G, van der Wal AC, Winters GL. 2011 consensus statement on endomyocardial biopsy from the Association for European Cardiovascular Pathology and the Society for Cardiovascular Pathology. Cardiovasc Pathol. 2012;21(4):245–74.
31. Hauck AJ, Kearney DL, Edwards WD. Evaluation of postmortem endomyocardial biopsy specimens from 38 patients with lymphocytic myocarditis: implications for role of sampling error. Mayo Clin Proc. 1989; 64(10):1235–45.
32. Stiermaier T, Föhrenbach F, Klingel K, Kandolf R, Boudriot E, Sandri M, Linke A, Rommel KP, Desch S, Schuler G, Thiele H, Lurz P. Biventricular endomyo-cardial biopsy in patients with suspected myocarditis: feasibility, complication rate and additional diagnostic value. Int J Cardiol. 2017;230:364–70.

27

Multiparametric cardiac magnetic resonance imaging (CMR) for the diagnosis of Loeffler's endocarditis

Mareike Gastl*, Patrick Behm, Christoph Jacoby, Malte Kelm and Florian Bönner

Abstract

Background: Endocarditis parietalis fibroplastica Löfflein (EPF) is a rare form of primary restrictive cardiomyopathy with poor prognosis. It is generally caused by hypereosinophilic syndrome with eosinophilic penetration of the heart. This leads to congestive heart failure in three different stages. As a frequent manifestation of neoplastic diseases, cardiac involvement means poor prognosis.

Case presentation: The present report deals with a case of EPF caused by non-specified T-cell lymphoma (T-NOS). Besides an elevated Troponin-T enzyme, the electrocardiogram and the transthoracic echocardiography did not show any characteristic results. Due to risk/benefit assessment and low thrombocyte amounts, endomyocardial biopsy and catheterization were discarded. Using cardiovascular magnetic resonance (CMR) with steady-state free precession sequences, T2-mappping, strain analysis and late gadolinium enhancement, we were able to clearly highlight cardiac involvement at different stages. These findings characterized T-NOS as a palliative situation.

Conclusion: Multiparametric CMR can not only identify EPF but also characterize the patchy disease state. This provides an individual prognosis assessment. Aside from prognosis estimation, it can also be used for therapy monitoring.

Keywords: CMR, Restrictive cardiomyopathy, Loeffler's endocarditis, Heart failure, Hypereosinophilic syndrome, Fibrosis, Case report

Background

Endocarditis parietalis fibroplastica (Loeffler's disease) (EPF) is a disease with poor prognosis, first described by Loeffler in 1936. A diagnosis requires blood eosinophilia and affection of the endocardium as key steps [1]. The EPF belongs to the hypereosinophilic syndromes (HES) with rare epidemiologic data. Spry et al. showed a prevalence of 1:200000 in general population [2]. In more recent studies, the prevalence of EPF is shown from 40 to 50% among patients with HES [3]. Eosinophils must be elevated over $1.5x10^9$ eosinophils per litre for about 6 months to lead to the diagnosis of hypereosinophilia, although blood levels may lack hypereosinophilia in later stages. HES syndrome can be idiopathic or correlated to clonal interleukin 5 (IL-5) over-production of T-helper cells. Once the heart is affected, the disease passes three steps: 1. Acute necrosis followed by 2. thrombosis and 3. end stage of fibrosis [4]. The underlying pathophysiology is a degradation of cytotoxic eosinophilic proteins, which may reveal endocardial thickening, ventricular obliteration by echogenic material, suggestive of fibrosis or thrombosis, atrial dilation, restrictive pattern in echo Doppler or coronary vessel alterations [5]. Still, diagnostic process is heterogeneous and is yet to be standardized. Electrocardiogram (ECG) and transthoracic echocardiography (TTE) are unspecific and these technologies have certain restrictions (i.e. insufficient acoustic window). Endomyocardial biopsy is supposed to be the gold standard of diagnostic tools, but exerts a considerable inherent sampling error and may thus suffer from insufficient diagnostic sensitivity. Cardiovascular magnetic resonance (CMR) might be able to characterize the specific stages of the disease

* Correspondence: Mareike.Gastl@med.uni-duesseldorf.de
Department of Cardiology, Pulmonology and Vascular Medicine, Heinrich-Heine University Düsseldorf, Düsseldorf, Germany

Table 1 Timeline

12/2012:	Diagnosis of non-specified T-cell lymphoma (T-NOS); Stage III B Ann Arbor
12/12 – 03/13:	CHOEP-14 protocol
03/13:	Massive progress of T-NOS (change from CHOEP to DHA, to vincristine and SDH in emergency)
04/13	Autogenic stem cell transplantation + Radiochemotheraphy (Cyclophosphamid)
06/13:	Allogenic stem cell transplantation
06/13:	Thrombosis Vena cava inferior/iliaca communis
10/13:	Remission of T-NOS
07/15:	Relapse of T-NOS
07/15 – 01/16:	IGEV-Therapy, bendamustine, DLI
01/16:	Change to everolimus
01/16:	Diagnosis of Loeffler's endocarditis

CHOEP-14 cyclophosphamide, doxorubicin, vincristine, etoposide and prednisone, *DHA* Docosahexaenoic acid, *SDH* Solu-Decortin, *IGEV* ifosfamide, gemcitabine, vinorelbine and prednisone, *DLI* donor lymphcyte infusion

due to its superior native soft tissue contrast and further tissue characterisation by contrast-enhanced sequences.

Case presentation

A 38-year-old man with a medical history of non-specified T-cell lymphoma (T-NOS) including immunosuppressive therapy regimes and a stem cell transplantation came to the emergency unit of the university hospital in Duesseldorf because of his uncontrolled nose bleeding (Table 1). Next to low thrombocyte amounts (less than 9000/µl), blood diagnostic showed an elevation of the Troponin-T enzyme up to 324 ng/l (normal cut-off at 14 ng/l). ECG revealed unspecific negative T-waves in leads II, III, aVF, V4 and V6. In TTE, only a slight hypertrophy of the interventricular septum and the left ventricular posterior wall was detected, while the global ventricular function was normal. Due to inadequate acoustic window, the quality of TTE images proved too poor for strain evaluation. The patient was transferred to the department of cardiology on suspicion of an acute myocarditis or coronary artery disease. Due to risk assessment (GRACE Score <140) and thrombocytopenia, invasive coronary angiography or endomyocardial biopsy (EMB) were initially discarded. In the meantime, a CMR examination for identification of myocardial lesions was conducted.

Cine steady state free precession (SSFP) images revealed normal left and right ventricular function (LV ejection fraction (EF) 61%, RV-EF 61%). As can be seen in Fig. 1a (*doubled arrows*), LV and RV walls were thickened and displayed subendocardial susceptibility artefacts (arrow). Despite normal LV-EF, myocardial feature tracking analysis (TomTec Imaging Systems, Unterschleißheim, Germany) revealed impaired systolic endocardial and epicardial global longitudinal strain (GLS) compared to literature standards (-17.7% vs. -22.2% for endocardial GLS; -14.5% vs. -20.4% for epicardial GLS) [6]. Peak early diastolic strain rate (SRe) was impaired in epi- and endocardium as well, indicating diastolic impairment (1.2 s^{-1} vs. 1.7 s^{-1} for endocardial diastolic SRe; 1.0 s^{-1} vs. 1.5 s^{-1} for epicardial diastolic SRe) (Fig. 1b).

Perfusion images showed an imbalance of transmyocardial perfusion already under resting conditions (Fig. 2a, *arrows*). This phenomenon was aggravated during regadenoson induced hyperaemia, that showed highly impaired perfusion in endocardial layers, indicating altered coronary microcirculation (Fig. 2b).

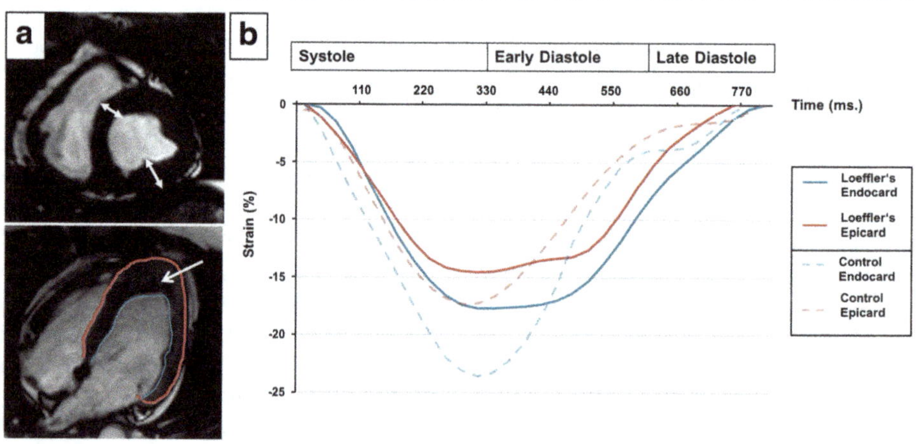

Fig. 1 *Functional characteristics of Loeffler's endocarditis.* **a** Cine steady state free precession images (SSFP) in two and four chamber views. Thickened myocardial wall is indicated by doubled arrows. Altered myocardium in terms of subendocardial susceptibility artefacts can be seen in native contrast (*arrow*). The blue line marks the endocardial, the red line the epicardial contour used for myocardial strain analysis. **b** Systolic endocardial and epicardial global longitudinal strains (GLS) were altered compared to literature standards and an age-matched control (*dotted blue line* vs. continuous *blue line* for endocardial GLS; *dotted red line* vs. continuous *red line* for epicardial GLS). Epi- and endocardial borders revealed diastolic dysfunction in terms of delayed diastolic relaxation

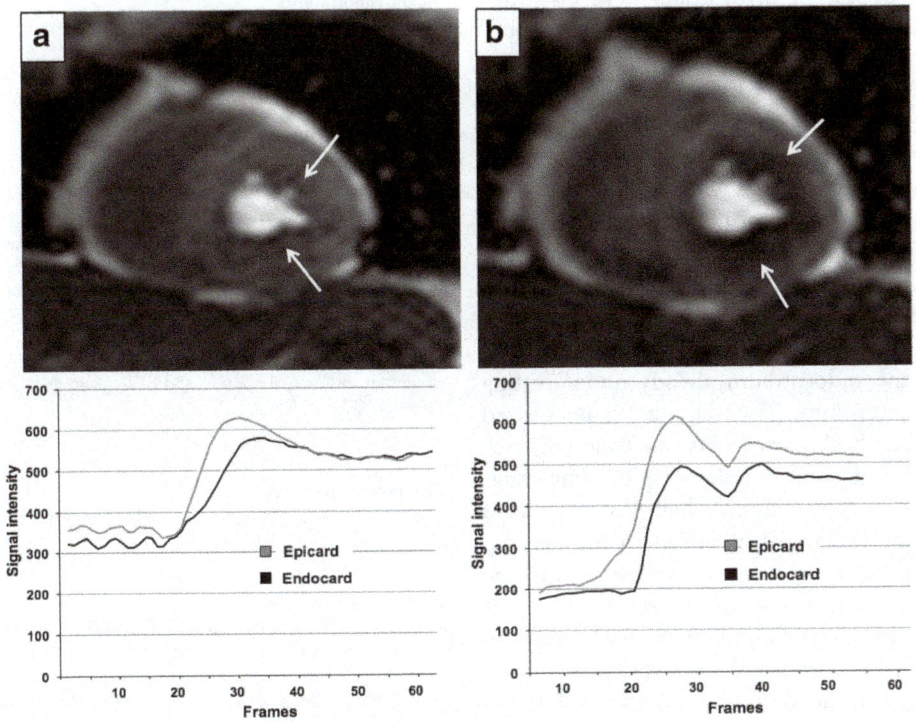

Fig. 2 *Coronary flow characteristics of Loeffler's endocarditis.* Myocardial perfusion at rest (**a**) and in hyperaemia state (**b**). At rest, a small lack of endocardial perfusion is present (*arrows*, **a**). The endocardial intensity-time curve shows a slower contrast agent uptake in comparison to the epicardial curve still reaching epicardial intensity at the end of the sequence. This phenomenon was intensified in regadenoson stress protocol (*arrows*, **b**). Endocardial intensity-time curve did not reach epicardial values throughout the sequence indicating impaired coronary microcirculation

To analyse myocardial tissue texture, a parametric CMR was conducted to separate oedema or acute necrosis to other tissue texture components with T2 mapping [7]. As shown in Fig. 3a, T2 mapping revealed a slightly reduced T2 time (55.0 ± 8.4 ms, arrows) compared to an age- and gender-matched control (56.4 ± 3.5), which was still in the normal value range according to current literature [8]. Epimyocardial T2 time was elevated compared to the control (69.6 ± 11.9 ms vs. 60.3 ± 4.6 ms, arrowheads) suspecting acute tissue oedema [8]. Diffuse subendocardial late gadolinium enhancement (LGE) was detected in both chambers in those areas of slightly reduced T2 time completing the previous findings (Fig. 3b, *arrows*).

Taking the localisation of fibrosis, the T2 map and the perfusion abnormalities into account, the hypotheses of

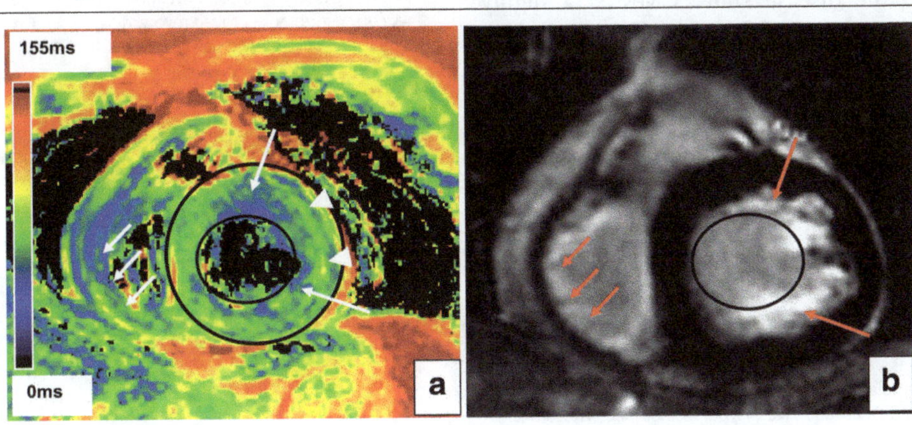

Fig. 3 *Myocardial texture of Loeffler's endocarditis.* **a** Parametric T2 mapping revealed a slightly reduced T2 time in subendocardial layers (*white arrows*). Interestingly, epicardial T2 time was elevated (*arrowheads*) indicative for acute tissue oedema. **b** Late gadolinium enhancement (LGE) in subendocardial layers (*red arrows*) of the left and right ventricle corresponded to reduced T2 time suspective of subendocardial fibrosis. However, epicardial layers were not affected with LGE, but with increased T2 time

vascular coronary disease or myocarditis were discarded since there was neither an endocardial lesion corresponding to a coronary territory nor an epicardial lesion. Additional details of the patient's history revealed a hypereosinophilia (max. 11.900/µl, normal value < 440/µl) for more than 6 months. On the basis of the CMR findings and the patient's history of T-NOS with hypereosinophilia, he was diagnosed to have Endocarditis parietalis fibroplastica Löfflein (EPF). Interestingly, the multiparametric CMR workup revealed different stages of myocardial involvement: reduced GLS, diffuse LGE, perfusion defect and slightly lower T2-time displayed fibrosis and reduced coronary flow of the endocardium already under resting conditions. The epicardium, however, was characterized by abnormal GLS with abnormal diastolic function, lack of LGE, preserved perfusion, but elevated T2 times suggesting an inflammatory stadium. A high-dose corticoid drug (Dexamethasone 40 mg) was added to the existing everolimus-therapy and the patient was transferred to the department of haematology for further diagnostics. His bone marrow showed elevated numbers of eosinophilia up to 10% during completion of diagnostic steps.

Cardiac involvement at different stages of EPF as shown by multiparametric CMR characterized T-NOS as a palliative situation, as recent therapeutic regimes such as immunosuppressive drugs and stem cell transplantation did not lead to a lasting remission.

Since multiparametric CMR workup could not only identify EPF but also characterize the patchy disease state (T2 map, LGE and myocardial strain) and stratify the patient's individual prognosis, invasive coronary angiography and endomyocardial biopsy were not conducted.

Discussion and Conclusion

The present case of EPF illustrates that multiparametric CMR can not only identify EPF, but also characterize EPF according to the disease state. CMR is a highly efficient tool for the process of diagnosis if invasive procedures are discarded due to risk/benefit assessment. In this particular case, myocarditis and coronary artery disease could be excluded without EMB or angiography due to multiparametric CMR. In addition, CMR detected advanced endocardial fibrosis with wall thickening as morphological hallmarks of the disease, while those features would have technically impeded adequate EMB.

Abbreviations

CMR: Cardiac magnetic resonance; ECG: Electrocardiogram; EF: Ejection fraction; EMB: Endomyocardial biopsy; EPF: Endocarditis parietalis fibroplastica Löfflein; GLS: Global longitudinal strain; HES: Hypereosinophilic syndromes; IL-5: Interleukin 5; LGE: Late gadolinium enhancement; LV: Left ventricle; RV: Right ventricle; SSFP: Steady state free precession; T-NOS: Non-specified T-cell lymphoma; TTE: Transthoracic echocardiography

Acknowledgments

Not applicable.

Funding

No funding has been received.

Authors' contributions

MG and FB have been involved in drafting the manuscript, have made substantial contributions to conception and presentation of the case and have revisited it critically for important intellectual content. They have given final approval of the version to be published. CJ has made substantial contributions to conception and design of the case. Together with PB and MK, they have been involved in revising the manuscript critically for important intellectual content and have given final approval of the version to be published.

Competing interests

The authors declare that they have no competing interests.

References

1. Löffler W. Endocarditis parietalis fibroplastica mit Bluteosinophilie. Ein eigenartiges Krankheitsbild. Schweiz Med Wochenschr. 1936;66:817–20.
2. Spry C. The hypereosinophilic syndrome: clinical features, laboratory findings and treatment. Allergy. 1982. http://onlinelibrary.wiley.com/doi/10.1111/j.1398-9995.1982.tb02339.x/epdf. Accessed 4 July 2016.
3. Parrillo J. Heart disease and the eosinophil. New Eng J Med. 1990. Retrieved from http://www.nejm.org/doi/pdf/10.1056/NEJM199011293232211. Accessed 19 Apr 2016.
4. Niemeijer ND, LA van Daele P, Caliskan K, Oei FB, Loosveld OJ, van der Meer NJ, Hicks G. Löffler endocarditis: a rare cause of acute cardiac failure. J Cardiothorac Surg. 2012;7(1):109. http://doi.org/10.1186/1749-8090-7-109.
5. Corssmit E, Trip M, & Durrer J. Löffler's endomyocarditis in the idiopathic hypereosinophilic syndrome. Cardiology. 1999;91(4):272–6.
6. Andre F, Steen H, Matheis P, Westkott M, Breuninger K, Sander Y, Lima J. Age- and gender-related normal left ventricular deformation assessed by cardiovascular magnetic resonance feature tracking. J Cardiovasc Magn Reson. 2015;17(1):25. http://doi.org/10.1186/s12968-015-0123-3.
7. Bönner F, Janzarik N, Jacoby C, Spieker M, Schnackenburg B, Range F, Kelm M. Myocardial T2 mapping reveals age- and sex-related differences in volunteers. J Cardiovasc Magn Reson. 2015;17(1):9. http://doi.org/10.1186/s12968-015-0118-0.
8. Bönner F, Spieker M, Haberkorn S, Jacoby C, Flögel U, Schnackenburg B, Westenfeld R. Myocardial T2 mapping increases noninvasive diagnostic accuracy for biopsy-proven myocarditis. JACC. 2016. http://doi.org/10.1016/j.jcmg.2015.11.014. Accessed 12 July 2016.

28

Use of speckle-tracking echocardiography–derived strain and systolic strain rate measurements to predict rejection in transplant hearts with preserved ejection fraction

Andrew S. Tseng[1], Umama S. Gorsi[2], Sergio Barros-Gomes[2], Fletcher A. Miller[2], Patricia A. Pellikka[2], Alfredo L. Clavell[2] and Hector R. Villarraga[2*]

Abstract

Background: Noninvasive diagnosis of allograft rejection in heart transplant recipients is challenging. The utility of 2-dimensional speckle-tracking echocardiography (2D-STE) to predict severe rejection in heart transplant recipients with preserved left ventricular ejection fraction (LVEF) was evaluated.

Methods: Adult heart transplant patients with preserved LVEF (> 55%) and severe rejection by biopsy (Rejection Grade ≥ 2R) or no rejection between 1997 and 2011 at the Mayo Clinic in Rochester, Minnesota were evaluated. Transthoracic echocardiography was performed within 1 month of the biopsy. LV global longitudinal and circumferential strain and strain rates (GLS, GLSR, GCS, and GCSR) were analyzed retrospectively.

Results: Of 65 patients included, 25 had severe rejection and 40 were normal transplant controls without rejection. Both groups had more men than women (64 and 75%, respectively). Baseline clinical variables were similar between the groups. Both groups had normal LVEF (64.3% vs 64.5%; $P = .87$). All non-strain echocardiographic variables were similar between the 2 groups. Strain analysis showed significantly increased early diastolic longitudinal strain rate ($P = .02$) and decreased GCS ($P < .001$) and GCSR ($P = .02$) for the rejection group compared with the control group. The area under the receiver operating characteristic curve for GCS was 0.77. With a GCS cutoff of – 17.60%, the sensitivity and specificity of GCS to detect severe acute rejection were 81.8 and 68.4%, respectively.

Conclusions: 2D-STE may be useful in detecting severe transplant rejection in heart transplant patients with normal LVEF.

Keywords: Echocardiography, Imaging, Rejection, Heart transplant, Strain

Background

Heart transplantation is the treatment of choice for many patients with end-stage heart failure. Improvement in long-term survival has been recognized in the past several decades as a consequence of careful recipient and donor selection, advances in immunosuppression, and management of opportunistic infections. A 2015 report by the Organ Procurement and Transplantation Network and the Scientific Registry of Transplant Recipients documented the overall survival rate after heart transplant in the United States as 82% after 1 year and approximately 69% after 5 years [1]. As such, detecting severe acute heart transplant rejection is imperative for increasing the survival of heart transplant patients. Currently, the diagnostic standard for organ rejection is myocardial biopsy, an invasive procedure that has numerous potential complications including carotid puncture, prolonged bleeding, arrhythmias, and myocardial

* Correspondence: villarraga.hector@mayo.edu
[2]Department of Cardiovascular Diseases, Mayo Clinic, Rochester, Minnesota, 200 First St SW, Rochester, MN 55905, USA
Full list of author information is available at the end of the article

perforation [2]. The risk of major complications from this invasive procedure is estimated to be between 0.09 and 5.2% [3].

Echocardiography is an important noninvasive tool to evaluate graft size and function, given its portability and availability. The use of 2-dimensional speckle-tracking echocardiography (2D-STE), in particular, to measure strain and systolic strain rate is important for evaluating myocardial mechanical dysfunction [4, 5]. 2D-STE determines strain and systolic strain rate from myocardial motion derived from the echocardiogram. In otherwise normal heart transplant patients, systolic strain indices obtained from 2D-STE were determined to be sensitive markers of myocardial dysfunction [6]. Left ventricular (LV) mechanical function in heart transplant patients and non-transplant patients has previously been analyzed using 2D-STE, which showed decreased strain in transplant patients. Saleh et al. [7] previously reported normal LV mechanical function and synchrony values by 2D-STE in transplanted hearts with preserved ejection fraction (EF). Previous studies using 2D-STE have shown that various indices of LV radial, circumferential, longitudinal and torsional strain may be useful in detecting heart transplant rejection [8–12].

The aim of this study was to evaluate the use of 2D-STE–derived strain measurements as a noninvasive clinical prediction tool in a specific subset of patients with severe acute rejection in heart transplant patients with preserved LVEF.

Methods

Study population

The study population consisted of adult patients (age greater than or equal to 18 years) who underwent heart transplantation at Mayo Clinic, Rochester, Minnesota, from January 1, 1997, through December 31, 2011. Patients were retrospectively identified by a search of our institutional patient database. All heart transplant patients during this time period who experienced severe biopsy-confirmed cell-mediated rejection (2R or greater) based on the 2004 International Society for Heart and Lung Transplantation (ISHLT) grading system [13] and who had LVEF greater than 55% were included in this study. Patients with known transplant vasculopathy were excluded. Transthoracic echocardiography was performed within 1 month prior to the biopsy. Control participants included heart transplant patients without transplant vasculopathy by angiography or intravascular ultrasonography, with no evidence of rejection by routine surveillance endomyocardial biopsy and normal echocardiography findings at one-year post-transplantation follow-up. Patients with abnormal renal function, significant valvular disease, or uncontrolled hypertension were excluded from the study. The electronic medical records were reviewed for demographic characteristics, along with clinical and echocardiographic data. Pertinent laboratory values, medications, and other clinical history were obtained at the time of echocardiography. All participants provided written informed consent. The study protocol was approved by the Mayo Clinic Institutional Review Board.

Standard echocardiography

Comprehensive 2D echocardiography was performed using a Vivid E9 Ultrasound System (GE Healthcare) with a 2.5- to 4.0-MHz transducer, as part of the recommendations from the American Society of Echocardiography [14]. The modified Quinones equation or volumetric biplane Simpson method, or both, as appropriate, was used to quantify LVEF. Offline 2D-STE analysis (Velocity Vector Imaging) was performed retrospectively. Clinical, survival, and echocardiographic data were masked to the reviewers.

Speckle-tracking echocardiography

Three consecutive heart cycles from each of the apical views (apical 4-chamber, 3-chamber, and 2-chamber) were obtained for longitudinal strain analysis, including global longitudinal strain (GLS), global longitudinal strain rate (GLSR), and early diastolic global longitudinal strain rate (GLSRe). Short-axis views at the midpapillary level were obtained for circumferential strain analysis, including global circumferential strain (GCS) and global circumferential strain rate (GCSR).

Strain measurements were performed offline and analyzed with syngo Velocity Vector Imaging software (Siemens Medical Solutions USA, Inc) after transthoracic echocardiography evaluation. The LV wall was divided into 17 segments, and the tracing was performed using a 1-beat cycle starting at mid or end systole. The region of interest was adjusted to cover at least 90% of the myocardial wall thickness. Visual analysis was done first for endomyocardial tracking and, if required, manually adjusted. The epicardial border was then traced to include the entire myocardial thickness and was readjusted as needed. No segments were excluded for 2D-STE analyses. Clinical, survival, and echocardiographic data were masked to the reviewers.

Statistical analysis

Continuous variables are presented as mean (SD); categorical variables are presented as number (percentage of total). Continuous data were analyzed with a *t* test or a Wilcoxon rank sum test when assumptions were not met. Paired *t* tests were used to compare means for GLS and segmental longitudinal strain between groups. Categorical variables were analyzed using either the Pearson χ^2 or Fisher exact test. Receiver operating characteristic analysis was used to evaluate accuracy of strain and systolic strain rates to detect rejection.

For interobserver variability, two independent investigators (A.S.T. and S.B.-G.) to whom the initial results were masked assessed strain in 6 randomly selected patients. For intraobserver variability, repeat assessment of 2D-STE examination in 6 randomly selected patients by the same investigator was performed. To assess agreement, the concordance correlation coefficient (CCC) and Bland-Altman analysis, and calculation of bias (mean [SD] difference between 2 measurements) and of differences in individual pairs of measurements (limits of agreement) were used. Spearman rank correlation coefficient was also calculated.

Statistical analysis was performed using 2 commercially available software packages: JMP 12.0 (SAS Institute Inc) and statistical software version 12 (MedCalc Software 5). All probability values were 2-sided, and a *P*-value <.05 was considered statistically significant.

Results

Study population

A total of 65 heart transplant patients were included, 25 with severe rejection and 40 controls without rejection. Baseline demographics, risk factors, and clinical variables are summarized in Table 1. The mean (SD) age was 48.5 (13.5) years in the rejection group and 53.2 (11.5) years in the control group. There were more men than women in both groups (64 and 75%, respectively). All baseline variables, including body mass index, body surface area, hypertension, low-density lipoprotein cholesterol, diabetes mellitus, hypertension, heart rate, and hyperlipidemia, were similar in both groups. There were no significant differences in medication usage, including immunosuppression, prior prednisone use in the preceding 12 months, angiotensin-converting enzyme inhibitors, beta-blockers and statins. Eighty percent of patients had non-ischemic dilated cardiomyopathy as their heart transplant indication. In regards to symptoms, of the patients with severe rejection, 19 patients (76%) were asymptomatic at the time of diagnosis of severe rejection. The most frequently reported symptoms included lower extremity edema, dyspnea, dizziness, fatigue and headaches.

Table 1 Patient characteristics

Characteristic	Group[a]		*P*
	Control (*n* = 40)	Rejection (*n* = 25)	
Age, y	53.2 (11.5)	48.4 (13.5)	.15
Time since transplant, y	0.98 (0.08)	1.13 (1.3)	.47
Men	30 (75)	16 (64)	.34
BMI, kg/m^2	25.96 (5.0)	25.96 (5.9)	.99
BSA, m^2	1.94 (0.26)	1.87 (0.25)	.26
Hypertension	17 (44)	12 (45)	.73
LDL cholesterol, mg/dL	103.0 (32.47)	104.9 (39.15)	.57
Diabetes mellitus	8 (20)	3 (12)	.40
SBP, mm Hg	126.3 (15.3)	126.5 (15.5)	.95
DBP, mm Hg	76.3 (11.3)	79.1 (10.0)	.30
Heart rate, beats/min	90.2 (11.2)	94.5 (11.4)	.15
Hyperlipidemia	20 (50)	16 (64)	.27
QRS duration, ms	106.6 (19.5)	103.7 (25.6)	.61
Cyclosporine, n (%)	16 (40)	14 (56)	.21
Tacrolimus, n (%)	7 (18)	5 (20)	.84
Sirolimus, n (%)	19 (48)	9 (36)	.34
Azathioprine, n (%)	8 (20)	4 (16)	.69
Mycophenolate mofetil, n (%)	25 (63)	21 (84)	.07
Prednisone in last 12 months, n (%)	38 (95)	21 (84)	.14
ACE-I/ARB, n (%)	16 (40)	6 (24)	.19
Beta-blocker, n (%)	5 (13)	2 (8)	.54
Statin, n (%)	20 (50)	16 (64)	.27

Abbreviations: BMI body mass index, *BSA* body surface area, *DBP* diastolic blood pressure, *LDL* low-density lipoprotein, *SBP* systolic blood pressure
[a]Values are mean (SD) or No. of patients (%)

Baseline echocardiographic and hemodynamic evaluation

Both groups had preserved and similar mean (SD) LVEF (64.3% [5.2%] rejection group vs 64.5% [3.7%] control; *P* = .87). LV end-diastolic diameter (45.9 [4.6] mm vs 46.3 [3.7] mm; *P* = .75), ratio of early and late diastolic waves of mitral inflow, or *E/A ratio* (2.21 [1.03] vs 1.97 [0.70]; *P* = .51), and deceleration time of mitral inflow, or *DT* (180.3 [25.5] ms vs 169.0 [27.7] ms; *P* = .23) were not significantly different between the rejection and control group, respectively. Table 2 summarizes the echocardiographic data for both groups.

Strain analysis

There were no significant differences in mean (SD) GLS (– 13.18% [3.32%] vs – 13.63% (2.35%); *P* = .52) and GLSR (– 0.86 [0.24] s^{-1} vs – 0.82 [0.15] s^{-1}; *P* = .46) between the rejection and control groups. Strain analysis showed significant differences in mean (SD) GLSRe (1.04 [0.28] s^{-1} vs 0.80 [0.21] s^{-1}; *P* = .02), GCS (– 15.74% [3.40%] vs – 19.90% [4.25%]; *P* < .001), and GCSR (– 1.09 [0.30] s^{-1} vs – 1.28 [0.30] s^{-1}; *P* = .02) between the rejection and control groups, respectively. The area under the receiver operating characteristic curve for GCS was 0.77. With values less negative than a cutoff of – 17.60%, the sensitivity and specificity of GCS to detect severe acute rejection were 81.8 and 68.4%, respectively (Fig. 1).

Interobserver variability analysis

Interobserver data between 2 independent researchers showed strong agreement for GLS and GCS. For GLS, the Bland-Altman plots showed statistically significant minimal bias (mean [SD], – 0.17 [3.6]; *P* < .05) with relatively narrower limits of agreement (– 7.3 to 6.9 [1.96SD]); CCC,

Table 2 Conventional and Strain Echocardiographic Variables

Variable	Group[a]		*P*
	Control (*n* = 40)	Rejection (*n* = 25)	
LVEF, %	64.5 (3.7)	64.3 (5.2)	.87
LV EDD, mm	46.3 (4.2)	45.9 (4.6)	.75
LV ESD, mm	29.1 (3.2)	28.7 (2.8)	.59
LV IVSd, mm	11.3 (1.8)	10.9 (1.3)	.33
LV PWd, mm	11.0 (1.5)	11.0 (2.1)	.96
Mean LVWT, mm	11.1 (1.5)	10.9 (1.5)	.65
LVMI 2D, g/m^2	95.3 (21.1)	98.0 (22.4)	.63
E/A ratio	1.97 (0.70)	2.21 (1.03)	.51
DT, ms	169.0 (27.7)	180.3 (25.5)	.23
e'_{sep}, cm/s	0.086 (0.023)	0.093 (0.022)	.26
E/e'_{sep} ratio	11.0 (4.3)	11.2 (2.7)	.89
GCS, %	−19.90 (4.25)	−15.74 (3.40)	< 0.001
GCSR, s^{-1}	− 1.28 (0.30)	− 1.09 (0.30)	.02
GLS, %	−13.63 (2.35)	−13.18 (3.32)	.52
GLSR, s^{-1}	−0.82 (0.15)	−0.86 (0.24)	.46

Abbreviations: DT deceleration time of mitral inflow, *E/A ratio* ratio of early and late diastolic waves of mitral inflow, *E/e'_{sep}ratio* ratio of early wave of mitral inflow and early diastolic tissue Doppler velocity at septal mitral annulus, *EDD* end-diastolic diameter, *ESD* end-systolic diameter, *e'_{sep}* early diastolic tissue Doppler velocity at septal mitral annulus, *IVSd* interventricular septal thickness, *LV* left ventricular, *LVEF* LV ejection fraction, *LVMI 2D* left ventricular mass index, *LVWT* LV wall thickness, *PWd* posterior wall thickness
[a]Values are mean (SD)

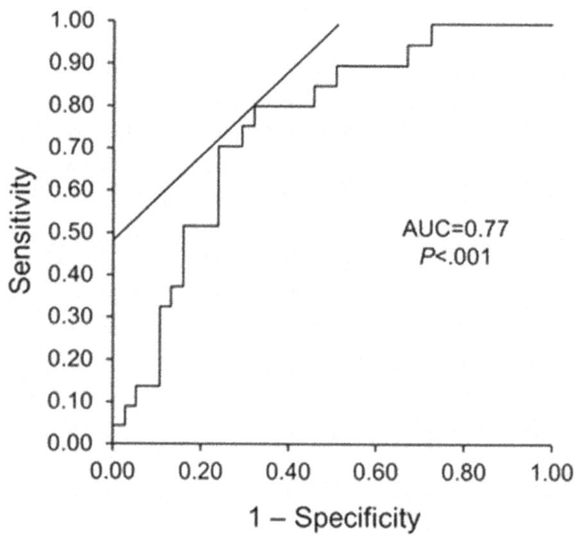

Fig. 1 Global Circumferential Strain Area Under the Receiver Operating Characteristic Curve. With values less negative than a cutoff of − 17.60%, the sensitivity and specificity of GCS to detect severe acute rejection were 81.8 and 68.4%, respectively. Area under the curve (AUC) of the receiver operating characteristic analysis for global circumferential strain is 0.77 ($P < .001$)

0.57 (95% CI, 0.19–0.80); Pearson ρ (precision), 0.57; and bias correction factor Cb (accuracy), 0.99. For GCS, the Bland-Altman plots showed statistically significant minimal bias (mean [SD], 0.14 [4.3]; $P < .05$) with relatively narrower limits of agreement (− 4.4 to 4.6 [1.96SD]); CCC, 0.66 (95% CI, − 0.11-0.93); Pearson ρ (precision), 0.69; and bias correction factor Cb (accuracy), 0.95. Intraobserver variability analysis for GCS and GLS also showed agreement: CCC of 0.85 (95% CI, 0.65–0.94) and 0.97 (95% CI, 0.81–0.99), respectively.

Discussion

The use of 2D-STE strain indices is becoming an important diagnostic tool in detecting acute rejection in heart transplant patients. We specifically evaluated the use of 2D-STE in a subset of patients who experienced severe acute rejection but had preserved LVEF. This group had decreased (ie, less negative) GCS as compared with heart transplant recipients without rejection. A cutoff value of–17.60% for GCS has a sensitivity and specificity of 81.8 and 68.4%, respectively (area under the receiver operating characteristic curve, 0.77), for its detection. GLS and GLSR were similar in both groups.

Our findings are consistent with those of previous animal and human studies. Pieper et al. [14] showed a decrease in GCS in the evaluation of cardiac transplant rejection in a rat model. Their study also showed that radial strain, peak systolic radial strain rate, and peak early diastolic radial strain rates were lower in rats with transplant rejection than in those without rejection. Using 2D-STE, they were able to detect LV dysfunction when conventional echocardiographic measures were unable to demonstrate a difference in systolic function between the 2 groups. Elied et al. [15] established the natural history of LV mechanics in transplanted hearts by 2D-STE and showed that persistently low GLS was a negative prognostic indicator in heart transplant patients. They also showed that failure of GLS to improve by 3 months after transplant is associated with a greater incidence of death and cardiac events. They demonstrated that heart transplant patients have LV regional and global dysfunction within the first 2 years of transplantation, which develops independently of transplant rejection, and that these findings are clinically detectable. In addition, significantly decreased circumferential strain was observed at 2 years after acute allograft rejection, as compared with those without rejection, although the values were comparable at the initial time of rejection [15].

Previously, our group showed that, in normal heart transplant patients without rejection compared with healthy persons without transplant, circumferential deformation indices were normal, but longitudinal deformation indices, including GLS (− 13.43% [2.39%] vs − 17.28% [2.30%];

$P < .001$) and GLSR (-0.83 [0.15] s^{-1} vs -0.96 [0.13] s^{-1}; $P < .001$), were decreased. From these results in normal transplant patients it appears that longitudinal strain impairment occurs early as a result of insults that lead to LV dysfunction, such as LV remodeling (eg, ischemia-reperfusion injury, allograft vasculopathy, and previous allograft rejection) [7]. Pichler et al. showed that deformation values remain stable if LVEF is preserved. Therefore, it is assumed that strain values in normal heart transplant patients are decreased soon after transplantation and stay constant as long as allograft rejection does not develop [16].

Knowing these dynamic changes that occur in normal heart transplant patients and in those with rejection, we postulate that longitudinal strain is the first strain variable to be decreased in cardiac dysfunction. We assume that preserved circumferential strain might be responsible for maintaining cardiac function in transplant patients and that during acute rejection this compensatory mechanism is impaired and leads to graft dysfunction despite preserved LVEF. Further investigation should be performed to elucidate the mechanism of longitudinal and circumferential strain mechanics during acute rejection.

Contrary to our findings, previous studies have showed that acute transplant rejection was associated with a decrease in GLS and not GCS [9, 10, 12] (citations). Few studies evaluated the role of GCS in acute severe rejection and those that did evaluate GCS generally had few patients in the severe rejection group (ISHLT grade 2R or greater). Furthermore, the time since transplantation during each rejection event was variable and study dependent. In our cohort, severe rejection events were identified approximately one year post-transplantation, on average. While other mean times since transplantations for acute severe rejection events in Clemmensen et al. and Mingo-Santos et al. were 3 years and 2.5 years, respectively [10, 12]. Therefore, it is possible that measurement of circumferential strain may provide incremental benefit in evaluating acute rejection to detect more severe rejection, possibly in newer transplant grafts. Further investigation is required to confirm the diagnostic utility of GCS in severe acute rejection.

With the advancements in medical technology, it is important to diagnose acute subclinical rejection when LVEF and other conventional 2D echocardiographic parameters are normal. We have shown that strain and strain rate indices derived from 2D-STE may assist in the evaluation of heart transplant patients, especially if acute rejection is suspected despite preserved LVEF.

Limitations

Our study has several limitations. The study population consisted of a small sample from a single center. Larger studies are necessary to further evaluate the validity of the use of strain and strain rate derived from 2D-STE in the evaluation of heart transplant graft function during severe acute rejection. Furthermore, significant variability between different image processing software exists. Therefore, there are limitations in creating universal cut-off values for strain parameters when different studies use different programs to perform tracings and calculate strain.. The retrospective study design without serial echocardiographic examinations limits the conclusions we were able to draw, particularly is it pertains to the longitudinal changes in strain parameters over time. Although we excluded patients with known transplant vasculopathy, we were unable to definitively ascertain whether patients had concomitant vasculopathy during the acute episode of rejection. Also, our study did not evaluate radial strain because higher interobserver variability has been previously reported in the literature [17]. Lastly, the present study also excluded pediatric heart transplant patients in whom the same mechanophysiology may not apply.

Conclusion

In our study, GCS, which is initially preserved in normal transplant patients, is significantly decreased in patients with preserved LVEF and severe acute rejection, defined as grade 2R or greater using the 2004 ISHLT rejection grading system. 2D-STE can be a useful clinical tool in monitoring heart transplant patients for acute rejection. With increasing evidence of its clinical utility, this non-invasive technique may be useful in detecting rejection in heart transplant patients.

Abbreviations

2D-STE: 2-dimensional speckle-tracking echocardiography; CCC: Concordance correlation coefficient; EF: Ejection fraction; GCS: Global circumferential strain; GCSR: Global circumferential strain rate; GLS: Global longitudinal strain; GLSR: Global longitudinal strain rate; GLSRe: Early diastolic global longitudinal strain rate; ISHLT: International Society for Heart and Lung Transplantation; LV: Left ventricular

Acknowledgements

Not applicable.

Funding

No funding was utilized.

Authors' contributions

AST collected, analyzed the data and wrote the manuscript, USG wrote the manuscript, SBG collected data, FAM edited the manuscript, PAP edited the manuscript, ALC edited the manuscript, HRV designed the study, analyzed the data and edited the manuscript. All authors read and approved the final manuscript.

Competing interests

The authors declare that they have no competing interests.

Author details
[1]Department of Internal Medicine, Mayo Clinic, 13400 E Shea Blvd, Scottsdale, AZ 85259, USA. [2]Department of Cardiovascular Diseases, Mayo Clinic, Rochester, Minnesota, 200 First St SW, Rochester, MN 55905, USA.

References

1. Lund LH, et al. The registry of the International Society for Heart and Lung Transplantation: thirty-second official adult heart transplantation report--2015; focus theme: early graft failure. J Heart Lung Transplant. 2015;34(10):1244–54.
2. Deckers JW, Hare JM, Baughman KL. Complications of transvenous right ventricular endomyocardial biopsy in adult patients with cardiomyopathy: a seven-year survey of 546 consecutive diagnostic procedures in a tertiary referral center. J Am Coll Cardiol. 1992;19(1):43–7.
3. Fiorelli AI, et al. Comparative analysis of the complications of 5347 endomyocardial biopsies applied to patients after heart transplantation and with cardiomyopathies: a single-center study. Transplant Proc. 2012;44(8):2473–8.
4. Sitia S, Tomasoni L, Turiel M. Speckle tracking echocardiography: a new approach to myocardial function. World J Cardiol. 2010;2(1):1–5.
5. Dandel M, et al. Strain and strain rate imaging by echocardiography - basic concepts and clinical applicability. Curr Cardiol Rev. 2009;5(2):133–48.
6. Syeda B, et al. Two-dimensional speckle-tracking strain echocardiography in long-term heart transplant patients: a study comparing deformation parameters and ejection fraction derived from echocardiography and multislice computed tomography. Eur J Echocardiogr. 2011;12(7):490–6.
7. Saleh HK, et al. Normal left ventricular mechanical function and synchrony values by speckle-tracking echocardiography in the transplanted heart with normal ejection fraction. J Heart Lung Transplant. 2011;30(6):652–8.
8. Sato T, et al. Utility of left ventricular systolic torsion derived from 2-dimensional speckle-tracking echocardiography in monitoring acute cellular rejection in heart transplant recipients. J Heart Lung Transplant. 2011;30(5):536–43.
9. Sera F, et al. Left ventricular longitudinal strain by speckle-tracking echocardiography is associated with treatment-requiring cardiac allograft rejection. J Card Fail. 2014;20(5):359–64.
10. Clemmensen TS, et al. Changes in longitudinal myocardial deformation during acute cardiac rejection: the clinical role of two-dimensional speckle-tracking echocardiography. J Am Soc Echocardiogr. 2015;28(3):330–9.
11. Dandel M, Hetzer R. Post-transplant surveillance for acute rejection and allograft vasculopathy by echocardiography: usefulness of myocardial velocity and deformation imaging. J Heart Lung Transplant. 2017;36(2):117–31.
12. Mingo-Santos S, et al. Usefulness of two-dimensional strain parameters to diagnose acute rejection after heart transplantation. J Am Soc Echocardiogr. 2015;28(10):1149–56.
13. Stewart S, et al. Revision of the 1990 working formulation for the standardization of nomenclature in the diagnosis of heart rejection. J Heart Lung Transplant. 2005;24(11):1710–20.
14. Pieper GM, et al. Speckle-tracking 2-dimensional strain echocardiography: a new noninvasive imaging tool to evaluate acute rejection in cardiac transplantation. J Heart Lung Transplant. 2010;29(9):1039–46.
15. Eleid MF, et al. Natural history of left ventricular mechanics in transplanted hearts: relationships with clinical variables and genetic expression profiles of allograft rejection. JACC Cardiovasc Imaging. 2010;3(10):989–1000.
16. Pichler P, et al. Two-dimensional speckle tracking echocardiography in heart transplant patients: three-year follow-up of deformation parameters and ejection fraction derived from transthoracic echocardiography. Eur Heart J Cardiovasc Imaging. 2012;13(2):181–6.
17. Nishimura K, et al. Direct measurement of radial strain in the inner-half layer of the left ventricular wall in hypertensive patients. J Cardiol. 2012;59(1):64–71.

Endomyocardial biopsy guided by intracardiac echocardiography as a key step in intracardiac mass diagnosis

Marco Zanobini[4], Antonio Dello Russo[1], Matteo Saccocci[4*], Sergio Conti[1], Elisa De Camilli[2], Giulia Vettor[1], Valentina Catto[3], Maurizio Roberto[4], Cesare Fiorentini[4,5], Giuseppe Viale[2,6], Claudio Tondo[1,5] and Michela Casella[1]

Abstract

Background: Based on a plenty of different applications, intracardiac echocardiography (ICE) is now a well-established technology in complex electrophysiological procedures. Recently, ICE has become the most widely used ultrasound-based imaging tool to guide diagnostic endomyocardial biopsy (EMB). EMB of cardiac mass guided by ICE is an interesting application of ICE. Allowing a correct positioning of the bioptome, ICE reduce the procedure-related risks and the need of a diagnostic open-chest procedure reserving the more invasive approach to selected cases.

Case presentation: Hereby we report a case series of right ventricular masses in which the EMB was safely and effectively performed under ICE guidance giving essential information for planning the therapeutic strategy.

Conclusions: The diagnosis of both metastatic and primary cardiac tumors relies on the histopathological analyses. The endomyocardial biopsy is a valuable tool for preoperative diagnosis and surgical planning of intracardiac masses suspected for tumors. In our experience, the use of ICE for right ventricle EMB of an intracardiac mass is an attractive modality thanks to the precise localization of the cardiac structures and the ability to guide bioptic withdrawal in the target area.

Keywords: Intracardiac echocardiography, Endomyocardial biopsy, Right ventricle, Intracardiac mass

Background

Intracardiac echocardiography (ICE) is a well-established imaging technology frequently used in complex electrophysiological procedures, such as atrial fibrillation and ventricular tachycardia ablation. As in other scenario, ICE can contribute in improving the efficacy and the safety of procedures. It allows a better definition of the anatomical structures involved in ablation procedures and permits a continuous monitoring of catheter-tissue contact avoiding procedure-related complications [1]. For these reasons, ICE is becoming the most widely used ultrasound imaging tool in diagnostic guidance endomyocardial biopsy (EMB). In addition, the use of ICE is an attractive modality also for EMB of intracardiac mass, in particular for right-sided structures. ICE-guided EMB allows a correct position of the bioptome in relation to the intracardiac mass permitting a reduction of procedure-related risks.

We describe three different cases of EMB of right ventricular masses performed under ICE guidance. In all cases, ICE imaging was performed using a 9F ViewFlex™ Xtra 64-element phased-array and 4-way steerable ultrasound catheter (St. Jude Medical, St. Paul, MN, USA) inserted via the right femoral vein or 8F Acunav 4-way steerable ultrasound catheter (Biosense Webster, Diamond Bar, CA, USA). The technique used by our operators to perform EMB guided by ICE is described in Additional file 1: Movie 1.

The study was conducted according to our Institutional Review Board and in adherence to the Declaration of Helsinki. A written informed consent was obtained from all patients or their closest relatives.

* Correspondence: matteo.saccocci@unimi.it
[4]Department of Cardiovascular Surgery, Centro Cardiologico Monzino IRCCS, Via Carlo Parea 4, 20138 Milan, Italy
Full list of author information is available at the end of the article

Case presentation

Case 1

A 65-year-old woman smoker with a long history of malignancy was referred to our Center due to the evidence of an intracardiac mass at transthoracic echocardiography (TTE). Her past medical history included pulmonary adenocarcinoma treated with right lobectomy and lymphadenectomy, right nephrectomy due to clear cell renal carcinoma and total gastrectomy for adenocarcinoma. The TTE revealed a hyperechogenic thickening at the apex of the right ventricle (RV) without clear evidence of pathological mass. CMR showed a 20 × 28 mm intramyocardial mass localized at the apex of the RV (Fig. 1a). Due to previous history of malignancy there was a high suspicion of cardiac metastatic secondarism. Patient underwent percutaneous EMB of the RV mass under fluoroscopic and ICE guidance. The RV apical mass was visualized and five biopsies were performed (Fig. 1b and c; Additional file 2: Movie 2). No pericardial effusion was present at the end of the EMB (Fig. 1d). Pathologic specimens demonstrated no evidence of malignancy permitting to avoid open-chest surgical removal of the mass. The patient was safely discharged the day after EMB procedure and followed-up in outpatient clinic.

Case 2

A 54-years-old male, with previous history of liver transplant related to hepatocellular carcinoma (HCC) and HBV-cirrhosis, presented to our center for severe dyspnea. TTE demonstrated a 23 × 27 mm multilobed mass in the right ventricular outflow tract (RVOT) involving the pulmonary trunk. CMR imaging and contrast-enhanced CT also confirmed the intracardiac mass detected by TTE (Fig. 2a and b). Patient was scheduled for EMB under ICE guidance. Clear visualization of the mass was rapidly obtained permitting accurate evaluation of size and intracardiac extension (Fig. 2c). Four biopsies were then taken from the right ventricular side under close ICE guidance (Fig. 2d and e; Additional files 3 and 4: Movie 3 and 4). Histopathological analyses showed a poorly differentiated carcinoma characterized by a highly cellular proliferation rate. The pleomorphic epithelioid cells organized in cords of variable thickness resembles dysmorphic hepatocytes with large amounts of cytoplasm. Immunohistochemically studies demonstrate the presence of cytocheratins MNF, Glutamine Syntetase and Heat-shock protein 70, confirming the diagnosis of a metastatic HCC. Successful complete

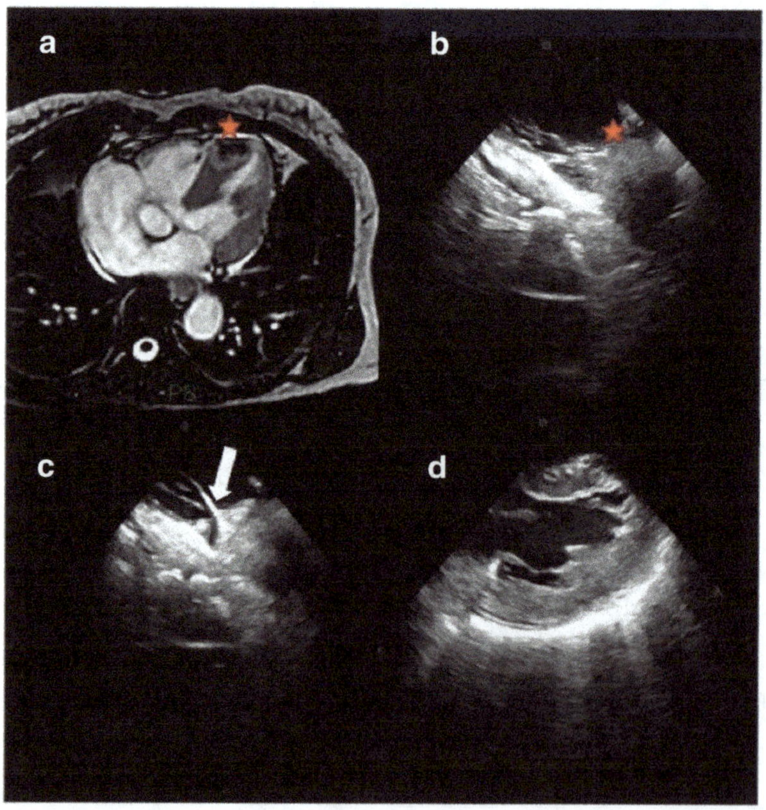

Fig. 1 Cardiac magnetic resonance imaging: a 20 × 28 mm intramyocardial mass localized at the apex of the right ventricle (RV) is showed in panel (**a**). ICE shows the RV apical mass, panel (**b**). The bioptome (white arrow) is clearly visualized and is possible to confirm the good contact between the catheter and the mass, panel (**c**). After obtained all the biopsies needed, ICE is useful to exclude the presence of pericardial effusion, panel (**d**)

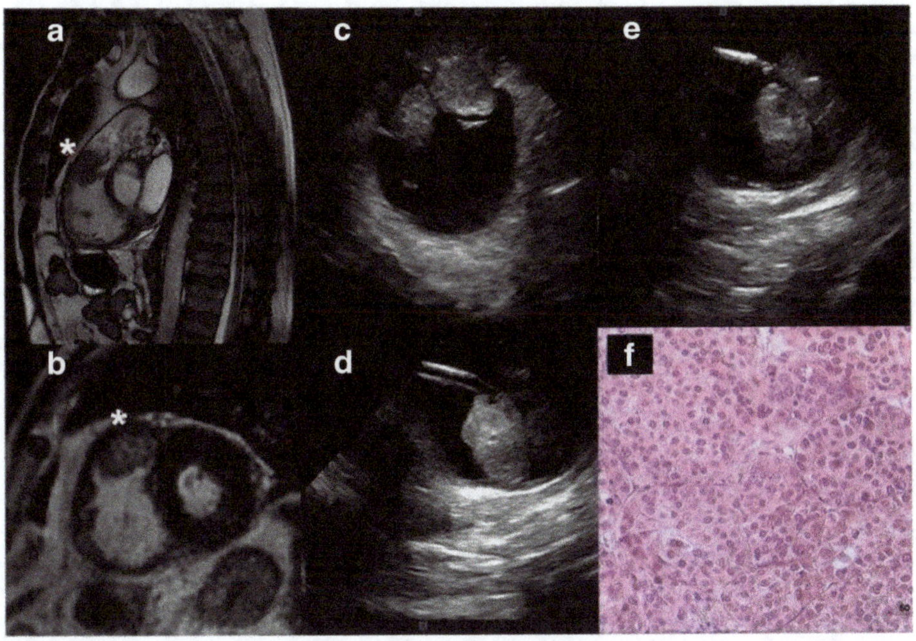

Fig. 2 Cardiac magnetic resonance imaging: a rounded 30 × 17 mm mass based in the anterior portion of the right ventricular outflow tract (RVOT) involving the pulmonary valve is showed in panel (**a** and **b**) (white star). ICE clearly shows the mass, panel (**c**), and is useful to guide the correct positioning of the long-deflectable sheath through which the bioptome is introduced, panel (**d**). ICE visualizes a good contact between the bioptome and the mass, panel (**e**). Histopathological diagnosis revealed a metastatic localization of hepatocellular carcinoma, panel (**f**)

surgical removal of the intracardiac mass confirmed the diagnosis of HCC metastasis.

Case 3

A 77-years-old male with history of diabetes, myocardial infarction with reduced left ventricular ejection fraction and cerebrovascular disease was referred for an occasional finding of right ventricular mass. TTE showed a dishomogeneous mass that infiltrates the RV from the base to the apex with the only exclusion of the RVOT. CT scanning and CMR highlighted an irregular and frayed voluminous mass of 12 × 7.6 cm with a thickness of 5.5 cm extending along the free wall of the RV to the tricuspid annulus (Fig. 3a and b). The heterogeneity nature of the intracardiac mass permitted to show the importance of ICE guidance in EMB procedures. Indeed, it was possible to selectively guide the bioptome into the different areas of the mass obtaining optimal samples (Fig. 3c-e). Histopathological analyses showed solid sheets and nests of large pleomorphic lymphoid cells, with abundant cytoplasm, conspicuous cleaved nuclei with multiple nucleoli, many atypical mitotic figures and apoptotic cells. Immunohistochemical analyses revealed a B-cell large lymphoma with strong expression of CD20, CD45 but negative for CD10 and CD3. The proliferation rate was approximately 95%, as shown in the Mib1 stain. A fluorescent in situ hybridization (FISH) study showed no evidence of MYC translocation ruling out Burkitt like lymphomas. All these findings confirm the diagnosis of diffuse large B cell lymphoma. After diagnosis the patient was scheduled for a multichemotherapy regimen and is currently under treatment.

Discussion and conclusions

Intracardiac masses are uncommon findings and can be distinguished as non-neoplastic and neoplastic. Non-neoplastic intracardiac masses include thrombi, pericardial cysts, and prominent anatomic structures. Primary cardiac tumors are rare, occurring with a prevalence ranging from 0.0017 to 0.28% in an autopsy series, while metastatic tumors are more common (2.3–18.3%) [2]. Intracardiac tumors rarely occurs in the RV and usually present with symptoms and manifestations of general malaise, unexplained fever, shortness of breath, right-sided heart failure or syncope. Most primary cardiac tumors are benign. Malignant tumors of the heart are rare and mostly metastatic. Primary cardiac lymphoma is a very rare malignancy, typically non-Hodgkin type with minimal extracardiac involvement [3].

Although clinical diagnosis of intracardiac masses could be mainly done by echocardiography, CT, and/or

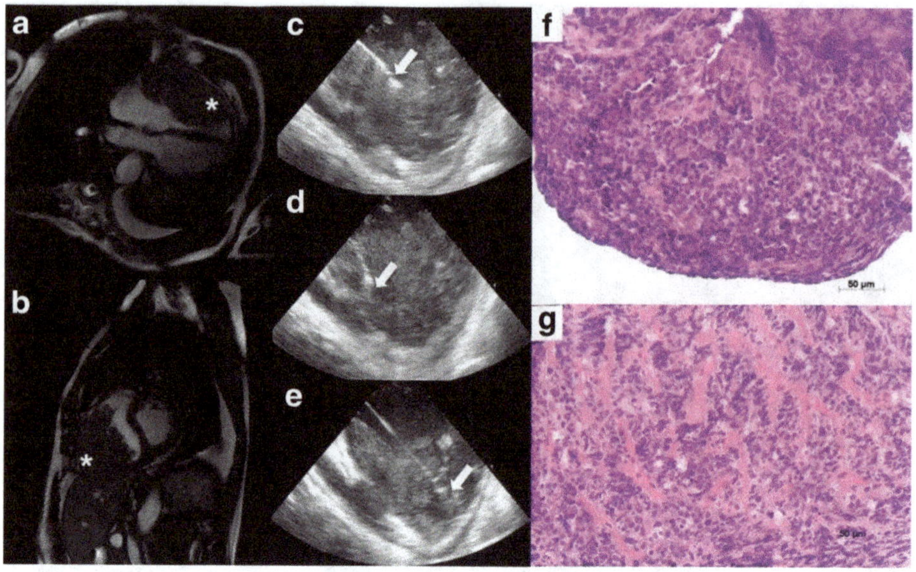

Fig. 3 Cardiac magnetic resonance imaging: an irregular voluminous mass (12 × 7.6 cm, thickness of 5.5 cm) extending along the free wall of the RV to the tricuspid annulus is showed in panel (**a** and **b**) (white star). ICE was extremely helpful to identify the heterogeneity of the mass and to selectively place the bioptome, panel (**c**, **d** and **e**) (white arrow). Hystopathological diagnosis revealed a diffuse large B cell non-Hodgkin lymphoma, panel (**f** and **g**)

CMR, histopathological analysis remains crucial for differential diagnosis. Histology provides critical information for treatment and prognosis, which are largely dependent upon tumor histotype and biological behavior. EMB is a valuable tool for diagnosis of intracardiac masses. It is mainly indicated for the investigation of right-sided masses showing an infiltrative or obstructive growth pattern and for the differential diagnosis of sarcomas, lymphomas, and metastatic tumors. Unresectable intracardiac masses may benefit from EMB to plan therapy or palliative treatment [4].

We demonstrated the usefulness of ICE guidance to perform EMB in different sites and pathologies involving the RV. In all cases, the histopathological diagnosis was made on samples obtained by EMB ICE-guided. Our approach was helpful not only for the final diagnosis but also to plan the optimal therapeutic strategy, reserving more invasive procedure only for selected cases. Indeed, the use of ICE eliminates the risks of a diagnostic open-chest procedure. According to this strategy, surgery is reserved only for patients who would benefit the most in terms of prognosis. Another approach to perform transvenous EMB is under fluoroscopic or 2D- or 3D–transesophageal echocardiography (TEE). However, the use of fluoroscopic guidance to perform right ventricular EMB has some drawbacks, in particular the inability to accurately guide the bioptome, the longer radiation exposure and some possible complications including myocardial perforation, tricuspid valve apparatus disruption and arrhythmias. On the other hand, 2D or 3D–TEE can be cumbersome, it requires general anesthesia and a skilled echocardiographist in the operating room [5].

Recently, the use of ICE has increased in many procedures in order to facilitate transseptal puncture, ablation of cardiac arrhythmias, percutaneous mitral valve intervention, interatrial septal abnormalities closure, and left atrial appendage closure. The capability to clearly show intracardiac structures makes ICE a safe and effective tool to guide transcatheter EMB of right side cardiac mass. Moreover, EMB can be performed under conscious sedation with direct visualization of the mass minimizing the risk for perforation. Of note, there are some drawbacks related to the use of ICE, such as the need of a venous approach, the risks of right chamber catheterization and some technical and economical aspects as the probe cost [6].

To the best of our knowledge, there are few reports of ICE-guided EMB of right atrial cardiac tumor [7–9], in contrast we are describing ICE-guided EMB of both metastatic and primary cardiac tumor in the RV for the first time. In all cases, ICE was safely and effectively used to provide precise localization of the mass and of the cardiac structures and to guide EMB. For these reasons, in our experience ICE can be considered an extremely useful tool in EMB of intracardiac mass.

Additional files

Additional file 1: Movie 1. The whole action of EMB is showed. Fluoroscopy image in RAO view: ICE probe is placed across the tricuspid valve and positioned in the right ventricular inflow tract to image the ventricles in the long axis view. Through a long-deflectable sheath (Agilis, St. Jude Medical, MN, USA) the bioptome is inserted and directed to the mass visualized by ICE. After checking carefully the placement of the bioptome, a sample is taken. (MOV 4285 kb)

Additional file 2: Movie 2. ICE imaging of EMB taken in the right ventricular apex. (MOV 4960 kb)

Additional file 3: Movie 3. ICE imaging of massive multi-lobed intracardiac mass in the right ventricular outflow tract. (MOV 4341 kb)

Additional file 4: Movie 4. EMB guided by ICE. ICE visualizes a good contact between the bioptome and the mass. (MOV 4225 kb)

Abbreviations

CMR: Cardiac magnetic resonance; EMB: Diagnostic endomyocardial biopsy; HCC: Hepatocellular carcinoma; ICE: Intracardiac echocardiography; RV: Right ventricle; RVOT: Right ventricular outflow tract; TEE: Transesophageal echocardiography; TTE: Transthoracic echocardiography

Acknowledge

n/a

Funding

Not applicable

Authors' contributions

MZ and MC equally collaborate to the work Data collection/analysis: MZ, ADR, MS, SC, EDC, GV, VC, MR, CF, GV, CT,MC Manuscript designing/drafting/ writing: MZ,MC,GV,VC,MS Revision: MZ, MC, MS. All authors read and approved the final manuscript.

Competing interests

The authors have no disclosure.

Author details

[1]Cardiac Arrhythmia Research Center, Centro Cardiologico Monzino IRCCS, Milan, Italy. [2]Division of Pathology and Laboratory Medicine, European Institute of Oncology, Milan, Italy. [3]Department of Cardiology, Centro Cardiologico Monzino IRCCS, Milan, Italy. [4]Department of Cardiovascular Surgery, Centro Cardiologico Monzino IRCCS, Via Carlo Parea 4, 20138 Milan, Italy. [5]Department of Cardiovascular Sciences, University of Milan, Milan, Italy. [6]Department of Oncology and Haemato-oncology, University of Milan, Milan, Italy.

References

1. Dello Russo A, Casella M, Pelargonio G, Bonelli F, Santangeli P, Fassini G, Riva S, Carbucicchio C, Giraldi F, De Iuliis P, Bartoletti S, Pintus F, Di Biase L, Pepi M, Natale A, Fiorentini C, Tondo C. Intracardiac echocardiography in electrophysiology. Minerva Cardioangiol. 2010;58:333–42.
2. Basso C, Rizzo S, Valente M, Thiene G. Prevalence and pathology of primary cardiac tumours. Cardiovascular Medicine. 2012;15:18–29.
3. Gowda RM, Khan JA. Clinical perspective of primary cardiac lymphoma. Angiology. 2003;54(5):599–604.
4. Leone O, Veinot JP, Angelini A, Baandrup UT, Basso C, Berry G, Bruneval P, Burke M, Butany J, Calabrese F, d'Amati G, Edwards WD, Fallon JT, Fishbein MC, Gallagher PJ, Halushka MK, McManus B, Pucci A, Rodriguez ER, Saffitz JE, Sheppard MN, Steenbergen C, Stone JR, Tan C, Thiene G, van der Wal AC, Winters GL. 2011 consensus statement on endomyocardial biopsy from the Association for European Cardiovascular Pathology and the Society for Cardiovascular Pathology. Cardiovasc Pathol. 2012;21:245–74.
5. Platts D, Brown M, Javorsky G, West C, Kelly N, Burstow D. Comparison of fluoroscopic versus real-time three-dimensional transthoracic echocardiography guidance of endomyocardial biopsy. Eur J Echocardiogr. 2010;11:637–43.
6. Sun BJ, Lee J-H. Intracardiac echocardiography for guiding biopsy of cardiac tumors: a novel noninvasive technique. Interv Cardiol. 2015;7(6):537–42.
7. Park KI, Kim MJ, Oh JK, Lee JH, Park JH, Choi SW, Jeong JO, Seong IW. Intracardiac echocardiography to guide biopsy for two cases of intracardiac masses. Korean Circ J. 2015;45(2):165–8.
8. Segar DS, Bourdillon PD, Elsner G, Kesler K, Feigenbaum H. Intracardiac echocardiography-guided biopsy of intracardiac masses. J Am Soc Echocardiogr. 1995;8(6):927–9.
9. Mitchell AR, Timperley J, Hudsmith L, Neubauer S, Bashir Y. Intracardiac echocardiography to guide myocardial biopsy of a primary cardiac tumour. Eur J Echocardiogr. 2007 Dec;8(6):505–6.

30

Deactivation vs. asynchronous pacing - prospective evaluation of a protocol for rhythm management in patients with magnetic resonance conditional pacemakers undergoing adenosine stress cardiovascular magnetic resonance imaging

Oliver Klein-Wiele[1*], Marietta Garmer[2], Gianluca Barbone[1], Rhyan Urbien[1], Martin Busch[2], Kaffer Kara[3], Harald Schäfer[1], Michael Schulte-Hermes[1,4], Birgit Hailer[1] and Dietrich Grönemeyer[2]

Abstract

Background: Cardiovascular Magnetic Resonance (CMR) imaging with adenosine stress is an important diagnostic tool in patients with known or suspected coronary artery disease (CAD). However, the method is not yet established for CAD patients with pacemakers (PM) in clinical practice. A possible reason is that no recommendations exist for PM setting (paused pacing or asynchronous mode) during adenosine stress. We elaborated a protocol for rhythm management in clinical routine for PM patients that considers heart rate changes under adenosine using a test infusion of adenosine in selected patients.

Methods: 47 consecutive patients (mean age 72.3 ± 10,0 years) with MR conditional PM and known or suspected CAD who underwent CMR in clinical routine were studied in this prospective observational study. PM indications were sinus node dysfunction (SND, $n = 19$; 40,4%), atrioventricular (AV) block ($n = 26$; 55.3%) and bradyarrhythmia in permanent atrial fibrillation (AF, $n = 2$; 4.3%). In patients with SND, normal AV-conduction and resting HR >45 bpm at the time of CMR and in AF the PM was deactivated for the scan. In intermittent AV-block a test infusion of adenosine was given prior to the scan. All patients with permanent higher degree sinuatrial or AV-block or deterioration of AV-conduction in the adenosine test were paced asynchronously during CMR, in patients with preserved AV-conduction under adenosine the pacemaker was deactivated. CMR protocol included cine imaging, adenosine stress perfusion and late gadolinium enhancement.

Results: The adenosine test was able to differentiate between mandatory PM stimulation during CMR and safe deactivation of the device. In patients with permanent sinuatrial or AV-block ($n = 11$; 23.4%) or deterioration of AV conduction in the adenosine test ($n = 5$, 10.6%) asynchronous pacing above resting heart rate did not interfere with intrinsic rhythm, no competitive stimulation was seen during the scan. 10 of 15 (66,7%) patients with intermittent AV-block showed preserved AV-conduction under adenosine. As in SND and AF deactivation of the PM showed to be safe during CMR, no bradycardia was observed.
(Continued on next page)

* Correspondence: o.klein-wiele@kk-essen.de
[1]Department of Cardiology, Katholisches Klinikum Essen, University of Witten/Herdecke, Hülsmannstraße 17, 45355 Essen, Germany
Full list of author information is available at the end of the article

(Continued from previous page)

Conclusion: Our protocol for rhythm management during adenosine stress CMR showed to be feasible and safe and may be recommended for pacemaker patients undergoing routine CMR.

Keywords: Pacemaker, MRI conditional, Cardiovascular magnetic resonance, CMR, Adenosine stress, Safety, Sinus node dysfunction, Atrioventricular block, Asynchronous pacing

Background

CMR as a non-invasive imaging modality is firmly established in the clinical workup for patients with known or suspected CAD. Beside cine imaging and scar detection with Late Gadolinium Enhancement (LGE) ischemia detection plays a major role in CAD [1, 2]. It has a class Ia level A recommendation in case of intermediate pre test probability of CAD in latest guidelines [2]. Hemodynamic relevance of stenoses in known CAD can be evaluated reliably [3].

In patients with cardiac conduction disorders underlying or concomitant CAD is common [4, 5]. However, while safety of CMR without stress agents in patients with MR conditional PM has been shown in a number of studies [6–8] no prospective data exists on rhythm management of those patients in adenosine stress CMR.

In MR conditional PM no inhibited mode can be chosen. Only deactivation (ODO-mode) or asynchronous pacing (DOO, AOO, VOO) [9] are available to avoid inhibition by electromagnetic interference or tracking of electromagnetic impulses. In SND and AV-block selecting an adequate pacing mode for routine adenosine stress CMR can be challenging because the effect of adenosine on heart rate (HR) has not been thoroughly studied in this entity of patients. Asynchronous mode (i.e. pacing at a fixed rate above baseline HR) could result in competitive pacing when HR accelerates under adenosine [10] reaching the pacing rate. This is due to the fact that sensing is deactivated in this mode and intrinsic rhythm cannot inhibit PM activity. PM stimuli falling in the vulnerable period of the cardiac cycle could then trigger arrhythmia [11]. On the other hand deactivation of the PM in patients with normal HR under resting conditions could result in bradycardia or asystole under adenosine administration [12].

We recently published first data on adenosine stress CMR in pacemaker patients in a small retrospective study and found no relevant complications under a predefined pacing protocol [13]. However, the number of patients with AV-block was limited and it remains unclear what pacing mode is preferable for patients with intermittent AV-block i.e. without higher degree AV-block at the time of CMR. To further investigate adenosine response and to decide whether the pacemaker can be deactivated during the scan we used a test infusion of adenosine for patients with intermittent AV-block and preserved AV-conduction at the time of CMR to screen for adenosine induced bradycardia.

In conclusion the diagnostic value of perfusion analysis by CMR in CAD is well known but still no recommendations exist for PM programming in MRI conditional devices during adenosine stress. We sought to test the safety of a protocol for rhythm management in those patients that is adapted to the adenosine response in PM patients with different underlying conduction disorders.

Methods

In this prospective observational study we analyzed 47 consecutive patients with MR conditional PM who underwent routine adenosine stress CMR including cine imaging, adenosine stress perfusion and LGE from april 2015 to december 2016. Inclusion criteria were presence of a MR conditional pacemaker system, indication for adenosine stress CMR for the evaluation of known or suspected CAD, age > 18 years. Exclusion criteria were implantation <6 weeks from the scan, epicardial or abandoned pacemaker leads, bronchial, asthma, impaired renal function, ejection fraction <35%, presence of an antitachycardia device.

General characteristics

Patients had a mean age of 72.1 ± 11.0 years. 19 (40.4%) had known CAD, 8 (17.0%) previous MI. All other patients had intermediate pretest probability of CAD [14]. Echocardiography had shown preserved systolic left ventricular (LV) function in all subjects. Pacemaker indications were sinus node dysfunction (SND, 19; 40.4%), second or third degree AV-block (n = 26; 55.3%) and bradyarrhythmia in permanent AF (n = 2; 4.3%). Eight patients (17.0%) were PM dependent (HR <30 bpm). Impulse generator/lead models were Advisa (n = 1; 2.1%) and Ensura (n = 46; 97.9%) MRI SureScan/CapSureFix 5076 Novus (atrial), CapSureSense 4074 (ventricular) (Medtronic Inc., Minneapolis, MA, USA). For detailed baseline characteristics see Table 1.

Pacemaker programming and adenosine test

CMR was performed more than six weeks after PM implantation in all individuals according to ESC guidelines [15]. Prior to and after CMR imaging battery status of the device, lead impedance, pacing capture thresholds and sensing amplitudes were measured. In patients with

Table 1 Baseline characteristics

Total patients	47	
Mean Age (years)	72.3 ± 10.0	
	N	%
Female	22	46.8
Pacemaker indication		
Higher degree AV Block	26	55.3
Sinus node dysfunction	19	40.4
Bradyarrhythmia in AF	2	4.3
Coronary artery disease	19	40.4
Previous MI	8	17.0
Paroxysmal atrial fibrillation	17	36.2
In AF at the time of CMR	2	4.3
Hypertension	40	85.1
Impaired renal function	2	4.3
Previous Stroke	7	15.0
Pacemaker		
Ensura MRI Sure Scan	46	97.9
Advisa DR MRI Sure Scan	1	2.1
Pacemaker dependent	8	17.0

AV, atrioventricular, AF, atrial fibrillation, MI, myocardial infarction, CMR, cardiovascular magnetic resonance

intermittent AV-block and preserved AV-conduction at the time of CMR PQ-interval was measured in resting ECG and the Wenckebach point was assessed by testing in AOO mode via the PM programmer. A Wenckebach point below 120 bpm was considered pathologic. Furthermore these patients received a test infusion of adenosine as 3-min infusion of 140μg/kg body weight/min according to the dose for CMR. The pacemaker was deactivated for the test (ODO). Possible deterioration of AV-conduction was recorded and classified in progression to second degree AV-block II Mobitz I, second degree AV-block Mobitz II and third degree AV-block. Reactivation of pacing was performed immediately in case of bradycardia. In SND the PQ interval and the Wenckebach point were measured to rule out occult AV-nodal disease; as in AF no adenosine test was performed prior to MR.

Devices were programmed to MR safe mode following manufacturer's instructions immediately prior to the scan and reprogrammed immediately thereafter. Programming was performed according to a predefined protocol: To avoid interference of intrinsic rhythm with PM-stimulation in patients with SND and resting heart rate HR > 45 bpm no pacing (ODO)-mode was engaged during the scan - also when atrial fibrillation (AF) was present. In individuals with SND and HR ≤ 45 bpm the pacemaker was set to asynchronous atrial stimulation (AOO, 60 bpm). All patients with permanent second or third degree AV block and those with deterioration of AV-conduction in the adenosine test were continuously paced in asynchronous mode. Pacing rate was set 10 bpm above spontaneous heart rate with a minimum of 60 bpm. VOO mode at 60 bpm was chosen in AV block with sinus rate > 45 bpm to avoid competitive atrial stimulation, DOO mode at 60 bpm in AV block with sinus bradycardia ≤45 bpm. In patients with intermittent AV-block and preserved AV-conduction (i.e. no progression to second or third degree AV-block in the adenosine test) the PM was deactivated as in SND. Patients in AF at the time of the scan were paced VOO at 60 bpm if resting heart rate was ≤45 bpm. Table 2 shows the protocol used to select pacing modes for specific clinical constellations.

Safety precautions

As previously described [13] patients were monitored during the scan with continuous electrocardiographic and visual supervision by a cardiologist present in the scanner room. Voice contact was maintained with the patient at all times of the scan. Advanced cardiac life support protocol was in effect. In the scanner the patient was placed on a carry sheet; medical staff was trained for rapid removal of the patient from the scanner room in the event of cardiopulmonary compromise. Thus immediate treatment of severe arrhythmia and reactivation of PM stimulation within seconds in non-paced patients was guaranteed. Atropine, adrenaline and theophylline injections were prepared ready for use in case of bradycardia. Two separate cubital venous cannulas were used for adenosine and gadolinium contrast agent respectively.

Cardiac magnetic resonance imaging

CMR scans were performed with a 1.5 T wide bore system (ESPREE – Siemens Healthcare, Erlangen, Germany) using a 4-channel body array and an 8-channel spine coil. Maximum gradient field was 33 mT/m (Z-Engine) with a slew rate of 100 T/m/S. *maximum* specific absorption rates were limited to 2.0 W/kg.

As previously published [13] our standard protocol meets the Society of Cardiovascular Magnetic Resonance (SCMR) guidelines for CMR [16]. Cine steady-state free precession (SSFP) gradient-echo images were obtained in 10 to 12 short axis slices depending on the size of the ventricles and in 3 long axis planes corresponding to two, three and four chamber views. For stress perfusion-imaging adenosine was administered as 3-min infusion of 140μg/kg body weight/min. First-pass perfusion imaging was carried out with intravenous bolus administration of gadolinium (0.2 mmol/kg body weight) in a fast low angle shot (FLASH) sequence (3 to 4 slices). Late Gadolinium Enhancement (LGE) images were acquired fifteen minutes after injection of gadolinium as phase-

Table 2 Protocol for the selection of pacing modes

Sinus node dysfunction without AV-block	ODO; AOO at 60 bpm when IHR <45 bpm
Atrial fibrillation at time of scan	VOO at 60 bpm when HR <45 bpm
AV-block >I° (present)	VOO at 10 bpm > IHR when SR > 45 bpm, minimum 60 bpm DOO at 10 bpm > IHR when SR < 45 bpm, minimum 60 bpm

Intermittent AV-block, preserved AV-conduction present

↓

Adenosine test (3 min. infusion at 140ug/kg body weight/min)

↙ ↘

Progression to AV-block II/III	preserved AV-conduction under adenosine
↓	↓
VOO at 10 bpm > IHR	ODO

AV, atrioventricular; bpm, beats per minute; IHR, intrinsic heart rate; SR, sinus rhythm

sensitive inversion-recovery (PSIR) in short (10 to 12 slices) and long axis (3 planes) views.

Results

Adenosine test prior to CMR

15 patients (31.9%) with intermittent AV-block and preserved AV-conduction at the time of CMR were tested. 5 of them (33.3%) showed deterioration of AV conduction with a drop of HR. All of those individuals had both prolonged PQ-interval (220 to 305 ms) and pathologic Wenckebach point (70 to 90 bpm). Two patients showed worsening of AV-conduction to AV-block II Mobitz II, three patients developed AV-block III. One patient had pathologic PQ-interval (230 ms) and normal Wenckebach point (130 bpm) and showed acceleration of HR from 70 to 85 bpm without progressive AV-block. One patient had normal AV-conduction (190 ms) and pathologic Wenckebach point (115 ms) and showed an increase in HR from 85 to 95 bpm. Seven of 15 patients with intermittent AV-block (46.6%%) had normal PQ-interval and normal Wenckebach point. None of them showed higher degree AV-block in the test, heart rate increased from 66 ± 8.6 to 75 ± 11.4 bpm ($p < 0.001$, paired t-test). Thus only in patients with both pathologic PQ-interval and pathologic Wenckebach point worsening of AV-conduction and drop of HR were observed. The adenosine test was well tolerated by the patients; no adverse reactions were seen. Figure 1 summarizes heart rate response under the test infusion of adenosine.

Effect and safety of adenosine administration for stress perfusion

There were no adenosine induced adverse events. Asynchronous stimulation of patients with permanent AV-block or progressive AV-block under adenosine 10 bpm above resting HR did not cause competitive pacing or arrhythmia during MR. Patients with preserved AV-conduction under adenosine and deactivated PM did not develop higher degree AV-block in CMR, HR increased from 67.6 ± 9.1 to 77.6 ± 11.3 bpm. Two patients with SND were in AF at the time of CMR. In patients with SND and normal AV-conduction i.e. normal PQ interval and normal Wenckebach point ($n = 17$; 36.2%) at the time of the scan with deactivated (ODO) pacemaker adenosine administration accelerated HR from 60.1 ± 9.1 to 76.0 ± 9.3 bpm ($p < 0.001$, Wilcoxon signed rank test). AV-conduction was not significantly influenced by adenosine; no higher degree AV block

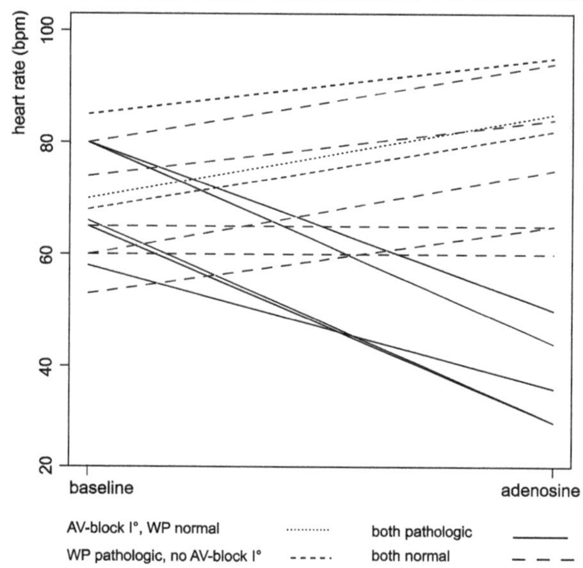

Fig. 1 Adenosine test in intermittent AV-block. Individual changes of heart rate in patients with intermittent AV-block and currently preserved AV-conduction under a 3 min infusion of adenosine at 140μg/kg body weight/min. PQ-interval and Wenckebach point was assessed before the test and is indicated by different lines. Progression to AV-block II/III was only observed in patients with both prolonged PQ-interval (AV-block I°) and pathologic Wenckebach point (< 120 bpm). AV, atrioventricular; WP, Wenckebach point; bpm, beats per minute

occurred. When sinus rate was <45 bpm (n = 1; 2.1%) AOO pacing at 60 bpm led to permanent capture, no acceleration of HR under adenosine was noticed. Of 4 patients in AF in 3 HR remained unchanged during stress perfusion, one patient had acceleration of HR from 110 to 125 bpm.

Device integrity

Device integrity was not compromised by the CMR scan. No patient showed relevant alterations of lead impedance, pacing capture threshold, sensing amplitude or battery voltage. Table 3 summarizes device parameters pre and post CMR.

Table 3 Comparison of device parameters before and after CMR

	before MR	after MR	P^a
P-wave amplitude (mV)	2.87 ± 1.86	3.10 ± 1.70	0.32
R-wave amplitude (mV)	12.27 ± 5.32	12.05 ± 5.44	0.59
Atrial lead impedance (Ohm)	469 ± 61	468 ± 65	0.65
Ventricular lead impedance (Ohm)	601 ± 120	603 ± 118	0.57
Atrial PCT (V@0.4 ms)	0.66 ± 0.25	0.66 ± 0.20	1.0
Ventricular PCT (V@0.4 ms)	0.63 ± 0.26	0.55 ± 0.28	0.1
Battery voltage (V)	2.97 ± 0.42	2.97 ± 0.42	n.a.

CMR, Cardiovascular Magnetic Resonance; PCT, pacing capture threshold, [a]Wilcoxon signed rank test

Discussion

Adenosine stress CMR in patients with MR conditional PM is complicated by the absence of an inhibited pacing mode in these devices. Choosing an adequate PM setting (deactivation vs. asynchronous pacing) in specific conduction disorders can be challenging due to possible alterations of HR and heart rhythm under adenosine. Until now no guidelines for clinical routine have been established addressing this issue. We therefore elaborated a protocol for rhythm management intending to minimize the risk of arrhythmia due to competitive PM stimulation on the one hand and possible bradycardia on the other. In this study our protocol proved to be safe and feasible. No complications of adenosine stress CMR related to the presence of a PM or the underlying cardiac conduction disorder occurred.

The present study is in line with our previous findings [13] that in SND with normal resting HR and normal PQ interval paused PM stimulation (ODO mode) is suitable for adenosine stress perfusion. We found predominance of the sympatho-excitatory effect of adenosine [17] that overrides cardiac inhibition comparable to patients without SND resulting in a significant increase in HR. We selected DOO pacing only in patients with sinusbradycardia <45 bpm to prevent competitive atrial stimulation which can induce AF [18], also considering the fact that adenosine may promote AF by shortening the atrial action potential and refractory period [19]. Avoiding competitive atrial stimulation by pacing above intrinsic HR is not useful due to the acceleration of HR under adenosine (up to 40 bpm in tis study). Pacing far above baseline HR for a longer time could cause discomfort or even circulatory compromise in PM patients adapted to relative bradycardia [20]. VOO mode was avoided because ventricular tachycardia can be induced by R-on-T PM stimulation [21]. The risk of proarrhythmia with asynchronous ventricular pacing for PM interrogation is considered low [22]. However, routine adenosine stress CMR in CAD requires a long period in MR conditional mode because sequences for localization, cine imaging, first pass perfusion and LGE are necessary. Asynchronous ventricular PM stimulation might be hazardous under these conditions. In patients with higher degree AV-block or bradycardia induced by adenosine in the preceding test the risk of R-on-T stimulation considered low because the patient is paced above intrinsic HR at rest and under adenosine. Prolonged asystole under adenosine stress imaging in occult SND has been reported [23], therefore immediate reactivation of the PM in case of persistent bradycardia must be guaranteed. For further clinical practice we recommend deactivation of the device under careful monitoring in SND without AV-block.

The adenosine test in patients with intermittent AV-block was useful to differentiate patients that can be examined with deactivated devices from those with mandatory PM stimulation. One could argue that asynchronous pacing for all patients with AV-block may be chosen. However, with intact AV-conduction under adenosine the risk of proarrhythmia due to competitive ventricular stimulation cannot be excluded. Deterioration of AV-conduction was only observed in patients with both prolonged PQ interval and pathologic Wenckebach point. Larger studies have to show if CMR can be performed without previous testing in patients without first degree AV-block at rest and normal Wenckebach point. We believe that screening for occult AV-dysfunction by measuring the PQ-interval and Wenckebach point prior to CMR in SND is useful because SND patients may develop binodal disease [24] that does not become clinically apparent due to the PM therapy. We recommend adenosine test for SND patients with pathologic AV-conduction at the time of CMR, however all individuals in this study had normal AV-conduction. Further studies have to show if adenosine testing is adequate for patients with SND and impaired AV-conduction unmasked prior to CMR.

The investigated pacing protocol showed to be feasible and safe. However, adenosine stress CMR has to be compared to other diagnostic strategies, namely when the high supervisory expense in this setting is considered. We encourage prospective randomized studies to clarify which imaging strategy is the best choice for PM patients in terms of safety and clinical value.

Limitations

This study is limited by the relatively sample size. Adverse effects may only appear in a larger cohort of patients. Furthermore we did not test a high dose adenosine protocol, which may be more effective in ischemia detection [25].

Conclusion

Our protocol for rhythm management in patients with MR conditional PM appears to be feasible and safe and may be used for adenosine CMR in clinical routine until larger studies exist.

Abbreviations

AV: Atrioventricular; BV: Battery voltage; CAD: Coronary artery disease; CMR: Cardiovascular Magnetic Resonance; ESC: European Society of Cardiology; FLASH: Fast low angle shot; HR: Heart rate; LGE: Late Gadolinium Enhancement; MI: Myocardial infarction; PCT: Pacing capture threshold; PM: Pacemaker; PSIR: Phase-sensitive inversion recovery; SCMR: Society for Cardiovascular Magnetic Resonance; SND: Sinus node dysfunction; SSFP: Steady-state free precession; STIR: Short-tau inversion recovery

Acknowledgements

We acknowledge Michael Pilz for editing the graphic content of the manuscript.

Funding

Not applicable.

Authors' contributions

OK conceived of the study, performed the PM interrogations and tests and wrote the manuscript. MG was involved in the conception of the study. GB and RU collected clinical data. MB helped in statistical analysis and literature review and revised the manuscript. KK helped in the conception of the study and in drafting the manuscript. HS was involved in the conception of the study and data analysis. MS was involved in the conception of the study. BH was involved in the conception of the study and revised the manuscript. DG helped in the coordination of the study and revised the manuscript. All authors read and approved the final manuscript.

Authors' information

OK: Cardiologist, member of the German Cardiac Society (DGK), SCMR and DGK Level III qualification for CMR, DGK-approved for interventional cardiology and special rhythmology. MG: Radiologist, member of the German Röntgen Society, Q2 certificate for CMR. GB: Doctorand, RU: Cardiologist, DGK member. MB: Physicists, research-, software-, and application specialist for MR. KK: Cardiologist, DGK member, approved for interventional cardiology. HS: Cardiologist, member of the German Cardiac Society (DGK), DGK-approved for interventional cardiology and special rhythmology. MS: Cardiologist, DGK-member, approved for interventional cardiology, SCMR and DGK level III qualification for CMR. BH: Cardiologist, DGK-member, approved for interventional cardiology and special rhythmology. DG: Radiologist, member of the German Röntgen Society, specialist in MR guided interventional therapy.

Competing interests

The authors declare that they have no competing interests.

Author details

[1]Department of Cardiology, Katholisches Klinikum Essen, University of Witten/Herdecke, Hülsmannstraße 17, 45355 Essen, Germany. [2]Department of Radiology, Grönemeyer Institut Bochum, University of Witten/Herdecke, Universitätsstraße 142, 44799 Bochum, Germany. [3]Cardiovascular Center, Josef Hospital, University of Bochum, Gudrunstr. 56, 44791 Bochum, Germany. [4]Department of Cardiology, Prosper-Hospital Recklinghausen, University of Witten/Herdecke, Mühlenstraße 27, 45659 Recklinghausen, Germany.

References

1. Nandalur KR, Dwamena BA, Choudhri AF, Nandalur MR, Carlos RC. Diagnostic performance of stress cardiac magnetic resonance imaging in the detection of coronary artery disease: a meta-analysis. J am Coll Cardiol. 2007;50:1343–53.
2. Authors/Task Force m, Windecker S, Kolh P, Alfonso F, Collet JP, Cremer J, et al. 2014 ESC/EACTS guidelines on myocardial revascularization: the Task Force on myocardial revascularization of the European Society of Cardiology (ESC) and the European Association for Cardio-Thoracic Surgery (EACTS) developed with the special contribution of the European Association of Percutaneous Cardiovascular Interventions (EAPCI). Eur Heart J. 2014;35:2541–619.
3. Li M, Zhou T, Yang LF, Peng ZH, Ding J, Sun G. Diagnostic accuracy of myocardial magnetic resonance perfusion to diagnose ischemic stenosis with fractional flow reserve as reference: systematic review and meta-analysis. JACC Cardiovasc Imaging. 2014;7:1098–105.
4. Alonso A, Jensen PN, Lopez FL, Chen LY, Psaty BM, Folsom AR, et al. Association of sick sinus syndrome with incident cardiovascular disease and mortality: the atherosclerosis risk in communities study and cardiovascular health study. PLoS One. 2014;9:e109662.
5. Hsueh CW, Lee WL, Chen YT, Ting CT. The incidence of coronary artery disease in patients with symptomatic bradyarrhythmias. Jpn Heart J. 2001;42:417–23.
6. Wollmann CG, Thudt K, Kaiser B, Salomonowitz E, Mayr H, Globits S. Safe performance of magnetic resonance of the heart in patients with magnetic resonance conditional pacemaker systems: the safety issue of the ESTIMATE study. J Cardiovasc Magn Reson. 2014;16:30.

7. Gimbel JR, Bello D, Schmitt M, Merkely B, Schwitter J, Hayes DL, et al. Randomized trial of pacemaker and lead system for safe scanning at 1.5 Tesla. Heart Rhythm. 2013;10:685–91.
8. Schwitter J, Kanal E, Schmitt M, Anselme F, Albert T, Hayes DL, et al. Impact of the Advisa MRI pacing system on the diagnostic quality of cardiac MR images and contraction patterns of cardiac muscle during scans: Advisa MRI randomized clinical multicenter study results. Heart Rhythm. 2013;10:864–72.
9. Bernstein AD, Daubert JC, Fletcher RD, Hayes DL, Luderitz B, Reynolds DW, et al. The revised NASPE/BPEG generic code for antibradycardia, adaptive-rate, and multisite pacing. North American Society of Pacing and Electrophysiology/British pacing and electrophysiology group. Pacing Clin Electrophysiol. 2002;25:260–4.
10. Biaggioni I, Killian TJ, Mosqueda-Garcia R, Robertson RM, Robertson D. Adenosine increases sympathetic nerve traffic in humans. Circulation. 1991; 83:1668–75.
11. Sweeney MO, Porkolab FL. Ventricular fibrillation induced by double premature ventricular pacing stimuli in a dual-chamber pacemaker with auto capture. Heart Rhythm. 2009;6:429–32.
12. Hesse B, Tagil K, Cuocolo A, Anagnostopoulos C, Bardies M, Bax J, et al. EANM/ESC procedural guidelines for myocardial perfusion imaging in nuclear cardiology. Eur J Nucl med Mol Imaging. 2005;32:855–97.
13. Klein-Wiele O, Garmer M, Urbien R, Busch M, Kara K, Mateiescu S, et al. Feasibility and safety of adenosine cardiovascular magnetic resonance in patients with MR conditional pacemaker systems at 1.5 Tesla. J Cardiovasc Magn Reson. 2015;17:112.
14. Task Force M, Montalescot G, Sechtem U, Achenbach S, Andreotti F, Arden C, et al. 2013 ESC guidelines on the management of stable coronary artery disease: the Task Force on the management of stable coronary artery disease of the European Society of Cardiology. Eur Heart J. 2013;34:2949–3003.
15. Brignole M, Auricchio A, Baron-Esquivias G, Bordachar P, Boriani G, Breithardt OA, et al. 2013 ESC guidelines on cardiac pacing and cardiac resynchronization therapy: the Task Force on cardiac pacing and resynchronization therapy of the European Society of Cardiology (ESC). Developed in collaboration with the European heart rhythm Association (EHRA). Eur Heart J. 2013;34:2281–329.
16. American College of Cardiology Foundation Task Force on Expert Consensus D, Hundley WG, Bluemke DA, Finn JP, Flamm SD, Fogel MA, et al. ACCF/ACR/AHA/NASCI/SCMR 2010 expert consensus document on cardiovascular magnetic resonance: a report of the American College of Cardiology Foundation Task Force on expert consensus documents. J am Coll Cardiol. 2010;55:2614–62.
17. Costa F, Biaggioni I. Adenosine activates afferent fibers in the forearm, producing sympathetic stimulation in humans. J Pharmacol exp Ther. 1993;267:1369–74.
18. Furman S, Cooper JA. Atrial fibrillation during A-V sequential pacing. Pacing Clin Electrophysiol. 1982;5:133–5.
19. Kanei Y, Hanon S, Van-Tosh A, Schweitzer P. Adenosine-induced atrial fibrillation during pharmacologic stress testing: report of eight cases and review of the literature. Int J Cardiol. 2008;129:e15–7.
20. Tops LF, Schalij MJ, Bax JJ. The effects of right ventricular apical pacing on ventricular function and dyssynchrony implications for therapy. J am Coll Cardiol. 2009;54:764–76.
21. Oupadia P, Ramaswamy K. Images in clinical medicine. "R-on-T" phenomenon. N Engl J med. 1998;338:1812.
22. Nowak B, Hemmer W, Israel CW, Kramer LI, Neuzner J, Pfeiffer D, et al. Statement of the working Group of the Germany Society on the safety of asynchronous ventricular pacemaker stimulation. Clin res Cardiol. 2006;95:57–60.
23. Pennell DJ, Mahmood S, Ell PJ, Underwood SR. Bradycardia progressing to cardiac arrest during adenosine thallium myocardial perfusion imaging in occult sino-atrial disease. Eur J Nucl med. 1994;21:170–2.
24. Rosenqvist M. Atrial pacing for sick sinus syndrome. Clin Cardiol. 1990;13:43–7.
25. Karamitsos TD, Ntusi NA, Francis JM, Holloway CJ, Myerson SG, Neubauer S. Feasibility and safety of high-dose adenosine perfusion cardiovascular magnetic resonance. J Cardiovasc Magn Reson. 2010;12:66.

Permissions

All chapters in this book were first published in CD, by BioMed Central; hereby published with permission under the Creative Commons Attribution License or equivalent. Every chapter published in this book has been scrutinized by our experts. Their significance has been extensively debated. The topics covered herein carry significant findings which will fuel the growth of the discipline. They may even be implemented as practical applications or may be referred to as a beginning point for another development.

The contributors of this book come from diverse backgrounds, making this book a truly international effort. This book will bring forth new frontiers with its revolutionizing research information and detailed analysis of the nascent developments around the world.

We would like to thank all the contributing authors for lending their expertise to make the book truly unique. They have played a crucial role in the development of this book. Without their invaluable contributions this book wouldn't have been possible. They have made vital efforts to compile up to date information on the varied aspects of this subject to make this book a valuable addition to the collection of many professionals and students.

This book was conceptualized with the vision of imparting up-to-date information and advanced data in this field. To ensure the same, a matchless editorial board was set up. Every individual on the board went through rigorous rounds of assessment to prove their worth. After which they invested a large part of their time researching and compiling the most relevant data for our readers.

The editorial board has been involved in producing this book since its inception. They have spent rigorous hours researching and exploring the diverse topics which have resulted in the successful publishing of this book. They have passed on their knowledge of decades through this book. To expedite this challenging task, the publisher supported the team at every step. A small team of assistant editors was also appointed to further simplify the editing procedure and attain best results for the readers.

Apart from the editorial board, the designing team has also invested a significant amount of their time in understanding the subject and creating the most relevant covers. They scrutinized every image to scout for the most suitable representation of the subject and create an appropriate cover for the book.

The publishing team has been an ardent support to the editorial, designing and production team. Their endless efforts to recruit the best for this project, has resulted in the accomplishment of this book. They are a veteran in the field of academics and their pool of knowledge is as vast as their experience in printing. Their expertise and guidance has proved useful at every step. Their uncompromising quality standards have made this book an exceptional effort. Their encouragement from time to time has been an inspiration for everyone.

The publisher and the editorial board hope that this book will prove to be a valuable piece of knowledge for researchers, students, practitioners and scholars across the globe.

List of Contributors

Ruixue Du, Wen-Xiu Leng, Peng Gao, Hong-Mei Wu and Ping Ye
Department of Geriatric Cardiology, Chinese PLA General Hospital, No. 28, Fuxing Road, Beijing 100853, China

Jianming Cai and Lin Ma
Department of Radiology, Chinese PLA General Hospital, No. 28, Fuxing Road, Beijing 100853, China

Xue-Qiao Zhao
Department of Medicine, Division of Cardiology, University of Washington, Seattle, WA, USA

Mohamed Faisal Lutfi
Department of Physiology, Faculty of Medicine and Health Sciences, Al-Neelain University, Mailbox: 12702, Khartoum 11121, Sudan

Ameen Mosa Mohammad
Department of Medicine, Division of Cardiology, Medical School, Faculty of Medical Sciences, Duhok University, Kurdistan, Iraq

Christian Fastner, Michael Behnes, Benjamin Sartorius, Ibrahim El-Battrawy, Ralf Lehmann, Stefan Baumann, Tobias Becher, Martin Borggrefe and Ibrahim Akin
First Department of Medicine, University Medical Center Mannheim, University of Heidelberg, DZHK (German Center for Cardiovascular Research), Mannheim, Germany

Mustafa Yildiz
Department of Cardiology, Istanbul University Cardiology Institute, Istanbul, Turkey

Kambis Mashayekhi
Internal Medicine Clinic II, Helios Vogtland Klinikum Plauen, Academic Teaching Hospital of Leipzig University, Leipzig, Germany

Karolina Dorniak, Marcin Hellmann, Dorota Rawicz-Zegrzda, Maria Wesierska and Maria Dudziak
Department of Noninvasive Cardiac Diagnostics, Medical University of Gdansk, Gdansk, Poland

Einar Heiberg and Erik Hedström
Lund University, Skane University Hospital, Department of Clinical Sciences Lund, Clinical Physiology, Lund, Sweden

Einar Heiberg
Department of Biomedical Engineering, Faculty of Engineering, Lund University, Lund, Sweden

Rafal Galaska
1st Department of Cardiology, Medical University of Gdansk, Gdansk, Poland

Agnieszka Sabisz and Edyta Szurowska
2nd Department of Radiology, Medical University of Gdansk, Gdansk, Poland

Erik Hedström
Lund University, Skane University Hospital, Department of Clinical Sciences Lund, Diagnostic Radiology, Lund, Sweden

Valentina Giacchi, Pietro Sciacca, Ileana Stella, Martina Filippelli, Patrizia Barone, Mario La Rosa and Salvatore Leonardi
Pediatric Pneumo-Allergology and Cystic Fibrosis Department, Pediatric Cardiology Clinic, AOU "Policlinico-Vittorio Emanuele", University of Catania, Catania, Italy

Esra Akyüz Özkan
Department of Pediatrics, Bozok University Medical Faculty, Yozgat, Turkey

Hashem E. Khosroshahi
Department of Pediatric Cardiology, Bozok University Medical Faculty, Yozgat, Turkey

Jehill D. Parikh, Kieren G. Hollingsworth, Vijay Kunadian, Andrew Blamire and Guy A. MacGowan
Institute of Cellular Medicine, Newcastle University, Newcastle upon Tyne, UK

Guy A. MacGowan
Institute of Genetic Medicine, Newcastle University, Newcastle upon Tyne, UK

Vijay Kunadian and Guy A. MacGowan
Cardiothoracic Centre, Freeman Hospital, Newcastle upon Tyne, UK

Andrea Ponsiglione, Marta Puglia, Carmine Morisco, Luigi Barbuto, Antonio Rapacciuolo, Mario Santoro, Letizia Spinelli, Bruno Trimarco, Alberto Cuocolo and Massimo Imbriaco
Department of Advanced Biomedical Sciences, University "Federico II", Via Pansini, 5, 80123 Naples, Italy

Ardan M Saguner, Sabrina Ganahl, Deniz Akdis, Arhan R Saguner, Thomas Wolber, Laurent M Haegeli, Jan Steffel, Nazmi Krasniqi, Thomas F Lüscher, Felix C Tanner, Corinna Brunckhorst and Firat Duru
Department of Cardiology, University Heart Center Zurich, Rämistrasse 100, CH-8091 Zurich, Switzerland

Andrea Kraus
Division of Biostatistics, Institute for Social and Preventive Medicine, University Zurich, Zurich, Switzerland

Samuel H Baldinger
Department of Cardiology, University Hospital Bern, Bern, Switzerland

Thomas Wolber, Thomas F Lüscher, Felix C Tanner and Firat Duru
Center for Integrative Human Physiology, University Zurich, Zurich, Switzerland

Annalisa Sechi, Andrea Dardis and Bruno Bembi
Regional Coordinator Centre for Rare Diseases, University Hospital Santa Maria della Misericordia, Udine, Italy

Gaetano Nucifora
Cardiothoracic Department, University Hospital Santa Maria della Misericordia, Udine, Italy

Gianluca Piccoli
Department of Diagnostic Imaging, University Hospital Santa Maria della Misericordia, Udine, Italy

Takao Konishi, Naohiro Funayama, Tadashi Yamamoto, Daisuke Hotta and Kenjiro Kikuchi
Department of Cardiology, Hokkaido Cardiovascular Hospital, 1-30, West 13, South 27, Chuou-ku, Sapporo 064-8622, Japan

Katsumi Ohori
Department of Cardiovascular Surgery, Hokkaido Cardiovascular Hospital, Sapporo, Japan

Takao Konishi, Hiroshi Nishihara and Shinya Tanaka
Department of Cancer Pathology, Hokkaido University, Graduate School of Medicine, Sapporo, Japan

Can Qian and Wen Zeng
Sichuan Industrial Institute of Antibiotics, Chengdu, China

Can Qian, Li Gong, Zunyuan Yang and Wen Zeng
Sichuan PriMed Shines Bio-Tech Co., Ltd, Chengdu, China

Wei Chen, Yushu Chen, Ziqian Xu, Bing Wu and Fabao Gao
Department of Radiology, West China Hospital, Sichuan University, Chengdu, China

Chungui Tang
Department of Radiology, Yaan People's Hospital, Yaan, China

Jonathan Yap, Ju Le Tan, Thu Thao Le, Fei Gao, Liang Zhong, Swee Yaw Tan and Ru San Tan
Department of Cardiology, National Heart Centre Singapore, 5 Hospital Drive, Singapore 169609, Singapore

Fei Gao, Reginald Liew, Swee Yaw Tan and Ru San Tan
Duke-NUS Graduate Medical School, Singapore, 8 College Rd, Singapore 169857, Singapore

Lei Zhao, Zhuang Tian and Quan Fang
Department of Cardiology, Peking Union Medical College Hospital, Peking Union Medical College and Chinese Academy of Medical Sciences, No.1 Shuaifuyuan, WangfujingDongcheng District, Beijing 100730, China

Rong-juan Li, Jiao Yang, Ya Yang, Ning Ma, Bo Jiang, Qi-wei Sun and Yi-jia Li
Department of Echocardiography, Beijing Anzhen Hospital, Capital Medical University, Beijing, China
Beijing Institute of Heart, Lung and Blood Vessel Disease, Beijing, China

Monika Bieseviciene, Jolanta Justina Vaskelyte, Vaida Mizariene, Rasa Karaliute and Raimonda Verseckaite
Department of Cardiology, Medical Academy, Lithuanian University of Health Sciences, Eivenių Str. 2, Kaunas 50009, Lithuania

Vaiva Lesauskaite
Institute of Cardiology at Lithuanian University of Health Sciences, Kaunas, Lithuania

Kai O. Hensel, Markus Roskopf, Francisca Abellan Schneyder and Andreas Heusch
HELIOS University Medical Center Wuppertal, Children's Hospital, Center for Clinical & Translational Research (CCTR), Faculty of Health, Center for Biomedical Education & Research (ZBAF), Witten/Herdecke University, Faculty of Health, Heusnerstr. 40, D-42283 Wuppertal, Germany

Kai O. Hensel
University of Cambridge, Addenbrooke's Hospital, Department of Paediatrics, Cambridge, UK

Roman Panovský, Věra Feitová, Petr Novotný, Vladimír Kincl, Tomáš Holeček, Jaroslav Meluzín, Ondřej Sochor
The Department of Cardiovascular Diseases, International Clinical Research Centre, St. Anne's Faculty Hospital, Brno, Czech Republic

Roman Panovský, Petr Novotný, Vladimír Kincl, Jaroslav Meluzín and Ondřej Sochor
The 1st Department of Internal Medicine/ Cardioangiology, International Clinical Research Centre - ICRC, St. Anne's Hospital, Masaryk University, Pekařská 53, 656 91 Brno, Czech Republic

Júlia Borová and Martin Pleva
The Department of Cardiology, Heart Centre, Hospital Podlesi, Trinec, Czech Republic

Věra Feitová and Tomáš Holeček
The Department of Medical Imaging, St. Anne's Faculty Hospital and Masaryk University, Brno, Czech Republic

Radka Štěpánová
International Clinical Research Centre, St. Anne's University Hospital Brno, Brno, Czech Republic

Juan Lacalzada-Almeida, María Manuela Izquierdo-Gómez, Carima Belleyo-Belkasem and Patricia Barrio-Martínez
Department of Cardiology, Hospital Universitario de Canarias, Ofra s/n, La Cuesta, 38320 La Laguna, Tenerife, Spain

Javier García-Niebla
Servicios Sanitarios del Área de Salud de El Hierro, Valle del Golfo Health Center, El Hierro, Spain

Roberto Elosua
Cardiovascular Epidemiology and Genetics Research Group, IMIM (Hospital del Mar Medical Research Institute), Barcelona, Catalonia, Spain
CIBER Cardiovascular Diseases (CIBERCV), Barcelona, Spain

Alejandro Jiménez-Sosa
Research Unit, Hospital Universitario de Canarias, La Laguna, Santa Cruz de Tenerife, Spain

Luis Alberto Escobar-Robledo and Antonio Bayés de Luna
Fundación Investigación Cardiovascular, Institut Català Ciències Cardiovasculars, Barcelona, Catalonia, Spain

Caroline Morbach, Diego Bellavia and Lissa Sugeng
Yale School of Medicine, Section Cardiovascular Medicine, 330 Cedar Street, New Haven, CT 06511, USA

Caroline Morbach and Stefan Störk
Comprehensive Heart Failure Center and Department of Internal Medicine I, University of Würzburg, Würzburg, Germany

Diego Bellavia
Istituto Mediterraneo per i Trapianti e Terapie ad Alta Specializzazione (IRCCS-ISMETT), Palermo, Italy

Tim Salinger, Kai Hu, Dan Liu, Sebastian Herrmann, Georg Ertl and Peter Nordbeck
Department of Internal Medicine I, University Hospital Würzburg, Würzburg, Germany

Tim Salinger, Kai Hu, Dan Liu, Sebastian Herrmann, Georg Ertl and Peter Nordbeck
Comprehensive Heart Failure Center (CHFC), University of Würzburg, Würzburg, Germany

Kristina Lorenz
Leibniz-Institut für Analytische Wissenschaften - ISAS, University Duisburg-Essen, Dortmund, Germany

Peter Nordbeck
Medizinische Klinik und Poliklinik I - Kardiologie, Universitätsklinikum Würzburg, Oberdürrbacher Str. 6, 97080 Würzburg, Germany

Xu Guo, Xiaoou Wang, Xinzhong Zhang, Ahmed O. Ahmed and Daqing Zhang
Department of Cardiology, Shengjing Hospital of China Medical University, #36 Sanhao Street, Heping district, Shenyang City, Liaoning Province 110004, People's Republic of China

David H. Hsi
Heart& Vascular Institute, Stamford Hospital, Stamford, CT 06904, USA

Joselyn Rwebembera, William Manyilirah, Zhang Wan Zhu, Juliet Nabbaale, Judith Namuyonga, Isaac Ssinabulya, Sulaiman Lubega, Peter Lwabi, John Omagino and Emmy Okello
Uganda Heart Institute, Kampala, Uganda

Judith Namuyonga, Isaac Ssinabulya, Peter Lwabi and Emmy Okello
School of Medicine Makerere University, Kampala, Uganda

Tomasz Plonek, Mikolaj Berezowski and Marek Jasinski
Department of Cardiac Surgery, Wroclaw Medical University, Borowska 213, 50-556, Wroclaw, Poland

Tomasz Plonek
Department of Cardio-Thoracic Surgery, Onze Lieve Vrouwe Gasthuis, Amsterdam, the Netherlands

Jacek Kurcz, Przemyslaw Podgorski and Marek Sąsiadek
Department of General and Interventional Radiology and Neuroradiology, Wroclaw Medical University, Wroclaw, Poland

Bartosz Rylski
Department of Cardio-vascular Surgery, Heart Centre Freiburg University, Faculty of Medicine, University of Freiburg, Freiburg, Germany

Andrzej Mysiak
Department of Cardiology, Wroclaw Medical University, Wroclaw, Poland

Sophie Mavrogeni, George Markousis-Mavrogenis and Genovefa Kolovou
Onassis Cardiac Surgery Center, 50 Esperou Street, 175-61 P.Faliro, Athens, Greece

Loukia Koutsogeorgopoulou and Sotiris Plastiras
Pathophysiology Department, Laikon Hospital, Athens, Greece

Georgia Karabela, Efthymios Stavropoulos and Gikas Katsifis
Athens Naval Hospital, Athens, Greece

John Raftakis
Asklipion Voulas Hospital, Athens, Greece

Michel Noutsias
Department of Internal Medicine III, Division of Cardiology, Angiology and Intensive Medical Care, University Hospital Halle, Martin-Luther-University Halle, Ernst-Grube-Straße 40, D-06120 Halle (Saale), Germany

Mareike Gastl, Patrick Behm, Christoph Jacoby, Malte Kelm and Florian Bönner
Department of Cardiology, Pulmonology and Vascular Medicine, Heinrich-Heine University Düsseldorf, Düsseldorf, Germany

Andrew S. Tseng
Department of Internal Medicine, Mayo Clinic, 13400 E Shea Blvd, Scottsdale, AZ 85259, USA

Umama S. Gorsi, Sergio Barros-Gomes, Fletcher A. Miller, Patricia A. Pellikka, Alfredo L. Clavell and Hector R. Villarraga
Department of Cardiovascular Diseases, Mayo Clinic, Rochester, Minnesota, 200 First St SW, Rochester, MN 55905, USA

Antonio Dello Russo, Sergio Conti, Giulia Vettor, Claudio Tondo and Michela Casella
Cardiac Arrhythmia Research Center, Centro Cardiologico Monzino IRCCS, Milan, Italy

Elisa De Camilli and Giuseppe Viale
Division of Pathology and Laboratory Medicine, European Institute of Oncology, Milan, Italy

Valentina Catto
Department of Cardiology, Centro Cardiologico Monzino IRCCS, Milan, Italy

Marco Zanobini, Matteo Saccocci, Maurizio Roberto and Cesare Fiorentini
Department of Cardiovascular Surgery, Centro Cardiologico Monzino IRCCS, Via Carlo Parea 4, 20138 Milan, Italy

Cesare Fiorentini and Claudio Tondo
Department of Cardiovascular Sciences, University of Milan, Milan, Italy

Giuseppe Viale
Department of Oncology and Haemato-oncology, University of Milan, Milan, Italy

Oliver Klein-Wiele, Gianluca Barbone, Rhyan Urbien, Harald Schäfer, Michael Schulte-Hermes and Birgit Hailer
Department of Cardiology, Katholisches Klinikum Essen, University of Witten/Herdecke, Hülsmannstraße 17, 45355 Essen, Germany

Marietta Garmer and Martin Busch and Dietrich Grönemeyer
Department of Radiology, Grönemeyer Institut Bochum, University of Witten/Herdecke, Universitätsstraße 142, 44799 Bochum, Germany

Kaffer Kara
Cardiovascular Center, Josef Hospital, University of Bochum, Gudrunstr. 56, 44791 Bochum, Germany

Michael Schulte-Hermes
Department of Cardiology, Prosper-Hospital Recklinghausen, University of Witten/Herdecke, Mühlenstraße 27, 45659 Recklinghausen, Germany

Index

www.ingramcontent.com/pod-product-compliance
Lightning Source LLC
LaVergne TN
LVHW080735210926
848485LV00003B/560